What Really Makes You Ill?

Why Everything You Thought You Knew About Disease is Wrong

Dawn Lester & David Parker

DISCLAIMER: Healthcare in the early 21st century is almost completely controlled by 'vested interests', which claim that their system, known as 'modern medicine', is the only genuine form of healthcare and that all other forms are to be regarded as pseudoscience and quackery. The consequence of this control is that we, the authors of this book, are under a legal requirement to state that we are not medical doctors. In addition, we are obliged to state that, even though its contents have been obtained from professional and reliable sources, this book is intended to serve as an informational guide; its core purpose is to assist people to make truly informed decisions about their healthcare.

This book is dedicated to all those who seek truth

"An error does not become truth by reason of multiplied propagation, nor does truth become error because nobody sees it."

Mahatma Gandhi

"Unthinking respect for authority is the greatest enemy of truth."

Albert Einstein

Contents

Contents

Contents

products, foods and drinks, as well as some lesser-known applications.

The medical establishment admits to not knowing the 'exact' causes of most, if not all, chronic health problems, more commonly referred to as noncommunicable diseases. The discussions in chapter seven examine a number of major noncommunicable diseases to expose the existence and extent of these 'knowledge gaps'; they also examine some of the known causal factors and reveal the existence of an underlying mechanism common to virtually all of them.

Health problems cannot be considered in isolation; they are invariably associated with other circumstances, most of which affect a significant proportion of people throughout the world, especially in countries referred to as 'developing'. International organisations, especially those within the UN system, claim to be able to resolve all of the problems that confront humanity in the 21st century; but this claim is unfounded. The discussions in chapter eight examine the most recent efforts to implement measures claimed to provide solutions to these problems, with particular emphasis on those that impact human health, whether directly or indirectly, and reveal that these measures are inappropriate as solutions, because they fail to address and thereby remove the real causes of these problems.

The reason that 'modern medicine' employs inappropriate solutions to the problem of 'disease', despite the unimaginably huge sums of money that have been, and continue to be, expended on the development of medicines and vaccines, is largely due to the influence of 'vested interests'. The existence and influence of these vested interests over key areas of human life, including the healthcare system operated by the medical establishment, are discussed in chapter nine.

Having revealed the problems with the explanations presented by the medical establishment in the previous chapters, the final chapter explains the real nature of 'disease'. It also discusses how illness is almost always the result of multiple causes and reveals the existence of a common mechanism. In addition to discussing the problems, chapter ten provides information about how people can reduce their exposures to these causal factors and take responsibility for, and control over, their own health.

The definition of each 'disease', referred to as the 'establishment definition', is taken from the 2007 edition of the Oxford Concise Medical Dictionary, unless otherwise stated.

All emphases in quoted statements are as they appear in the original.

All articles and web pages from which extracts have been quoted are listed in the References section at the end of the book, unless the web page has been deleted or the website is no longer active.

The dynamic nature of the internet means that web pages and fact sheets are often updated; the information used in this book was correct at the time of writing.

All quoted extracts from the published books listed in the Bibliography are considered to be consistent with Fair Usage.

Chapter One

A Prescription for Illness: Dying to be Healthy

"Physicians who are free with their drugging keep themselves busy treating the effects of the drugs."

Herbert Shelton ND DC

The word 'medicine' has two applications, the establishment definitions for which are,

"the science or practice of the diagnosis, treatment or prevention of disease."

And,

"any drug or preparation used for the treatment or prevention of disease."

The various drugs and preparations that are referred to as 'medicines' are considered to be essential, core components of the 'healthcare' provided by medical practitioners to their patients. The inclusion in the definition of the word 'science' conveys the impression that the practice of medicine has a solid foundation that is based on and fully supported by scientifically established evidence. The definition also conveys the impression that the use of drugs and preparations is similarly science-based, and that 'medicines' are both appropriate and effective for the purposes for which they are employed.

Unfortunately, however, nothing could be further from the truth; any healthcare practice that employs the use of 'drugs and preparations' in the treatment and prevention of disease has no basis in 'science', nor is it capable of restoring patients to health.

This statement will no doubt be considered by many to be outrageous; but that does not deny its veracity, as will be demonstrated by the discussions in this chapter about the use of medicines for the treatment of disease. The use of vaccinations for the prevention of disease is discussed in the next chapter.

The medical establishment claims that there are many hundreds of different diseases, each of which is recognisable by its unique set of symptoms and each of which is treatable with the appropriate 'medicine'. The purpose of the 'medicine' is to achieve the cessation of symptoms; an outcome that is interpreted to mean that the disease has been successfully conquered by the treatment.

This, at least, is the theory; but in practice, in the real world, it is not uncommon for a wide variety of different outcomes to be experienced by patients, even though they have all been diagnosed with the same disease and treated with the same medicine. The existence of such widely varying outcomes presents a direct challenge to the theory. Furthermore, although some patients may experience a complete cessation of their symptoms, this successful outcome cannot be attributed to the medicine, nor does it mean their health has been restored, for reasons that will be explained in later chapters.

An interesting feature of the definition of medicine is the reference to the 'treatment' rather than the 'cure' of disease; the reason for this is because the medical establishment states that many diseases are 'incurable'. For these diseases, they claim that the appropriate treatments will 'manage' the patients' conditions; which means that their symptoms will only be alleviated rather than eliminated.

It is widely acknowledged that all medicines produce 'side effects', which are effectively new symptoms that are the direct result of the treatment. The significance of this fact is inadequately reported and therefore insufficiently appreciated by most people; it is, however, a core problem of the prevailing medical system because the production of new symptoms is essentially the creation of a new health problem.

It is clear that the wide variation in the efficacy of medicines used as treatments for disease, as well as the additional symptoms they cause, raise serious questions about the ability of these 'treatments' to restore a patient to a state of health; which ought to be the fundamental purpose and function of a 'healthcare' system.

The website of the WHO (World Health Organisation) provides a definition of health that states,

> "Health is a state of complete physical, mental and social well-being and not merely the absence of disease or infirmity."

This definition has remained unaltered since first declared in their constitution when the WHO was founded in 1948. The WHO is the agency of the UN (United Nations) assigned to be the 'authority' for health matters for all of the people in all of the countries that have ratified the WHO constitution. In other words, the WHO directs health policies for implementation by virtually every country around the world. Yet the WHO policy recommendations with respect to disease treatment almost exclusively refer to the use of 'medicines' that are acknowledged to alleviate symptoms but not cure disease.

The WHO's policies are clearly inconsistent with their objective to achieve better health for everyone, everywhere; especially in the context of their own definition of 'health'.

Science is a process; it is a process that involves the study of different aspects of the world in order to expand the level of human knowledge; it also entails the creation of hypotheses and theories to explain the various phenomena observed during the course of those scientific investigations. As the various studies progress and the body of knowledge increases, they may reveal new information or they may expose anomalies and contradictions within existing hypotheses and theories. In such instances, it is essential for scientists, in whichever field they study, to reassess those hypotheses and theories in the light of the new findings; a process that may necessitate revisions or adaptations to be made to prevailing theories. Sometimes the new information may indicate a need to abandon existing theories and replace them with entirely new ones, especially when new theories provide better and more compelling explanations for the observed phenomena.

The theories underlying the use of 'medicine' to treat disease can be shown to contain many anomalies and contradictions; they are clearly in need of a thorough reassessment. However, and more importantly, other theories exist that present far more credible and compelling explanations for human illness and its causes. These explanations also offer the means by which people can address the causes of their illness, which can assist a full recovery from most conditions of ill-health and help restore people to the state of good health, in the true meaning of the word.

It is neither intended nor necessary to provide a history of 'medicine'; it is far too vast a topic. Nevertheless, it is necessary to refer to certain aspects of this history to identify the origins of the use of 'medicine' and outline its progression to the situation that prevails in the early 21st century, especially in view of the dominance of the healthcare system recommended by the WHO for adoption by all Member States.

In various parts of the world and throughout history, a variety of ideas have arisen about the causes of illness and the appropriate measures to be taken to treat these conditions and restore health to the patient. However, all systems of 'medicine' operate from the same basic principle, which is that a person who is ill requires 'treatment' with a certain substance that is said to have 'curative properties' in order for the patient to recover their health.

Some of the ancient customs and traditions relating to the treatment of people exhibiting symptoms of illness were based on beliefs in the existence of malevolent, supernatural influences, rather than earthly ones, and these invariably involved the use of 'remedies' of a similarly supernatural nature; they may have included spells or incantations or the use of special tokens to ward off evil spirits. Other ancient customs and traditions employed an approach towards illness and its treatment of a more earthbound variety; many of the remedies employed by these systems involved the use of various natural substances, such as plants and similar materials that could be found locally and were claimed to have curative properties.

The medicinal use of plants has been documented in many regions of the world and recorded to date back many thousands of years. For example, Ayurveda, the ancient Indian system of medicine, is claimed to be approximately 5,000 years old. Similarly, TCM (Traditional Chinese the harm that they can cause; this topic is discussed in more detail in the next section.

Pharmaceutical 'medicines' are, however, harmful; the reason for this is due to the nature of the chemicals used in their manufacture, many of which are inherently toxic and all of them are physiologically incompatible with the human body.

One extremely useful document that explains the manufacturing processes and the ingredients used by the pharmaceutical industry is called *Pharmaceutical Waste Analysis*. This document was produced in 2006 by the Blacksmith Institute and is available from their website (blacksmithinstitute.org); the Institute changed its name in 2015 to Pure Earth (pureearth.org).

One of the pharmaceutical manufacturing processes, called 'fermentation', is employed in the production of antibiotics and steroids; two of the most widely used drugs. The process of fermentation involves the use of solvents, some of which are discussed in the *Pharmaceutical Waste* document that states,

"...the solvents most often used in fermentation operations are acetone, methanol, isopropanol, ethanol, amyl alcohol and MIBK."

All of these solvents are toxic. MIBK stands for methyl isobutyl ketone, which is claimed to be of 'low toxicity', although the document states that it may damage the liver, which clearly refutes the claim of 'low' toxicity.

Another pharmaceutical manufacturing process is called 'chemical synthesis', which is the production method used for most of the active ingredients in a wide variety of drugs; this process also involves a number of highly toxic substances as the *Pharmaceutical Waste* document explains,

"A variety of priority pollutants are used as reaction and purification solvents during chemical synthesis."

The document provides a list of some of the 'priority pollutants' that are used in the process of chemical synthesis; they include,

"...benzene, chlorobenzene, chloroform, chloromethane, o-dichlorobenzene, 1,2-dichloroethane, methylene chloride, phenol, toluene and cyanide."

The term 'priority pollutants' means that these substances are known to be extremely hazardous chemical compounds.

The processes described above are not the only ones used in the production of 'medicines'; but they serve as examples to demonstrate that the manufacture of drugs involves the use of highly toxic substances. The concern expressed by the document refers to the hazardous nature of the waste produced by the industry and the effects of these wastes on the environment; this topic is discussed in detail in chapter six.

The information contained within the document clearly identifies the toxic nature of the substances used in the manufacturing processes, as well as the ingredients utilised by the pharmaceutical industry in the production of 'medicine', and provides supportive evidence for the claim that medicines are inherently harmful. This fact has also been identified by Herbert Shelton who states that,

"All so-called medicines, in doses of any size, are poisons."

It is therefore unsurprising that all drugs are recognised to produce 'side effects'; but the degree of harm is invariably understated and mostly hidden, for reasons that will become increasingly obvious throughout this book. The scale of harm they cause is the subject of the next discussion.

Iatrogenesis

Iatrogenesis, which is derived from the Greek word for doctor, is a recognised phenomenon, the establishment definition of which refers to a condition that,

> "...has resulted from treatment, as either an unforeseen or inevitable side-effect."

The 'medicines' of the early 21st century are perceived to be a 'modern miracle' for their ability to combat the many hundreds of different diseases to which humans are able to succumb. A substantial part of this 'miracle' is regarded as having been achieved through advances in 'medical science' coupled with the use of highly sophisticated technologies. But, as outlined in the previous two discussions, 'modern medicine' was not established from a basis in science and the effects of drugs have not been proven to be beneficial for health. The existence of the phenomenon of iatrogenesis demonstrates that medical treatments can, and do, have serious consequences.

Dr Carolyn Dean is one of the many physicians who have recognised the failings of the orthodox medical system in which they were trained. In *Death by Modern Medicine*, she refers to the history of the use of chemicals in 'medicine' and states that,

> "From the beginning, chemical drugs promised much more than they delivered. But far beyond not working, the drugs also caused incalculable side effects."

The establishment definition of a 'side-effect' refers to,

> "an unwanted effect produced by a drug in addition to its desired therapeutic effects. Side-effects are often undesirable and may be harmful."

The description of an iatrogenic condition as a 'side effect' is clearly misleading, because it is a condition that is recognised to have resulted from a 'treatment'; in other words, it is a direct effect of treatment. An iatrogenic condition is obviously not the intended effect of any treatment, but to relegate it to the label of 'side effect' is disingenuous; especially since all drugs are recognised to produce effects, many of which are far more harmful than the original disease.

No 'side effect' is desirable, but the fact that they occur and are described as 'unforeseen', 'unwanted' and 'undesirable' is a clear demonstration of a woefully inadequate level of knowledge within pharmacology, and especially within pharmacodynamics.

The reason that patients are prescribed the same pharmaceutical drugs for the same condition is based on a mistaken idea about the processes that result in 'disease'. This fallacy assumes that all human responses to the same disease will be uniform, because it is claimed that a 'disease' is an independent entity that 'attacks' all people alike, and therefore the appropriate treatment is one that will fight the disease entity. This fallacy is also the basis for the use of tissues or 'disease molecules' in laboratory

19

Although the pharmaceutical industry is clearly reluctant to admit that their products are toxic, there is undeniable evidence of the harm they cause, as documented by the many drugs that have been withdrawn from the market due to their adverse effects, as Dr Dean explains,

"Fully half the drugs prescribed are eventually pulled from the marketplace due to undeniable side effects."

Her statement is based on the US GAO report referred to in the previous section. However, because pharmaceutical drugs are not officially recognised as being inherently toxic, the true scale of the problem is not only unknown, but unknowable. An added complication that further masks the magnitude of the problem is that the 'effects' of drugs are not always immediately obvious and can take months or even years to develop, which means it is highly unlikely that an illness will be associated with the prior use of any medication.

It is abundantly obvious that iatrogenesis has far more victims than has been acknowledged or reported, but this situation is predominantly due to the suppression of facts about the toxicity of pharmaceutical products, which is the direct result of the toxic chemicals used in the manufacturing processes.

'Medicines' are supposed to heal not harm; yet, as Dr Dean states,

"How modern medicine has come to be the number one killer in North America is as incredible as it is horrifying. Doctors certainly don't think of themselves as killers but as long as they promote toxic drugs and don't learn non-toxic options, they are pulling the trigger on helpless patients."

This is a dire situation; but it is not unique to North America; it will exist within all countries that adopt the WHO-led medical establishment system.

It is clear that expensive 'healthcare' does not result in better health for people; it does however, provide healthy profits for the pharmaceutical and medical technology industries. The existence of iatrogenesis demonstrates that a health system based on the use of toxic pharmaceutical 'medicines' is unable to deliver healthcare, no matter how much money is spent, how sophisticated the technology or how new and innovative the drugs that are used.

Health is not something that will improve by merely increasing healthcare budgets or by spending larger amounts of money on the development of new 'medicines', as the American system has proved. Health can only be improved by identifying and addressing the real causes of illness.

Psychiatric Medications

The establishment definition of psychopharmacology refers to,

"the study of the effects of drugs on mental processes and behaviour, particularly psychotropic drugs."

The chemical compounds that are used in 'medicines' affect many parts of the body including the brain; this means that the brain can be affected by 'medicines' prescribed for conditions other than those referred to as 'mental health' problems.

The reason that a branch of 'science' studies the effects of pharmaceutical drugs on 'mental processes and behaviours' is because certain 'behaviours' are considered to be 'abnormal' and therefore people who exhibit such behaviours are deemed to have a 'mental illness', also referred to as a 'mental disorder'; as indicated by the April 2018 WHO fact sheet entitled *Mental Disorders* that states,

> "There are many different mental disorders, with different presentations. They are generally characterized by a combination of abnormal thoughts, perceptions, emotions, behaviour and relationships with others."

The problem with this statement is that it relies on a highly subjective analysis of what is perceived to be 'abnormal' with reference to all the criteria by which a diagnosis is made. Yet nowhere is there a definitive definition of 'normal'; it is neither a medical nor a scientific term. Nevertheless, when a person's thoughts or behaviours are considered to be 'abnormal' and they are diagnosed with a 'mental disorder' they are frequently prescribed 'medications' which, like all 'drugs', are made using toxic chemicals. The fact sheet suggests that insufficient numbers receive such treatments and states,

> "Health systems have not yet adequately responded to the burden of mental disorders. As a consequence, the gap between the need for treatment and its provision is wide all over the world."

The definition of 'health' as declared in the WHO constitution, includes reference to mental as well as physical well-being, which further demonstrates the disparity between the ideas they promote and the practices they recommend. It is another example of the contradictions that pervade the medical establishment system.

The use of drugs for the treatment of people diagnosed with a mental disorder is based on the theory that people with such conditions have developed a 'biochemical imbalance' within their brain. Despite its frequent use, the phrase 'chemical imbalance in the brain' is based on yet another unproven theory, as psychiatrist Dr Peter Breggin MD has explained many times during the course of his long and distinguished career. His website contains a great deal of useful material and articles, including his June 2015 article entitled *Rational Principles of Psychopharmacology for Therapists, Healthcare Providers and Clients*, in which he refers to the theory of 'biochemical imbalance' as being both false and a myth. In his article, he states that,

> "...the evidence for any biological basis for 'psychiatric disorders' is utterly lacking."

In his 1991 book entitled *Toxic Psychiatry*, Dr Breggin explains the situation in more detail and states that,

> "...no causal relationship has ever been established between a specific biochemical state of the brain and any specific behaviour and it is simplistic to assume it is possible."

He further explains that,

> "There's little evidence for the existence of any such imbalances and absolutely no way to demonstrate how the drugs would affect them if they did exist."

One fact that is rarely highlighted by the medical establishment is that patients undergo no tests that are able to determine whether they have a biochemical imbalance in their brains. Dr Breggin states that the only tests capable of determining the existence of any biochemical imbalance would only be carried out during an autopsy!

In his June 2015 article Dr Breggin explains why drugs appear to have an effect,

"All drugs that impact on the brain and mind 'work' by partially disabling the brain and mind."

He further explains that,

"The so-called therapeutic effect is always a disability."

He describes these disabilities as always representing a diminished quality of life. Dr Breggin's comments clearly add further credence to the discussion in the previous section, in which it was shown that all drugs produce adverse effects; the interpretation of these effects as 'therapeutic' is not only highly subjective, it has no basis in 'science'.

One of the most common types of 'mental disorder' is depression, the establishment definition of which is,

"a mental state characterized by excessive sadness."

The problem with this definition, as should be immediately obvious, is that it too is based on a subjective interpretation of the level of sadness that would constitute 'excessive'. It is highly likely that different physicians will have differing interpretations of the meaning of 'excessive', which means that the 'treatments' offered to patients can vary amongst physicians according to their particular and personal interpretations. Not only does this highlight the absence of a standardised healthcare system, but also refutes any idea that physicians are in possession of a clear definition of 'normal' by which they can determine what is 'abnormal'.

The WHO regards depression as a distinctive condition that differs from ordinary emotional responses to the everyday challenges of life; the definition in the March 2018 WHO fact sheet entitled *Depression* claims that,

"Depression is a common mental disorder."

The WHO estimates that depression affects more than 300 million people around the world, which clearly represents a huge potential market for the products of the pharmaceutical industry. Yet the distinction made by the WHO between emotional responses and depression relies purely on duration and severity. Both of these criteria are similarly subjective and unhelpful in providing a method for determining any clear distinctions between an ordinary emotional response to the difficulties of life and depression; if any genuine distinctions do exist. Dr Breggin suggests that there are no such distinctions and that emotions are normal aspects of being human. He expands on this point in *Toxic Psychiatry* and states that,

"Depression and elation are among the most common human experiences."

In this context, depression should not be considered as 'abnormal' and as an illness or disorder that requires a patient to be medicated so that they can return to 'normal'. Depression frequently follows a tragic and distressing event in a person's life, such as the death of a loved one, for example. It should be recognised that people are different in many ways and that these differences include the way they respond to the emotional challenges of life. The theory that a certain level of emotional response is 'abnormal' has no basis in science; it is a social construct.

Dr Breggin explains the origin of the idea that a certain level of emotion is to be considered as a 'mental health problem' that requires treatment and states that,

"Psychiatry and the pharmaceutical industry have been marketing depression as a 'real disease' in need of medical treatment."

Despite the absence of a genuine biochemical theory of depression and associated 'behaviours', as well as the lack of any test to determine the existence of a 'chemical imbalance', millions of people around the world have been regularly prescribed drugs to treat their alleged 'mental disorder'. This is a highly lucrative market for the pharmaceutical industry, especially in view of the WHO claim that there is an 'under-provision' of treatment. In addition, the WHO fact sheet claims that,

"There are effective psychological and pharmacological treatments for depression."

Pharmacological treatments include antidepressants, the establishment definition of which is,

"a drug that alleviates the symptoms of depression."

There is however, a large and growing body of evidence which demonstrates that antidepressants do not genuinely alleviate the symptoms of depression. Although patients may perceive that their symptoms have abated due to the drugs, Dr Breggin explains that this is often a mistaken perception, and that changes in the symptoms people experience tend to mask the existence of the disabling effects of the drugs.

It is widely acknowledged that all drugs produce 'effects', some of which are extremely harmful; the same applies to antidepressants. Some of the dangerous effects of antidepressants are revealed by Dr Peter Breggin and David Cohen PhD in their book entitled *Your Drug May Be Your Problem*, in which they state that,

"At public hearings in 2004 the FDA presented re-evaluations of antidepressant clinical trials for children and youth under age eighteen documenting that the suicide risk was doubled in children taking antidepressants compared to similar individuals taking a sugar pill."

The result of these hearings was a limited action, which was that,

"The FDA published a new required label for all antidepressants on January 26, 2005 including a black box headlined 'Suicidality in Children and Adolescents'."

Whilst 'increased suicidality' is a more than adequate reason to be extremely concerned about these drugs, they are associated with many other 'side effects'. The acknowledged 'side effects' of antidepressants include the following symptoms: anxiety, agitation, panic attacks, insomnia, irritability, hostility, aggressiveness, impulsivity, akathisia (psychomotor restlessness), hypomania, and mania. These symptoms are often similar to, and in some cases the same as, the symptoms for which the drug would have been originally prescribed.

Dr Russell Blaylock MD, a former neurosurgeon, discusses the use of antidepressants in his book entitled *Health and Nutrition Secrets*, in which he refers to many of the 'side effects' of 'psychiatric medications' and particularly the effects that they have produced in young people,

> "It is also interesting to note that in virtually all of the school shootings, the kids responsible for the violence were taking SSRI medications, which are known to produce suicidal and homicidal side effects. It is also known that these medications increase brain levels of the neurotransmitter serotonin, which in high concentrations can also act as an excitotoxin."

There has, however, been a recent change in the approach of the medical establishment towards the use of SSRI (selective serotonin reuptake inhibitor) medications for children and teenagers. The WHO fact sheet about depression refers to antidepressants and states that,

> "They should not be used for treating depression in children and are not the first line of treatment in adolescents, among whom they should be used with extra caution."

This is clearly a better approach but it should have been implemented many decades ago, as it would have saved countless children and young people from being damaged by these drugs; although the best approach would be one that avoids drugs entirely.

One drug that is still prescribed for young children is Ritalin, which is one of the trade names of a compound called methylphenidate that is referred to as a central nervous system stimulant. Ritalin is described as 'amphetamine-like', which is the reason it was previously referred to as one of the legal drugs that are similar to 'illegal' ones. Ritalin is used for 'behavioural disorders' such as 'ADD' and 'ADHD', which are conditions claimed to be suffered by some young children who are considered to have problems paying attention, particularly in school. Some of the 'side effects' of this drug include: loss of appetite, mood swings and stomach aches. Dr Breggin comments on the effects of Ritalin in *Toxic Psychiatry* and states,

> "It seems to have escaped Ritalin advocates that long-term use tends to create the very same problems that Ritalin is supposed to combat – 'attentional disturbances' and 'memory problems' as well as 'irritability' and hyperactivity."

The reduction or alleviation of symptoms is perceived to be a successful outcome of treatment, which means that any reduction in the feeling of depression will be similarly perceived to be a successful outcome; but, as with all drug treatments, they do not address the real causes of the strong emotions that many people experience.

Dr Breggin summarises his own approach to depression in *Toxic Psychiatry*, in which he states that,

> "Despite all of this biopsychiatric propaganda ...depression is a readily understandable expression of human despair that is frequently responsive to psychosocial help."

The topic of stress is discussed in detail in chapter ten.

NOTE: It must be emphasised that anyone who takes psychiatric medications must seek competent professional advice if they wish to consider or to undertake a withdrawal programme, as there are many potential effects that withdrawal from these drugs can produce. In his 2015 article, Dr Breggin states that,

> "Withdrawing from psychiatric drugs can be emotionally and sometimes physically dangerous. It should be done carefully with experienced supervision."

Antihypertensives

The establishment definition of hypertension refers to,

> "high blood pressure i.e. elevation of the arterial blood pressure above the normal range expected in a particular group."

There is a great deal of concern within the medical establishment about elevated blood pressure, because it is said to force the heart to work harder in its efforts to pump blood through the arteries and around the body. This extra work is said to cause excess strain on the heart and blood vessels and lead to health problems, especially heart disease. It is claimed that elevated blood pressure above the range considered to be 'normal' is a reliable indicator of an increased risk for the occurrence of a heart attack or a stroke.

The medical establishment clearly considers high blood pressure to be synonymous with hypertension; as also indicated by the May 2019 WHO fact sheet entitled *Hypertension*, which states that,

> "Hypertension – or elevated blood pressure – is a serious medical condition that significantly increases the risks of heart, brain, kidney and other diseases."

Dr Richard D Moore MD PhD, however, disagrees with this view and states in his book entitled *The High Blood Pressure Solution* that,

> "There is a lot more to hypertension than just elevated blood pressure. The increased blood pressure is a marker, or a sign that something is out of balance."

A salient point made by Dr Moore is that a stroke can occur in the absence of elevated blood pressure, which means that the relationship is not as direct as the medical establishment claims it to be.

The May 2017 WHO fact sheet entitled *Cardiovascular diseases* states that,

> "Cardiovascular diseases (CVDs) are a group of disorders of the heart and blood vessels..."

The fact sheet refers to the scale of the problem and states that,

> "CVDs are the number 1 cause of death globally..."

In addition, the *Hypertension* fact sheet states that,

> "Hypertension is a major cause of premature death worldwide."

It is clear that diseases of this nature are indicative of extremely serious health problems; but, like all other diseases, their nature is misunderstood by the medical establishment. CVDs are discussed in greater detail in chapter seven.

The original theory about blood pressure claimed that an elevated level was the underlying health problem; an idea that arose as the result of observations in which elevated blood pressure correlated with certain ill-health conditions. These observations were developed into the theory that

27

elevated blood pressure was a causal factor for various health problems, such as heart attacks and strokes.

The medical establishment solution for raised blood pressure, as with virtually all other health problems, inevitably involves the use of drugs that are intended to lower blood pressure to a 'normal range'. The achievement of a blood pressure reading within that normal range is perceived to be a successful outcome of the treatment and one that is able to reduce or even eliminate the risks of the associated health problems. The original theory about blood pressure was, however, based on a mistaken assumption, as Dr Moore explains,

> "But we now know that rather than being the primary problem, high blood pressure is a *symptom* of an unhealthy imbalance in the cells and tissues throughout the body."

Unfortunately, the 'we' of Dr Moore's statement does not refer to the medical establishment, which continues to maintain the position that elevated blood pressure requires medication so that it can be lowered to fall within the range regarded as 'normal'; as indicated by the information provided by the WHO fact sheet.

The ranges of blood pressure readings considered to be 'normal' for each age group have undergone a number of revisions since they were first created; at each revision the 'normal' range has been reduced. The basis for these changes is the continuing, but erroneous, assumption that elevated blood pressure is the cause of health problems and that the reduction of a person's blood pressure reading will also reduce the risks of the health problems associated with it.

The medical establishment claims that the most effective method for lowering blood pressure to the 'normal range', is through medication with antihypertensive drugs to be taken over the course of long periods of time; and often become lifelong. The continual downward revisions of the 'normal' ranges result in an ever-greater proportion of the population perceived to have elevated blood pressure and therefore 'at risk'; this results in an ever-increasing number of people who are prescribed antihypertensive drugs and also, inevitably, in vastly increased profits for the pharmaceutical industry.

The most recent large study that has been undertaken to investigate the problems associated with high blood pressure, indicates that another revision to an even lower 'normal' range is likely to occur in the near future. This study, called SPRINT (Systolic Blood Pressure Intervention Trial), was designed to answer certain questions, as explained on the website. One of the questions was,

> "Will lower blood pressure reduce the risk of heart and kidney diseases, stroke, or age-related declines in memory and thinking?"

This question indicates that the study intended to investigate other health problems in addition to heart disease and stroke, the two that are most often associated with elevated blood pressure. The UK NHS suggests that kidney disease is one of a number of conditions that can cause high blood pressure.

The SPRINT study involved more than 9,300 people aged 50 or older, who had a blood pressure reading that was higher than a certain designated figure and who were regarded as having at least one 'risk factor'. These participants were divided into two groups, one of which received the 'standard' blood-pressure-lowering treatment with the aim of achieving a certain target level of blood pressure. The other group received 'intensive' blood-pressure-lowering treatment with the aim of reducing their blood pressure to an even lower target level. The purpose was to determine if there were any benefits to be gained by achieving the lower blood pressure levels.

In September 2015, the NIH (National Institutes of Health), which had provided funding for the study, prepared a Press Release stating that the study had been ended a year early because the results were felt to be sufficiently significant. The Press Release begins with the statement that,

> "More intensive management of high blood pressure, below a commonly recommended blood pressure target, significantly reduces rates of cardiovascular disease, and lower risk of death in a group of adults 50 years and older with high blood pressure."

This statement would tend to suggest that the study has produced good news; but this would be a mistaken interpretation. One of the findings reported within the initial results was that the 'intensive treatment' group experienced significantly higher rates of serious adverse events than the 'standard treatment' group. This result ought to have been expected by those people who know that all drugs produce 'side effects' and that the use of multiple drugs increases the number of adverse health events.

Dr Moore explains the nature of some of the adverse health effects that result from antihypertensive drugs,

> "Besides lowering blood pressure, all antihypertensive drugs can produce undesirable side effects. This is not surprising since they alter basic body functions not only in the blood vessels but in the nervous system and kidneys as well."

This indicates that kidney disease can be the result of antihypertensive drugs, rather than the cause of high blood pressure, as suggested by the NHS.

Drugs, by definition, are intended to interfere with the normal functions of a living organism. The existence of effects in the blood vessels, nervous system and kidneys indicate that antihypertensive drugs interfere systemically; their effects are not restricted to the lowering of blood pressure. This further corroborates the statement in the previous section that drugs produce effects in parts of the body that are not the targeted, 'diseased' area.

The belief that the body is comprised of separate parts, each of which can be 'fixed' without reference to any other parts, perpetuates the idea that the adverse effects of drugs are 'risks' worth taking as they 'fix' the diseased part; but this is a false belief. Furthermore, patients are rarely advised of the full extent of the risks associated with the drugs they have been prescribed.

The failure of the medical establishment to acknowledge the toxicity of pharmaceutical drugs continues to endanger lives on a daily basis.

In his book, Dr Moore discusses the different types of drugs that are used for the treatment of hypertension and explains their 'action' in the body. The first type of treatment that is usually offered to a patient is a diuretic, which 'works' by stimulating the kidneys to increase their production and excretion of urine. The purpose of this is to encourage a reduction in the level of sodium in the body, because an increased level of sodium in the body is believed to be a major factor that can cause hypertension.

But, as Dr Moore reveals, it is not the absolute level of sodium in the body that is a problem; instead, the key factor is the comparative level of sodium with respect to the level of potassium. Cells require both sodium and potassium, but they must be in the correct balance with respect to each other for the cells to function properly.

It is not uncommon that diuretics will fail to achieve an adequate reduction in blood pressure, which leads to the recommendation of other more powerful drugs to continue the process. There are a number of drugs in this category, for example, adrenergic inhibitors, ACE inhibitors and calcium channel blockers. As indicated by their names, all of these drugs are designed to inhibit, block or otherwise interfere with the body's normal functions; which means that adverse effects are inevitable as Dr Moore explains,

"All these drugs have undesirable side effects because they act at several locations and tend to upset the body's normal balance."

Although referred to as 'side effects', the fact that all drugs enter the bloodstream means that they are able to, and invariably do, interfere systemically; causing a wide variety of adverse effects.

A worrying consequence of the SPRINT study is that, in addition to the possibility that it may generate a new lower 'range' for blood pressure readings for all age groups, it will generate a drive for increasing numbers of people to undergo regular blood pressure monitoring, even if they have no existing ill-health problems. The idea that blood pressure increases with age and that this is inevitably associated with increased 'risks' to health, already impacts many people over the age of 50, who are encouraged to have regular blood pressure checks. The UK NHS recommends that people aged 40 and older should have their blood pressure monitored annually.

The causes of elevated blood pressure are admitted to be poorly understood by the medical establishment; the UK NHS claims that it can result from certain conditions or as the result of certain medications. The CVD fact sheet suggests that there are some 'behavioural factors' that can increase the risk of developing heart disease and states,

"The most important behavioural risk factors of heart disease and stroke are unhealthy diet, physical inactivity, tobacco use and harmful use of alcohol."

Although hypertension is usually associated with increased age, it is not a condition that is only experienced by people over a certain age, whether 50 or even 40. It is reported that high blood pressure is becoming an increasingly common phenomenon in young people and even children; especially in association with obesity. Yet, despite the recognition that an unhealthy diet is a factor that increases the 'risk' of heart disease, for which the WHO recommends that people reduce their salt intake and increase their consumption of fruit and vegetables, the use of blood-pressure-lowering drugs remains a key aspect of the recommended solution.

Three of the four 'behavioural risk factors' listed by the WHO are certainly relevant to health, but they by no means provide a complete explanation of cardiovascular health problems, therefore addressing these factors alone will not solve the problem. Furthermore, 'health' is a full body issue; it cannot be achieved by only addressing the functioning of an individual organ or system in the body; even if that organ is the heart, which is vital for life itself.

One of the listed 'risk' factors, namely physical inactivity, is not the cause of any disease and so increasing physical activity can neither prevent nor solve any condition of ill-health; this topic will be discussed further in chapter ten.

In the attempt to provide a solution to the problem of CVDs, the WHO fact sheet recommends treatments that include aspirin and beta-blockers, as well as those previously mentioned. Aspirin is discussed in the final section of this chapter on the topic of OTC drugs.

The focus of this discussion has been on the use of 'medicine' to address the problem of hypertension based on the idea that the human body is solely biochemical in nature. But this idea is misleading as the human body is also bioelectrical in nature; an attribute that applies particularly to the heart, which is one of the major organs that function electrically. Therefore, any factors that produce electrical interference can have adverse effects on the cardiovascular system and especially the heart.

A 2013 article entitled *Earthing (Grounding) the Human Body Reduces Blood Viscosity: a Major Factor in Cardiovascular Disease* explains that red blood cells have a negative electrical charge and this maintains their separation from each other in the bloodstream through electrostatic repulsion. The article also states that if the negative charge on the red blood cells is reduced, the electrostatic repulsion is reduced and this leads to the inability of blood cells to remain sufficiently separated. The result of this impaired functioning is that the cells 'clump' together and that blood viscosity increases; the article explains the consequences,

> "Blood viscosity and aggregation are major factors in hypertension and other cardiovascular pathologies, including myocardial infarction."

Myocardial infarction is the medical term for a heart attack.

The article clearly supports Dr Moore's claim that hypertension is more than just elevated blood pressure and provides an explanation for one of the causes of the condition; unfortunately, the medical establishment is largely oblivious of the body's bioelectrical nature and therefore ignorant of a significant causal factor of ill-health. The bioelectrical nature of the body and the health consequences of electrical interference are discussed in greater detail in later chapters.

Statins

The establishment definition of a statin refers to,

> "any one of a class of drugs that inhibit the action of an enzyme involved in the liver's production of cholesterol."

31

The reason that drugs are required to inhibit the production of cholesterol is claimed by the NIH, on the *Resources* web page entitled *High Blood Cholesterol: What You Need to Know*, to be because,

"High blood cholesterol is one of the major risk factors for heart disease."

The medical establishment theory, which claims that a high level of cholesterol is dangerous and needs to be reduced, is, however, flawed. Interestingly, the establishment definition of cholesterol highlights one of the flaws in this theory because it includes the statement that,

"Cholesterol and its esters are important constituents of cell membranes..."

Despite the plethora of recommendations by the medical establishment that people should lower their intake of cholesterol, the total level of cholesterol within the body is not regulated by dietary intake. The overwhelming proportion, approximately 85%, of the body's requirement for cholesterol is produced by the liver; it is only the remaining 15% approximately that is obtained through the diet. If, for some reason, the diet provides the body with insufficient cholesterol, the liver will increase its production to compensate for that dietary deficiency. It is clear therefore, that it is the body that regulates the level of this vital substance.

Cholesterol is not solely an important constituent of cell membranes; it is also an important constituent of the brain and essential for its proper functioning; as indicated by a 2010 article entitled *The Effects of Cholesterol on Learning and Memory*, which states that,

"Cholesterol is ubiquitous in the central nervous system (CNS) and vital to normal brain function including signaling, synaptic plasticity, and learning and memory."

The recognition that cholesterol is vital for the proper functioning of many of the body's vital organs directly contradicts the information promulgated by the medical establishment that cholesterol is 'dangerous', and that high levels in the body pose a serious 'risk' to health.

An April 2016 article entitled *Re-evaluation of the traditional diet-heart hypothesis*, published in the *BMJ*, explains that the original hypothesis about levels of cholesterol stemmed from a study called the *Minnesota Coronary Experiment* that was conducted between 1968 and 1973; but the results of this study were not published. This experiment was a controlled study that, for the participants of one of the groups, involved the replacement of saturated fats with vegetable oils rich in linoleic acid, a polyunsaturated fat. This dietary intervention was shown to reduce serum levels of cholesterol and assumed to be beneficial.

The documents and data from this original study have recently been re-analysed and the results published in the *BMJ*. The reason that the original study was not published is claimed to be because the researcher did not believe the results he had obtained. The *BMJ* article states that,

"In meta-analyses, these cholesterol lowering interventions showed no evidence of benefit on mortality from coronary heart disease."

In addition to the lack of evidence that any benefits accrued from the lowering of cholesterol levels, the *BMJ* article reports that the evidence,

"...suggests the possibility of an increased risk of death for the intervention group..."

This is not the only study that has discovered that low cholesterol correlates with an increased risk of mortality, not a reduced risk, as the medical establishment claims.

It is stated that there are two types of cholesterol; LDL (low-density lipoproteins), which is regarded as 'bad' and HDL (high-density lipoproteins), which is regarded as 'good'; but these labels are completely misleading. The idea that cholesterol can be either good or bad is based on a misunderstanding that arose from another study that investigated the effects of cholesterol on laboratory animals. The misunderstanding occurred because it was not recognised at the time that the cholesterol used in the study had been oxidised; it is the oxidation of cholesterol that causes health problems. In his book entitled *Health and Nutrition Secrets*, Dr Russell Blaylock explains the mistaken perception about the different types of cholesterol,

"The reason LDL cholesterol is bad is that it is much easier to oxidize than HDL cholesterol. But oxidized HDL cholesterol is just as dangerous as oxidized LDL cholesterol."

Oxidation of the cholesterol that constitutes cell membranes will inevitably, adversely affect the cell's function and, likewise, oxidation of the cholesterol in the brain will affect brain function. These detrimental effects are the direct result of the process of oxidation; a process that produces 'free radicals', which are highly reactive particles that can cause damage to any part of the body with which they make contact. Oxidised cholesterol has been shown to cause damage to blood vessels; although free radicals cause damage wherever they are produced in the body.

On the basis of the flawed idea that it is a high level of cholesterol in the body that is the problem, the pharmaceutical industry developed drugs called statins to inhibit the production of this vitally important substance. Inevitably, there are many dangers associated with the use of statins, which, by intention, are designed to interfere with the body's normal production of cholesterol. The consequences of inhibiting the enzyme in the liver to reduce the production of cholesterol are discussed by Dr Carolyn Dean in *Death by Modern Medicine*,

"That enzyme, however, does much more in the body than just make cholesterol, so when it is suppressed by statins there are far-ranging consequences."

Statins are proclaimed by the medical establishment to be both safe and effective, yet, like all other drugs, they produce a number of severely detrimental effects, some of which are explained by Dr Dean,

"Since the brain has the highest concentration of cholesterol in the body, it's no wonder that the constant demand for lower and lower cholesterol counts is going to impinge on brain function. Previous studies have shown that statins can result in polyneuropathy, which causes numbness, tingling, and burning pain. Researchers showed that people taking statins were 4 to 14 times more likely to develop polyneuropathy than those who did not take statins."

Statins are intended to inhibit the production of cholesterol; they are not intended to address the problem of oxidised cholesterol, which means that they fail to address the underlying cause of the problem. There are a number of factors that can cause the oxidation of cholesterol and they include many toxic chemicals that are ubiquitous to the environment, as Dr Dean explains,

"In addition, chlorine, fluoride in water, pesticides and other environmental pollutants can also oxidize cholesterol in the body."

The problems with these chemicals and other environmental pollutants are discussed in more detail in chapter six. Oxidised cholesterol can also be found in processed and 'fast' foods, which are also discussed in more detail in chapter six.

In addition to their increased use as treatments for patients with high levels of cholesterol, statins are increasingly prescribed as preventives on the basis of the idea that this will reduce the risk of developing a CVD. As demonstrated by the study published in the *BMJ*, there is no evidence that high levels of cholesterol constitute a health problem or even increase the risk of developing health problems. The study in fact revealed the opposite; that low levels of cholesterol produce adverse health consequences and that statins increase the level of harm to health.

The harm that they have been shown to cause is demonstrated by the withdrawal of certain statin drugs from the market following reports about a number of severe 'side effects', and even death in some cases. Nevertheless, many statin drugs remain on the market, including some that are known to produce many serious adverse effects, as has been reported by many patients who have taken these drugs. This would seem to be another instance of the benefit being claimed to outweigh the risk; but this is clearly not the case.

One of the serious adverse effects that can result from the use of statins is reported in a December 2015 article entitled *Statin Use and the Risk of Kidney Disease With Long-Term Follow-Up (8.4-Year Study)* published in the *American Journal of Cardiology*. This study acknowledges that there had been few studies on the long-term use of statins, especially with respect to the effects on kidney disease. The conclusion to the study states that,

"...statin use is associated with increased incidence of acute and chronic kidney disease."

The reason that these serious health problems were not discovered from the original clinical trials is also explained by the article that states,

"These findings are cautionary and suggest that long-term effects of statins in real-life patients may differ from shorter term effects in selected clinical trial populations."

Yet again, the medical establishment's lack of knowledge about the human body has created more problems than it has solved in the attempt to reduce the incidence of heart disease. Cholesterol is not responsible for heart disease, therefore attempts to reduce the body's production of cholesterol will not reduce the risk of heart disease.

Over-The-Counter (OTC) Medicines

The establishment definition of an over-the-counter medicine refers to, "a drug that may be purchased directly from a pharmacist without a doctor's prescription."

This means that people can 'self-medicate'; which has many implications. One major anomaly that is rarely raised in discussions on the subject relates to the idea that the use of OTC drugs is deemed acceptable to reduce the burden on the 'health system', because it means that people do not need to see a 'qualified' physician. But all professional medical associations claim that anyone who 'treats' illness other than a suitably qualified physician is a 'quack'. Yet the medical establishment deems 'ordinary' people to be sufficiently competent to treat their own aches, pains and fevers with OTC 'medicines'.

The use of OTC drugs is justified on the basis that they are able to treat 'minor' conditions, such as headaches and fevers, and that the cessation of these symptoms indicates that the illness has been conquered and the person is now 'well'. However, pain and fever can occur as the result of a number of underlying factors, including the use of prescription drugs, that are not addressed by the OTC drugs, which only alleviate symptoms or sometimes stop them, albeit temporarily.

Although the drugs that are available without prescription are limited to certain types and only available in restricted strengths and quantities, the inherent problems with pharmaceutical ingredients and manufacturing processes demonstrate that OTC drugs are similarly toxic by nature and therefore similarly harmful. Their potential dangers are indicated by the fact that these drugs are available in restricted quantities to avoid the adverse effects from the 'wrong' dose.

There is a limited recognition by the medical establishment of the potential harm from OTC drugs, as described in an April 2013 article entitled *Over-the-counter medicine abuse – a review of the literature* published in the *Journal of Substance Abuse*. The emphasis in the article is clearly with reference to the abuse of OTC drugs, but it does include an acknowledgement of the potential for addiction and of the harm they can cause. A particularly relevant comment in the article is that,

"OTC medicine abuse is a recognised problem internationally but is currently incompletely understood."

This statement shows yet another facet of 'healthcare' that is poorly understood, but it also fails to address a fundamental question, which is why 'medicines' that are supposed to 'heal' can cause 'harm'; especially those of the restricted types that are allowed to be purchased without a prescription.

In addition to any 'effects' caused by each individual drug is a lesser known problem, which is the effects that result from interactions between different drugs. It is a sad fact of life in the early 21st century that a large number of people take multiple prescription medications as well as many OTC drugs; this is known by the term 'polypharmacy'.

The medical establishment recognises the existence of interactions and some information may be printed on the package inserts of OTC drugs, which is usually available and accessible after the purchase has been made, unless the customer has consulted the pharmacist, who may be able to provide some information about contraindications.

The scale of OTC drug manufacture alone is huge; the FDA web page entitled *Drug Applications for Over-the-Counter (OTC) Drugs* states that,

"...there are over 300,000 marketed OTC drug products..."

The total number of drug products available on the market is therefore clearly enormous. However, the full extent of the potential interactions between all drugs, both prescription and OTC, is entirely unknown, because, although some drug-drug interactions have been investigated, the overwhelming majority of drugs remain untested for their interactions with all other available drugs, both prescription and OTC.

The failure to address the problem of unknown drug-drug interactions is only in a very small part due to the fact that new drugs of all kinds are constantly being introduced onto the market, even though some drugs are removed. The major reason for the lack of full knowledge about the interactions between drugs is because, as previously mentioned, many 'treatments' have not been exhaustively tested or independently assessed.

The easy availability of OTC 'medicines' suggests that they would have been thoroughly tested for their efficacy and safety; but this is not the case. On the web page about OTC drug applications, the FDA states that they only review the active ingredients, not the individual drugs. But, as previously cited, the FDA only conducts reviews of reports prepared by the pharmaceutical company that manufactured the drug; they do not conduct their own independent tests to determine the safety and efficacy of the active ingredients of the drugs they approve.

This is a major problem within the medical establishment 'system', which is increasingly controlled by the pharmaceutical industry, as will be discussed in chapter nine. The general public is therefore completely in the hands of the pharmaceutical industry with respect to all of the 'medicines' they may take.

A few examples of common OTC drugs will demonstrate some of the hazards associated with their use.

Aspirin

The establishment definition of aspirin refers to,

"a widely used drug that relieves pain and also reduces inflammation and fever."

Aspirin (acetylsalicylic acid) is a common OTC drug; it is an NSAID (nonsteroidal anti-inflammatory drug). It is also used as a 'preventive' for heart attacks and strokes; although for this preventive purpose it is recommended to be taken at a 'low dose' and usually under the direction of a physician. Although all 'experts' within the medical establishment are generally in agreement on topics relating to appropriate treatments, the Mayo Clinic web page entitled *Daily aspirin therapy: Understand the benefits and risks* makes the interesting revelation that,

"...there's some disagreement among experts about whether the benefits of aspirin outweigh its potential risks."

This statement illustrates two points, one of which is the intriguing idea that 'experts' do not always agree, thus challenging the ridiculous notion that science is always the result of a 'consensus'. The other, more salient, point is that it highlights the contradictory notion that a substance can be both beneficial for and pose risks to health.

Some of the 'side effects' of aspirin include gastrointestinal problems such as nausea, vomiting and abdominal pain; more serious effects include gastrointestinal bleeding. These effects, which are not 'side effects' but directly result from the ingestion of aspirin, should not be surprising because aspirin is recognised to irritate the stomach lining.

It was once quite common for doctors to recommend aspirin for children with a fever. But it was later discovered that when children were diagnosed with conditions such as chickenpox or 'flu', the use of aspirin to treat the fever could cause a condition called Reye's syndrome, which affects the brain and liver and is often fatal.

The 'active ingredient' in aspirin is salicylic acid, which is synthesised from a substance found in willow bark that has long been regarded as an effective pain relief agent; it is claimed that Hippocrates used it. Previous discussions have indicated however, that a long history of the use of any substance to alleviate symptoms does not prove that it is beneficial or safe. Some of the substances used as remedies 'worked' due to their toxic nature; an emetic is a pertinent example.

It is also important to emphasise that the suppression of symptoms, such as pain or fever, with drugs will never 'cure' the problem because they do not address or remove the underlying cause.

Paracetamol/Acetaminophen

The establishment definition of paracetamol refers to,

"an analgesic drug that also reduces fever."

Paracetamol, or acetaminophen as it is also called, became a popular replacement for aspirin when detrimental effects, such as Reye's syndrome, were discovered to result from its use. However, paracetamol is also associated with a number of detrimental effects and has been officially cited as a major cause of liver failure. It is likely that most people who take this OTC drug for their aches, pains and fevers are completely unaware of its potential danger to their health.

The definition does include a limited recognition of the potential harm that paracetamol can cause in the statement that,

"...overdosage causes liver damage."

Paracetamol is a glutathione-exhausting drug, which is one of the reasons that it is dangerous because glutathione is an essential element for proper functioning of the body and glutathione depletion can result in hepatic and renal failure, hence the statement that it is a cause of liver failure.

Paracetamol can also result in death, which is why it is sometimes used in large quantities by people who have tried, and occasionally succeeded, in taking their own lives. Whilst people believe the maxim that it is the dose that makes a substance a poison, they will continue to assume that small doses are 'safe'; but this is a false and dangerous assumption, because an accumulation of paracetamol resulting from many small doses over the course of a long period of time can be similarly dangerous.

Codeine

The establishment definition of codeine refers to,

"an opioid analgesic derived from morphine but less potent as a pain killer and sedative and less toxic."

Codeine is an example of a powerful drug that can nevertheless be purchased and used without a prescription. As the definition states, it is a member of the opiate family of drugs that includes morphine and heroin and, like them, can be addictive. Although the definition states that dependence on codeine is 'uncommon', there is adequate evidence to demonstrate that it has caused addiction, a fact that is stated in the previously cited article about OTC medicine abuse.

In addition to the possibility of addiction, there are distinct symptoms associated with withdrawal from codeine, which, if people are unaware of them, can be confused with a new kind of health 'problem'.

It has also been established that codeine is metabolised in the body into morphine, which can be passed by a breastfeeding mother to her baby.

The 'side effects' of codeine include symptoms that range from headaches and vomiting to hallucinations, mood changes and impotence. These are extremely unpleasant 'effects' from a medicine that is supposed to relieve pain. Most people will, however, be unaware that these new symptoms are the result of the codeine they have taken and may assume it is a new health problem for which they may seek relief from the use of other OTC medicines.

Antacids

The establishment definition of an antacid refers to,

"a drug that neutralizes the hydrochloric acid secreted in the digestive juices of the stomach."

Antacid drugs are another very popular group of over-the-counter medications. They are used for the relief of heartburn or indigestion, which are assumed to be the result of the production of too much acid in the stomach. The stomach normally produces acid as part of the digestive processes and usually does so in the correct volume to fully process the food that has been consumed. However, antacids disrupt the natural level and balance of acid in the stomach, which therefore needs to produce more acid to counteract the effects of the antacid in order to process the food.

The frequent use of antacids will inevitably result in digestive problems and can lead to more serious conditions; the continual consumption of antacids will intensify digestive problems rather than relieve them.

The real problem that causes the symptoms associated with indigestion is that the stomach contains too much food for the digestive juices to be able to process all of it efficiently. Antacids therefore produce the completely opposite effect from the one they are claimed to produce.

The examples discussed above are clearly only a few of the drugs available without prescription. There are of course many more, all of which can be viewed in the same way: in other words: they do not address the underlying causes of the symptoms; they do not result in the return to a state of 'health'; and they invariably cause additional health problems, some of which are more serious than the original problem they were intended to remedy.

In Summary

It should be abundantly obvious from the discussions in this section that drugs are not only ineffective, but are also harmful. This statement, although challenging to the information promulgated by the medical establishment, can be corroborated by the physicians quoted in this chapter, to which can be added the following remarks.

First from Dr Carolyn Dean in *Death by Modern Medicine*,

> "Loss of confidence in drug companies is inevitable when drugs are pulled from the market due to dangerous side effects. Numerous recent examples include hormone replacement therapy, causing heart disease and cancer; suicides on antidepressants, Vioxx causing heart attacks; diabetes drugs causing heart disease; statin drugs to lower cholesterol causing heart disease, impotence, and muscle disease; and osteoporosis drugs causing jaw bone destruction."

There are two pertinent quotes by Herbert Shelton ND DC from his book, *Natural Hygiene: Man's Pristine Way of Life*, the first of which states that,

> "It is necessary, if they [the public] are to be rescued from drug induced degeneracy and death, that the truth about drugs shall be made known. It must become common knowledge that there are no good drugs and that even their apparent beneficial effects are illusions. The symptomatic relief afforded by drugs is as illusory as the snakes the alcoholic sees in his boots."

The second states that,

> "...so long as the medical profession and the drug industry...continue to teach the stultifying doctrine that poisons are the proper means with which to build, maintain and restore health, the public can have no different attitude towards drugs than the traditional one which it now holds."

NOTE: Withdrawal from any drug should always be undertaken with appropriate supervision from a practitioner who is aware of the potential withdrawal reactions that can occur.

Chapter Two

Vaccinations: Ineffective and Dangerous

"An error does not become truth by reason of multiplied propagation, nor does truth become error because nobody sees it."

Mahatma Gandhi

The definition of 'medicine' cited in the previous chapter refers to the prevention of disease. The medical establishment claims that one of the most effective methods by which certain diseases can be prevented is vaccination, which the establishment definition refers to as,

> "a means of producing immunity to a disease by using a vaccine, or a special preparation of antigenic material, to stimulate the formation of appropriate antibodies."

The presence of the appropriate antibodies is therefore deemed to be synonymous with immunity.

Vaccination is widely acclaimed as one of the finest achievements of 'modern medicine'; a view that is encapsulated by the WHO on the web page entitled *Vaccines: A global health success story that keeps us on our toes*, which asserts that,

> "It's no secret that vaccines are considered one of the greatest global health achievements."

To this statement is added the claim that,

> "Every year they avert an estimated 2 to 3 million deaths."

Nothing could be further from the truth; these claims and assertions are entirely unfounded.

The quote attributed to Mahatma Gandhi that opens this chapter is particularly pertinent to vaccination, which is a practice based on theories that have never been proven to be true. It is for this reason that vaccination must be understood as an 'error'. It is, however, an error of such a

40

fundamental nature that it cannot be made into 'truth' no matter how fervently the medical establishment asserts otherwise.

The idea that vaccination is an error will be viewed as highly controversial; nevertheless, there is an abundance of evidence to demonstrate that, contrary to the claims promulgated by the medical establishment, vaccines are not one of the greatest health achievements; they do not confer immunity to disease; they do not save lives; and, most importantly, they are neither safe nor effective.

These assertions can be substantiated; but to do so requires more detailed discussions about the theories on which the practice of vaccination is based.

As indicated by the definition, the main theory involves the concept of 'immunity'. This theory claims that exposure to an infectious disease stimulates the body to produce the appropriate antibodies, the presence of which is said to indicate that the body has acquired 'natural immunity' to that disease. There is however, a problem with this theory, because people can and do experience repeated episodes of the same infectious disease; this means that they have failed to acquire 'immunity' from their first exposure to the disease. The theory is clearly flawed as it is not supported by empirical evidence.

The practice of vaccination is based on the same assumption about immunity with the additional claim that vaccines are more effective in stimulating the body to produce the appropriate antibodies. However, vaccinated people also experience repeated episodes of the infectious diseases against which they have been vaccinated; they too have failed to acquire 'immunity'. Vaccinated people who fail to produce the appropriate antibodies are called 'non-responders'.

In an attempt to offer an explanation for vaccine 'non-responders', the WHO web page entitled *Adverse Events Following Immunization (AEFI)*, in a series of pages on the topic of *Global Vaccine Safety*, makes the following revealing statement,

> "There is no such thing as a 'perfect' vaccine which protects everyone who receives it AND is entirely safe for everyone."

This statement clearly contrasts with the generally accepted view that vaccines are fundamentally safe and effective; if this were the case, they would be safe and effective for everyone. Nevertheless, the WHO fails to explain the reason that the 'greatest global health achievement' is unable to protect or be safe for everyone.

However, the mechanism by which some people become 'non-responders' is unknown; an anomaly that is acknowledged in an August 2013 article entitled *When vaccinations fail to cause response: Causes vary with vaccine and person*, which states that the reasons that some people do not respond to vaccines,

> "...have remained unidentified up to now."

This admission undermines the assurances of the medical establishment prior to 2013 that vaccines stimulate the body to produce antibodies that confer immunity to disease; there are clearly a number of knowledge gaps with respect to vaccines and especially to how they 'work'. However, despite the claim in the article that the reasons that some people are non-responders have now been identified, the explanation offered does not provide any real clarity on the subject; the article continues,

"...there is no standard pattern to this but that the causes vary according to vaccination and group of people..."

The underlying assumption is that all human bodies are alike, which means that people should all respond in exactly the same manner to vaccines. This assumption is clearly flawed because people do not all respond in the same way to vaccines, but this does not mean that some vaccines are effective for some people.

In reality, no vaccine is effective for anyone; none of them is capable of producing immunity and therefore providing protection from disease.

The previously cited WHO statement about vaccines also revealed that they are not 'entirely safe for everyone'; an admission that, although significant, fails to acknowledge the true scale of the problem of 'unsafe' vaccines.

As this chapter will demonstrate, no vaccine is safe for anyone; they are all fundamentally harmful.

Some of the evidence of harm caused by vaccines is acknowledged by the medical establishment itself; for example, the establishment definition of vaccination also states that,

"Vaccination is often carried out in two or three stages, as separate doses are less likely to cause unpleasant side effects."

The most common vaccine 'side effects' are recognised by physicians, who generally warn their patients about the possibility of a fever or of soreness and inflammation at the site of the injection. The previous chapter demonstrated that the term 'side effect' is a misnomer when used to refer to the effects of pharmaceutical drugs; it is also a misnomer when used to refer to the effects of vaccines. There are many 'effects' that are the direct result of vaccination and some of them are far more serious than fever, soreness or inflammation.

The topic of vaccine injury is discussed in more detail later in this chapter.

The assertion that vaccines are not only ineffective but positively dangerous is also substantiated by Herbert Shelton who, with reference to the smallpox vaccine, states in *Natural Hygiene: Man's Pristine Way of Life* that,

"In addition to being a failure as a preventive, the vaccine produces a whole train of evil side effects and iatrogenic diseases."

The discussion about iatrogenesis in the previous chapter indicated that the term is used to refer to illness and death from pharmaceutical drugs and medical procedures. The *Death by Medicine* report also referred to in that discussion does not include vaccines as a source of iatrogenic illness and death; which indicates that the real tragedy of iatrogenesis is far worse than has been reported.

The adverse effects of vaccines are seriously underreported for a number of reasons, one of which is that revelations of their truly harmful nature would undermine the WHO claim that vaccines are a great health achievement that saves lives; a procedure that causes harm to health cannot be one that simultaneously save lives. Another reason is that, in order to eradicate 'deadly infectious diseases', it is claimed that a high percentage of the population needs to be vaccinated; this is referred to as 'herd immunity', the erroneous nature of which is discussed later in this chapter. This high level of 'vaccine coverage' will however, be jeopardised by widespread public awareness of the harmful nature of vaccines, because it is highly likely that large numbers of people will refuse to submit themselves and their families to vaccination.

It is asserted that a failure to achieve herd immunity within a specified population will have a detrimental impact on efforts to eradicate deadly diseases, but this is not the case; the only detrimental impact from the failure to reach the requisite percentage of 'vaccine coverage' will be on the profits of vaccine-producing pharmaceutical companies.

Although admitted to be estimated, the number of lives alleged to be saved by vaccines varies widely according to the source of the estimate. In marked contrast to the statistics provided by the WHO are those provided by UNICEF (United Nations Children's Emergency Fund) in a 1996 article entitled *Vaccines bring 7 diseases under control*, which makes the bold statement that,

> "Two hundred years after the discovery of vaccine by the English physician Edward Jenner, immunization can be credited with saving approximately 9 million lives a year worldwide."

The discrepancy between the claims of the WHO and those of UNICEF is significant but unexplained; nevertheless, neither of these claims can be substantiated.

It is possible, however, to substantiate the assertion that vaccines are ineffective and harmful; the supportive evidence for this statement has been gleaned from the work of many eminently qualified medical practitioners, some of whom raised valid objections to vaccination from its inception. These people and their work are usually referred to in derisory terms by the medical establishment, but that does not deny the veracity of their reasons for opposing the practice of vaccination; the statements they have made in opposition to vaccination were the result of their own independent investigations.

England was the country in which the practice of vaccination was first introduced, courtesy of Edward Jenner; it was also the first country to introduce mandatory vaccination. It is for these reasons, plus the substantial documentation and statistical information available on the topic, that the situation in England provides much of the material for this discussion.

One of the many medical practitioners who raised objections to vaccination was Dr Walter Hadwen MD MRCS LRCP, who had qualified in England under both the Royal College of Surgeons and the Royal College of Physicians. In 1896 Dr Hadwen addressed a meeting, at which he stated,

> "As a medical man I look upon vaccination as an insult to common sense, as superstitious in its origin, unscientific in theory and practice, and useless and

dangerous in its character."

The 1853 and subsequent Vaccination Acts made infant vaccination compulsory in England, although at the time only the smallpox vaccine was mandatory. Dr Hadwen's objection to vaccination was so strong that he refused to allow his own children to be vaccinated, despite this refusal earning him a total of nine prosecutions.

Dr Charles Creighton MD, another qualified English physician, was so highly regarded by the medical establishment that in 1884 he was asked to write the vaccination entry for the ninth edition of the *Encyclopaedia Britannica*. At the time he was fully supportive of vaccination; but, before writing the required text, he decided to investigate the subject thoroughly. The result of his investigation is explained by Eleanor McBean PhD ND in her book, *The Poisoned Needle*,

> "He agreed to do so, but instead of contenting himself with the usual stock statements he went right back to Jenner's own writings and to contemporary documents. He searched the pro- and anti-vaccination literature of many countries and came to the conclusion that vaccination is a 'grotesque superstition'."

Dr Creighton's vaccination entry, although accepted by the editor of the *Encyclopaedia*, was considered totally unacceptable to those in positions of authority within the medical establishment, because it contradicted the prevailing view on the topic. Despite the high esteem in which he was held by most of his medical colleagues, Dr Creighton received no further requests to contribute to *Encyclopaedia Britannica*.

Another English physician who opposed the practice of vaccination was Dr M Beddow Bayly MD MRCS LRCP, who had also qualified under both the Royal College of Surgeons and the Royal College of Physicians. In 1936 Dr Beddow Bayly wrote a booklet entitled *The Case Against Vaccination*, in which he states that,

> "Of scientific basis or justification for the practice there is none, and the history of vaccination is the record of a superstitious rite pursued by a series of methods each in turn abandoned when experience proved its danger, and presenting a trail of extravagant claims not one of which has stood the test of time."

Clearly by 1936 the scientific basis of and justification for the practice of vaccination were still conspicuous by their absence; a situation that remains unchanged at the beginning of the 21st century.

It may be suggested that the criticisms cited in this discussion are out of date, but this would be an insufficient argument. It is inappropriate, as well as illogical, to refute the words of qualified physicians who refer to vaccination as unscientific, unjustified and a superstition purely on the basis that they lived during an earlier period of time. The main reason that this is an entirely inappropriate argument is because the theory underlying the practice of vaccination is far older; it is based on ideas that date back to much earlier periods of history, long before the 18th century work of Edward Jenner, all of which substantially predate the writings of the vaccination critics cited above.

It may also be suggested that 21st century vaccinations are different, that the practice now operates from the basis of 'evidence-based science';

however, as shown by the work of Drs Hadwen, Creighton and Beddow Bayly, objective investigations into the history of the practice have revealed that there is no science or evidence on which this practice was originally based; nor has any new 'scientific theory' been developed since that of Edward Jenner. There is still no scientific basis or justification for the practice of vaccination.

The subject of vaccination is also discussed within the 'alternative health' community, many of whom argue for 'safer', fewer or more widely-spaced vaccinations and for the vaccine schedules to be limited to only those that are necessary. The discussions in this chapter will demonstrate that this view is also mistaken; there are no safe vaccines and no necessary vaccines.

Some History

The belief that people can become 'immune' to a disease after an exposure to that disease dates back many centuries. For example, the Greek historian Thucydides, who was a contemporary of Hippocrates, is reported to have claimed that people who survived the plague of Athens were not later re-infected by the same disease.

This early belief developed into the idea that a mild form of any disease provides 'protection' against a more serious 'attack' of the same disease; it also inspired the creation of different methods to induce the 'mild' form of the disease; one of these methods was the practice of 'inoculation', or variolation as it was also called.

Although credited as the originator of 'vaccination', Edward Jenner is not to be credited as the originator of inoculation, which was practised in various places around the world many centuries before he was born. Some sources credit the Chinese as the originators of the practice of variolation during the 10th century.

Inoculation, the precursor of vaccination, was introduced into England in the early 18th century, which was a period when illness was often interpreted by reference to local traditions or superstitions and invariably 'treated' with a wide variety of crude methods and toxic substances as discussed in the previous chapter.

The practice of inoculation involved taking some 'matter', in other words 'pus', from the pustules or sores of a person suffering from the disease and introducing that 'matter' into the bloodstream of a healthy person via a number of deliberately made cuts on their arms or legs. However, prior to inoculation, patients had to undergo other procedures, such as 'dieting, purging and bleeding', that were administered by physicians. At that period of time, inoculation was exclusively a custom of the middle and upper classes, as they were the only people who could afford the services of a physician.

The following extract is from the 1885 book entitled *The Story of a Great Delusion* by William White; it provides a revealing description of the state of 'medicine' in the early 18th century in England when inoculation was first introduced.

"Those who fancy there could be any wide or effective resistance to inoculation in 1721 misapprehend the conditions of the time. There was no scientific knowledge of the laws of health; diseases were generally regarded as mysterious dispensations of Providence over which the sufferers had little control; and a great part of medicine was a combination of absurdity with nastiness. It would not be difficult to compile a series of recipes from the pharmacopoeia of that day which would alternately excite amusement, surprise, and disgust, and to describe medical practice from which it is marvellous that ever patient escaped alive; but so much must pass without saying. Suffice it to assert, that to inoculation there was little material for opposition, rational or irrational; and that what we might think the natural horror of transfusing the filth of smallpox into the blood of health, was neutralised by the currency of a multitude of popular remedies which seemed to owe their fascination to their outrageous and loathsome characteristics."

The practice of inoculation also appeared in America in the early 18th century, courtesy of Cotton Mather. It is reported that he learned of the practice from his Sudanese slave.

The English medical establishment of the 18th century was generally supportive of inoculation, despite the complete absence of any 'scientific evidence' for its efficacy or safety. Dr Beddow Bayly explains in his booklet, *The Case Against Vaccination*, that inoculations frequently caused the disease they were supposed to prevent. He also discusses the introduction in 1721 of inoculation, which,

"...being acclaimed by the Royal College of Physicians as 'highly salutary to the human race', was assiduously carried out until 1840, when, on account of the disastrous spread of smallpox which resulted, it was made a penal offence."

The Royal College of Physicians was considered a prestigious organisation, but those who were responsible for their policies had clearly failed to undertake a genuine scientific investigation of the practice of inoculation. As Dr Beddow Bayly explains, inoculation was discontinued in England in 1840; it was however, fully replaced by vaccination. But vaccination was based on exactly the same unproven theory, which is that the introduction of noxious matter into the bloodstream of an otherwise healthy person would provide 'protection' from smallpox.

The influence of Paracelsus and his belief that 'poisons' can create health is clearly discernible.

The only difference between inoculation and vaccination is that the former introduced 'matter' taken from the pustules of a person suffering with smallpox and the latter introduced 'matter' taken from the pustules of a cow suffering with cowpox.

The origin of the word vaccinate is from the Latin for cow.

The practice of vaccination originated from the work of Edward Jenner, who, in the late 18th century, discovered a belief amongst dairymaids that an attack of 'cowpox', which is an ulceration of the cow's udder and believed to be transmissible to humans, was said to provide a certain degree of relief from 'smallpox'. It was also believed that cowpox and smallpox were related diseases, which explains the belief that any attack of smallpox that occurred subsequent to an attack of cowpox would only be very mild.

It is reported that Edward Jenner accepted the dairymaids' belief about cowpox, but there is a further twist to this tale because at one time he held a different view, which is explained by William White in *The Story of a Great Delusion*,

> "Cows in Gloucestershire were milked by men as well as by women; and men would sometimes milk cows with hands foul from dressing the heels of horses afflicted with what was called grease. With this grease they infected the cows, and the pox which followed was pronounced by Jenner to have all the virtue against smallpox which the dairymaids claimed for cowpox."

William White further states that Jenner published a paper on his horse-grease theory, but as it was not well-received, he returned to his cowpox theory. Whilst this may seem to be merely a minor detail, it is relevant to a full appreciation of Edward Jenner's true contribution to humanity; the introduction of methods of poisoning the bloodstream in the name of 'protection' from disease.

Dr John W Hodge MD, an American physician, also began his medical career as a supporter of vaccination. However, he later conducted his own investigation into the subject and this led him to became aware that vaccinations did not prevent disease, but instead, were harmful. His investigation inspired him to write a booklet entitled *The Vaccination Superstition*, in which he lists his objections to the smallpox vaccination. These objections include the following,

> "After a careful consideration of the history of vaccination and smallpox .... I am firmly convinced:
>
> That vaccination is not only useless but positively injurious;
>
> That there is no evidence worthy of the name on record to prove that vaccination either prevents or mitigates smallpox."

In his role as the originator of the practice of vaccination, Edward Jenner is regarded by the medical establishment as a 'hero'; but he is a false hero and his accolades are undeserved. Although referred to as a physician, it is documented that he did not study for or pass the medical examinations that would have been necessary for him to qualify as a physician. It is also documented that Edward Jenner purchased his medical degree, although this was not an entirely uncommon practice of the time in which he lived. These are facts, however, that are invariably omitted from the mainstream histories of his life, as they would certainly tarnish his reputation.

Furthermore, his qualification as a fellow of the Royal Society was not the result of any work that related to medical matters, but the result of his study on the life of the cuckoo. The only paper about vaccination that he submitted to the Royal Society was rejected on the basis that it lacked proof. Other than this rejected paper no further 'scientific' work was submitted by Edward Jenner to the Royal Society for approval on the topic of vaccination, as Herbert Shelton explains,

> "Neither Jenner nor any of his successors ever re-presented the claims for this vaccine, together with proofs, to the Royal Society..."

During the 19th century there was a great deal of opposition in England to the practice of vaccination and this led to the creation in 1866 of an anti-vaccination movement, particularly after the enactment of the compulsory Vaccination Acts. The movement gained momentum after further and more stringent compulsory Vaccination Acts had been passed and larger numbers of people became aware of the dangers of vaccines. This movement would eventually include a number of eminent physicians of the time; two of whom are cited by Dr Hadwen in *The Case Against Vaccination*,

> "...Dr Crookshank and Dr Creighton...have knocked the bottom out of this grotesque superstition and shown that vaccination has no scientific leg to stand on..."

At the time Dr Edgar Crookshank MD was professor of pathology and bacteriology at Kings College. He, like Dr Creighton, was originally supportive of vaccination but, after conducting his own independent investigation into the subject, he too changed his professional opinion. He is recorded to have stated that the medical profession should give up vaccination.

In 1896 the movement was re-named 'The National Anti-Vaccination League of Great Britain'. Its members included some of the qualified physicians whose work is quoted in this chapter, in addition to the two eminent physicians referred to above, who supported the movement once they had investigated the matter for themselves and discovered the complete absence of any scientific evidence for its use. Other notable supporters of the British anti-vaccination movement were the scientists Alfred Russel Wallace and Herbert Spencer and the author George Bernard Shaw.

The attitude of the medical establishment towards the 'anti-vaccination movement' in the 19th century was extremely derogatory, despite the eminent physicians and scientists who were supportive of their efforts. This disparaging attitude has continued and remains firmly in place in the early 21st century. It is illustrated by an article in the February 2008 Bulletin of the WHO entitled *Vaccination greatly reduces disease, disability, death and inequity worldwide* that provides a suggestion of how to address people who question vaccines,

> "The best way in the long term is to refute wrong allegations at the earliest opportunity by providing scientifically valid data."

The genuine 'scientifically valid data' to be used to refute the wrong allegations with respect to the efficacy and safety of vaccines, can be demonstrated by the scientific investigations conducted by physicians such as Drs Creighton, Crookshank, Hodge and Hadwen, to name just a few, all of whom concluded that vaccines have no basis in science, nor are they safe or effective. The 'wrong allegations' are therefore those that claim otherwise.

Inoculation and vaccination were both introduced on the basis of the same beliefs and superstitions, not on the basis of science, and they both generated an increased incidence of and mortality from the disease known as smallpox.

Unfortunately, however, although inoculation was abolished, the 'grotesque superstition' that is vaccination has yet to be subjected to the same fate.

Smallpox

The establishment definition of smallpox refers to it as,

"an acute infectious disease causing high fever and a rash that scars the skin."

Smallpox is the only human disease that the medical establishment claims to have successfully eradicated; this is said to have occurred as the result of a vaccination campaign during the 1960s and 1970s.

'Pox', in whichever form, refers to a disease that is characterised by skin sores, pustules and fever. The occurrence of diseases like smallpox results from a combination of factors that include poor living conditions, as described by Dr Hadwen in his previously cited 1896 address, in which he states that,

"It was a time when, to take London for instance...Sanitary arrangements were altogether absent. They obtained their water from conduits and wells in the neighbourhood, Water closets there were none, and no drainage system existed. It was in London especially that smallpox abounded..."

Unfortunately, the statistics relating to the incidence of smallpox in London were extrapolated to the rest of the country under the assumption that the incidence was the same everywhere. This was a mistaken assumption because smallpox was far more rampant in overcrowded towns and cities with no sanitary arrangements than in rural areas, which made the problem of smallpox seem far worse than it was. The greatest problem was that the mistaken ideas about disease causation promulgated by the medical establishment and taught in medical schools, prevented most physicians from recognising that the dreadful conditions in which many people lived were directly related to their poor health.

These dreadful living conditions also existed in a number of European countries in the early 18th century; they were not restricted to England, nor were mistaken ideas about disease causation restricted to that country either. As indicated in the previous chapter, erroneous notions of health and disease have existed in various countries around the world for millennia.

It is quite clear from books and documents written during the 19th century that a number of physicians were aware that poor living conditions, which included a lack of sanitation and drainage, as well as a lack of fresh water and personal cleanliness, were important factors in the causation of smallpox. There is irrefutable evidence to support this assertion; such evidence includes two examples of courses of action implemented that were both successful in achieving substantial reductions in the incidence of and mortality from smallpox. In both examples, the actions taken included the abolition of existing vaccination programmes, as well as the implementation of sanitary reforms.

The first example refers to the situation in Cleveland, Ohio as explained by Dr John Hodge, who wrote in 1902 that,

"To Dr Friedrich, in charge of the Health Board of Cleveland, Ohio, is due the credit of furnishing the civilized world with an example of a large city being absolutely free from smallpox, and it would be well to note that one of the first means that he adopted in producing this result was to abolish vaccination absolutely."

death cannot result from the use of any pharmaceutical drug. The training doctors undergo inculcates a strong belief in the Hippocratic Oath that they should 'do no harm', which makes doctors understandably reluctant to attribute harm to any of the procedures they have used for their patients. This reluctance is acknowledged by Professor George Dick who states in an article in the June 1971 edition of the *British Medical Journal* that,

"...few doctors like to attribute a death or complication to a procedure which they have recommended and in which they believe."

Although understandable, this reluctance should not blind doctors to the increasing volume of empirical evidence that vaccines do cause harm. Many brave physicians, as discussed in previous sections of this chapter, have overcome many of the fallacies of their medical training and recognised the failings within the theories about vaccination.

Despite accumulating evidence to the contrary, medical training programmes preserve the dogma that vaccinations are effective and a safe method of preventing disease; with the proviso that some people 'may' react badly to them. There are reasons that some people react more strongly to vaccines than others, but those reasons are not understood by the medical establishment that denies the relevance of toxic vaccine ingredients as contributory factors.

The denial that vaccines cause harm, except in allegedly 'rare' circumstances, is illustrated by the NHS *Vaccine side effects* page that states,

"Not all illnesses that occur following vaccination will be a side effect. Because millions of people every year are vaccinated, it's inevitable that some will go on to develop a coincidental infection or illness shortly afterwards."

The claim that an ensuing illness is 'coincidental' is unscientific; illness following vaccination is rarely a 'coincidence' and is invariably a direct effect of the vaccine. The idea that a subsequent illness can be an 'infection' is also erroneous, as the discussions in the next chapter will demonstrate. Although some effects occur within a short period after the administration of a vaccine, some effects take longer to become noticeable, as Dr Buchwald explains,

"Vaccine damage is generally not recognised immediately after vaccination, but in many cases only after weeks, months or – in certain circumstances – also years later."

Eleanor McBean wrote *The Poisoned Needle* in 1957, which was a time when the standard infant vaccination schedule contained far fewer vaccines than in the early 21st century. However, she reports that many medical doctors were beginning to observe an increase in the incidence of cancer and other serious health problems as the vaccination coverage in the population increased. Many of these physicians were fully convinced that vaccines were substantial contributing factors to these diseases. One of the physicians referred to in her book is Dr Forbes Laurie MD, who had been Medical Director of the Metropolitan Cancer Hospital (London); Eleanor McBean quotes his statement that,

"I am thoroughly convinced that the increase in cancer is due to vaccination."

The claim that there is a connection between vaccination and cancer may be perceived as yet another outrageous statement but that does not make it untrue or even impossible. As the detailed discussion about cancer in chapter seven will show, one of the main factors that contribute to its development is the accumulation of toxins, especially those that are carcinogenic. It should be noted that mercury and formaldehyde are both recognised carcinogens.

The above statement should not be interpreted to mean that vaccination is the sole cause of cancer; nevertheless, vaccines are likely to be major contributory factors, even though this is rarely acknowledged. The fact that the vast majority of the population has been subjected to vaccination means that it is virtually impossible to perform comparison studies between vaccinated and unvaccinated populations, that may be able to indicate if the incidence of cancer in the former group exceeds that of the latter group. There are reasons that epidemiological studies are unable to establish the existence of a clear link between vaccines and cancer and these are discussed in chapters six and seven. However, the use of carcinogenic substances as ingredients of vaccines indicates that a causal link cannot be dismissed.

When the practice of vaccination was originally introduced, Edward Jenner claimed, without any evidence to support his claim, that a single vaccination against smallpox would be protective for life. However, the increased incidence of smallpox that occurred, despite the increased numbers of people who had been vaccinated, indicated that 'protection' was clearly not life-long. Instead of recognising that vaccines did not work as believed, the medical establishment instituted the practice of re-vaccination throughout people's lives to ensure continuing 'protection'; a practice that completely contradicts the basic theory that vaccines confer immunity to disease.

The idea that people needed to be regularly revaccinated is also a complete contradiction of the claim by the NHS that the early vaccines were 'crude' but 'worked'. They certainly were crude, but it is abundantly obvious that they did not 'work'.

The 20th century smallpox vaccine that is claimed to have been successful against the disease was similarly crude but also ineffective. In her book, Lily Loat provides information from the July 1947 edition of the *British Medical Journal* that published a question referring to the recommended frequency of re-vaccination in areas where smallpox was endemic. She reports the reply to have been that,

> "Re-vaccination every ten to twelve months should be carried out in areas where smallpox is endemic."

This advice was published approximately 20 years before the introduction of the worldwide smallpox vaccination campaign that is claimed to have eradicated the disease.

It has been a continuing practice of the medical establishment to suppress the failure of vaccines; one of the methods used to achieve this has been the reclassification of illness subsequent to vaccination. This has led to a range of new disease names; for example, the creation of AFP to replace 'polio'.

As previously mentioned, the author George Bernard Shaw was a member of the Anti-Vaccination League of Great Britain; he was also a member of a London health committee and attended their meetings. As a result of this work, he encountered the technique of re-naming post-vaccine illnesses and wrote about his experiences; some of his writings on the topic are quoted by Eleanor McBean in *The Poisoned Needle* including his statement that,

> "...I learned how the credit of vaccination is kept up statistically by diagnosing all the re-vaccinated cases (of smallpox) as pustular eczema, varioloid or what not – except smallpox."

Although no longer called 're-vaccination', it is still claimed that certain vaccines need to be repeated at various stages of people's lives because the 'protection' conferred is not life-long; these are referred to as 'booster shots'. It should be obvious, however, that if the theory that vaccines confer immunity were correct, re-vaccination or booster shots would never be necessary.

The establishment definition of vaccination claims that vaccines are administered in separate doses in order to minimise 'unpleasant side effects'; however, it is increasingly common for infants to receive combination vaccines, also referred to as multivalent vaccines, such as the trivalent vaccines for MMR (measles, mumps and rubella) and DTP (diphtheria, tetanus and pertussis). However, as more vaccines have been added to the standard infant vaccination schedules, they have been increasingly aggregated; pentavalent and hexavalent vaccines have become commonplace. The medical establishment view of combination vaccines has clearly changed since the 2007 definition that referred to the use of 'separate shots' to prevent 'unpleasant side effects'. The current view, according to the CDC web page entitled *Multiple Vaccines and the Immune System*, is that,

> "Scientific data show that getting several vaccines at the same time does not cause any chronic health problems."

Empirical evidence from the real world, however, proves otherwise.

Furthermore, many of the multiple vaccines are administered in multiple stages; for example, in the UK the '5-in-1' vaccine is administered at 8, 12 and 16 weeks of age. A schedule of this nature is not unique; it is typical of most infant vaccination schedules that are applied in most countries around the world, in accordance with the WHO policy recommendations.

These multiple vaccines introduce a substantial volume of toxic materials into the tiny and vulnerable bodies of very young babies; inevitably there will be consequences, none of which will be beneficial and all of which will be detrimental to health. Some of these consequences involve effects that can prevent children from leading a 'normal' life and can include debilitating impairments that affect a child's cognitive skills, which is indicative of harm caused to the brain; a situation that has resulted in a number of conditions that are labelled as 'behavioural problems'.

Dr Buchwald refers in his book to behavioural symptoms that he calls 'unrecognisable vaccine damage', which he describes as follows,

"These behavioural disturbances are marked by unmotivated aggression, hyperactivity, uncontrolled behaviour, lack of concentration and lessened or lacking inhibition threshold."

Yet, as shown by the CDC statement cited above, the medical establishment denies that vaccines cause 'chronic health problems', and therefore refuses to acknowledge that injecting neurotoxic materials into babies will have detrimental effects on their still developing brains. These conditions, which may be diagnosed with labels such as ADD, ADHD or autism, are invariably the result of a number of factors, but vaccines need to be recognised as major contributing factors.

For a variety of reasons, it is impossible to prove a direct causal relationship between a specific effect and a specific vaccine, but the fact that many 'effects' occur subsequent to the administration of a vaccine indicates that, at the very least, the vaccine was the 'trigger' for the reaction and subsequent health problems. The tragedy is that behavioural disturbances that can be triggered by vaccines are frequently treated with toxic psychiatric drugs; but, as discussed, these drugs will only exacerbate the problem.

The reluctance of the medical establishment to properly acknowledge vaccine damage is demonstrated by an article in the May 2011 Bulletin of the WHO entitled, *No-fault compensation following adverse events attributed to vaccination: a review of international programmes*. The title of the article is noteworthy by the description of the compensation as 'no-fault' and by the adverse events being 'attributed' to vaccines rather than caused by them. The article begins with the claim that,

"The public health benefits of vaccination are clear."

Although unwilling to openly admit that vaccines cause harm, the article nevertheless acknowledges that,

"...vaccines are not without risks and it is commonly accepted that adverse events occur following vaccination."

The general view held by the medical establishment is that treatments must be assessed according to the perceived 'risks' and 'benefits'; with respect to vaccination, it is believed that the risks of adverse events are worth taking for the alleged benefits they confer. The reason for this view is summarised in the article that states,

"At a population level, it is considered that these small risks are balanced by the benefits of widespread population immunization."

This view is based on the concept of 'herd immunity', which claims that the spread of an infectious disease can be contained, provided that a certain percentage of the population is vaccinated and has therefore been made 'immune' to the disease. The fallacy of this concept is exposed by the statistics, which showed that the compulsory smallpox vaccination programme in England resulted in a substantially increased incidence of illness and death; despite the fact that almost the entire population had been vaccinated.

There are clearly many problems with the concept of 'herd immunity', not least of which is that vaccination has never been proven to confer immunity;

the topic of immunity is discussed further in the next chapter.

However, a point that deserves particular attention is that the 'small risk' referred to in the WHO Bulletin article is not 'small' for the baby or child that suffers vaccine damage; the risk for them is total. The article acknowledges this point and states that,

> "…this means that an individual occasionally bears a significant burden for the benefit to the rest of the population."

This is a fallacy; the 'significant burden' suffered by any individual has no ability to confer any benefit whatsoever on the rest of the population; their suffering has no purpose and, as discussed in the section about cervical cancer, it has been entirely unnecessary. This is the real tragedy of the unproven and erroneous concept of 'herd immunity'.

There is, however, one form of immunity that does require further discussion; this is the immunity conferred on the vaccine industry by the US National Childhood Vaccine Injury Act of 1986. As a result of this legislation, manufacturers are not held liable for injuries caused by any vaccines that are mandated by the US government.

This is an outrage!

The WHO Bulletin article acknowledges that 'adverse events' can follow the administration of vaccines and refers to compensation funds that have been established in some countries around the world; most notably the US.

The US fund is called the National Vaccine Injury Compensation Program (VICP), details of which can be found on the website of the US Department of Health and Human Services. This website provides useful information about the programme including the Vaccine Injury Table, which lists various vaccines and their possible adverse events. The Table shows that there are very specific time periods during which reactions must occur in order for compensation to be considered. In other words, if a particular reaction does not occur within the specified time then it is not accepted as vaccine damage.

These conditions are totally inappropriate because damage from a vaccine should not be restricted in this way. Adverse effects can occur over a varying period of time, which, as Dr Buchwald explained, can extend to weeks, months or even years. The denial of damage as vaccine-related because it does not occur within a specified time period indicates the disingenuous nature of this programme.

Further revealing information is available from the May 2019 Data report on the US website about the VICP; the latest statistics refer to the period to the end of 2017; the report states that,

> "Since 1988, over 20,629 petitions have been filed with the VICP. Over that 30-year time period, 17,875 petitions have been adjudicated, with 6,551 of those determined to be compensable, while 11,324 were dismissed."

These statistics show that only a little over 36 per cent of all claims that have been adjudicated have been successful. The total compensation paid to successful applicants has, however, involved a huge sum of money,

> "Total compensation paid over the life of the program is approximately $4.1 billion."

Unfortunately for the American public, the US vaccine compensation programme is funded from taxes levied on the sale of vaccines; it is therefore American taxpayers who are funding the compensation paid to victims of vaccine damage. It should, however, be the vaccine manufacturers that are held responsible for the injury caused by their products and made liable for the compensation due to those who have been injured.

The existence of this situation, in which vaccine manufacturers are exonerated from responsibility for the adverse health effects of their products, exposes the heart of the problem; which is that the pharmaceutical industry is not in the business of producing healthcare products that benefit the public. Instead, it is in the business of making profits that benefit their shareholders.

The words of Herbert Shelton are wholly appropriate to conclude this discussion,

> "The vaccinating and inoculating program is merely a commercial one. While it nets huge profits to the traffickers in vaccines and serums, it provides no health for the people."

The Future

Until the existing situation changes, the error of vaccination will continue to cause untold suffering, because the medical establishment continues to promulgate the fallacy that vaccines are safe and effective. The evidence to the contrary is overwhelming; it is only a fraction that has been included in this relatively brief discussion.

Unless it can be stopped, the future direction of the practice of vaccination is one of continual expansion; the agenda of the medical establishment, led by the WHO, is to ensure that everyone is vaccinated. This very real agenda has been formulated by the United Nations and is encapsulated within its latest incarnation called the 2030 Agenda, which was adopted by all UN member states in September 2015. Goal number 3 of this agenda refers to,

> "...safe, effective, quality and affordable medicines and vaccines for all."

The goals of the 2030 Agenda that relate to health matters are discussed in greater detail in chapter eight.

The GVAP (Global Vaccine Action Plan) 2011-2020 Report is another document intended to contribute to the expansion of the vaccination programme; in this instance, the claim is made that it is a 'human right' to be vaccinated. The introduction to this report includes the statement that,

> "Immunization is, and should be recognized as, a core component of the human right to health and an individual, community and governmental responsibility."

The human right to health should include the human right to refuse to be poisoned on the basis of an unproven and erroneous theory.

The use of the term 'community responsibility' is intended to refer to the concept of 'herd immunity', which has been discussed. The reference to 'governmental responsibility' indicates the potential for the introduction of mandatory vaccination laws.

The suffering and mortality that ensued after smallpox vaccination became compulsory in England should have provided a salutary lesson against the implementation of mandatory vaccination programmes.

The pharmaceutical industry obviously plays a major role in promulgating the belief that vaccines are safe and effective, and they achieve this mainly through their substantial influence over the medical establishment; this influence is discussed more fully in chapter nine.

A significant proportion of the pharmaceutical industry is based in the US, and PhRMA (Pharmaceutical Research and Manufacturers of America), as the name suggests, is the industry organisation for American pharmaceutical companies. In 2013 PhRMA produced a report, which documented that almost 300 new vaccines were in development. Although the majority of these vaccines are being developed to combat 'infectious diseases', others are being developed to combat a variety of other illnesses. Disturbingly, some of the new vaccines under development are intended for the treatment of some 'neurological disorders', particularly Alzheimer's disease and MS (multiple sclerosis), and of other conditions including diabetes and asthma.

The discussions in chapter seven demonstrate that conditions of illness that are categorised as noncommunicable are poorly understood by the medical establishment. In virtually all of the diseases discussed, the medical establishment admits to not knowing their causes. This means that they therefore cannot know the correct methods by which the diseases can be 'treated'; what is certain is that no disease can be prevented by a vaccine.

The reference in the GVAP report to 'individual responsibility' is intended to suggest that an individual has the right to demand a vaccine to protect them; it should be clear from the discussions in this chapter that individuals should also have the right to be fully informed about the hazardous nature of vaccines and to be able to assert the right not to be vaccinated.

The human right to health does require 'individual responsibility', but this should be interpreted as the right of an individual to take personal responsibility for their health, and for all decisions that pertain to matters that will affect their own health. The concept of herd immunity is a fallacy that should not be used to coerce people into being poisoned against their will.

In order to make informed decisions, people need all of the information that relates to the subject. It is for this reason that people need to understand that vaccination is not based on any scientific theory; it is wholly unable to prevent or eradicate any disease. Vaccines have never been proven to be safe or effective; on the contrary, they have been proven to be both ineffective and dangerous.

There are a number of reasons that the vast majority of doctors are reluctant to publicly challenge the claim that vaccines are safe and effective, despite the growing body of evidence that they cause harm. These reasons are discussed in more detail later in the book, especially in chapters seven and nine.

It is imperative that, in order to protect human health, the harmful practice of vaccination is eradicated as soon as possible.

Chapter Three

The Germ Theory: A Deadly Fallacy

"Germs as a cause of disease is a dying fallacy."

Dr John H Tilden MD

The information promulgated by the medical establishment about infectious diseases is based on the 'germ theory', the fundamental assertion of which is that germs invade the body and cause disease. The establishment definition describes a 'germ' as,

"any microorganism, especially one that causes disease."

Disease-causing microorganisms are referred to as pathogens; however, although it is widely believed that all 'germs' are pathogenic, this is not the case.

The NIH (National Institutes of Health) is a US government agency that conducts and supports biomedical research; as one of the key members of the medical establishment, the NIH is, inevitably, a proponent of the 'germ theory'. The NIH website is a vast repository of information that includes more than 5 million archived medical journal articles; it also contains various educational materials, including books and teacher's guides. One of the online books in the *Curriculum Supplement* series of teacher's guides is entitled *Understanding Emerging and Re-emerging Infectious Diseases*. This book, which will be referred to as the *Infectious Diseases* book, describes microorganisms as the agents that cause infectious diseases, but adds the interesting comment that,

"Although microorganisms that cause disease often receive the most attention, it is important to note that most microorganisms do *not* cause disease."

With reference to the microorganisms that do cause disease the book states that,

"A true pathogen is an infectious agent that causes disease in virtually any susceptible host."

The idea that a host must be susceptible before even a 'true' pathogen can cause disease indicates that other factors must be involved; an idea that is

71

inconsistent with the information about 'infectious diseases' promulgated to the general public. It is, however, only one of the many anomalies, inconsistencies and contradictions that are exposed by a genuine investigation of the medical establishment's statements with respect to 'pathogens' and the 'infectious diseases' they are claimed to cause.

Scientists state that the word 'theory' does not refer to 'an idea', but that it has a much more specific meaning. The first phase of a scientific investigation involves the creation of a general hypothesis, which is a suggested explanation for the subject under investigation. Experiments are then devised and conducted in order to discover more information about and gain a better understanding of the phenomenon under review. The results of these experiments usually lead to the creation of a theory, which is intended to provide a more comprehensive and compelling explanation for the phenomenon than the explanation provided by the hypothesis.

References by the medical establishment to the 'germ theory' would therefore tend to suggest the existence of a number of established facts, which are: that all 'germs' have been thoroughly investigated and identified; that their ability to cause disease has been scientifically proven beyond doubt; and that the 'theory' furnishes a comprehensive and compelling explanation for 'germs' and the mechanisms by which they cause disease.

Nothing could be further from the truth.

It is a fundamental principle that the burden of proof lies with those who propose a theory. Yet in the case of the 'germ theory' that 'proof' does not exist; there is no original scientific evidence that definitively proves that any 'germ' causes any specific infectious disease.

Although this statement will be regarded as highly controversial and even outrageous, its veracity will be demonstrated by the discussions in this chapter.

There are a number of sources that provide a corroboration of the assertion that the 'germ theory' lacks any original scientific proof. One of these sources is Dr M.L. Leverson MD, who, in May 1911, gave a lecture in London in which he discussed his investigations that had led him to the conclusion that,

> "The entire fabric of the germ theory of disease rests upon assumptions which not only have not been proved, but which are incapable of proof, and many of them can be proved to be the reverse of truth. The basic one of these unproven assumptions, wholly due to Pasteur, is the hypothesis that all the so-called infectious and contagious disorders are caused by germs."

Corroboration is also provided by Dr Beddow Bayly, who, in addition to exposing the lack of any scientific basis for vaccination, also exposed the lack of any scientific basis for the 'germ theory'. In 1928 he wrote an article that was published in the journal *London Medical World*; in this article Dr Beddow Bayly states that,

> "I am prepared to maintain with scientifically established facts, that in no single instance has it been conclusively proved that any microorganism is the specific cause of a disease."

It is clear that evidence to support the 'germ theory' remained conspicuous by its absence more than half a century after it had been proposed by Louis

Pasteur in the early 1860s. The situation has not been rectified in the intervening decades since 1928; the germ theory of disease remains unproven, with overwhelming evidence to demonstrate that it also remains a fallacy.

Another critic of the prevailing ideas about disease in the 19th century was Florence Nightingale. During her long nursing career, she took care of many thousands of patients; an experience that proved to her that diseases were not individual entities with separately identifiable causes. In her 1860 book entitled *Notes on Nursing*, she writes that,

"I have seen diseases begin, grow up and pass into one another."

She records that when the wards were overcrowded, the ordinary 'fevers' with which patients suffered would change and worsen to become 'typhoid fever' and worsen again to become 'typhus'. These diseases are regarded as specific conditions caused by distinctly different 'pathogens', but Florence Nightingale reports that no new 'infection' occurred; that the worsening of the 'diseases' were the natural result of the unhealthy conditions that the patients endured. Typically, these conditions included overcrowding, poor sanitation, lack of fresh air and lack of hygiene, which are strikingly similar to the conditions in which smallpox thrived.

The idea that each specific pathogen causes a distinct disease is further explored in the next chapter, in which a number of different 'infectious diseases' are discussed.

It was shown in the previous chapter that the practice of vaccination was not originally based on the idea that 'germs' were the causal agents of disease; instead, it was based on the claim that a mild form of 'disease' would provide a degree of protection against a more serious attack of 'disease'. However, after Louis Pasteur's version of the germ theory gained increased popularity in the late 19th century, the idea of 'germs' as the causal agents of disease became an extremely useful tool to justify the introduction of different vaccines to combat different 'infectious diseases'.

In the early 21st century, vaccinations are still justified on the basis that they prevent 'infectious diseases'; the 'germ theory' and the practice of vaccination are therefore inextricably interconnected. Together they provide the foundation for a large proportion of medical establishment practices and consequently account for a large proportion of pharmaceutical industry profits.

It is Louis Pasteur who is generally hailed as the 'father' of the germ theory; however, he was not the originator of the basic idea that diseases were caused by external 'infectious agents'. Prior to the 19th century, a variety of ideas had been proposed that attempted to explain the nature of disease; many of these ideas involved the existence of disease-causing 'entities'. The earliest theory is reported to have been that of the Italian physician Girolamo Fracastoro, who, in 1546, proposed that disease is caused by minute entities that can transmit 'infection'. His theory included the idea that these 'entities' become pathogenic through heat. But Fracastoro was unable to observe the entities whose existence he had proposed; microscopes with sufficient lens magnification were not available until more than a century later.

It is reported that, in 1676, Antonius van Leeuwenhoek constructed a sufficiently powerful microscope to be able to view the small entities that are now recognised as bacteria; however, he proposed no theories about these entities or their functions, he merely observed them and wrote extensively about his observations in a correspondence he held with the Royal Society in London. It was almost another century later, in 1762, that Dr M Plenciz, a Viennese physician, proposed a 'germ theory of infectious disease'; a full century earlier than the theory attributed to Louis Pasteur.

These historical facts have been extracted from the book *Pasteur: Plagiarist, Imposter* written by R B Pearson, whose source is a textbook entitled *Historical Review of Microbiology*, which was written by F Harrison, who was principal Professor of Bacteriology at McGill University.

The long-held beliefs, customs and traditions that evolved into the various ideas about diseases and their causes are also discussed by Herbert Shelton in his July 1978 article entitled *Disease is Remedial Action*, in which he states that,

"This very old idea that disease is an entity that attacks the body and wreaks as much havoc therein as possible has taken several forms through the ages and is incarnated in the germ theory that holds sway today."

William White explains in *The Story of a Great Delusion* that many of the old attitudes from ancient times persisted into the 18th century; although an extract from his book was quoted in the previous chapter, one part of that extract deserves repetition,

"There was no scientific knowledge of the laws of health; diseases were generally regarded as mysterious dispensations of Providence over which the sufferers had little control; and a great part of medicine was a combination of absurdity with nastiness."

The old beliefs were gradually replaced by 'scientific theories', although the latter varied little from the ideas they replaced. The 'theories' were often no more than variations on the basic ideas, which were: that an external entity invades and 'infects' the body; that this 'infection' causes illness; and that sufferers have little control over their illness. More importantly, these 'scientific theories' did not represent a significant advance in medical knowledge about disease or health; as Herbert Shelton states,

"A hundred years ago it was freely admitted that the nature and essence of disease was unknown."

Unfortunately, the nature and essence of disease remains largely unknown to the medical establishment of the 21st century; the reason for this situation is mainly, but not exclusively, due to their rigid adherence to the 'germ theory'.

As demonstrated throughout this book, many medical establishment practices are based on erroneous and unproven theories, the problems with which are manifested by empirical evidence that demonstrates worsening rather than improving health for virtually the entire population of the world. Yet, despite the obvious contradictions between the theory and the empirical evidence, the medical establishment exhorts the public to believe their pronouncements about disease epidemics caused by dangerous 'germs', on the basis that they are the 'authority' on matters pertaining to health.

In his book entitled *Confessions of a Medical Heretic*, Dr Robert Mendelsohn MD indicates that belief in the 'authority' of the medical establishment is misplaced. He expands on his discussion of the problems with 'modern medicine' by reference to similarities between beliefs, religion and 'modern medicine'. He describes the medical establishment as 'the church of modern medicine' and justifies this description with the statement that,

> "Modern medicine can't survive without our faith, because modern medicine is neither an art nor a science; it's a religion...Just ask 'why' enough times and sooner or later you'll reach the chasm of faith."

Science is an ongoing process of enquiry and discovery; this means that scientists should reassess theories that have been found to be flawed and generate more compelling explanations for the phenomena under review. Yet the 'germ theory', which can be shown to be fundamentally flawed, has not been subjected to any rigorous reassessment. If it had been, scientists would have discovered that the theory is contradicted by a significant volume of empirical evidence, which is normally regarded as paramount. The intransigence of the scientific community on this topic has turned the 'germ theory' into dogma, not science.

Dr Mendelsohn recommends that people ask the question 'why'; but the problems with the 'germ theory' require that people also ask the question 'how'; were they to do so, they would soon encounter the 'chasm of faith', which is likely to manifest as the familiar phrase, 'trust me, I'm a doctor'.

Although it is firmly believed by the medical establishment that Louis Pasteur's 'germ theory' was scientifically proven beyond any doubt, it has been revealed that the 'science' he used in his experiments was not as meticulous as has been claimed. In his 1995 book entitled *The Private Science of Louis Pasteur*, historian Dr Gerald Geison refers to his investigation of Louis Pasteur's work that involved a comparison of his personal notebooks with his published papers. Journalist Torsten Engelbrecht and physician Dr Claus Köhnlein MD provide extracts from Dr Geison's book in their own book, *Virus Mania*; one of the extracts states that,

> "During his lifetime, Pasteur permitted absolutely no one – not even his closest co-workers – to inspect his notes."

Another extract from Dr Geison's book quoted by the authors of *Virus Mania* states that Pasteur,

> "...arranged with his family that the books should also remain closed to all even after his death."

Although ideas about his possible motive for making this request can only be speculative, this arrangement does raise the question of why Louis Pasteur would not have wanted the basis of his world-famous work to be widely known. Torsten Engelbrecht and Dr Köhnlein provide a possible motive in the extremely revealing quote from Dr Geison's book in summary of the situation that states,

"The conclusion is unavoidable; Pasteur deliberately deceived the public, including especially those scientists most familiar with his published work."

It is clear that Louis Pasteur, like Edward Jenner, has failed to earn the right to be revered or to be cited as a 'hero' of modern medicine. The facts show that they both contributed a great deal towards the sum of human illness, misery and suffering, all of which have resulted from the adoption of their theories by the medical establishment.

It is unnecessary to provide full details of the history of the 'germ theory' in order to be able to expose the flaws on which it has been based. One of those flaws arises from the basic assumption about 'infectious diseases' and the meaning of the word 'infection', the establishment definition of which refers to,

"invasion of the body by harmful organisms (pathogens)..."

It is clear from this definition that an infection is considered to be synonymous with an invasion by microorganisms and subsequent disease; but this is misleading, as the body's endogenous microorganisms are also claimed to be able to cause disease; as indicated by the Mayo Clinic web page entitled *Infectious Diseases*, which states that,

"Many organisms live in and on our bodies. They're normally harmless or even helpful, but under certain conditions, some organisms may cause disease."

This statement is highly anomalous. Although the Mayo Clinic web page offers no further information about the conditions deemed necessary for otherwise harmless microorganisms to become pathogenic, it is suggested that 'germs' constantly mutate to overpower the immune system and cause disease.

Another explanation is offered by the *Infectious Diseases* book, which states that the body's 'normal flora',

"... do not cause disease because their growth is kept under control by the host's defense mechanisms and by the presence of other microorganisms."

The book claims that endogenous and invading microorganisms compete with each other but that, in normal circumstances, the invaders are successfully suppressed. However, if its defence mechanisms are weak, the body may be overwhelmed by 'opportunistic pathogens', which are described as,

"...potentially infectious agents that rarely cause disease in individuals with healthy immune systems."

The medical establishment acknowledges that they possess a poor level of understanding about either the mechanisms involved, or the conditions that cause endogenous organisms to be activated and become pathogenic; this is discussed in more detail in the section about bacteria.

However, reliance on the immune system to prevent an invading pathogen from causing disease is problematic; as discussed in the previous chapter, it is claimed that the function of the immune system is to attack and destroy pathogens. This means that a strong and fully functioning immune system would be able to destroy all invaders and that anyone with a strong immune system should therefore have no 'infectious agents', potential or otherwise, within their bodies; microorganisms claimed to be 'pathogenic' have, however, been found in the bodies of healthy people. One explanation for this situation is that some pathogens can exist in the body in a 'dormant' state. But a strong immune system should not permit the presence of any pathogen, even in a so-called 'dormant' state, that can subsequently be 'activated' when the immune system has become weakened.

The explanations offered by the medical establishment fail to genuinely address all of the anomalies within their explanations relating to the 'germ theory'; this will become increasingly obvious as each type of 'germ' is discussed in this chapter; the immune system is also discussed in more detail later in this chapter.

Unfortunately, in their attempts to address these anomalous situations, the medical establishment creates even more complex explanations that do not provide clarification, but instead, introduce further anomalies, inconsistencies and contradictions.

The 'germ theory' has become deeply embedded not only within modern medicine, but also within the 'alternative health' community. The belief in 'germs' is so pervasive that virtually all physicians have accepted the ideas contained within the 'germ theory'; this includes many of the physicians whose work is referenced in this book due to the valid criticisms they have raised about the mainstream medical system.

The efforts of the medical establishment to promote and emphasise the dangers of so-called 'infectious diseases' is demonstrated by the WHO in the *World Health Report 2007*, which includes the statement that,

"...infectious diseases are emerging at a rate that has not been seen before."

There is no explanation within the context of the 'germ theory' for an accelerated rate of proliferation of germs; whether they are known germs that cause diseases believed to have been mostly conquered, or newly discovered germs that cause previously unknown diseases.

There are, however, many reasons for the 'germ theory' to be perpetuated as if it has been scientifically established and proven to be true; some of those reasons relate to economics, politics and geopolitics, which are discussed in chapter nine.

Other reasons relate to the need to justify the use of vaccines and medicines, but, as this chapter will demonstrate 'germs' do not cause disease; a fact that adds further to the weight of evidence that vaccines and medicines are ineffective as methods to prevent or treat any so-called 'infectious disease'.

Scientific Experimentation

Science and technology have generated many innovations that have profoundly changed the way people live; these changes have accelerated substantially over the past three centuries since, and largely as the result of, the Industrial Revolution.

The consequences of these changes have not always been beneficial; many have been positively detrimental. One of the main consequences has been the almost total obeisance to 'science' in the belief that it is the only method

escapes from the host cell if it is 'not motile'. It also fails to explain how the 'virus' is able to find and 'hitch' itself to the appropriate particle that is going to be ejected from the body during a sneeze or a cough.

The second question requires an explanation of the method by which a virus is claimed to be able to 'infect' a cell. The web page of UCMP (University of California Museum of Paleontology) Berkeley entitled *Introduction to Viruses*, states that,

> "When it comes into contact with a host cell, a virus can insert its genetic material into its host..."

The purported mechanism is described in a little more detail in a July 2007 article entitled, *Imaging Poliovirus Entry in Live Cells*, the abstract of which begins,

> "Viruses initiate infection by transferring their genetic material across a cellular membrane and into the appropriate compartment of the cell."

This 'insertion' or 'transfer' assumes that the virus takes an active part in these mechanisms, but the idea that a virus can be active is contradicted by Dr Margulis and others who state categorically that a virus is inert outside of a living cell. The 2007 article makes the highly revealing statement that,

> "The mechanisms by which animal viruses, especially non enveloped viruses, deliver their genomes are only poorly understood."

The article also reveals that,

> "How non enveloped viruses, such as poliovirus, enter target cells is not well understood."

These statements are not only profoundly revealing but also astounding, considering that the idea of 'viral infection' rests on the theory that viruses enter cells in order to cause disease. These statements clearly demonstrate how little is actually known about viruses and their alleged mechanism of action in causing an 'infection'. It should be obvious that a great deal of the 'information' about viruses promulgated by the medical establishment is based on a collection of unproven assumptions and suppositions.

The lack of known facts about viruses can be demonstrated by the example of a cold 'virus' that is claimed to be transmitted via saliva or mucous particles when a person sneezes or coughs. These particles are said to be inhaled by another person, who then becomes 'infected' by the virus, which travels through the person's body to the appropriate cells of their lung tissues. The transmission of any viral particle attached to saliva or mucous travelling through the air has never been observed; viral particles are only ever observed in a laboratory under an electron microscope. The transmission of viruses in the air is an assumption; as is their ability to travel through a human body.

A further contradiction of the theory that viruses are transmitted between people can be seen from another common 'infectious disease', namely, influenza or 'the flu'. The worst outbreak of this disease is reported to have occurred during 1918 and to have killed many tens of millions of people. The number of people reported to have died as the result of this epidemic varies widely from about 20 million to about 100 million people, which raises many questions about the veracity of these claims and about the number of genuine casualties from the flu rather than from the effects of WWI. There are also many reports that claim the real duration of the 'epidemic' to have been far longer than a single year. The reason that a huge number of people died during this period is claimed to be because the disease was highly contagious; there are however, many problems with such claims; the '1918 Flu' is discussed in greater detail in the next chapter.

The epidemic of 1918 is usually referred to as a 'viral' disease, although initially there were ideas that it was caused by a bacterium. Herbert Shelton describes some of the early experiments conducted on volunteers from the US Naval Detention camp to determine the alleged bacterial cause and to test the transmission of the disease. In his book entitled *The Hygienic System: Vol VI Orthopathy*, he describes one of the experiments conducted to test the transmission of the disease and explains that,

"Ten other men were carried to the bedside of ten new cases of influenza and spent 45 minutes with them. Each well man had ten sick men cough in his face."

He records that the results of these experiments were that,

"None of these volunteers developed any symptoms of influenza following the experiment."

It may be suggested that 10 is too small a number to be a statistically significant sample size, but this argument would miss the salient point, which is that each healthy man had ten sick men cough in his face and none of them became ill; a fact that contradicts the idea that viral particles 'hitchhike' onto saliva or mucous that is ejected from the body during a sneeze or cough. According to the 'germ theory', all of the healthy men should have been 'infected' by the viruses and become ill. The fact that they did not fall ill poses a direct and serious challenge to the basic assumption that 'flu' is infectious.

Exceptions to any rule is an indication that the 'rule' is flawed and needs to be re-examined; the empirical evidence is primary.

The lack of understanding by the medical establishment about the mechanism for the viral 'infection' of cells has not improved since the publication of the 2007 poliovirus article previously referred to; there remain both a lack of understanding about and an absence of proof of the mechanism involved. This lack of progress is indicated by an August 2015 article entitled *A Non-enveloped Virus Hijacks Host Disaggregation Machinery to Translocate across the Endoplasmic Reticulum Membrane*, which states that,

"How non-enveloped viruses penetrate a host membrane to enter cells and cause disease remains an enigmatic step."

Dr Hillman identified the 'endoplasmic reticulum' as one of the artefacts that are generated as the result of the preparation procedures necessary to view viruses under an electron microscope.

The website of the *Encyclopedia of Life* (EoL), a project that promotes the medical establishment view, contains a page about 'viruses' and refers to them as 'microscopic organisms', which demonstrates the efforts to present the case that viruses are 'alive'. To further promote this view, the EoL web page provides information about the stages in a 'viral life cycle', the first stage of which is claimed to be one in which a virus attaches itself to a cell; the page states that,

"Attachment is the intermolecular binding between viral capsid proteins and receptors on the outer membrane of the host cell."

The problem with this explanation is that Dr Hillman also identified 'receptors' as cellular artefacts that are generated by the preparation procedures used in such experiments.

It is claimed that once a virus has penetrated the cell, it will replicate, which is said to initiate the 'disease' process. The EoL web page refers to numerous mechanisms involved in this process that include cell lysis and the ultimate death of the cell. The page makes the significant statement that,

"In multicellular organisms, if sufficient numbers of cells die, the whole organism may suffer gross metabolic disruption or even mortality."

There is a huge problem with this statement, which is that many billions of human cells die every day; 'cell death' is a normal part of the processes of human life. The idea that cell death is synonymous with 'disease' is therefore highly misleading; it completely contradicts known biological functions of the human body.

The reason that cell death is perceived to be a 'disease process' is because this is what is likely to have been observed during laboratory experiments. However, there are genuine reasons for cells to die after tissue samples have been subjected to the various preparation procedures used in laboratory experimentation; as explained by Torsten Engelbrecht and Dr Köhnlein in *Virus Mania*,

"This phenomenon is particularly virulent in bacterial and viral research (and in the whole pharmaceutical development of medicines altogether) where laboratory experiments on tissue samples which are tormented with a variety of often highly reactive chemicals allow few conclusions about reality. And yet, conclusions are constantly drawn – and then passed straight on to the production of medications and vaccines."

This explanation exposes the fundamental error in conducting laboratory research without an adequate understanding of the living organism that is the human body. It also clearly supports the conclusions drawn by Dr Hillman, that laboratory procedures affect the samples being investigated to the point that they bear no resemblance to 'reality'.

Yet most scientific information about viruses is derived from laboratory experiments of this nature. In these experiments 'viruses' are reported to have replicated inside a cell, after which the cell dies. This process does not prove that the 'virus' killed the cell nor does it prove that the 'virus' initiates any disease processes; it merely proves that the cell died after the processes used in the experiments. These points are also raised in *Virus Mania*, in which the authors state that,

"Another important question must be raised: even when a supposed virus does kill cells in a test-tube (in vitro) ... can we safely conclude that these findings can be carried over to a living organism (in vivo)?"

The assumption that a particular 'viral particle' causes a particular 'infection' is solely based on the claim that certain antibodies have sometimes been found in samples extracted from some people exhibiting certain symptoms; in other words, there appears to be a correlation between symptoms and antibodies. It should be noted that viruses are not detected directly.

However, many people are diagnosed as suffering from a 'viral illness' without any investigations or tests having been conducted to ascertain whether they have been infected by an allegedly pathogenic virus. A diagnosis is frequently based on the different symptoms that a patient experiences and reports to their doctor. People can also be discovered to have a 'virus' in their bodies without exhibiting the specific symptoms of the disease it is alleged to cause; this is claimed to represent the 'dormant' stage of the virus, as discussed on the EoL web page that states,

"Although viruses may cause disruption of normal homeostasis resulting in disease, in some cases viruses may simply reside inside an organism without significant harm."

Although the virus may be 'dormant' and therefore harmless, it is claimed that there is a potential for the virus to be 'activated' and to initiate the relevant disease. In their efforts to justify the existence of an allegedly 'dormant' virus in the body, the medical establishment has created the term 'latent infection'. The following extract from the Yale Medical group website page entitled *All About Viruses* shows how the medical establishment attempts to explain what is clearly an anomaly,

"Varicella viruses are examples of viruses that cause latent infections. The varicella-zoster virus remains in the body after causing the initial infection known as chicken pox. If it is re-activated, it travels through nerves to the skin, where it causes the blister-like lesions of shingles. The virus then returns to its dormant state."

Despite the claim that they explain 'all about viruses', these statements are made without any supportive evidence; there is no explanation for any of these stages of an allegedly 'latent infection'; nor is there any explanation for the mechanisms by which a virus becomes 'dormant' or is re-activated. Yet the 'germ theory' is still claimed to have been scientifically proven, and to provide a comprehensive and compelling explanation for 'viruses' and the 'infectious diseases' they are alleged to cause.

There are only a very few brave scientists who have been prepared to contradict the medical establishment and acknowledge publicly that viruses are not pathogenic. One such scientist is Dr Lynn Margulis, who states in *Symbiotic Planet* that,

"The point that bears mentioning, however, is that viruses are no more 'germs' and 'enemies' than are bacteria or human cells."

Another of these brave scientists is Dr Stefan Lanka PhD, a German biologist who studied virology as well as molecular biology, ecology and marine biology.

An interview with Dr Lanka was conducted in 2005 for the online German newspaper *Faktuell*. The interview, which has fortunately been translated into English, reveals that the topics of discussion included bird flu and vaccination. During the interview Dr Lanka referred to his studies in molecular biology and made the bold claim that,

"In the course of my studies, I and others have not been able to find proof of the existence of disease-causing viruses anywhere."

He continues to discuss his research and further explains that,

"Later we have discoursed on this publicly and have called on people not to believe us either but to check out themselves whether or not there are disease causing viruses."

He also stated in the interview that he and a number of other people had been questioning the German authorities for the 'proof' of pathogenic viruses. He reports that the result of their efforts revealed that,

"...the health authorities are no longer maintaining that any virus whatsoever purportedly causing a disease has been directly proven to exist."

This statement that no 'disease-causing' virus has been directly proven to exist highlights another crucial fact, which is that the 'presence' of a virus in the body is not determined directly, but only through the detection of antibodies that the body is alleged to have produced against the virus; there is no test that is able to directly detect the presence of a 'whole virus'. The real purpose and function within the human body of these particles of genetic material contained within a protein coating are unknown; the claim that they cause disease remains entirely unproven.

Dr Lanka was also interviewed in April 2016; this time by David Crowe for his internet programme, *The Infectious Myth*, on the *Progressive Radio Network*. In this interview Dr Lanka again asserted that there is no evidence that proves any virus to be the cause of any disease, and that the theories about infectious diseases are wrong. He also discussed the details of his recent court case that arose from a challenge he had set a number of years earlier. This challenge was that a certain sum of money would be paid to anyone who produced genuine scientific 'proof' of the existence of the measles virus. The purpose of this challenge was to expose the fallacy of the claim that measles is caused by a virus.

In 2015 a German doctor accepted the challenge; the basis of his 'proof' was a set of six published papers that he claimed provided the necessary evidence. Dr Lanka, however, claimed that the papers did not contain the required evidence, and refuted the doctor's claim to the 'reward' money. This dispute resulted in a court case that found in favour of the German doctor. The court's decision that the papers provided the required 'proof' and that Dr Lanka had therefore 'lost' his case were widely reported in many media outlets, some of which also contained disparaging comments about Dr Lanka personally.

However, Dr Lanka maintained his claim that the papers did not provide the required proof and appealed against the court's decision. The appeal was heard in early 2016 and the decision this time found in favour of Dr Lanka; in other words, it was found that the papers failed to provide the necessary 'proof'. The mainstream media, however, were noticeably silent about the result of the appeal. The lack of media coverage of Dr Lanka's successful appeal is revealing, especially as it coincided with reports about a number of 'outbreaks' of measles cases in the early months of 2016. But these reports studiously avoided making any reference to the court case that had demonstrated that no evidence exists that proves measles to be caused by a virus.

It should be clear from this discussion that no disease is caused by a virus.

In his interviews, Dr Lanka urges people to investigate for themselves if there is any genuine evidence for any 'disease-causing viruses'. The authors of this book make the same request and ask people to investigate for themselves whether any 'virus' has been conclusively proven to be the cause of any infectious disease. Any investigation of this nature should involve contact with the organisations that claim viruses to be the cause of disease to ask them the following questions:

Is there an electron micrograph of the pure and fully characterised virus?

What is the name of the **primary** specialist peer reviewed paper in which the virus is illustrated and its full genetic information described?

What is the name of the **primary** publication that provides proof that a particular virus is the sole cause of a particular disease?

It is vitally important that any documents referred to by the organisation, should they reply, must be primary papers; textbooks or other reference materials that are not primary documents are not acceptable; they must provide primary evidence.

It should be noted that investigations of this nature, including those undertaken by virologists such as Dr Lanka, have failed to unearth any original papers that conclusively prove that any virus is the cause of any disease. In addition, as this discussion has demonstrated, the functions attributed to viruses in the causation of disease are based on assumptions and extrapolations from laboratory experiments that have not only failed to prove, but are incapable of proving, that viruses cause disease. The inert, non-living particles known as viruses do not possess the ability to perform such functions because they lack the necessary mechanisms.

The real nature and causes of diseases claimed to be 'viral' are discussed in greater detail in chapters four and ten.

Bacteria

Bacteria, unlike viruses, are living organisms.

However, like viruses, bacteria are erroneously accused of being pathogens.

It first became possible to observe microorganisms when Antonie van Leeuwenhoek invented his powerful microscope in 1676; however, as discussed, his study of these tiny entities did not involve an investigation of their possible connection with diseases.

The first 'germ theory of disease' was proposed by Dr Plenciz in 1762, but it was not until the 19th century that the Italian entomologist, Agostino Bassi performed experiments that are alleged to be the first to provide 'proof' for the theory. His initial investigations were in connection with a silkworm disease; it is claimed that he discovered the cause of this disease to be a microscopic fungus. This study led to further investigations, the result of which was that in 1844 he proposed the theory that human diseases were also caused by microorganisms; his theory therefore precedes that of Louis Pasteur.

During the 17th, 18th and 19th centuries, many diseases were rife throughout Europe; these diseases include typhus, cholera, tuberculosis and smallpox. It is claimed that smallpox alone was responsible for nearly half a million deaths each year during the 18th century. It was during this period that treatments for these diseases involved the use of measures that were described by William White as 'a combination of absurdity with nastiness'. It must be noted that the insanitary conditions that existed in many of the towns and cities in England were also prevalent in many of the towns and cities throughout Europe.

However, this was also the period in which 'science' began its meteoric rise. The Scientific Revolution, which is said to have begun in the middle of the 16th century, saw many significant discoveries and inventions that overturned long-held ideas and beliefs about the world and how it worked.

Unfortunately, scientific investigations in the field of 'medicine' did not succeed in overturning the old belief that disease was the result of an attack by external entities. Instead, this basic assumption was retained and appeared to be supported by the discovery of microorganisms; a discovery that exerted, and continues to exert, a powerful influence on the direction of medical research. However, appearances can often be deceptive; a maxim that has proven to be entirely applicable to bacteria.

Although Louis Pasteur is regarded as the father of the germ theory, it is Dr Robert Koch who is regarded as the founder of modern bacteriology; nevertheless, like Louis Pasteur, Dr Koch is falsely venerated as a hero. It is widely claimed that Dr Koch provided the necessary 'proof' that certain diseases were caused by certain bacteria; but this is a mistaken claim, as will be demonstrated.

In order for him to test his theory that bacteria were the causes of disease, Dr Koch developed four Postulates that continue to bear his name. The first Postulate, which is the most crucial for determining a causal agent of disease, comprises two criteria, the first of which is that the microbe alleged to cause a specific disease must be found in all people suffering from that disease. The second criterion is that the microbe should not be found in anyone who does not have the disease it is claimed to cause. The logic of this first postulate is undeniable; any exception to either criterion means that the 'microbe' could not be the causal agent of the disease in question. This logic is recognised by Dr Peter Duesberg, who states in his book entitled *Inventing the AIDS Virus* that,

> "A single exception would be enough to pronounce the microbe innocent of creating that disease."

However, investigations of bacteria and their relationship to different diseases reveal the existence of exceptions to both criteria of Koch's first postulate; bacteria have been found in the bodies of people who do not have the disease they are alleged to cause, and the relevant bacteria have not been found in all people with the disease they are alleged to cause. The significance of these exceptions is that they utterly refute the basic assumption that bacteria cause disease. These exceptions should have persuaded scientists like Dr Koch to reassess the 'germ theory', if not completely abandon it.

There was, and still is, a great reluctance to abandon or even reassess the theory; instead, efforts have been made to solve the anomalies raised by these exceptions by making adaptations to the theory. But these adaptations do not resolve the underlying anomalies; on the contrary, they introduce additional anomalies. The main problem is that the adapted theory retains the underlying assumption that 'bacteria' are pathogens; but it is precisely this assumption that is fundamentally flawed.

The adapted theory claims that people who have been found to 'house' bacteria, but not to have the disease they are alleged to cause, are 'asymptomatic carriers'. The implication of this label is that carriers can transmit their bacteria to other people, who will then become 'infected' and fall ill with the disease; but this label fails to clarify the situation and only raises further questions.

There are many aspects of the original and adapted theories that remain unexplained; for example, there are no explanations for the mechanism by which bacteria are 'transferred' from the bodies of the 'carrier' to another person, or for the basic mechanism by which bacteria produce the variety of symptoms of an infectious disease. There is also no explanation for the fact that 'asymptomatic carriers' do not become ill; it is merely asserted that these people have a 'latent infection'. But this assertion offers no explanation for the situation; the concept of a 'latent infection' directly contradicts the core assertion of the 'germ theory' that bacterial infections cause disease.

One alleged 'pathogen', that falls into the category of those that are said to produce 'asymptomatic carriers', is the common bacterium called *Staphylococcus*. It is widely reported that a 'Staph infection' causes illness; it is nevertheless acknowledged that this bacterium can be found on the skin of healthy people. This anomalous situation fails Koch's first postulate; the bacterium cannot therefore be regarded as a 'pathogen'. The significance of this bacterium is further discussed in the next section, because it is claimed to be a 'superbug' that causes a serious 'MRSA infection'.

Another example that demonstrates the fallacy of the claim that specific bacteria cause specific diseases, or any disease at all, is that of Dr Max Pettenkofer MD, who Eleanor McBean reports to have swallowed, on more than one occasion, the contents of a glass containing millions of cholera bacilli in full view of a class of his students; yet it is reliably reported that Dr Pettenkofer failed to succumb to the disease.

Although it has been suggested by certain sections of the scientific community that Koch's postulates are flawed, out-of-date and need to be revised, such a suggestion ignores the central point, which is that allegedly 'pathogenic' bacteria can be found in abundance in and on the bodies of healthy people. These bacteria cannot therefore be regarded as pathogens merely on the basis that they are sometimes found in some people who are ill. Dr Peter Duesberg states the logical conclusion succinctly,

"Simply finding a microbe is not enough to convict it of causing a disease."

The analogy of discovering firemen at the scene of a fire and inappropriately accusing them of being the cause is yet again pertinent.

As discussed above, investigations also discovered a problem with the other criterion of Koch's first postulate, which states that the bacterium must always be present in people with the disease it is alleged to cause; many exceptions to this 'rule' have also been found. In *Orthopathy*, Herbert Shelton provides some examples, one of which is from an article published in the journal *The Lancet* in 1898, which states that,

> "Dr Beddow Bayly says that the diphtheria bacillus is missing in 14 per cent of cases of clinical diphtheria."

Herbert Shelton cites a further example in which it had been found that 50 per cent of TB (tuberculosis) cases had failed to exhibit the tubercle bacillus and quotes Dr Hadwen's words that,

> "Nobody has ever found a tubercle bacillus in the early stages of tuberculosis."

If the tubercle bacillus were the cause of TB, it would always be present at the very earliest stages of the disease. The significance of this example is that TB is one of the main diseases that Dr Koch is reputed to have 'proven' to be caused by a bacterium, and specifically by the tubercle bacillus. However, unlike the anomaly with the other component of the first postulate, there has been no adaptation of the theory to explain the absence of the bacterium in people with the disease it is alleged to cause. The subject of TB is discussed in more detail in chapters four and eight, as it remains a disease of significance.

It is important to refer again to the work of Dr Hillman in respect of observations of samples under a microscope, especially in view of the fact that bacteria are almost always fixed and stained before they are examined under a microscope; these procedures are said to be able to make bacteria easier to observe. It is reliably reported by many mainstream scientific sources that in his investigations and observations of bacteria within 'diseased tissue', Dr Koch used both fixing and staining preparation procedures. Whilst these procedures may assist the observation of bacteria, it is inappropriate to make assumptions about the actions of bacteria in a living human body, merely from observations of their presence in diseased tissue samples viewed under a microscope, after they have been subjected to fixing and staining processes. As Dr Lipton's work showed, the condition of their environment has a direct effect on living samples, whether they are cells or bacteria.

In addition to the observation of bacteria under microscopes, many experiments have been conducted that are claimed to have 'proved' that bacteria are transmitted between people and that they are capable of causing the same disease after transmission. But the evidence, which shows that in many cases the 'germ' is absent when it should be present or present when it should be absent, means that there are fundamental flaws in the theory that cannot be 'proved' by experimentation. The monkey experiments used to 'prove' the transmission of polio is a pertinent example of flawed experimental methods that do not 'prove' what they are claimed to prove.

The assumption that bacteria are fundamentally pathogenic is continually challenged by discoveries about their real nature and functions.

One of the acknowledged facts is that bacteria live in a variety of habitats; as recognised by the establishment definition that states,

"Some live in soil, water or air..."

However, the definition makes the additional claim that,

"...others are parasites of humans, animals and plants."

It is an error to refer to any bacterium as a parasite, the establishment definition of which refers to an organism that contributes nothing to the welfare of the host. Recent discoveries about bacteria show that some of the actions they perform include a number of vitally important functions that substantially contribute to the welfare of a variety of hosts.

Although the definition states that bacteria live in soil, their range of habitats in the ground extends beyond merely the soil; these habitats include, for example, the roots of certain plants in which they 'fix' the nitrogen from the atmosphere and convert it into the appropriate form for the plant to absorb. Bacteria also inhabit the digestive systems of animals, including humans; their functions in these habitats include processing foods to allow the release of vital nutrients for absorption into the body.

It has been estimated that the human body contains approximately 50 trillion cells; it has also been estimated that the human body contains a similar number of bacteria. It is abundantly clear that the human body is one of their natural habitats; which means it is therefore totally inappropriate to refer to bacteria as 'invaders' or as parasites of humans, or of any other living organism.

The discussion earlier in this chapter about the microorganisms that normally live in and on the body is particularly relevant to this section, as bacteria are by far the most common endogenous microorganisms; they are also the most often claimed to be simultaneously harmless and harmful. This anomaly is demonstrated by a July 2017 article entitled *Commensal-to-pathogen transition: One-single transposon insertion results in two pathoadaptive traits in Escherichia coli-macrophage interaction*, which states that,

"*Escherichia coli* is both a harmless commensal in the intestines of many mammals, as well as a dangerous pathogen."

The article claims that genes are one of the factors that contribute to the bacteria's ability to 'switch' from harmless to harmful; but it also exposes the poor level of understanding about the processes involved in such a 'switch' in the comment that,

"Our understanding of how often and by which mechanisms bacteria transit from a commensal to a pathogenic lifestyle is still far from complete."

This lack of a complete understanding raises questions about the underlying assumption that bacteria make such a transition; the discussions in this section will demonstrate that there is no evidence that any bacterium is or becomes a 'dangerous pathogen'.

Bacteria are extremely hardy; they live under some of the most extreme conditions, from extreme cold to extreme heat; they also live in some of the most hostile environments, such as deep-sea hydrothermal vents. Some types of bacteria require oxygen for their survival, others cannot survive in the presence of oxygen. Some even have the ability to become dormant, if the conditions require it.

Bacteria can therefore be said to be truly ubiquitous.

It has been shown that bacteria are one of the most ancient 'life-forms' on Earth; their single-celled ancestors appeared at least three and a half billion years ago. Dr Peter Duesberg, a molecular biologist and also a member of the prestigious NAS, makes the comment in *Inventing the AIDS Virus* that,

> "Microbes lived on this planet long before humans. We coexist with a sea of microbes and benefit from many, including those that naturally reside in the human body."

There is, in reality, a very fundamental relationship between bacteria and all other life-forms on Earth; biologist Dr Lynn Margulis explains this relationship in her 1998 book, *Symbiotic Planet*,

> "All life, we now know, evolved from the smallest life-forms of all, bacteria."

Although this is an acknowledged fact within biology, the 'information' promulgated by the medical establishment remains focused on the idea that bacteria are pathogens; even though it has been recognised that most microorganisms are not pathogenic.

This is an inconsistency that continues to have serious consequences; it is therefore extremely important to expose the fallacy of the claim that any bacterium is a pathogen.

From the earliest investigations of bacteria, they have always been categorised as 'germs' and therefore as primary causal agents of disease. To the scientists of the 19th century, it seemed that the only relevant investigations to conduct were those that would discover which specific bacterium was the cause of which specific disease. Although shown to be erroneous, this approach has persisted throughout the field of medical research and has continued into the early 21st century.

There have, however, been some scientists who have investigated bacteria from a different perspective and realised that 'science' had misunderstood these microorganisms. One such scientist is Dr Ivan Wallin PhD, a microbiologist, who investigated the behaviour and functions of bacteria; the result of his work led him to state in 1927 that,

> "Above all, it must be emphasised that our knowledge of the behaviour of bacteria is decidedly limited."

Unfortunately, the vast majority of Dr Wallin's peers were firmly of the opinion that bacteria were fundamentally pathogenic and refused to consider any other view.

Although knowledge about the behaviour and functions of bacteria has expanded since 1927, the medical establishment retains its intransigence. There is a continuing reluctance to relinquish the 'germ theory', for a variety of reasons, many of which are discussed in chapter nine; however, these reasons obviously include the fact that to do so would necessitate fundamental changes to the prevailing 'healthcare system'.

Erroneous ideas about bacteria are slowly being changed as the result of new discoveries, and replaced with knowledge of their real functions, some of which are:

Bacteria are saprotrophic, which means that they feed on and break down dead organisms and release the nutrients back into the environment to be utilised by other organisms.

Bacteria break down waste products and are used in sewage treatment plants for just such a purpose.

Bacteria are involved in the cycles of important elements such as oxygen, nitrogen and carbon.

The discovery that bacteria are saprotrophic has profound implications, one of which is that it provides the most plausible explanation for their presence within diseased tissue. It is fully acknowledged within the wider field of science that bacteria are part of the community of 'decomposers' that break down dead organic matter, which includes the bodies of animals and humans. Their ability to decompose dead organic matter, which results in the release of nutrients into the 'environment', should not be considered to be a function that is performed solely on the death of an animal or human and only occurs in the external environment.

Human cells die every day; it is part of the normal processes of 'life', which include the processes necessary for the elimination of dead cells from the body. In addition to the dead cells that require removal is the added burden of damaged cells; this damage can occur as the result of different factors, but is mainly the result of exposures to toxins. The fact that bacteria act as saprotrophs means that they perform the function of decomposing damaged as well as dead materials within the body; a function that is similar to the break-down of food in the digestive system that results in the release of nutrients in the appropriate form for the body to absorb.

Another erroneous idea maintained by the medical establishment relates to blood and the bloodstream; as indicated by a December 2002 article entitled, *Are There Naturally Occurring Pleomorphic Bacteria in the Blood of Healthy Humans* which states that,

"In our search for spirochetes involved in Alzheimer's disease, we observed pleomorphic bacteria in the blood of healthy human subjects..."

The article reports that the observation of bacteria in the blood of healthy human subjects was 'surprising'; the reason that this is described as a surprise is because the bloodstream has long been believed to be a 'sterile' environment; but this is a mistaken belief. The medical establishment claims that the presence of bacteria in the blood represents an 'infection' or blood poisoning, also known as sepsis or septicaemia; but this too is erroneous; bacteria do not 'infect' or 'poison' the blood.

Although the article refers to the search for a spirochete, a type of bacterium, in Alzheimer's disease, there is a great deal of evidence that demonstrates a far closer association between this disease and neurotoxins, particularly aluminium; the neurotoxic effects of aluminium were discussed in chapter two. However, the idea that bacteria may be involved in Alzheimer's disease demonstrates just how deeply embedded the 'germ theory' is in the search for the causal agents of a wide variety of diseases, despite the huge volume of evidence demonstrating the existence of other and far more plausible causal factors.

Bacteria are single-celled organisms that, over the course of many billions of years of evolution, have developed into many forms. It has been discovered that the development of larger life-forms has occurred through a process called symbiosis. Dr Ivan Wallin PhD was one of the first proponents of the idea of symbiotic relationships; he was the first to recognise combinations of single-celled bacteria and their development into more complex multicellular life-forms.

In his 1927 book entitled *Symbionticism and the origin of species*, Dr Wallin explains the idea of symbiotic relationships and how, as the title suggests, they have played a significant role in the development of new species. His ideas were, unfortunately, rejected by his peers, who remained committed to the dogma that bacteria are fundamentally pathogenic. Fortunately, his ideas have not been totally ignored; one scientist who has followed and expanded upon his work is Dr Lynn Margulis, who has also recognised the erroneous theories about bacteria, as she explains in *Symbiotic Planet*,

"Microbes, especially bacteria, are touted as enemies and denigrated as germs."

Unfortunately, Dr Wallin abandoned his research because of the attitude of his peers; a situation that substantially impeded the progress of scientific investigation in this field until Dr Margulis began to research his work and further develop his ideas. Whilst the evolution of new species, a major aspect of her research, is extremely interesting, it is not pertinent to the current discussion.

One of the most important aspects of Dr Wallin's work is that it demonstrates that bacteria are the foundation of all 'life', which thoroughly refutes the claim that any of them can be 'pathogenic'. One of Dr Wallin's most profound discoveries was in respect of mitochondria, which are organelles that are present within most cells of animals, the main exception being red blood cells. Dr Wallin discovered that mitochondria are bacterial in origin and that,

"...mitochondria are living organisms, symbiotically combined within the cells of animals."

Plants have similar organelles, called plastids, which, like the mitochondria of animals, are also bacterial in origin.

The fact that mitochondria and plastids are bacterial in origin is acknowledged within mainstream cell biology, as indicated by the 2002 textbook entitled *Molecular Biology of the Cell*, which states that,

"It is widely accepted that mitochondria and plastids evolved from bacteria..."

What is most surprising, considering the ramifications of this discovery, is that the idea that these organelles were produced from symbiotic relationships with bacteria is no longer controversial, as Dr Margulis explains,

"Acceptance of symbiotic origin for mitochondria and plastids was finalised with the discovery that both these kinds of organelles contain distinct DNA, separate from that of the nucleus and unequivocally bacterial in style and organization."

Unfortunately, this information is not widely promulgated to the general public, who are constantly 'informed' that bacteria are dangerous pathogens, despite the fact that most cells in the human body contain mitochondria that are bacterial in origin.

Mitochondria perform an extremely important function, which is that of generating energy for the cell; this energy is in the form of a chemical called adenosine triphosphate (ATP), without an adequate production of which cells in the living organism would fail to function properly. The bacterial origin of mitochondria demonstrates the erroneous nature of the idea that bacteria are fundamental parasites that contribute nothing to the welfare of the host. There are serious consequences from the failure of the medical establishment to recognise the scientifically established facts about bacteria; the main consequence relates to the continuing use of antibiotics to 'kill' allegedly pathogenic bacteria; antibiotics are discussed in the next section.

The significance of bacteria to all forms of 'life' is indicated by Dr Margulis, who states in *Symbiotic Planet* that,

"We evolved from a long line of progenitors, ultimately from the first bacteria. Most evolution occurred in those beings we dismiss as 'microbes'."

Recognition of the importance of bacteria to all 'life' obviously poses a serious and direct challenge to the 'germ theory'; the sums of money invested in the applications derived from it are far too large to readily permit a revelation that the theory is fatally flawed. The influence of 'vested interests', which is discussed in detail in chapter nine, is a major deterrent to any scientific investigation that would pose a challenge to their dominance; this means that investigations likely to question the 'consensus' view require efforts that are rarely acknowledged or appreciated, as Dr Margulis indicates,

"Our culture ignores the hard-won fact that these disease 'agents', these 'germs', also germinated all life."

It is a commonplace within science for new ideas to be 'hard-won', but it is becoming increasingly difficult for certain new ideas to be accepted, especially if they do not accord with the 'consensus' view. The problems with the requirement for all scientists to accept and support the 'consensus' are also discussed in chapter nine.

One of the many fascinating attributes of bacteria is their ability to change their form; an attribute referred to as pleomorphism. Science orthodoxy almost exclusively teaches bacterial monomorphism, which means that all forms with the same shape belong to the same species but do not change into other forms. It has, however, been acknowledged that there are some exceptions to the rule of bacterial monomorphism, but that these exceptions are restricted to only a few types of bacteria and occur in only specific circumstances.

Pleomorphism is not, however, a newly recognised phenomenon. In his 1938 book entitled *Impaired Health: Its Cause and Cure*, Dr John Tilden MD discusses the changes that bacteria can undergo and, although he does not use the term 'pleomorphism', it is clear that this is the phenomenon he refers to in the following statement,

"That the explorers of the microscopic world have some excuse for the infinite number of varieties already discovered, there is no question; for these infinitely small beings have the habit of taking on an individuality, or personality, in keeping with the chemic changes of the medium with which they are correlated."

The phenomenon of pleomorphism was discussed even earlier by Dr Ivan Wallin in his 1927 book, in which he states that,

"It has further been established that the morphology of a microorganism may be altered by changing the environmental factors."

Dr Wallin refers to pleomorphism exhibited by mitochondria, which is not surprising considering that the genetic material of mitochondria is bacterial in nature. However, he refers to experiments that had investigated the effects of phosphorus poisoning on mitochondria, which were discovered to have undergone pleomorphic modifications. These experiments clearly corroborate the assertion that bacteria are affected by the chemical nature and composition of their environment.

Unfortunately, the scientific community has great difficulties in accepting pleomorphism as a phenomenon exhibited by most, if not all, bacteria; a situation that Dr Milton Wainwright PhD discusses in his 1997 article entitled *Extreme Pleomorphism and the bacterial life cycle: a forgotten controversy*, in which he states that,

"Nearly all modern microbiologists belong to the monomorphic school..."

Although he states that most microbiologists reject pleomorphism, it is nevertheless, a genuine phenomenon; the demand for scientific consensus denies the emergence of new ideas, which impedes scientific progress. Fortunately, there is a growing recognition of pleomorphism, even if of a limited nature, as Dr Wainwright indicates,

"Reports of the existence of limited pleomorphism continue to appear somewhat infrequently in the modern literature."

One group of bacteria that are acknowledged to be 'highly pleomorphic' are *Rickettsiae*, which include the bacterium claimed to be the causal agent of typhus, which Florence Nightingale claimed was not caused by a 'new infection' but by the worsening conditions within the hospital wards.

Another bacterium known to be pleomorphic is *Deinococcus radiodurans*; which, interestingly, has not been claimed to be the causal agent of any disease. A 2009 article entitled, *Nutrition induced pleomorphism and budding mode of reproduction in Deinococcus radiodurans* states that the researchers,

"...observed different forms of the bacterium morphology by varying the culture medium concentration."

Although the researchers only varied the concentration of the culture medium, these changes nevertheless resulted in the bacteria altering their forms according to the nature of the environment in which they were placed. The observation of different morphologies demonstrates that bacteria are highly adaptable and that they adapt their form according to the conditions of the environment they inhabit.

The article also provides an interesting revelation in the admission that,

> "The conflicting aspect of the true morphology of the bacterium in natural environment and observed morphology in laboratory conditions always posed questions to microbiologists."

This 'conflict' demonstrates that bacteria exhibit different behaviours within the confines of the laboratory from those within their natural environment; it also emphasises the serious consequences that can arise from assumptions made from the results of laboratory experiments that are extrapolated to 'nature' and to situations in the real world. The article reveals that most microbiologists do not have an adequate level of knowledge about bacteria in one of their 'natural' habitats; the living human body.

Although pleomorphism is acknowledged to exist, most medical establishment sources interpret the phenomenon to refer to changes that merely involve a 'variation' in the shape or size of bacteria rather than a complete change in their form. This denial of the existence of full pleomorphism is another situation that can be attributed to the rigid adherence to the dogma that bacteria are 'germs'; that they cause disease and therefore need to be killed by antibiotic medicines or prevented by vaccines. Dr Wainwright was certainly aware of the difficulties of gaining acceptance by the medical establishment for the concept of full or 'extreme' pleomorphism; he states that,

> "While claims for such limited pleomorphism offend no one, modern reports of extreme pleomorphism are likely to suffer derision, or more usually just be ignored."

Deriding claims and ignoring evidence do not constitute a scientific method of disproving the veracity of claims about any phenomena.

It is obvious that pleomorphism does not fit the existing 'consensus' view of bacteria; but it does provide a compelling explanation for the variety of bacterial forms that are often mistakenly believed to be distinctly different entities, each of which is claimed to be the causal agent of a distinctly different disease.

It is the contention of some people, particularly in the 'alternative health' community, that bacteria only become pathogenic under certain conditions; that they only play a secondary role in disease. This view claims that bacteria are not the original cause of disease, but that they proliferate as the direct result of disease. It is further claimed that it is the proliferation of the bacteria that directly contributes to the worsening of the disease due to the 'toxins' released by these 'bad' bacteria.

The idea that 'bacterial toxins' are the causes of many illnesses is fundamentally flawed; the main reason is due to the normal presence in the body of many trillions of bacteria. If only a tiny percentage of the trillions of bacteria in the body produced 'toxins' people would always be ill, from the moment of birth and throughout their entire lives. If any of these toxins were truly 'deadly', it raises the question of how life could ever have begun, considering that bacteria are one of the earliest 'life-forms'.

In his book entitled *Food Is Your Best Medicine*, Dr Henry Bieler MD discusses the role of bacteria and explains why they are found in diseased tissue,

"After the cells have been damaged by toxic wastes, it is easy for bacteria, as scavengers, to attack and devour the weakened, injured and dead cells."

His use of the word 'scavenger' and his description of bacterial activity as an 'attack' may appear misleading, but Dr Bieler does not accuse bacteria of causing disease; he is expressing recognition of their function as decomposers of dead and damaged cells.

The idea that bacteria play a secondary role in disease has also been claimed to have been proved by experiments in which examination of diseased tissue in its early stages revealed no bacteria, but that later stages of the disease revealed the presence of bacteria. A suggestion of this kind ignores the acknowledged fact that bacteria are saprotrophic; a fact that fully explains their presence at the site of severely damaged tissue, which is to be 'decomposed' and eliminated from the body.

Organic materials are acknowledged to be decomposed through 'biodegradation', which refers to the processes carried out by microorganisms, especially bacteria; this clearly demonstrates that the scientific community recognises that bacteria are saprotrophic. A number of investigations have discovered that many different materials can be biodegraded by different organisms.

The use of microorganisms to biodegrade environmental pollutants is known by the term 'bioremediation'; as indicated by a July 2010 article entitled *Microbial Degradation of Petroleum Hydrocarbon Contaminants: An Overview*, which discusses bioremediation and states that,

"Many indigenous microorganisms in water and soil are capable of degrading hydrocarbon contaminants."

Bacteria are not the only decomposers, other organisms have also been recognised to be saprotrophic; however, bacteria are particularly effective in the biodegradation of important environmental pollutants, as the article states,

"Bacteria are the most active agents in petroleum degradation... Several bacteria are even known to feed exclusively on hydrocarbons."

This therefore demonstrates an extremely useful and beneficial property of bacteria, but their usefulness in the processes of bioremediation should not be used to justify the continued production and use of petrochemical products that pollute and contaminate the environment; as will be discussed in greater detail in chapter six.

Bacteria are also capable of biodegrading many other pollutants, such as heavy metals, as indicated by a 1998 article entitled *Physical properties and heavy metal uptake of encapsulated Escherichia coli expressing a metal binding gene*. This article is extremely revealing because *E. coli* are regarded as a major cause of food poisoning, but it is also widely recognised that *E. coli* normally reside in the intestines of healthy people. These bacteria are regarded as both commensal and pathogenic; the anomalous nature of this claim was previously mentioned. The fact that they are found in healthy people who do not suffer from 'food poisoning' is a situation that fails to meet Koch's first postulate, which means that *E. coli* cannot be the cause of any disease, including 'food poisoning'.

The CDC website provides information about *E. coli* on a page entitled *What are Escherichia coli?* which includes the following surprising admission,

"It does get a bit confusing – even to microbiologists."

The idea that microbiologists are confused about any bacterium demonstrates that there are serious and fundamental problems with the 'germ theory' on which they base their work, and also corroborates the assertion that the medical establishment possesses a poor level of understanding about these microorganisms.

There is certainly a great deal of information about bacteria still to be discovered. Nevertheless, the knowledge that has accumulated since Dr Koch conducted his experiments in the late 19th century demonstrates that his theory that they are the causes of disease needs to be abandoned. The growing weight of evidence shows that the real functions of bacteria are far from 'disease-causing'; their role is an important one that is vital for the continuing existence of life on Earth.

Dr Margulis, in particular, recognised the amazing attributes of bacteria and was able to contemplate them from a completely different perspective than that of most scientists, as indicated by her comment that,

"Life is an incredibly complex interdependence of matter and energy among millions of species beyond (and within) our own skin."

Life is indeed complex and interdependent. The world is not a battleground, in which the germs must be killed, because clearly what kills the germs will surely kill all life-forms.

Dr Stefan Lanka provides an eloquent summary in his 2005 interview for *Faktuell*,

"The basis of biological life is togetherness, is symbiosis, and in this there is no place for war and destruction."

Antibiotics, Resistance and 'Superbugs'

The establishment definition of an antibiotic refers to it as,

"a substance, produced by or derived from a microorganism, that destroys or inhibits the growth of other microorganisms."

Antibiotics are used primarily in the treatment of 'bacterial infections'; they are considered to be ineffective for 'viral infections'.

The first antibiotic to be developed was penicillin, which is widely acclaimed as one of the greatest achievements of 'modern medicine'.

Nothing could be further from the truth.

The discussion in the first section of this chapter revealed that the medical establishment is fully aware of the fact that most bacteria are harmless. The discussion in the previous section revealed that the medical establishment is fully aware of the fact that many trillions of bacteria normally reside within the human body. These revelations demonstrate that the use of antibiotics to destroy bacteria in the name of 'healthcare' is an error of idea that external entities invade and infect the body thereby causing disease; but the refutation of the 'germ theory' means that diseases cannot be the result of 'infections'. This, in turn, means that the entire concept of 'immunity' needs to be re-examined from a completely different perspective.

The definition of immunity refers to the presence of antibodies, the establishment definition of which refers to,

> "a special kind of blood protein that is synthesized in lymphoid tissue in response to the presence of a particular antigen and circulates in the plasma to attack the antigen and render it harmless."

An antigen is defined by the establishment as,

> "any substance that may be specifically bound by an antibody molecule."

It is clear therefore, that antibodies and antigens are interdependent 'entities'; but these definitions do not explain the processes involved. Antigens are also defined by the *Medical Encyclopedia* on the NIH website; this definition provides some examples and states that,

> "An antigen may be a substance from the environment, such as chemicals, bacteria, viruses, or pollen."

The definition of an antibody states that it is produced in response to the presence of antigens; it also states that antibodies attack antigens, which include pathogens. This definition suggests therefore, that the human body is a permanent battleground of antibodies, pathogens and antigens.

Nothing could be further from the truth.

It is alleged that during an 'infection', the body produces a specific 'antibody response' within the immune system to the pathogen. Once the antibody has been produced, it is said to remain in the body to recognise and to provide protection against any future 'infection' by that pathogen. It is also claimed that the existence of the appropriate antibodies provides 'proof' of a prior infection, and that they can be detected by means of certain antibody tests.

The discussion about viruses indicated that many people are diagnosed with an infectious disease, such as a cold, without any tests having been conducted to determine the nature of the alleged 'infection' or identify the causal agent.

It is abundantly clear that there are many problems with these ideas, not least of which is the fact that tests do not detect the actual microorganism; instead, they only detect 'antibodies', which are proteins, not living organisms.

Another major problem is that most of the microorganisms claimed to be pathogenic are endogenous; they are normal components of the human microbiota. This therefore raises the question of why the body would produce 'antibodies' with the specific purpose of attacking endogenous microorganisms; in other words, why would the body seek to attack its normal inhabitants, which are part of itself?

Although there is no explanation for this phenomenon, the medical establishment has generated another adaptation of the 'germ theory' that introduces the idea that the body can, and indeed does, attack itself. This idea is claimed to provide an 'explanation' for a category of diseases referred to as 'autoimmune diseases', a number of which are discussed in chapter seven. The inclusion of pollen as one of the many types of antigen introduces the notion that the immune system is implicated in 'allergies', which are also discussed in chapter seven.

The refutation of the 'germ theory' means that there is no need for the body to protect itself against any 'pathogens'; this therefore requires a further discussion about the concept of 'immunity', which is claimed to exist in two forms, referred to as 'natural immunity' and 'acquired immunity'.

The medical establishment claims that 'natural immunity' is passed during pregnancy from a mother to her baby. It is also claimed that babies retain a certain level of immunity after birth whilst their own immune system develops. However, despite these claims, newborn infants are the primary targets of the vaccine industry on the basis that they need to be 'protected' from the large number of so-called 'infectious diseases' to which they could succumb.

The other form of immunity, called 'acquired immunity', is claimed to be conferred through vaccination; the discussions in chapter two demonstrate that vaccines confer no immunity whatsoever.

In addition to the natural immunity passed by mother to baby during pregnancy, is the immunity passed during breast-feeding. This is recognised by a 1998 article on the website of the NIH, entitled *Breastfeeding provides passive and likely long-lasting active immunity*; the title is self-explanatory.

Nevertheless, there are no exemptions from the vaccination schedule for breastfed babies; a situation that is highly anomalous, although unsurprising. It is clear that the medical establishment disregards important aspects of scientifically-established facts that contradict their core message, which is that vaccines and drugs are essential to prevent and treat disease.

There are many contradictions that arise as the result of the poor level of understanding the medical establishment possesses about many of the functions of the human body; this includes a poor level of knowledge about the immune system.

This can be demonstrated by a 2011 article entitled *The Bodyguard: Tapping the Immune System's Secrets*, published on the website of Stanford Medicine. The article refers to Dr Garrison Fathman MD, a professor of immunology, and states that he regards the immune system as a 'black box', in the context that there is not a great deal of knowledge about its internal 'workings'. This is an astounding admission considering the strenuous efforts of the medical establishment to promote the idea that the immune system protects people from 'infectious diseases'.

The article also reports that, if asked by a patient about the state of their immune system, Dr Fathman is quoted to have stated that he would have difficulty in responding,

> "I would have no idea how to answer that, and I'm an immunologist. *None* of us can answer that."

Chapter Four

'Infectious' Diseases: Dispelling the Myths

"The practice of poisoning a person because he is ill is based on erroneous notions of the essential nature of disease."

Herbert Shelton

The medical establishment claims that there are two types of disease, infectious and non-infectious; those of the latter type, which are also known as noncommunicable diseases, are discussed in chapter seven.

Infectious diseases, also called communicable diseases, are said to possess two defining features that differentiate them from 'non-infectious' diseases. The first is that they are claimed to be caused by 'pathogens', as indicated by the WHO web page entitled *Infectious diseases* which states that,

"Infectious diseases are caused by pathogenic microorganisms, such as bacteria, viruses, parasites or fungi..."

The second feature is that they are claimed to be transmissible between people, as indicated by the establishment definition of 'communicable disease' that refers to,

"any disease that can be transmitted from one person to another."

It is clear that these features are inextricably interconnected. The claim that infectious diseases are transmitted between people is totally dependent on the claim that they are caused by pathogenic microorganisms. It is these 'microorganisms' that are claimed to be the 'infectious agents' that are spread, both directly and indirectly, between people, who become 'infected' with the 'pathogen' and develop the disease they are alleged to cause. However, as revealed in the previous chapter, the claim that microorganisms are pathogenic is erroneous; the claim that diseases are transmissible between people is therefore equally erroneous.

The logical conclusion to be drawn from this is that the term 'infectious disease' is a misnomer, because, in reality, there is no such phenomenon as an 'infectious disease'.

The assertion that no diseases are 'infectious' will inevitably be considered highly controversial, because it contradicts information promulgated by the medical establishment about 'infectious diseases'; but its controversial nature does not deny its veracity.

One of the main reasons that this assertion will be considered controversial is because it conflicts with a common experience, which is that diseases appear to behave as if they are infectious. It is therefore appropriate to quote the maxim that 'appearances can be deceptive'; the appearance of infectiousness is indeed deceptive. It is not unusual for people to be ill at the same time and to have the same or very similar symptoms; this is often assumed to mean that they have the same disease that has been 'spread' by some kind of 'germ'. Although it is not surprising that the overwhelming majority of people make this assumption, it is nevertheless an entirely erroneous one.

Within all forms of research, it is the evidence that is primary; this means that if a prevailing theory fails to adequately explain empirical evidence, it is the theory that requires reassessment. Prevailing theories may even need to be totally abandoned, especially when other theories exist that offer more compelling and comprehensive explanations for the available evidence. The increasing efforts to achieve 'consensus' within the field of 'medicine' have ensured that certain theories, especially the 'germ theory', form the 'consensus' view; but this is entirely inappropriate as it hampers researchers from formulating more compelling theories that better explain the evidence. The purpose of research is encapsulated by a statement attributed to Dr Albert Szent-Györgyi PhD,

> "Research is to see what everyone else has seen and to think what nobody else has thought."

Dr Peter Duesberg echoes this sentiment in his comment that,

> "Many pivotal contributions to science throughout history have consisted less of new observations than of new explanations for old data."

Although the medical establishment continues to make 'new observations' from laboratory experimentation, it fails entirely to provide plausible explanations for certain 'old data'; especially data about 'infectious diseases'. There is clearly a consensus view with respect to these diseases, but that does not mean it is a correct view.

One of the reasons for the perpetuation of the fallacy that 'germs' cause 'infectious diseases' is to support the pharmaceutical industry, which is a key member of the medical establishment, and to promote the need for medicines and vaccines to combat these diseases. However, despite the seemingly best efforts of the industry, modern medicine has been unable to contain 'infectious diseases', which are reported to be proliferating; as indicated by a July 2013 article entitled *Emerging Infectious Diseases: Threats to Human Health and Global Stability* which states that,

> "Today, however, despite extraordinary advances in development of counter measures (diagnostics, therapeutics and vaccines), the ease of world travel and increased global interdependence have added layers of complexity to containing

these infectious diseases that affect not only the health but the economic stability of societies."

The idea that infectious diseases can threaten 'economic stability' is based on the notion that ill people are not productive members of society; the problems with this idea and its global implications are discussed in chapters eight and nine.

Although the article refers to 'extraordinary advances' in the measures employed to contain infectious diseases, it fails to explain the distinct lack of success these measures have had in achieving their objective. The reference to 'layers of complexity' is wholly inadequate as an explanation for the failure of medicines and vaccines to be effective against infectious diseases. The real reason they are ineffective is because diseases are not caused by germs; they cannot be treated with toxic medicines or prevented by toxic vaccines. The many and very real threats to human health are discussed in chapter six.

The article states that infectious diseases have been emerging and re-emerging for millennia and that the emergence of new infectious diseases is inevitable. In addition, it suggests that the vast majority of new infections are 'likely' to have originated in animals, particularly rodents and bats; the use of the word 'likely' indicates that this idea remains unproven. The idea that animals harbour 'germs' that can be spread to humans is unfounded, as demonstrated by the discussions in the previous chapter. A number of animal diseases are discussed in the next chapter to demonstrate that they are also not caused by pathogens.

The article does however, acknowledge that the emergence and re-emergence of so-called 'infectious diseases' are driven by numerous factors, which include: technology and industry; poverty and social inequality; war and famine. Many of these factors are certainly relevant to health, or rather to ill-health, but the article relegates them to being of lesser significance than 'germs', which are claimed to pose the greatest threat.

The fact that 'infectious diseases' are not caused by 'germs' and are not transmissible, inevitably raises questions about the real nature of the illnesses referred to as 'infectious', and about their ability to appear to simultaneously affect large numbers of people with very similar symptoms.

The definition of each individual infectious disease lists a number of different symptoms that a person 'may' experience when they are deemed to have that 'disease'. However, because many symptoms are common to a number of diseases, a 'correct' diagnosis may require people to undergo additional tests that are claimed to be able to identify the pathogen, and therefore the disease. The most common types of test involve the examination of blood or urine samples; but, as previously stated, such tests do not detect the actual 'pathogen'; instead, they detect proteins, referred to as 'antibodies', that will help to identify the pathogen responsible for the infection, because each antibody is specific to each type of 'germ'.

Yet the medical establishment interprets the presence of antibodies in the body in two entirely different ways. One interpretation is that the production of antibodies claimed to be specific to a pathogen, indicates that the person has immunity to the disease it is said to cause. The other interpretation is that the presence of antibodies means that the person has been 'infected' by a pathogen and has the disease it is said to cause. These interpretations are mutually exclusive; nevertheless, they are both promulgated by the medical establishment as 'information' about infectious diseases, antibodies and immunity. It should be obvious, however, that neither interpretation is correct.

It is claimed that 'infectious diseases' are collectively responsible for the loss each year of many millions of lives and that these numbers are sporadically augmented by a virulent 'outbreak' of disease. Some of the most frequently cited 'deadly outbreaks' are the Black Death, the 1918 Flu and HIV/AIDS, all of which are discussed in this chapter.

The situation in which very large numbers of people become ill and suffer very similar symptoms is usually referred to as an 'epidemic', which Herbert Shelton describes as 'mass sickness' and explains that,

"In all epidemics, the so-called epidemic disease is but one among several symptom complexes presented by the sick."

Although it may appear that people display the same symptoms, it is rare that everyone will experience exactly the same set of symptoms with exactly the same intensity and for exactly the same duration. It is clear therefore, that people only ever experience varying 'symptom complexes'.

There are reasons that large numbers of people may be ill at the same time and display similar symptoms, as will be explained in the discussions in this chapter; but these reasons do not include infections with 'germs' that have been transmitted between people.

The refusal to recognise the fundamentally flawed nature of the 'germ theory' continues to present a serious obstacle to the implementation of genuine solutions to the many real threats to human health. This situation will continue to worsen whilst the medical establishment remains intransigent and continues to perpetuate flawed theories, especially through medical training. Although previously cited, Dr Carolyn Dean's statement is again pertinent and deserves repetition,

"In fact, we were told many times that if we didn't learn it in medical school it must be quackery."

It is this arrogant attitude that prevents progress towards the achievement of a better understanding about human health and illness; but the failings of the medical establishment do not invalidate other research studies and investigations that present far more compelling explanations of a number of so-called 'infectious' diseases; as the following discussions will demonstrate.

Smallpox

Smallpox has been previously discussed at some length; the reason for returning to this disease is to dispel the popular belief that claims smallpox to have been responsible for the devastating loss of life suffered by the indigenous peoples of America, because it was 'carried' there by Europeans. Variations of this story also refer to other diseases carried to the New World by the Spanish initially and later by the Portuguese and the British. These diseases include measles, influenza, bubonic plague, diphtheria, typhus, cholera, scarlet fever, chicken pox, yellow fever and whooping cough; it is commonly asserted, however, that smallpox was responsible for the greatest loss of life.

Within this 'myth' are a number of interrelated assertions, one of which is that none of these diseases had previously existed in the New World. Another is that, because these diseases were 'new' to them, the indigenous people had no immunity and were therefore unable to offer resistance to 'infection' with the germs carried by the Europeans. The inevitable conclusion, according to the myth, is that millions of people became 'infected' and therefore succumbed to, and even died from, the diseases the germs are alleged to cause.

However, yet again, nothing could be further from the truth.

Although the main reason this myth is false is because it is based on the fatally flawed 'germ theory', its assertions can also be shown to be in direct contradiction of a number of the claims made by the medical establishment about 'infectious' diseases.

One of these contradictions arises because few of the diseases alleged to have been 'carried' to the New World are regarded as inherently fatal, but they are claimed to have caused millions of deaths. Yet, if these diseases were so deadly to the indigenous peoples, how were any of them able to survive; as there clearly were survivors.

It is claimed that the crews of the ships that arrived in the New World spread their diseases easily because they are highly contagious. It is also claimed that these sailors remained unaffected by the germs they 'carried' throughout the long voyages across the Atlantic Ocean. Although some people are claimed to be 'asymptomatic carriers', it is highly improbable, if not impossible, that every crew member of every ship that sailed to the New World would have merely carried the 'germs' without succumbing to the diseases.

The most common explanation offered for the failure of the crews to succumb to these diseases is that they had developed immunity to them; but this explanation is highly problematic. According to the medical establishment, a healthy, competent immune system is one that contains antibodies that will destroy pathogens. Therefore, if the European sailors were 'immune' to all these diseases due to the presence of the appropriate antibodies, their bodies would not contain any 'germs'. If, on the other hand, the European sailors did carry 'germs' they could not have been 'immune'.

It is not the purpose of this discussion to deny that millions of people died, but to refute the claim that they died from 'infectious diseases', especially smallpox, because they had no 'immunity' to the 'germs' transmitted to them by Europeans. This refutation means therefore, that they must have died from other causes.

Fortunately, historical research has uncovered evidence of the existence of a number of causal factors that would have contributed to the devastating loss of life in the New World after 1492. One source of research is the work of historian Dr David Stannard PhD, who studied contemporary writings during his investigation of the history of the discovery of the New World. This research is documented in his book entitled *American Holocaust: The Conquest of the New World*, in which he reveals many pertinent factors, not least of which relates to the conditions in which most Spanish people lived during the period prior to the first voyages to the New World; he explains,

> "Roadside ditches, filled with stagnant water, served as public latrines in the cities of the fifteenth century, and they would continue to do so for centuries to follow."

These conditions are strikingly similar to those that prevailed in many European countries during the same period. The majority of the people lived without sanitation or sewers; they lived with their own waste and sewage. Those who lived in towns and cities had limited, if any, access to clean water, which meant that they drank polluted water and rarely washed themselves. The majority of the populations of these countries were also extremely poor and had little to eat. In his book, Dr Stannard quotes the words of J H Elliott, who states,

> "The rich ate, and ate to excess watched by a thousand hungry eyes as they consumed their gargantuan meals. The rest of the population starved."

Insufficient food that leads to starvation is certainly a factor that contributes to poor health, but eating to excess can also be harmful to health; which means that the rich would not have been strangers to illness either. It is not merely the quantity of food, whether too little or too much, that is the problem; of far greater significance to health is the quality of the food consumed.

The conditions in which the native populations of the New World lived were, by comparison, strikingly different; as Dr Stannard relates,

> "And while European cities then, and for centuries thereafter, took their drinking water from the fetid and polluted rivers nearby, Tenochtitlan's drinking water came from springs deep within the mainland and was piped into the city by a huge aqueduct system that amazed Cortes and his men – just as they were astonished also by the personal cleanliness and hygiene of the colourfully dressed populace, and by their extravagant (to the Spanish) use of soaps, deodorants and breath sweeteners."

One of the most significant contributions to the substantial reduction in morbidity and mortality from disease, especially smallpox, in Europe was the implementation of sanitary reforms. It is therefore wholly inappropriate to claim that people who lived in such clean and hygienic conditions would have been more susceptible to disease. In reality, the people who lived in such clean and hygienic conditions would have been far healthier than any of the colonists, all of whom lived in countries where most people lived in squalid conditions, amidst filth and sewage and rarely, if ever, bathed.

The original objective of the first voyage led by the Italian, Christopher Columbus, is said to have been to find a western route to Asia; however, the main purpose of the voyages to new lands was to seek and obtain valuable resources, such as gold and silver. When the conquistadors observed the golden jewellery worn by indigenous peoples, they assumed that the land was rich with such treasures and this resulted in atrocious behaviour, as Dr Stannard describes,

"The troops went wild, stealing, killing, raping and torturing natives, trying to force them to divulge the whereabouts of the imagined treasure-houses of gold."

Using these methods, the Spanish 'acquired' the gold and jewellery they desired, but when no more could be collected directly from the people, they proceeded to utilise other methods. One of these methods was to establish mines, using the local population as the work force, to extract the precious metals from the ground. In addition to being forced to work, the indigenous peoples endured appalling conditions within the mines, as Dr Stannard explains,

"There, in addition to the dangers of falling rocks, poor ventilation and the violence of brutal overseers, as the Indian labourers chipped away at the rock faces of the mines they released and inhaled the poisonous vapours of cinnabar, arsenic, arsenic anhydride and mercury."

To add insult to injury, the lives of the Indians were viewed by the Spanish purely in commercial terms, as Dr Stannard again relates,

"For as long as there appeared to be an unending supply of brute labor it was cheaper to work an Indian to death, and then replace him or her with another native, than it was to feed and care for either of them properly."

Mining was not the only type of work they were forced to perform; plantations were also established, with the local population again comprising the total labour force. The appalling conditions and the violence they suffered led to their lives being substantially shortened; as Dr Stannard further relates,

"It is probable, in fact, that the life expectancy of an Indian engaged in forced labor in a mine or on a plantation during those early years of Spanish terror in Peru was not much more than three or four months..."

The number of deaths that resulted from such brutal work and treatment is unknown, but clearly substantial, as indicated by author Eduardo Galeano, who describes in his book entitled *Open Veins of Latin America*, that,

"The Caribbean island populations finally stopped paying tribute because they had disappeared; they were totally exterminated in the gold mines..."

It is hardly surprising that so many died in the gold mines considering the conditions they were made to endure; these included exposures to many highly toxic substances, as described above.

There was a further and even more tragic reason that many people died, but this did not involve brutal work and appalling working conditions. It is reported that some of the native people refused to be enslaved and forced to work; instead they took their fate into their own hands, the tragic consequences of which are explained by the words of Fernandez de Oviedo as quoted by Eduardo Galeano in *Open Veins*,

"Many of them, by way of diversion took poison rather than work, and others hanged themselves with their own hands."

The number of people who died this way is also unknown, because these events were mostly unrecorded. Dr Stannard writes that there was a considerable level of resistance by the native people that often led directly to their deaths at the hands of the conquistadors, but the number of people who died this way is also unknown.

Dr Stannard states that 'diseases' were also a factor that caused the deaths of many of the indigenous people. Unfortunately, in this claim, like the overwhelming majority of people, he has clearly accepted the medical establishment claims about infectious disease. Although this reference to diseases must be disregarded, Dr Stannard's research is otherwise based on documented evidence; for example, he refers to eyewitness accounts written by people such as Bartolomé de Las Casas about the atrocities that devastated the native population. Dr Stannard also refers to documented reports, which state that many tens of thousands of indigenous people were directly and deliberately killed; he refers to these as massacres and slaughters.

Dr Stannard records that many native people attempted to retaliate but were invariably unable to overpower the conquistadors who had superior weapons; many of them died as the result of these battles. Others chose not to fight but instead attempted to escape, the result of which was that,

> "Crops were left to rot in the fields as the Indians attempted to escape the frenzy of the conquistadors' attacks."

Starvation would no doubt have accounted for many more deaths.

The enormous scale of the loss of life can be illustrated by statistics that relate to the indigenous population of Hispaniola, which Dr Stannard reports to have plummeted from 8 million to virtually zero between the years 1496 to 1535. He indicates that this devastation in Hispaniola was not unique; but represents a typical example of the almost total annihilation of the indigenous populations that occurred throughout the land now known as America.

The Spanish were not the only 'conquerors' of the New World; the Portuguese established themselves in Brazil soon after the Spanish had arrived in Hispaniola. The consequences for the indigenous population of Brazil were, however, virtually the same as those for Hispaniola, as Dr Stannard records,

> "Within just twenty years...the native peoples of Brazil already were well along the road to extinction."

The arrival of British settlers, beginning in 1607, saw no reprieve for the indigenous peoples; although the confrontations were initially of a more 'military' nature; Dr Stannard relates that,

> "Starvation and the massacre of non-combatants was becoming the preferred British approach to dealing with the natives."

The medical establishment has a clear vested interest in perpetuating the myth that it was the 'germs' that killed many millions of people who had no immunity to the diseases the germs are alleged to cause.

Unfortunately, this myth has distorted history, as it has succeeded in furthering the 'germ theory' fallacy, and failed to bring to light the real causes of the deaths of many millions of people; but, as the work of people like Dr David Stannard, Eduardo Galeano, and others, have shown, there is ample evidence to support other and more compelling explanations for that enormous death toll, all of which may eventually succeed in overturning the myth.

Childhood Diseases

The medical establishment view with respect to 'childhood diseases' is indicated by a 2008 article entitled *Childhood Diseases – What Parents Need to Know*, which states that,

"Children encounter many infectious diseases, especially in the early months and years of life. Some upper respiratory viral or bacterial infections – such as colds, bronchiolitis, or croup – are quite common and difficult to avoid."

The article does not explain why 'infectious' diseases are common nor why they mainly affect babies and young children; its main purpose is to advise parents about vaccines, which are claimed to be,

"...incredibly effective in preventing childhood diseases and improving child mortality rates."

Although many childhood diseases are claimed to be 'vaccine-preventable', there is one notable exception, namely the 'common cold', that continues to baffle modern medicine. The alleged reason that no vaccine has been produced to combat the common cold is due to the theory that it can be caused by more than 200 different viruses.

This clearly cannot be the case; however, the alleged existence of hundreds of different 'viruses' that can cause a cold raises the question of why these viruses do not attack people simultaneously. The medical establishment theory alleges that infections weaken the immune system and that this weakened state permits 'germs' to take advantage and attack the body. This situation should mean that people would have many concurrent infections and diseases.

The medical literature does refer to instances of concurrent infections, but they are not considered to be commonplace; this is clearly another anomaly that defies the tenets of the 'germ theory', which claims that 'germs' may cause 'opportunistic infections'.

One of the main reasons that babies are recommended to have vaccines is claimed to be because they are extremely vulnerable due to their immature immune systems. If this were true, babies and small children would be far more prone to illness from multiple concurrent infections with 'germs', against which they have not been vaccinated, including the 200 or more cold viruses.

This too is clearly not the case.

The US immunisation schedule involves vaccines against fourteen diseases, because, according to the CDC web page entitled *Vaccinate Your Baby for Best Protection*,

"Diseases that vaccines prevent can be very serious – even deadly – especially for infants and young children."

It is unnecessary to discuss all fourteen diseases, but they include chickenpox, measles and German measles (rubella), all of which are regarded as 'viral' infections that particularly affect children. All three of these diseases produce very similar symptoms, the most common of which are a fever and a rash.

It is claimed that the replication of a 'virus' in a cell causes cell death; yet there is no explanation by the medical establishment for the mechanism by which the death of a cell is able to induce a fever or a skin rash, or any of the other symptoms of a so-called 'viral' disease.

The medical establishment view of disease contains many flaws, one of which relates to the nature of symptoms; this is discussed in more detail in chapter ten. Another flaw is the belief that the human body possesses no inherent mechanisms that affect health. These flaws have been exposed by various pioneers who have been dissatisfied with the teachings of the medical establishment system and have conducted their own investigations. For example, in chapter one reference was made to the experience of Dr John Tilden MD who changed his practice from a drug-based one to a drugless one.

One of the discoveries that has resulted from these investigations is that the body does possess the ability to self-heal, which it performs through mechanisms that expel and eliminate substances that are toxic and therefore injurious to the body. One of those mechanisms utilises the skin, one of the major organs of the body. The elimination of toxins through the skin produces 'eruptions' that may be described as rashes, spots or pustules. The body's efforts to eliminate toxins may also involve a fever. These symptoms are, however, usually interpreted, albeit erroneously, as 'bad' and to require medicine to suppress them; but pharmaceutical drugs only increase the level of toxins in the body. In his book *Impaired Health Vol 2*, Dr Tilden explains the elimination process involved in measles,

"Measles is the manner in which a child's body throws off toxemia."

Dr Tilden mainly refers to toxins resulting from poor eating habits. The diet of most children in the 21st century is very different from that of children who were patients of Dr Tilden, who died in 1941. However, as will be discussed in chapter six, this does not mean that children's diets in the 21st century are better than those of the mid-20th century; in many instances, they are far worse.

Diet is clearly a significant factor as digestive problems are associated with a variety of ill-health conditions. Dr Tilden explains in his book that many diseases often begin with,

"...a decided derangement of the gastrointestinal canal..."

It is for this reason that a child with a fever and a rash will usually have no appetite; the digestive system needs to eliminate the accumulated toxins; a further intake of food will only worsen the problem. Dr Robert Mendelsohn MD indicates in *Confessions of a Medical Heretic* that one of the main 'problem foods' for young babies and small children is cow's milk. He regards human breast-milk as the only suitable food for a baby and refers to bottle-feeding with cow's milk as,

"...the granddaddy of all junk food..."

He expands on the health problems likely to arise for a baby that is not fed breast milk,

to the devastating resurgence of the disease. The article makes yet another astonishing admission which is that,

"Leprosy (or Hansen's disease) is one of the most renowned, but least understood diseases of man."

The article also highlights the flawed nature of the underlying theory relating to infectious diseases in the revealing statement that,

"*M. leprae* infection does not always cause disease, and it is estimated that anywhere between 30-75% of infections are spontaneously cleared without causing significant symptoms."

This revelation demonstrates that *M. leprae* fails to meet the criteria of Koch's first postulate, and provides unequivocal evidence that this bacterium cannot be the cause of the condition called 'leprosy'. Furthermore, *M. leprae* is recognised to be a pleomorphic bacterium, which means that its morphology is very likely to be dependent on the conditions of its environment.

The most recognisable symptoms associated with leprosy are the disfiguring skin eruptions, but the label of 'leprosy' was not always applied to a specific type of skin problem, as Herbert Shelton explains,

"For ages the term leprosy was applied to a wide variety of skin diseases..."

The previous discussion demonstrated that skin eruptions occur when the body is attempting to eliminate 'toxins', which can involve those arising from unhygienic and insanitary living conditions. This point is highlighted by Dr Gerhard Buchwald in *Vaccination: A Business Based in Fear*, in which he provides details of the living conditions people endured when leprosy was a commonly diagnosed disease,

"Leprosy was a constant guest in the times when increasing numbers of people lived together in the most cramped spaces as the city walls made the expansion of cities difficult. As soon as the cities grew beyond the city walls and people had more space available, leprosy disappeared."

There is a very clear association between certain factors, especially insanitary living conditions, and an 'eruptive' disease. Herbert Shelton provides another description of the results of sanitary reforms and improved living conditions,

"Europe was once a hot bed of leprosy. Even as far west as England it was a serious problem. It has practically disappeared from Europe and this has not been due to any vaccine or serum drug that has wiped it out. The improved social conditions — sanitation, diet, personal cleanliness, better housing, and other healthful factors—that have evolved in Europe, with no aid from the medical profession have eliminated this disease."

It is abundantly clear that unhygienic living conditions were major contributory factors for diseases such as smallpox and leprosy; it is equally clear that the implementation of sanitation measures was a substantial contributory factor for the reduction in morbidity and mortality due to these diseases.

Skin eruptions, whether diagnosed as leprosy or smallpox, are manifestations of the body's elimination processes, as explained by Dr Henry Bieler in *Food is Your Best Medicine*,

"In the same way, if the bile poisons in the blood come out through the skin, we get the various irritations of the skin..."

However, although skin eruptions can manifest as a variety of symptoms that are claimed to indicate the presence of certain diseases, it is a mistake to regard them as separate disease entities. The different kinds of lumps, bumps, spots, rashes and pustules are manifestations of the body's efforts to expel toxins through the skin.

There is very little recognition within the mainstream medical literature of the sanitary reforms that substantially reduced the incidence of leprosy. Unfortunately, neither is there sufficient recognition within the medical establishment literature of one factor that has been shown to produce leprosy. Fortunately, there is adequate evidence from other sources; for example, Eleanor McBean explains in her book entitled *Swine Flu Exposé* that,

"Many vaccines also cause other diseases besides the one for which they are given. For instance, smallpox vaccine often causes syphilis, paralysis, leprosy, and cancer."

The dangers of the smallpox vaccine have been discussed; although it is significant that leprosy is identified as one of the possible 'diseases' it can cause. But this should not be surprising considering that vaccines contain a variety of toxic ingredients that require elimination from the body. Further evidence of the link between vaccines and leprosy is provided by William Tebb in his book *Leprosy and Vaccination*,

"According to all the evidence which I have been able to obtain, leprosy was unknown in the Sandwich Islands until many years after the advent of Europeans and Americans, who introduced vaccination; and there is no aboriginal word in the Hawaiian language for this disease."

Clearly, the symptoms diagnosed as leprosy had existed long before the introduction of vaccines, but it is equally clear that vaccines contribute to many health problems.

Although the disease is considered to have greatly declined, it is not thought to have been eradicated; it is claimed to still exist in the parts of the world that are referred to as 'developing' countries, as will be discussed further in chapter eight.

Syphilis

The establishment definition of syphilis refers to,

"a sexually transmitted disease caused by the bacterium *Treponema pallidum*, resulting in the formation of lesions throughout the body."

The word syphilis is reported to have originated in 1530 with the Italian Girolamo Fracastoro, who was one of the early proponents of the idea that 'germs' cause disease. His introduction of the word syphilis was initially in a poem, in which he used the word to refer to both a character and the disease with which the character was suffering. In the poem Fracastoro seems to be of the opinion that the illness was the result of a pollution of the atmosphere.

The exact origin of the disease referred to as 'syphilis' is said to be unknown; although two hypotheses have been proposed. One hypothesis suggests that syphilis was 'carried' to Europe in the late 15th century by the Spanish, who had been 'infected' in the New World and transmitted the disease on their return to their native country. The other hypothesis suggests that it was not 'new', but had not been previously recognised.

A December 2015 article entitled *The Return of Syphilis*, on the website of The Atlantic, which will be referred to as the Atlantic article, refers to a quote from the book *Guns, Germs and Steel*, in which the author, scientist Jared Diamond, provides a description of the early form of syphilis,

"Its pustules often covered the body from head to the knees, caused flesh to fall from people's faces and led to death within a few months."

This description would seem to be more applicable to leprosy than syphilis; it clearly refers to a very different disease from the one that is now referred to as 'syphilis'; as acknowledged by Herbert Shelton who states that,

"The original 'syphilis' and what is called 'syphilis' today are not the same symptom-complex at all."

A major flaw in the hypothesis that syphilis originated in the New World, is that 15th and 16th century eyewitness accounts do not describe any of the indigenous peoples as being covered in pustules or with their flesh hanging from their faces. The evidence referred to in the discussion about smallpox, reveals that the documented accounts describe the indigenous people as scrupulously clean. As also cited in the smallpox discussion, Dr Stannard refers to incidents in which the Spanish conquistadors committed rape, but this fails to provide 'evidence' that syphilis either originated in the New World or that it is sexually transmitted.

The hypothesis that syphilis was previously unrecognised also fails to provide a clear explanation for its origin, or for the notion that it is sexually transmitted. There is, in fact, no evidence that definitively demonstrates syphilis to be sexually transmissible; it is certainly not caused by a bacterium.

The discussion about leprosy indicated that the label had been used for a variety of skin problems that were usually treated with mercury. However, the dangers of mercury remained unknown and mercury ointments became the standard treatment for syphilis as well as leprosy; as Dr Carolyn Dean explains,

"When syphilis appeared in Europe, around 1495, those same ointments were used for its skin manifestations. Its side effects slowly became known and were listed openly centuries later in old medical texts, but mercury and its side effects were tolerated because the effects of untreated syphilis were felt to be much more dangerous than the side effects of the 'cure'. Syphilis was responsible for keeping mercury ostensibly viable for 400 years..."

The recognised symptoms of mercury poisoning include the shedding and peeling of the skin, symptoms that may have been diagnosed as syphilis, leprosy or even smallpox. The symptoms that are now associated with syphilis are substantially different; although mercury remained a 'treatment' until the early 20th century.

One of the main methods for diagnosing any disease relies on the symptoms or symptom-complex displayed by the patient. However, in the case of a diagnosis of syphilis, the symptoms are not always specific and therefore not easily recognisable. This point is acknowledged in the Atlantic article cited above that discusses the problem with the identification of syphilis, because,

"...the symptoms of syphilis often mimic those of other diseases."

The article also states that,

"...syphilis can be difficult to prevent and to recognise..."

Syphilis has long been referred to as 'the great imitator', as Herbert Shelton explains in detail in his 1962 book entitled *Syphilis: Is it a Mischievous Myth or a Malignant Monster*,

"Let us take the paradox that 'syphilis' not only imitates every other known disease, so that no man, in the absence of reliable serologic tests, can possibly diagnose the 'disease' from its symptoms and pathology alone (a fact that makes it difficult to understand how physicians of the past ever discovered that there is such a disease), but also imitates health."

It was the discovery in 1905 of the bacterium *Treponema pallidum*, the alleged 'pathogen', that instigated the changes to both the diagnosis and treatment of syphilis. One of the main changes was the introduction of the Wassermann test, which was claimed to assist a correct diagnosis of syphilis by the detection of antibodies to the bacterium. The interpretation of the test was that the presence of the 'right' antibodies was claimed to prove 'infection'. The conflicting interpretations of the presence of antibodies have been discussed.

One of the problems with the Wassermann test was that the results were not specific to syphilis. In his book, Herbert Shelton refers to a number of diseases that could produce a positive test result; interestingly they include leprosy as well as malaria and diabetes.

He also states that pregnancy was able to produce a positive Wassermann test result; a situation that clearly demonstrates the test was not specific to any 'disease' and therefore a totally inappropriate method of diagnosing syphilis.

Unfortunately for Americans during the early 20th century, a negative Wassermann test result was a prerequisite for the issuance of a marriage licence. A positive test result could, and in many instances did, have serious and even tragic consequences, an example of which is related by Herbert Shelton,

"A few years ago, Walter Winchell told of a prospective groom who received a notice that his blood was 'positive'. This meant that he would be denied a license to marry. He was now a branded man. He committed suicide. Several days after his suicide, the laboratory forwarded a corrected 'negative' report with an apology for the error it had made."

The Wassermann test was not restricted to adults prior to marriage; it was also used to test all members of a family, including children of all ages, in the event of a positive test result for one parent. The reason that children were tested was not due to any suspicions about sexual abuse; it was due to a belief that children born to parents with syphilis would have hereditary 'defects'. This belief, which had not been based on any scientific evidence, was later proven to be totally unfounded.

The origin of the belief in an association between sexual activity and syphilis remains elusive; there is no evidence that syphilis is a sexually transmitted disease. The only plausible explanation for the original belief is that it was a remnant of long-held superstitions that 'disease' was a punishment from the gods for sins committed; and that syphilis was therefore the punishment for the sin of sexual activity.

What is most significant is that syphilis is first recognised during the time when the vast majority of the population of Europe lived in highly insanitary conditions, which included a lack of clean water for either bathing or for washing clothes. The eruption of pustules as a method of eliminating toxins can occur anywhere on the body, including the genitals; especially when this area of the body is rarely washed. However, the people rarely washed any parts of their bodies and often wore the same items of apparel, which were infrequently changed and rarely washed.

The improvements in sanitation and personal hygiene during the past century, indicate that, in the 21st century, skin eruptions in the genital area must have other causes, none of which relates to a bacterial 'infection' or to sexual activity.

Syphilis is no longer diagnosed using Wassermann tests, but the tests that have replaced them are no more reliable or accurate because the disease remains admittedly difficult to recognise. There are some tests that are said to be able to detect the presence of the bacterium when viewed with dark-field microscopy, but detection of the presence of a bacterium does not prove it is the cause of the condition. As previously discussed, the presence of bacteria in the body is entirely normal.

Although, as indicated by its title, the Atlantic article suggests that there is a resurgence of this disease, it states that,

> "Syphilis had become relatively rare in developed countries since the discovery of penicillin..."

The discussions in the previous chapter demonstrate that penicillin cannot be claimed to be responsible for the reduction in the incidence of any disease.

However, although sanitation and personal hygiene habits have improved, they have failed to completely eradicate this 'disease'; this means that other factors must be involved. One of the factors that have been shown to contribute substantially to the body burden of toxins is vaccination, which has also been shown to be associated with the development of many diseases. Although previously cited, the words of Eleanor McBean bear repetition,

> "Many vaccines also cause other diseases besides the one for which they are given. For instance, smallpox vaccine often causes syphilis, paralysis, leprosy, and cancer."

Vaccines have also been shown to produce other effects, as Herbert Shelton explains,

> "It was discovered that smallpox vaccination will give a positive Wassermann

reaction..."

This provides further evidence that this test is unable to detect any specific 'disease'.

The resurgence of syphilis is reported in the Atlantic article to be based on statistics from 2014 produced by the CDC. These statistics have been updated and are reported in an October 2016 Press Release entitled *2015 STD Surveillance Report Press Release* on the CDC website. The press release claims that all STDs, not just syphilis, have increased in incidence, and adds the comment that,

"Most STD cases continue to go undiagnosed and untreated..."

Unsurprisingly, the CDC also claims that,

"Widespread access to screening and treatment would reduce their spread."

Unfortunately, the recommended treatment includes antibiotics, the problems with which were discussed in the previous chapter.

It is clear that reports about the increased incidence of syphilis, whether true or not, serve the interests of the medical establishment and support their efforts to continue to generate fear. The trend to continually increase the use of antibiotics is a complete contradiction of the acknowledgement that they are vastly overused; the medical establishment cannot justify both views.

It is also clear that there is no need to invoke the existence of a 'germ' or to blame sexual activity as an explanation of the disease that has been named syphilis. The same applies to any other so-called 'sexually transmitted disease'.

1918 Flu

The establishment definition of influenza refers to,

"a highly contagious virus infection that affects the respiratory system."

It is claimed that influenza, or 'the flu', is often a seasonal illness, the symptoms of which are described by the November 2018 WHO fact sheet entitled *Influenza (Seasonal)*,

"Seasonal influenza is characterized by a sudden onset of fever, cough (usually dry), headache, muscle and joint pain, severe malaise (feeling unwell), sore throat and a runny nose."

Although it is not regarded as an inherently dangerous illness, the fact sheet adds that,

"...influenza can cause severe illness or death especially in people at high risk."

The sectors of the population considered to be at 'high risk' are children younger than the age of 5, adults older than the age of 65, pregnant women and people with certain chronic medical conditions.

The influenza epidemic of the early 20th century that is generally referred to as the '1918 Flu' is claimed to have been responsible for the loss of many millions of lives. In marked contrast with other outbreaks of 'influenza', seasonal or otherwise, this epidemic had a far greater impact on a completely different demographic, as it mainly affected adults between the ages of 20 and 40. Furthermore, contemporary sources indicate that the symptoms of this epidemic bore very little resemblance to the usual the time. But its dangers have since been recognised and aspirin has been shown to cause respiratory problems; as indicated by a November 2009 article entitled *Salicylates and Pandemic Influenza Mortality, 1918-1919 Pharmacology, Pathology and Historic Evidence* that states,

> "Pharmacokinetic data, which were unavailable in 1918, indicate that the aspirin regimens recommended for the 'Spanish influenza' predispose to severe pulmonary toxicity."

The article refers to pathology findings reported during 1918 and states that they are,

> "...consistent with aspirin toxicity."

The symptoms described by the previously cited Stanford University article are strikingly similar to symptoms that are recognised to result from a high intake of aspirin. This does not mean that it is the 'dose' that makes aspirin a poison; instead, it means that very serious and often fatal effects are the result of a high intake of aspirin. Low doses are also toxic, but their effects are less severe and may even remain undetected.

One of the consequences of the war was the need for a constant supply of new recruits to replace the soldiers who had been injured or killed. This need for additional troops meant that entry requirements for admittance to the military were, by necessity, lowered. The inevitable result of this was that the new recruits were not necessarily as fit and healthy as the men they replaced, and they were therefore more vulnerable to the effects of the toxic vaccines and medicines and to the appalling conditions they had to endure.

In addition to providing aspirin as treatment for 'influenza', the medical establishment also attempted to develop vaccines to combat as well as prevent the disease, which was originally believed to be caused by a bacterium. These vaccines are discussed in a 2009 article entitled *The fog of research: Influenza vaccine trials during the 1918-19 pandemic* which states that,

> "Bacterial vaccines of various sorts were widely used for both preventive and therapeutic purposes during the great influenza pandemic of 1918-19. Some were derived exclusively from the Pfeiffer's bacillus, the presumed cause of influenza, while others contained one or more other organisms found in the lungs of victims. Although initially most reports of the use of these vaccines claimed that they prevented influenza or pneumonia, the results were inconsistent and sometimes contradictory."

Although it is now firmly believed that the 1918 pandemic was due to viral influenza, in 1918 it was firmly believed that the disease was pneumonia, or a combination of influenza and pneumonia, and that it was caused by a bacterium called Pfeiffer's bacillus.

A 2010 article entitled *The State of Science, Microbiology and Vaccines Circa 1918* further explains the uncertain nature of those early vaccine trials,

> "Many vaccines were developed and used during the 1918-1919 pandemic. The medical literature was full of contradictory claims of their success; there was apparently no consensus on how to judge the reported results of these vaccine trials."

The vaccines were clearly recognised to have been of dubious efficacy, yet the underlying theory, that the cause was a bacterium, was not questioned; the idea that the disease was infectious also remained unquestioned. Chapter three refers to a description by Herbert Shelton of an experiment that had failed to demonstrate the infectious nature of the '1918 Flu'. In his article entitled *Contagion*, he describes a number of other experiments that attempted to determine the alleged bacterial agent that caused the disease,

> "Several groups of volunteers were inoculated with pure cultures of Pfeiffer's bacillus, with the secretions of the upper respiratory passages and with blood taken from typical influenza cases. About 30 of the men had the germs sprayed and swabbed in the nose and throat. The Public Health Report sums up the results in these words: 'In no instance was an attack of influenza produced in any one of the subjects'."

As previously cited, Herbert Shelton refers to epidemics as 'mass sickness', to which he adds the comment,

> "For example, in the 1918-19 influenza-pneumonia pandemic, there were great numbers of cases of mumps, of measles, of typhoid fever, of sleeping sickness, and more cases of colds than influenza."

Inexplicably, despite these other diseases, the pandemic is only ever referred to as one of 'influenza'. The incidence of other diseases indicates that people were not all suffering from the same symptom-complex; which means that they were not all suffering from the same 'disease' that had a single causal agent; whether viral or bacterial.

Two of the other diseases that Herbert Shelton reports as coinciding with the 'flu pandemic' require further discussion, because they provide additional evidence for some of the factors that contributed to the illness that is labelled as 'flu'.

According to some contemporary reports, there were many cases of typhoid fever within the military; however, this was one of the diseases against which the soldiers had been vaccinated. It would therefore be extremely inconvenient for the medical establishment, and especially for the vaccine industry, if soldiers were reported to be suffering from a disease against which they had been vaccinated and therefore seemingly 'protected'. It would not be unreasonable to assume, therefore, that certain illnesses were re-classified as 'influenza'. The medical establishment practice of renaming conditions has been shown to be a not uncommon one; the re-classification of polio as AFP is only one example of the practice.

Sleeping sickness is more often called sleepy sickness in order to differentiate it from African sleeping sickness, or trypanosomiasis. However, sleepy sickness has another name; it is also called 'lethargic encephalitis' (LE), which is claimed to be the result of a viral or bacterial infection. It is reported that an epidemic of LE occurred during the period between 1916 and 1930. This was a singular event; LE had never previously erupted as an epidemic, nor has it ever done so since that time, although it is still claimed to exist. It is significant that this epidemic of LE is synchronous with the epidemic of 'influenza'.

Dr Peter Breggin MD refers to LE in his 2008 article entitled *Parallels between Neuroleptic Effects and Lethargic Encephalitis* and states,

> "Lethargic encephalitis (LE) was identified by von Economo in the winter of

The Black Death

The establishment definition of 'plague' refers to,

> "an acute epidemic disease of rats and other wild rodents caused by the bacterium *Yersinia pestis*, which is transmitted to humans by rat fleas."

According to the October 2017 WHO fact sheet entitled *Plague*,

> "People infected with plague usually develop acute febrile disease with other non-specific systemic symptoms after an incubation period of one to seven days, such as sudden onset of fever, chills, head and body aches, and weakness, vomiting and nausea."

The fact sheet claims that there are two main forms of plague; bubonic and pneumonic.

It is reported that, in the past there have been three major outbreaks of 'plague', although a number of minor outbreaks have also occurred.

The first of the major epidemics occurred in the 5th century BCE and is often referred to as the Plague of Athens. An article entitled *The Plague* on the website (livius.org), refers to the writings of Thucydides, a Greek historian of the period. The article contains excerpts from his work that refer to the epidemic and describe a wide range of symptoms experienced by people who had been affected; they include violent spasms, bleeding mouth and a sensation of internal burning.

The second epidemic occurred in the 6th century CE and is often referred to as the Plague of Justinian, who was the Roman Emperor of the period. An article entitled *Justinian's Plague* on the website (ancient.eu), refers to the writings of Procopius, a Byzantine historian of the period. The article states that few details are known about the symptoms, but that they are reported to have included delusions, fever and coma.

A significant feature of both epidemics is the suddenness of the onset of symptoms that were of a far more serious nature than those described by the 'plague' fact sheet.

The third major epidemic occurred in the 14th century CE and is usually referred to as the Black Death. Fortunately, several contemporary eyewitness accounts have survived and these enable a better understanding of the prevailing conditions that, in turn, offer a better explanation than that of an 'infectious' bacterial disease, which, in view of the refutation of the 'germ theory', cannot be the case.

It is generally claimed that the Black Death erupted spontaneously; that it spread rapidly around the world; and that it caused millions of deaths; the WHO fact sheet claims the total mortality to have been an estimated 50 million people.

The mainstream narrative about the epidemic states that the fleas, which are said to normally live on rats, suddenly became 'infected' with dangerous bacteria that cause a deadly form of 'plague'. These infected fleas are said to have spread their dangerous bacteria to vast populations of rats, which succumbed to the deadly disease and died in incredibly huge numbers. It is also claimed that when their rat hosts died, the 'infected' fleas moved to new, mostly human, hosts.

The transfer of infected rat fleas to human hosts is claimed to be the mechanism by which many millions of people 'caught' the disease, became ill and died in devastatingly large numbers. It is also claimed that the reason so many people died is because they had no 'immunity' to the disease.

Yet again; nothing could be further from the truth.

Although the above is only a brief overview, it nevertheless illustrates the main points in the mainstream narrative. There are, however, a number of serious flaws in this narrative; as this discussion will demonstrate.

One of the main problems is that 14th century records do not refer to vast hordes of dead rats, which, if the mainstream narrative were correct, ought to have littered the streets of all the countries that are claimed to have been affected by the Black Death. Equally problematic is the incredibly rapid speed with which the disease is reported to have spread; a circumstance that cannot be accounted for by the 'rat-flea' story. A further point that remains entirely unexplained is how the fleas were completely unaffected by the disease-causing bacteria they are alleged to have carried.

The first of these flaws has been recognised by British archaeologist, Barney Sloane, who has claimed that the 'Black Death' could not have been transmitted by rats; as reported in an August 2011 article entitled *Can We Stop Blaming Rats for the Black Death*. The article refers to archaeological work that has been conducted in London and states that,

> "...excavations in the city have turned up little evidence of a massive rat die-off coinciding with the plague."

The article also refers to an alternative theory that has been posited; this theory suggests that the conditions of the 14th century would have been more favourable to gerbils than to rats. However, there is no evidence to support this theory; the archaeological excavations failed to uncover evidence of a massive gerbil die off; but this is unsurprising as gerbils are not native to England.

There has been a slight amendment to the establishment theory about the Black Death since the 2007 edition of the dictionary that is used for the disease definitions in this book. The WHO fact sheet refers to 'small animals' rather than rodents as the vectors of transmission. However, this explanation is equally invalid, because there is no evidence from the archaeological site in London that there had been a massive die off of any type of small animal.

The rapid speed with which the disease is claimed to have been spread has been recognised as problematic by scientists and archaeologists involved in the London excavations. The lack of an obvious animal 'carrier' has led to the proposal of other hypotheses, one of which is that the 'infection' was airborne, rather than animal-borne, and that transmission occurred through the atmosphere and via human contact. But this hypothesis fails to explain the basic mechanism by which a virulent and deadly 'disease' suddenly erupted, prevailed for a number of years and then suddenly disappeared. The reported duration of the epidemic varies between 3 and 8 years.

These anomalies highlight serious flaws in the explanations about the purported mechanisms of diseases described as 'infectious'.

The previous discussion about the '1918 Flu' demonstrated that the sudden onset of 'disease' and the resulting widespread morbidity and mortality are related to multiple factors that often act synergistically; these factors do not include any so-called 'germ'.

There is an inherent tendency to view historical events in the light of prevailing theories. It is therefore unsurprising that, with the 'germ theory' firmly entrenched in medical establishment thinking, the 'Black Death' continues to be reported as an 'infectious disease' caused by bacteria, which, according to the WHO fact sheet, are,

"...usually found in small mammals and their fleas."

The archaeological evidence has not yet persuaded the medical establishment to alter their obviously incorrect theory.

It sometimes requires a scientist from an entirely different scientific discipline to view evidence from a new perspective, and thereby produce a more compelling explanation for that evidence. In this instance, a new hypothesis about the likely causes of the Black Death has been developed by a dendrochronologist, a scientist who studies tree-rings to identify different growth patterns.

The dendrochronologist in this instance is Professor Mike Baillie, whose study of tree-ring data of the 14th century led him to discover some interesting tree growth patterns, and to undertake further investigations that included the study of ice-core data, as well as contemporary 14th century accounts of the event. Professor Baillie has recorded the results of his research and the basis for his hypothesis in his book entitled *New Light on the Black Death*, in which he includes extracts from some contemporary documents. One of the extracts he quotes includes the statement that,

"There have been masses of dead fish, animals and other things along the sea shore and in many places trees covered in dust .... and all these things seem to have come from the great corruption of the air and earth."

Contemporary writers were sufficiently observant to be aware of, and write about, 'masses of dead fish, animals and other things along the sea shore', as well as 'trees covered in dust'. They would, therefore, also have been sufficiently observant to have noticed, and specifically written about, masses of dead rats or even gerbils, had there been any to observe. Such reports are conspicuous by their absence; a situation that supports the archaeological findings.

An even more significant aspect of the quoted extract is the reference to 'the great corruption of the air and earth'. In addition to these documents, Professor Baillie obtained evidence from his examination of tree rings that led to his statement that,

"The Black Death sits in a clear environmental trough visible in smoothed tree ring chronologies from around the world."

The corruption of the atmosphere certainly must have been extremely severe to have been able to generate a 'clear environmental trough'; it was sufficiently severe to have been able to cause death from respiratory problems; as Professor Baillie states,

"The most likely mechanism would be through affecting their respiration system in some catastrophic way. After all, writer after writer on the Black Death makes the point that it is the 'pulmonary' form of the disease that was the dominant killer."

It is clear therefore that 'something' must have occurred to have caused such a severe corruption of the atmosphere over a large portion of the world. One interesting and undisputed fact is that a major earthquake erupted in Europe on 25th January 1348. Professor Baillie reveals however, that this was not a singular event, but part of a series of earthquakes that occurred during the mid-14th century, both before and after the January earthquake.

Another interesting piece of the puzzle is that an unusually high level of ammonium has been discovered from the examination of ice core data. A higher than normal level of ammonium has also been discovered in ice cores that have been dated to periods in which other epidemics of 'plague' occurred. The result of his investigation of the evidence led Professor Baillie to conclude that,

> "There really is enough information about comets, earthquakes and ammonium to permit the quite serious suggestion that the Black Death was due to an impact by comet debris on 25th January 1348 as witnessed by the major earthquake on that day."

Investigations and analysis of the toxic chemicals found within comets and comet debris have produced further supportive evidence for this conclusion; Professor Baillie explains,

> "Apart from ammonium, it is now known that a range of unpleasant, toxic and evil-smelling chemicals, including hydrogen sulphide and carbon disulphide, have been detected in recent comets."

The presence of 'evil-smelling chemicals' would certainly explain the documented reports about the 'corruption of the atmosphere'; their toxicity also explains how these chemicals would have caused severe respiration problems and rapid death from asphyxiation for those people in close proximity to the dense atmospheric poisoning.

Herbert Shelton provides further documentary evidence of 14th century earthquakes and the subsequent pollution of the atmosphere, in his 1967 article entitled *Pestilence and Plagues* that states,

> "Hecker's Epidemics of the Middle Ages says of the Plague that 'mighty revolutions in the organism of the earth, of which we have credible information, had preceded it. From China to the Atlantic the foundations of the earth were shaken, throughout Asia and Europe the atmosphere was in commotion, and endangered by its baneful influence, both vegetable and animal life'."

In the same article, Herbert Shelton also quotes from Berdoe's *Origins and Growth of the Healing Art* that provides further information about the prevailing conditions,

> "In 1337, four millions of people perished by famine in China in the neighbourhood of Kiang alone. Floods, famine and earthquakes were frequent, both in Asia and Europe. In Cyprus a pestiferous wind spread a poisonous odor before an earthquake shook the island to its foundations, and many of the inhabitants fell down suddenly and expired in dreadful agonies after inhaling the noxious gases. German chemists state that a thick stinking mist advanced from the East and spread over Italy in thousands of places, and vast chasms opened

The main characteristics of tuberculosis are respiratory problems that result from the alleged bacterial 'infection' of the lungs and produce symptoms that enable the disease to be 'spread'; as described by the WHO fact sheet that states,

"When people with lung TB cough, sneeze or spit, they propel the TB germs into the air. A person needs to inhale only a few of these germs to become infected."

The cough associated with TB usually results in the production of sputum, which is one of the means by which a diagnosis can be made; as also described by the fact sheet,

"Many countries still rely on a long-used method called sputum smear microscopy to diagnose TB."

The sputum samples are examined to detect the presence of bacteria and then cultured to determine the exact type of bacteria in the sample. These tests have not always been successful in detecting the alleged 'pathogen', as related by Nicholas Ashford and Dr Miller in *Chemical Exposures*,

"During the late nineteenth century, researchers collected sputum from patients with tuberculosis but were unsuccessful in culturing any organism."

Dr Koch was one of those 'researchers' who is reported to have had difficulties with culturing the bacteria; however, an appropriate culture medium was eventually discovered that proved to be useful, as further reported in *Chemical Exposures*,

"...the tubercle bacillus was fastidious and would grow out only after many weeks on a specialized culture medium."

The nature of the 'specialised culture medium' is not specified, although the culture medium used by Dr Koch is reported to have been agar, which is derived from algae and therefore not a natural constituent of the human body. The assumption that the ability to 'grow' the bacteria demonstrates their pathogenicity is highly flawed; it fails to recognise the phenomenon of bacterial pleomorphism.

The bacterium alleged to be the cause of TB has been recognised to be pleomorphic; this recognition is indicated by a 2010 article entitled *Pleomorphic appearance in Mycobacterium tuberculosis* that states,

"This organism exhibits extreme pleomorphism in certain circumstances..."

Despite the scientific evidence, the medical establishment continues to deny the existence of pleomorphism, except in certain limited circumstances. The main consequence of this refusal to fully recognise pleomorphism is the failure to recognise that the substances chosen for use as a culture medium will directly influence the morphology of the bacteria under investigation.

It should be clear that the 'success' attributed to Dr Koch's experiments is unfounded. However, in addition to the anomalous situation in which the 'germ' is absent from the bodies of people diagnosed with TB, is the further anomaly in which there is an absence of illness in people who are claimed to have been 'infected' by the 'TB germ'. The WHO fact sheet claims that,

"People infected with TB bacteria have a 5-15% lifetime risk of falling ill with TB."

The discussion about bacteria in chapter three referred to 'asymptomatic carriers' and to 'latent infection', both of which refer to 'infection' in the absence of illness. However, asymptomatic carriers are deemed to be able to transmit the bacteria, and therefore the disease, whereas those with latent infection are claimed not to be able to do so. This is highly anomalous; yet the medical establishment fails to offer an explanation for their claim that a bacterial 'infection' can have two entirely different outcomes. It should be obvious that, if TB bacteria were 'pathogens', they should always cause disease and that, if TB were an 'infectious disease', it should always be transmissible.

These anomalies and contradictory statements invalidate the claims made about the infectiousness and transmissibility of the TB 'germ'; nevertheless, the fact sheet makes an extravagant claim, which is that,

"About one-quarter of the world's population has latent TB, which means people have been infected by TB bacteria but are not (yet) ill with the disease and cannot transmit the disease."

The use of the word 'yet' is intended to suggest that illness with TB is inevitable, but this suggestion is in complete contrast to the claim that, in 85 to 95 per cent of cases, people 'infected' with TB bacteria do not develop tuberculosis.

For those people who do become ill, it is claimed that the TB bacteria had changed their status from 'latent' to 'active'; but, yet again, no explanation is offered for the mechanism by which this change of status occurs. Nevertheless, 'active TB' is regarded as synonymous with 'disease', for which the medical establishment offers 'treatment', which inevitably takes the form of antibiotics, as indicated by the fact sheet that states,

"Active, drug-susceptible TB disease is treated with a standard 6 month course of 4 antimicrobial drugs..."

The purpose of these drugs, as with all antibiotics, is to kill as many bacteria as possible; the reasons for using multiple drugs are that they attack the bacteria in different ways and that they help to avoid 'drug resistance'. Antibiotics for most 'bacterial infections' are usually prescribed for a short period of approximately 7-10 days. A 6-month course of highly toxic drugs is therefore an extremely aggressive measure against the disease. These drastic treatment measures inevitably exacerbate the problem of antibiotic overuse; the fundamental problems with antibiotics and their dangerous consequences have been discussed.

One of the main antibiotics used in the treatment of TB is isoniazid, some of the more minor 'side effects' of which include nausea, vomiting, stomach upset, constipation, dry mouth, fever, and skin reactions. Isoniazid is also associated with more serious effects that can include dizziness, inflammation of the nerves, psychotic episodes, blood disorders, raised blood sugar levels, and peripheral nerve damage. The most serious effect is severe and sometimes fatal liver damage, which is indicative of a systemic poisoning and a clear demonstration that the drug is highly toxic. These effects, which pose a serious threat to health, are considered to be 'worthwhile' risks to take in the effort to control the spread of TB 'infection', despite the low percentage of people 'at risk' of developing the disease.

The drive to 'eradicate TB' includes the recommendation that treatment should be extended to people diagnosed with 'latent TB'. Based on the WHO claim that this group represents about one quarter of the world population, currently estimated to be approximately 7 and a half billion, the manufacture of antibiotics for almost 2 billion people would provide the pharmaceutical industry with a phenomenal boost to their profits. More importantly, however, it would create a major tragedy of inestimable proportions for the people who receive these toxic treatments.

The discussion in the previous chapter showed that the overuse of antibiotics is claimed to be the cause of a loss of drug effectiveness, because bacteria have developed 'drug resistance'. The problem of 'resistance' is also associated with the drugs used as treatments for TB and has led to the creation of an allegedly new 'form' of the disease, called multidrug-resistant TB (MDR-TB), which is described by the fact sheet as,

> "...a form of TB caused by bacteria that do not respond to isoniazid and rifampicin, the 2 most powerful, first-line anti-TB drugs."

The 'side effects' of rifampicin are reported to include nausea, vomiting, headache, drowsiness and dizziness.

As discussed, the real effect in the body from antibiotics is an increased level of activity in the effort to eliminate substances the body recognises as toxic. The increased activity occurs mainly in the endocrine glands but, if the antibiotics are ingested, effects can also be produced in the digestive system, as demonstrated by the 'side effects' of both isoniazid and rifampicin that include nausea and vomiting.

This increased level of activity within the body may succeed in achieving a reduction in intensity or even the cessation of symptoms; a result that is often mistakenly credited as being due to the action of the drugs. However, the continuation of any antibiotic drug 'treatment' over a long period of time will gradually exhaust the endocrine glands, damage the digestive system and create a number of serious health problems, which are very likely those that are interpreted as 'drug resistance'. The rigid adherence of the medical establishment to the 'germ theory' means that the only solution available for people diagnosed with MDR-TB, is a further cocktail of even more toxic drugs that will only exacerbate their existing health problems.

Antibiotics are the main, but not the only, method by which the medical establishment attempts to control TB; they have also developed a vaccine, known as the Bacillus Calmette-Guérin (BCG) vaccine, which is claimed to provide protection against TB. Many, but not all, countries include this vaccine in their standard infant immunisation schedule. One notable exception is the US; a situation that is extremely surprising considering the fervour with which vaccines are normally promoted in that country; the CDC explains on their website that the reason for this policy is because,

> "BCG does not always protect people from getting TB."

The poor level of efficacy of the BCG vaccine is also recognised by the UK NHS on a page entitled *Who should have the BCG (TB) vaccine?* that states,

> "There's no evidence the BCG vaccine works for people over the age of 35."

It has however, been proven that the BCG vaccine is ineffective for all age groups. This was demonstrated by a large field trial to test the vaccine conducted between the years 1968 and 1971 by the WHO in India; a country in which TB was, and still is, regarded as endemic. In one area comprising 309 villages, about 364,000 people were vaccinated against TB, whilst people in another area of roughly the same size remained unvaccinated. The results however, caused the vaccination 'experts' considerable concern, because more cases of TB occurred in the vaccinated area than in the unvaccinated area. The incidence of TB in 'developing' countries is discussed further in chapter eight.

Despite the recognition that the BCG vaccine is not always effective, it remains widely used on the basis that TB is regarded as a major worldwide problem, as indicated by the WHO fact sheet that states,

"Tuberculosis (TB) is one of the top 10 causes of death worldwide."

The fact sheet also provides statistics of worldwide morbidity and mortality from TB,

"In 2017, 10 million people fell ill with TB and 1.6 million died from the disease."

Although TB is considered to be a serious disease, the vast majority of people survive, because, according to the fact sheet,

"TB is a treatable and curable disease."

This claim cannot be substantiated; the treatments that are used do not cure TB.

The reason that treatments fail to cure TB is due to a lack of understanding about the functions of the human body and its self-regulating mechanisms. Previous discussions have referred to the liver as one of the main organs that eliminate toxins; the kidneys also perform a similar function. If either of these organs becomes congested and unable to work efficiently, toxins can build up in the body and the blood; a situation that would be extremely dangerous and potentially fatal. Fortunately, the body's self-regulating mechanisms include other organs that provide assistance in the processes of elimination; this assistance is called 'vicarious elimination' as explained by Dr Henry Bieler in *Food is Your Best Medicine*,

"Toxic blood must discharge its toxins or the person dies, so nature uses substitutes. The lungs and skin help the kidneys and liver respectively."

He expands on the function performed by the lungs and states,

"From the irritation caused by the elimination of poison through this vicarious channel, we get bronchitis, pneumonia or tuberculosis, as is determined by the particular chemistry of the poison being eliminated."

The 'poisons' that require elimination can include substances consumed within the diet; for example, chemical food additives that are used in the manufacture of processed food products consumed by a large proportion of the world population. As the discussions in chapter six will demonstrate, most food additives are toxic. The greater the intake of these toxic substances, the greater will be the body's efforts to eliminate them. Dr John Tilden explains the connection between tuberculosis and all of the factors that may constitute what he refers to as a 'faulty diet',

"I recognize the disease as coming from perverted nutrition brought on from crowded digestion..."

TB is not necessarily the result of 'crowded digestion' due to over-eating; it can be due to the accumulation of substances, such as food additives, that the body regards as 'toxins' but may not be easily able to eliminate. This may be one reason that certain so-called 'developed' countries are reporting increases in the incidence of TB. However, TB also occurs in conjunction with poor living conditions, poverty and malnutrition; this is an indication that 'crowded digestion' is not the only factor that contributes to the disease.

Unfortunately, the preoccupation with the 'germ theory' means that, instead of addressing the real problems that cause tuberculosis, the medical establishment concentrates on the use of toxic drugs and vaccines, both of which exacerbate illness.

A matter of increasing concern with respect to TB is that, according to one of the key 'facts' in the WHO fact sheet, a strong association exists between TB and HIV, which is the subject of the next discussion. The fact sheet claims that,

"HIV and TB form a lethal combination, each speeding the other's progress."

As the following discussion will demonstrate; yet again, nothing could be further from the truth.

HIV/AIDS

The establishment definition of AIDS refers to,

"a syndrome first identified in Los Angeles in 1981; a description of the causative virus – the human immunodeficiency virus (HIV) – was available in 1983."

The definition also states that,

"AIDS is essentially a sexually transmitted disease..."

The mainstream media reports during the early 1980s about a new disease called AIDS (Acquired Immune Deficiency Syndrome) were highly dramatic. They gave the impression that the world was on the verge of a new and deadly 'plague' that threatened to decimate the global population, and that anyone who contracted this disease was doomed to suffer horribly and die. This new 'plague' seemed to have the potential to rival the Black Death and the 1918 Flu and be destined to become one of the most deadly scourges humankind had ever faced.

The media reports made a number of claims, which were: that 'infection' with the virus could not be cured; that progression to 'full-blown AIDS' would occur for an exceptionally high proportion of people infected with the virus; that there was no cure for AIDS; and that once a patient had progressed to AIDS they would become seriously ill and succumb very quickly to an early death.

These predictions of impending doom were not fulfilled. The fact that this 'deadly plague' failed to materialise prompted a revision to the medical establishment definition of AIDS, which states,

"Until recently, AIDS has been considered to be universally fatal, although the type and length of illness preceding death varies considerably."

Although less deadly than first predicted, 'infection' with the 'virus' called

HIV is still regarded as a serious health problem, as indicated by the July 2018 WHO fact sheet entitled *HIV/AIDS* that claims,

"HIV continues to be a major global public health issue, having claimed more than 35 million lives so far."

Yet again, nothing could be further from the truth.

The claims made by the medical establishment about the virus called HIV and the syndrome called AIDS are erroneous; not only because they are based on erroneous notions about 'germs' and 'infectious diseases', but also because they are based on fallacies; as this discussion will demonstrate.

The discovery of 'AIDS' began in 1981 when a number of men in the San Francisco area were diagnosed with two relatively rare diseases, Kaposi's sarcoma (KS), a type of cancer, and Pneumocystis carinii pneumonia (PCP). Although rare, KS and PCP were not new diseases, nor were either of them claimed to be caused by a virus; nevertheless, they became the first 'AIDS-defining' diseases.

The early research into these cases, which represented an abnormally high incidence of two otherwise rare diseases, indicated that they occurred almost exclusively within two 'risk groups', one of which comprised gay men with an extremely active sex-life. Their sexual activities, the details of which are unnecessary for this discussion, were often accompanied by the use of 'poppers' and antibiotics.

'Poppers' are a type of drug that is inhaled; they are made from alkyl nitrites, which are a group of chemical compounds that can be metabolised within the body to form nitrosamines, most types of which are recognised carcinogens. An article entitled *AIDS and Poppers* on the Virus Myth website (virusmyth.com) explains the connection,

"Kaposi's is a blood vessel tumor, and nitrites act on blood vessels."

The article states that the majority of the early cases of KS were gay men who regularly inhaled 'poppers' and had done so for a significant period of time. The previous discussion about TB referred to the lungs as a 'vicarious channel' for the elimination of toxins; the inhalation of toxic nitrites will cause damage to the respiratory system, including the lungs. The long-term toxic irritation of the lungs will produce a variety of symptoms that could also lead to a diagnosis of either pneumonia or PCP.

Although antibiotics were often taken as treatments for existing 'infections', they were also taken prophylactically over a significant period of time. The adverse health effects from the long-term use of antibiotics have been discussed.

The other main 'risk group' comprised drug addicts, most of whom were intravenous drug users; the adverse health effects from the injection of toxic substances into the bloodstream have been discussed in connection with vaccinations; the injection of toxic 'illegal' drugs will also produce serious adverse health effects.

It should be noted that many drugs now categorised as 'illegal' were originally manufactured by the pharmaceutical industry for use as 'medicines'. As previously discussed, many pharmaceutical medicines have been synthesised from the 'active ingredients' of plants; for example, retrovirus particle called 'HIV' is part of normal human body functioning and harmless; and, as such, it cannot cause any disease let alone the allegedly deadly disease known as 'AIDS'.

Amongst the many thousands of scientists who refute the 'HIV causes AIDS' dogma is Dr Kary Mullis PhD, the recipient of the 1993 Nobel Prize for his invention of the polymerase chain reaction (PCR). Dr Mullis' refutation of the orthodox theory was the result of his research during 1988 whilst he was engaged by the NIH to set up analyses for HIV testing. During the course of this work, he needed to cite the original research papers that contained the 'proof' that HIV caused AIDS. However, he was unable to find any such papers; as he has explained in his interviews with the London Sunday Times and with Spin Magazine. On the home page of the Virus Myth website is the statement made by Dr Mullis in 1993 that,

> "If there is evidence that HIV causes AIDS, there should be scientific documents which either singly or collectively demonstrate that fact, at least with a high probability. There is no such document."

In the Foreword he wrote for *Inventing the AIDS Virus*, Dr Mullis states that, according to his research,

> "No one had ever proved that HIV causes AIDS."

Nothing has occurred in the intervening decades to alter this fact; there is still no scientific proof that a virus called 'HIV' causes the illness referred to as 'AIDS'.

The scientific papers produced by Gallo and his colleagues that were finally published in May 1984 in the journal *Science*, have been found to only demonstrate a weak correlation of the 'virus' with AIDS patients. Whatever these papers contained; they clearly did not provide the unequivocal 'proof' that HIV causes AIDS; otherwise Dr Mullis would have acknowledged their existence.

In *Inventing the AIDS Virus*, which was published in 1996 and therefore more than a decade after the press conference announcement, Dr Duesberg referred to the continuing absence of any evidence that AIDS was, or could be, a deadly infectious disease,

> "Despite projections of wild spread, HIV infection has remained virtually constant throughout the industrialized world ever since it could be tested in 1985, whether in the United States or Europe; the estimated incubation period between infection and disease has been revised from ten months to more than ten years; and the predicted heterosexual explosion has failed to materialize."

A substantial increase in the incubation period is not the only revision to the orthodox AIDS theory; there have been many, including a substantial expansion of the conditions that are regarded as 'AIDS-defining'. According to the CDC, the conditions also include cervical cancer, tuberculosis and a number of 'bacterial infections'. PCP has also undergone a slight change in its definition; it is now claimed to be caused by a yeast-like fungus called *Pneumonia joveci*.

It is clear that many of the 'AIDS-defining' conditions listed by the CDC are not viral diseases; which contradicts the claim that a virus called 'HIV' is the cause of 'AIDS'; the original theory has also undergone a revision. The explanation offered for the classification of non-viral diseases as 'AIDS-defining' is that 'HIV' weakens the immune system and that this weakness permits an 'opportunistic infection' (OI) caused by another 'germ'. According to a page entitled *Opportunistic Infections* on the CDC website,

"Opportunistic infections (OIs) are infections that occur more frequently and are more severe in individuals with weakened immune systems, including people with HIV."

This point is of particular significance for TB, as indicated by the WHO TB fact sheet that states,

"TB is a leading killer of HIV-positive people."

The WHO *HIV/AIDS* fact sheet claims that TB is,

"...responsible for more than 1 of 3 HIV-associated deaths."

These claims are highly anomalous; the majority of TB cases are claimed to occur in India, whereas the majority of HIV/AIDS cases are claimed to occur in Sub-Saharan Africa.

The orthodox theory of HIV/AIDS would seem to have been revised, as indicated by the CDC web page about opportunistic infections that states,

"When a person living with HIV gets certain infections (called opportunistic infections, or OIs), he or she will get a diagnosis of AIDS, the most serious stage of HIV infection."

It is clear therefore that HIV is no longer regarded as the sole cause of AIDS.

A diagnosis of 'AIDS' does however require confirmation of the presence of 'HIV', which is alleged to be detectable by a test, as indicated by the fact sheet that claims,

"HIV infection is often diagnosed through rapid diagnostic tests (RDTs), which detect the presence or absence of HIV antibodies."

The discussion in the first section of this chapter explained that the presence of antibodies is interpreted in two completely different and mutually exclusive ways. One interpretation is that antibodies indicate 'protection'; the other is that they indicate 'infection'. The presence of 'HIV' antibodies as detected by HIV tests is interpreted to indicate 'infection'.

The discussion about syphilis explained that the Wassermann test was unable to identify antibodies specific to the 'germ' alleged to cause syphilis; the same is true of the HIV test. Antibodies are proteins, certain types of which are deemed to be specific to each 'pathogen'. Some of the proteins deemed specific to 'HIV' include those labelled p24 and p41. However, in his article entitled *HIV Tests Are Not HIV Tests*, Professor Henry Bauer PhD states that,

"Far from being specific to HIV or AIDS patients...p24 and p41 are not even specific to illness."

He makes the point quite clearly that HIV tests are not able to specifically identify 'HIV antibodies'; furthermore, he comments that,

"Tests for human immunodeficiency virus (HIV) do not detect HIV..."

In another similarity with the Wassermann tests, 'HIV tests' can also produce 'positive' results due to a number of other conditions; these are

Chapter Five

Animals & Diseases: More Medical Myths

"Those who can make you believe absurdities can make you commit atrocities"

Voltaire

The establishment definition of the term 'zoonosis' refers to,

"an infectious disease of animals that can be transmitted to humans."

The significance of zoonoses is that, according to the WHO web page entitled *Managing public health risks at the human-animal-environment interface,*

"Zoonoses comprise a large percentage of all newly identified infectious diseases as well as existing infectious diseases."

In an effort to address the problems due to zoonoses, the WHO has partnered with the OIE (World Organisation for Animal Health) and the FAO (Food and Agriculture Organization) to form a collaboration, which, in April 2010, produced a document that reports the 'vision' of this partnership to be,

"A world capable of preventing, detecting, containing, eliminating and responding to animal and public health risks attributable to zoonoses and animal diseases with an impact on food security through multi-sectoral cooperation and strong partnerships."

The causal agents of zoonoses are claimed to be mainly bacteria, viruses and parasites, although of different species from those claimed to cause 'infectious diseases' exclusive to humans; fungi are not considered to be significant causes of zoonoses. However, as demonstrated by the discussions in the two previous chapters, bacteria, viruses, parasites and fungi are not pathogens, they do not cause human 'infectious diseases'; this means therefore, that they cannot be the causal agents of 'infectious diseases of animals', whether zoonotic or non-zoonotic.

On the basis of the erroneous belief that 'germs' do cause zoonoses, the measures employed to address them are very similar to, if not the same as, those employed to address human infectious diseases. These measures, which were shown to be harmful to humans, will inevitably be harmful to animals. In addition, there are serious ramifications for human health, as a result of the harmful measures employed directly in the treatment of animals destined for the human food chain.

Although the FAO-OIE-WHO document does not discuss the recommendations in detail, it claims to ensure 'food security' through the prevention of 'food-borne pathogens'. It is clear that this is intended to refer to the use of chemical compounds that are inevitably toxic by nature because their intended purpose is to kill the pathogens. However, food is not made 'safe' by the addition of toxic, antimicrobial chemicals; as will be discussed in greater detail in chapter six.

It is therefore extremely important to expose the serious and far-reaching consequences of the rigid adherence to the 'germ theory' with respect to animal 'infectious diseases' and the measures employed to combat them.

It is claimed that zoonoses are transmitted in a number of ways, one of which is through direct contact, an animal bite, for example; another method of transmission is said to occur through the air via 'infected droplets'. It is also claimed that the 'pathogens' can be transmitted via a 'vector' or 'carrier'. A vector is usually an insect that carries and is therefore able to transmit a 'parasite'; the most common vectors are mosquitoes, many species of which are claimed to carry various parasites said to be the causes of a number of diseases. The best-known example of a 'vector-borne' disease is malaria, which is discussed in more detail in chapter eight.

Like human 'infectious diseases', each zoonosis is said to be caused by a distinct species of pathogen; however, unlike human pathogens, animal pathogens are said to have the ability to infect more than one host; as indicated by a 2002 article entitled *Identifying Reservoirs of Infection: A Conceptual and Practical Challenge*, which states that,

"...77% of livestock pathogens and 91% of domestic carnivore pathogens infect multiple hosts."

The term 'reservoir host' refers to an animal that is claimed to harbour and be the natural 'home' of a particular pathogen. Some sources claim that 'reservoir hosts' do not succumb to the disease the pathogen is alleged to cause, even though they are said to transmit infection; these animal 'reservoir hosts' are therefore comparable to human 'asymptomatic carriers'. It is clear however, that, like the theories about human 'infectious diseases', the theories about animal diseases contain many anomalies and contradictions; they are also similarly erroneous.

An erroneous theory of disease causation inevitably generates a flawed theory of disease eradication; a situation that clearly applies to all so-called 'infectious diseases'. However, according to a 2008 article entitled *Zoonoses – With Friends Like This, Who Needs Enemies*, only infectious diseases that exclusively affect humans are capable of eradication on the basis that it is only possible to achieve adequate vaccination coverage of the human population. The existence of multiple animal 'reservoir hosts' is said to make the eradication of zoonoses much more difficult, as the article states,

"...zoonotic infections (those that have an animal reservoir) can probably never be eradicated..."

This idea clearly applies to all animal diseases, but is disproven by claims about the 'eradication' in 2011 of rinderpest, which, although non-zoonotic, is a disease that was reported to have affected many different animals, both domestic and wild; it is the only animal disease claimed to have been eradicated.

Although the eradication of smallpox and rinderpest are widely acclaimed as representing major 'successes' in the fight against disease, many hundreds of 'infectious diseases' are said to exist; the eradication of only two of them cannot be regarded as a cause for celebration. On the contrary, these alleged 'successes' must be contrasted with the many reports that suggest the number of infectious diseases is increasing, rather than decreasing; a point that is demonstrated by a 2014 article entitled *Emerging zoonotic viral diseases*, which states that,

"The last 30 years have seen a rise in emerging infectious diseases in humans and of these over 70% are zoonotic."

The failure to successfully control the increasing incidence of 'infectious diseases' is largely due to the incessant search for 'pathogens' to the exclusion of almost any other factors that may cause or contribute to illness. The result of this focus on 'germs' has been the alleged 'discovery' of vast numbers of so-called 'pathogens', as described in a 2001 article entitled *Risk factors for human disease emergence* that states,

"A comprehensive literature review identifies 1415 species of infectious organism known to be pathogenic to humans..."

The article adds the comment that,

"The majority of pathogen species causing disease in humans are zoonotic..."

As mentioned above, the measures employed to combat animal 'diseases' include the use of pharmaceutical drugs and vaccines, both of which adversely affect the health of animals, including those reared for human consumption. The vaccination schedule for some animals is similar to that for humans, as indicated by the page entitled *Badgers* on the website of The Wildlife Trusts, which states that,

"Cattle are already vaccinated for up to 16 diseases..."

The implications for human health from the consumption of meat from vaccinated animals are, however, poorly understood; as acknowledged by a 2003 article entitled *Human Illness Associated with Use of Veterinary Vaccines*, which states that,

"The extent to which veterinary vaccines pose a health hazard to humans is unclear."

Unfortunately, the article regards the main human health hazard to be from exposure to the 'germs' contained within animal vaccines, rather than their toxic ingredients. Although the human body is able to process and excrete ingested toxins through the digestive system, the level of toxins consumed from the meat of vaccinated animals is poorly recognised and rarely studied due to the belief that vaccines are 'safe'.

The pharmaceuticals used in animal husbandry include antibiotics and growth hormones; although the latter are obviously not used to combat 'germs'. However, the safety of the drugs administered to animals reared for human consumption has not been conclusively established. A 2010 article entitled *Risk Assessment of Growth Hormones and Antimicrobial Residues in Meat* acknowledges that the use of these drugs has,

> "...provoked much debate on the safety of livestock products for human consumption."

In order to determine the correct 'dose', the risk assessment procedures for veterinary drugs require the setting of ADIs (Acceptable Daily Intakes) and MRLs (Maximum Residue Limits). The problem with these 'safety' procedures is that they only assess the 'dose' of each substance individually. The claim that there is a 'safe' dose of each individual substance ignores the fact that many different veterinary drugs and vaccines are used; it also fails to recognise the synergies that may occur from interactions between drugs and vaccines used in various combinations.

Animals reared for food are subjected to a wide variety of 'treatments' that are claimed to assure their 'safety' for human consumption, but, in reality, these treatments achieve the complete opposite; they cause a great deal of harm. The article refers to the use of growth hormones and states that,

> "The hormonal substances used for growth promotion in cattle are the naturally occurring steroids..."

The substances produced by the pharmaceutical industry, whether preparations derived from natural hormones or completely synthesised substances, are not equivalent to hormones that are produced naturally by an animal. Although referred to as 'naturally-occurring', that does not mean these hormonal substances are 'safe' or that specific hormones only produce a single specific effect within the animal's body. The article claims that these 'hormonal substances' have a negligible impact on human health, but a 'negligible impact' is not equivalent to 'no impact'. The use of hormonal substances in animals reared for food is discussed in a 2015 article entitled *Hormone Use in Food Animal Production: Assessing Potential Dietary Exposures and Breast Cancer Risk*, which refers to hormone drugs approved by the FDA for use in food animals and states that,

> "There is concern that these drugs or their biologically active metabolites may accumulate in edible tissues..."

Although these drugs are claimed to have a 'negligible impact' on human health, this has not, however, been fully established; as the article also states,

> "To date, the potential for human exposure to residues of these compounds in animal products, as well as the risks that may result from this exposure, is poorly understood."

The previously cited 2010 *Risk Assessment* article refers to the use of 'antimicrobials'; however, although bacteria are not the only zoonotic pathogen, antibiotics are one of the most commonly used drugs in animal husbandry. Significantly, their use for animals is on a scale that positively dwarfs their use in the treatment of human 'infections'.

Furthermore, the use of antibiotics in animal husbandry is not limited to the treatment of 'infections'; as indicated by a 2012 article entitled *A Review of Antibiotic Use in Food Animals: Perspective, Policy and Potential*, which states that they are used,

"...to treat clinical disease, to prevent and control common disease events, and to enhance animal growth."

The article acknowledges the widespread use of antibiotics for animals reared for human consumption; however, although it may be assumed that this means there have been extensive studies performed to evaluate and determine the safety and efficacy of these drugs, the article indicates otherwise,

"Furthermore, in existing studies, neither the risks to human health nor the benefits to animal production have been well studied."

Nevertheless, despite the lack of adequate studies, animal husbandry involves a wide variety of antibiotics, as the article also indicates,

"Twelve classes of antimicrobials – arsenicals, polypeptides, glycolipids, tetracyclines, elfamycins, macrolides, lincosamides, polyethers, betalactams, quinoxalines, streptogramins, and sulfonamides – may be used at different times in the life cycle of poultry, cattle and swine."

This huge volume of antibiotic drugs, all of which are toxic by nature, as well as by intention, is virtually ignored in the reports issued by the medical establishment on matters of animal health. Instead, it is invariably claimed that the main problem posed by the overuse of antibiotics is 'drug-resistance'; a claim that is also made on the WHO web page about 'managing public health threats', which states that,

"Antimicrobial resistance in human pathogens is another major public health threat which is partly impacted by use of antibiotics in animal husbandry and agriculture."

The real problem caused by the overuse of antibiotics has been discussed. The harm caused by antibiotics is not restricted to humans; it should be clear that they are equally harmful for animals.

The real causes of human diseases include environmental pollutants, many of which are discussed in chapter six; it should be clear however, that these environmental pollutants will also have a serious and detrimental impact on animal health.

Nevertheless, the 2014 article about emerging diseases suggests that the emergence of new zoonoses is the result of increased contact between humans, livestock and wildlife. Expanding populations of humans and livestock have certainly resulted in substantial changes to land use; these changes include the development of huge monoculture farms, whether for rearing livestock or for growing crops. This expansion of agriculture has had an impact of varying severity on wildlife populations and brought many wild animals into close contact with farmers and their livestock. The result of this closer contact is that wild animals have been increasingly exposed to the many chemical compounds used in most agricultural practices; but these chemicals are ignored in theories about animal diseases, including those claimed to affect wild animals.

Instead, it is claimed in the article that 'new zoonoses' have emerged because increasingly close contact between humans, livestock and wildlife has permitted the spread of 'pathogens' that seek new hosts to 'infect', and facilitated their transmission between animal and human 'hosts'. This claim is unfounded; as the previous discussions have demonstrated, there is no evidence to support the assumption that so-called 'pathogens' cause disease, transmit infection or even travel between 'hosts'.

The importance of exposing the fallacy of the 'germ theory' cannot be over-stated. The continuing belief in this fatally flawed theory continues to pose increasingly serious hazards to the health of all people and all animals. The potential for a substantially heightened danger for wild animals in particular is indicated by a very worrying prediction in the article that states,

> "The WHO and most infectious disease experts agree that the source of the next human pandemic is likely to be zoonotic and wildlife is emerging as the primary source."

Chapter three demonstrated that the dire predictions about HIV/AIDS failed to materialise; that the 1918 Flu was not caused by a bacterium or a virus; and that rats and their fleas have been exonerated as the causes of the Black Death. Although some reports claim that 'HIV' evolved from a monkey virus that 'escaped' from Africa, this is an erroneous claim, as demonstrated by the discussion in the previous chapter.

The failure of the medical establishment to acknowledge the fallacy of the 'germ theory' raises serious questions about the prediction of a new pandemic, the consequences of which have the potential to be disastrous, not only for the wild animals deemed to be the 'source', but for all animals, including humans. These consequences will not be due to any 'pathogen', but to the measures that are likely to be introduced to address or even prevent the predicted 'problem'. These measures will almost inevitably involve the introduction of toxic chemicals intended to kill the 'germs' alleged to cause the 'disease'. It is possible that the solutions may even involve the deliberate destruction of wild animals; a practice that has been implemented in certain situations.

The first step in any genuine effort to 'eradicate disease' must be the eradication of the belief in the 'germ theory'; until this is accomplished, all animals, and humans, will continue to face real threats to health from the inappropriate and dangerous measures introduced by the medical establishment and the animal health community to address so-called 'infectious diseases'.

The following sections discuss a few animal diseases to demonstrate the serious consequences of the erroneous assumptions about their causation, and of the inappropriate measures used to control them. The final section discusses vivisection to demonstrate the reason that animal experiments should cease.

As the discussions refer to animal diseases, the definitions used in this chapter are those provided on the OIE website.

Rabies

The OIE definition of rabies refers to,

"...a viral disease that affects the central nervous system of warm-blooded animals, including humans."

Rabies is classified as a zoonotic disease; as the definition explains,

"Rabies is one of the most deadly zoonoses. Each year, it kills nearly 60,000 people worldwide, mostly children in developing countries."

It is claimed that rabies is present throughout all continents of the world, with the sole exception of Antarctica; however, the May 2019 WHO fact sheet entitled *Rabies* states that,

"Rabies is one of the neglected tropical diseases that predominantly affects poor and vulnerable populations who live in remote rural locations."

It is claimed that rabies is transmitted via an animal bite and that the overwhelming majority of cases occur due to a dog bite, which exposes a person to 'infected' saliva. But this explanation does not seem to be consistent with the above statements that rabies mainly affects 'poor and vulnerable' children in 'developing' countries.

The OIE information sheet makes the interesting comment that the rabies virus is not immediately active after the bite but instead,

"...will generally remain at the entry site for a period of time before travelling along the nerves to the brain."

The WHO fact sheet refers to some of the symptoms associated with the disease. Although the initial symptoms are mild and include pain at the wound site and a fever, far more serious symptoms are said to develop later; the fact sheet explains,

"As the virus spreads to the central nervous system, progressive and fatal inflammation of the brain and spinal cord develops."

The discussion in chapter three demonstrated that the particles called 'viruses' are inert outside of a host cell; which means they cannot 'travel' around the body.

According to the fact sheet there are two forms of the disease, one of which is called 'furious' rabies because it is said to produce 'hyperactive behaviour'. This behaviour may include hydrophobia, which is an alternative term for 'fear of water' and also the original name for rabies. The other form of the disease is called paralytic rabies, because it is claimed that the virus can induce paralysis.

The bite from an 'infected' animal is said to require prompt 'treatment', which rather unusually involves the administration of the rabies vaccine. The vast majority of vaccines are administered prior to 'exposure' as a preventive measure; but the rabies vaccine can be administered both before and after 'exposure'. However, this vaccine is not routinely administered prophylactically, except for people who are considered to be 'at risk' from rabies; which mainly refers to people who work with animals, vets and animal researchers, for example.

The rabies vaccine is used for both animals and people, although the first rabies vaccine was produced only for human use. Its development is credited to the French chemist, Louis Pasteur, and it is considered to be another of his 'achievements'. As discussed in chapter three, Dr Geison's research revealed that the 'science' of Louis Pasteur was not as meticulous as it is believed to have been; his formulation of the rabies vaccine was equally flawed.

Prior to Louis Pasteur's study of rabies, the 'treatments' used for patients diagnosed with this disease were of a most bizarre nature; they owed their existence more to superstition than to 'science'. In her book *The Poisoned Needle*, Eleanor McBean presents an extract from an essay entitled *Rabies Past/Present in Scientific Review*, written by physician and surgeon Dr Millicent Morden MD. The essay includes reference to examples of the pre-Pasteur treatment of rabies,

> "In 1806 a Mr. Kraus was awarded $1000, by the then rulers of New York temtory for his scientific discovery which had kept rabies out of New York for over twenty years. His formula is a matter of record and consisted of the groundup jaw bone of an ass or dog, a piece of colt's tongue and the green rust off a penny of George the First reign."

These treatments would be more appropriately described using the previously cited words of William White that refer to 'a combination of absurdity with nastiness'. In view of the absurdity of these treatments, it is not surprising that the medical establishment regards it as 'fortunate' that Louis Pasteur decided to turn his attention to a study of rabies. But it has not been fortunate; the experiments he conducted were similar to the previously described gruesome monkey experiments, which were claimed to demonstrate the transmission of polio. In his book entitled *The Blood Poisoners*, Lionel Dole describes the nature of Louis Pasteur's experiments,

> "The manner in which Pasteur made rabbits "rabid" by boring holes in their skulls and inserting filth into their brains was not science but simply brutal quackery."

Nevertheless, it was on the basis of this brutal quackery that Louis Pasteur developed his rabies vaccine. The medical establishment references to this vaccine indicate that it was a resounding success; contemporary reports however, tell a very different story and one that again speaks of Louis Pasteur's fundamental errors and even of fraud.

In her essay, Dr Morden refers to two medical practitioners who were contemporaries of Louis Pasteur but outspoken in their criticism of his work; as the following extracts demonstrate. The first extract refers to Dr Bruette's exposure of the fraud of the rabies vaccine,

> "Dr William A. Bruette, former assistant chief of the Bureau of Animal Industry in Washington, was also a contemporary of Pasteur and gave many proofs of Pasteur's incorrect findings. Dr Bruette has proved, as a matter of fact, that rabies vaccine is not only a fraud, but harmful. He scorns the use of rabies vaccine and states that 'inoculation spreads disease.' He goes as far as to call the sale of rabies vaccine an out and out racket."

Although 21st century vaccines are different from those used in the 19th century, they are all based on the same flawed theory. The second extract

for the pharmaceutical industry but extremely detrimental to the health of both humans and animals.

Bovine TB

The OIE definition of bovine TB refers to,

> "...a chronic disease of animals..."

It is claimed that bovine TB is caused by *Mycobacterium bovis*, which suggests it is a disease that is exclusive to cattle, but the OIE definition indicates otherwise,

> "This disease can affect practically all mammals, causing a general state of illness, coughing and eventual death."

Although human TB is said to be caused by a different bacterium, *M. tuberculosis*, it is nevertheless claimed that bovine TB is zoonotic, which indicates that humans are also able to contract this disease. One of the main routes by which transmission to humans is said to occur is through drinking raw milk from allegedly 'infected' cows; a situation that is claimed to occur more frequently in 'developing' countries, in which the pasteurisation of milk is not a common practice. It is claimed that the pasteurisation process makes milk 'safe' because it kills bacteria; but this is yet another disastrous legacy of the 'germ theory' and the flawed science of Louis Pasteur.

Cattle are a major source of food for people throughout most parts of the world; a serious and potentially fatal cattle disease is, therefore, understandably a matter of grave concern for cattle farmers; but they are misled about the real causes of animal diseases, including bovine TB.

One of the major concerns of the medical establishment is the lack of success in the attempts to control and eradicate this disease; this concern is expressed by a 2007 article entitled *Tuberculosis: a reemerging disease at the interface of domestic animals and wildlife*, which states that,

> "As many countries attempt to eradicate M. bovis from domestic livestock, efforts are impeded by spill back from wildlife reservoirs."

The term 'reservoir host' was briefly discussed in the opening section of this chapter, in which it was explained that it is used to refer to animals that naturally 'harbour' a pathogen. Although the discussion in chapter three referred to bacteria as part of the human microbiota, it should be obvious that the human body is not their only natural habitat; bacteria are acknowledged to inhabit the bodies of most, if not all animals, and certainly all mammals. It is therefore unsurprising that *M. bovis* should have been 'found' in the bodies of a number of different mammals.

The OIE information sheet about bovine TB claims that *M. bovis* has been 'isolated' from a very wide range of animals, including, but not limited to: sheep, goats, equines, buffaloes, bison, camels, pigs, deer, antelopes, dogs, cats, foxes, mink, badgers, ferrets, rats, primates, elephants, otters, hares, moles, raccoons, lions, tigers, leopards and lynx. The 'isolation' of a bacterium from any of these animals does not prove they are 'reservoir hosts' or that they can facilitate the transmission of infective agents. Significantly, however, it is not claimed that these animals are necessarily 'diseased'. Nevertheless, the 2007 article claims that,

"It will not be possible to eradicate *M. bovis* from livestock until transmission between wildlife and domestic animals is halted."

The priority given to livestock can have disastrous consequences for wild animal species claimed to be 'reservoirs' of allegedly 'pathogenic' bacteria. This is a situation that has arisen in the UK, where the badger is claimed to be the main 'reservoir' of *M. bovis* and held responsible for the existence of TB in cattle herds; but this claim is unproven, as the article acknowledges,

"...although most of the evidence is indirect, it is hypothesized that badgers are a source of infection for cattle and responsible for the increase in tuberculosis among domestic cattle herds."

The basis for this 'hypothesis' is that *M. bovis* has been 'isolated' from badgers; a correlation that has been assumed to mean causation; but this is a mistaken assumption. Furthermore, it should be obvious that, even if bacteria were transmitted between animals, they could just as easily be transmitted in the opposite direction; in other words, from cattle to badgers. The main problem is the erroneous belief that bacteria are pathogens that can transmit disease between animals.

There are claimed to be two possible solutions to the bovine TB problem in the UK; badgers should be either vaccinated or culled, even though neither of these measures would be able to genuinely reduce the incidence of TB in cattle. Nevertheless, a badger vaccination programme was implemented, but halted in 2015 due to a shortage of the BCG vaccine. However, the result of this programme was described in a December 2015 article entitled *UK Badger vaccination projects threatened by global BCG shortage* on the website of the Farmers Guardian that states,

"The latest report from the vaccination area concludes there has been no meaningful change in TB levels."

The shortage of the BCG vaccine inevitably resulted in the implementation of badger culling programmes, as indicated by a December 2015 article entitled *Badger cull kills more than 10,000 animals in three months*; the title is self-explanatory.

In April 2018, the UK Government remained committed to the eradication of bovine TB and, according to their website,

"The Government is committed to eradicating bovine TB and sees badger culling as central to this."

The Wildlife Trusts disagrees with this view and instead claims that badgers have been made the scapegoats for bovine TB; on their web page entitled *Bovine Tuberculosis (bTB)*, is the statement that,

"The scientific evidence demonstrates that culling is likely to be ineffective in fighting the disease..."

Unfortunately, they recommend that cattle should receive the TB vaccine, together with all of the other vaccines administered to them.

However, as demonstrated by the discussions in chapter two, no vaccine is effective; this inevitably applies to animal vaccines as well as those used for humans. The OIE acknowledges that animal vaccines are of questionable efficacy and states that the animal TB vaccine,

"...is not widely used as a preventive measure in animals: the efficacy of existing vaccines is variable and it interferes with testing to eliminate the disease."

The comment that the vaccine 'interferes with testing' is significant because both the test and the vaccines are made using bacterial antigenic material. Nevertheless, a reaction to a vaccine is claimed to indicate 'immunity', whereas a reaction to the test is claimed to indicate 'infection'. This is an inconsistency that is entirely inexplicable within the context of the 'germ theory', and raises serious questions about the 'science' used to determine the health, or otherwise, of animals reared for human consumption.

Advice about TB testing for cattle farmers in the UK is provided by TB Hub, which is described as a joint industry initiative and is supported by DEFRA (Department for Environment, Food and Rural Affairs), a UK Government department. Under the heading *How does it work?* on the page entitled *Tuberculin skin testing*, is the statement that,

> "...the skin test in cattle relies on measuring the immune response of the animal to injections of tuberculin. Tuberculin is a complex mix of proteins extracted from cultures of *M. bovis* grown in the laboratory and killed by heat."

The page provides further details about the testing procedure and how the results are interpreted to determine which cattle have been 'infected' with bovine TB,

> "The skin test is comparative as the animal's immune response to injections of both bovine and avian (bird) tuberculin is measured and compared. By simultaneously injecting two types of tuberculin into the deep layers of the skin of the neck, the test can better distinguish between animals infected with *M. bovis* and animals previously exposed to or infected with other types of mycobacteria found in the environment which do not cause bovine TB."

It is claimed that an animal 'infected' with the TB bacterium will produce a reaction at the site of the bovine tuberculin injection, as indicated by the statement that,

> "Cattle that are infected with *M. bovis* tend to show a greater reaction to bovine tuberculin than avian tuberculin."

The animals deemed to be infected undergo further procedures to confirm the extent of their reaction; however, the general process is described succinctly by the OIE that states,

> "The standard control measure applied to TB is test and slaughter."

Fortunately, this measure is not applied to humans who test positive on a TB skin test.

The slaughter of animals regarded as 'infected' due to a significant reaction to the test is a relatively new phenomenon. In her book *Animal Research Takes Lives*, Bette Overell cites an article entitled *Animal health without vaccines* written by F Newman Turner, editor of the magazine *The Farmer*. An extract from the article states,

> "Tuberculosis has also been treated effectively, and animals rejected by the Ministry of Agriculture as tubercular have, after natural treatment, subsequently been readmitted to the herd by the same Ministry, as sound, and have continued to pass the tuberculin test regularly. I have even taken the discharges of cows badly suffering from mastitis and applied the virulent bacteria to the udders of healthy cows, with no ill-effect whatever to the healthy cow."

It is clear therefore, that a reaction to the test is not indicative of 'infection' with a 'dangerous' disease that is always fatal.

The establishment obsession with the idea that microorganisms are the major causes of disease, has effectively denied attention to any other theories about the causes of health problems in cattle, or to alternative treatments that are not based on pharmaceutical products.

One of the factors rarely considered as relevant to animal TB is the effect of the huge quantities of drugs and chemicals that are used in modern day farming practices and agriculture generally; antibiotics in particular, are used in immense quantities, as discussed in the opening section of this chapter.

Furthermore, if the 'germ theory' were correct, the routine use of antibiotics in cattle farming would ensure that all animals were continually protected and none of them would succumb to any 'bacterial infection'. However, far from being protective of their health, antibiotics are harmful to animals as well as humans; this is discussed by Heinrich Kremer in his book entitled *The Silent Revolution in Cancer and AIDS Medicine,*

> "The treatment of animals or man with antibacterial drugs can have harmful effects on mitochondrial function, especially in tissues that have a high proliferation rate."

Antibiotic drugs are harmful for animals; but they are not the only toxic substances to which livestock can be exposed. Although many environmental pollutants and contaminants can adversely affect the health of animals, certain farming practices are contributory factors to animal illness, even though they are implemented in the name of animal welfare, as the next discussion will demonstrate.

BSE (Bovine Spongiform Encephalopathy)

The OIE definition states that,

> "BSE is a progressive, fatal disease of the nervous system of cattle."

Bovine Spongiform Encephalopathy is usually referred to by the abbreviation BSE, but it is also known as 'mad cow disease', which is said to be an apt description of an animal with this condition.

BSE is not the only form of Spongiform Encephalopathy; there are other types that affect other animals, and these are referred to under the general heading of Transmissible Spongiform Encephalopathy, or TSE, the causes of which are explained by the OIE information sheet about BSE that states,

> "BSE, like other TSEs, is characterized by the presence of an abnormal infectious protein called a prion in nervous tissue."

The information sheet also states that,

> "The subsequent spongy degeneration of the brain results in severe and fatal neurological signs and symptoms."

Although referred to as 'transmissible', one form of TSE only affects sheep and goats; this disease is more commonly known as 'scrapie', which is also an apt description of the behaviour of animals with this condition, as they often scrape their fleeces against stationary objects. However, scrapie is also described as a fatal degenerative disease that involves more than fleece scraping.

The characteristic of the 'infectious protein' that is claimed by the OIE to be 'abnormal' and the cause of TSEs is that it is 'misfolded'. It is also claimed that the misfolding of a protein induces other proteins to become 'misfolded' and it is this process that is claimed to activate the 'disease'. However, despite these claims, the establishment information about TSEs shows that the actual mechanism of action, by which the proteins become misfolded and produce disease, is poorly understood.

It is not only animals that are claimed to be affected by diseases claimed to be caused by misfolded proteins known as prions. A well-known example is CJD (Creutzfeldt-Jakob disease), which is claimed to be the human version of BSE and is described as an incurable fatal neurodegenerative condition. One form of CJD, referred to as vCJD (variant Creutzfeldt-Jakob disease), is claimed to be acquired from animals, which has led to the classification of BSE as a zoonotic disease.

Interestingly there are a number of human neurodegenerative diseases that are also claimed to be associated with misfolded proteins; these diseases include Alzheimer's disease, Parkinson's disease and ALS (Amyotrophic Lateral Sclerosis).

Although BSE is claimed to be caused by an 'infectious agent', the source of this 'pathogen' is unknown; as the OIE information sheet indicates,

> "Scientists believe that the spread of this disease in cattle is caused by feeding rendered material from infected cattle or sheep back to other cattle."

The statement that 'scientists believe' demonstrates that this idea has not been conclusively proven; although the OIE claims that,

> "...dairy herds are fed concentrate rations that contain meat-and-bone meal..."

The idea that a feed product containing 'meat and bone meal' is the cause of BSE was refuted by Mark Purdey, who, in his book entitled *Animal Pharm*, relates his research and experiences as a farmer during the first BSE outbreak in the 1980s in England,

> "As a working livestock farmer and TSE researcher with firsthand experience of BSE erupting in cattle that had been purchased into my organic farm, I was struck by the fact that no cases of BSE had ever emerged in cows that had been born and raised on fully converted organic farms, despite those cattle having been permitted access to the feed that contained the incriminated meat and bone meal (MBM) ingredient - as part of their 20% conventional feeding stuff allowance decreed in the organic standards at that time."

Although Mark Purdey demonstrated that MBM was not the cause of BSE, it should be noted that cattle are herbivores, not omnivores. The natural diet of cattle is grass, which is rich in cellulose; the digestive systems of cattle consist of four stomach compartments that are able to process grass and obtain the required nutrients from it. The use of meat and bone meal as a 'feed' for cattle was clearly inappropriate.

The types of MBM alleged to have been the cause of BSE have since been banned, but cases of BSE continue to be reported, which demonstrates that MBM could not have been the sole or even the main cause of this disease.

Through his research, Mark Purdey discovered that a much more likely cause of BSE was phosmet, a chemical insecticide used as a cattle 'wash' in the control of warble fly, an insect pest common to cattle. This insecticide, which contains a chemical compound made from phosphorus, is applied directly onto the animals, usually over their necks; the neurotoxic properties of phosphorus-based chemicals is discussed in chapter six.

However, cattle in the UK suffered a significantly greater degree of neurological effects than cattle in the many other countries that also used this insecticide; the reason for this is explained by Mark Purdey, who states that,

> "In 1982 measures were passed that enforced twice annual application of a uniquely concentrated dose (20 mg/kg bodyweight) of a systemic acting organo-dithio-phosphate insecticide for the control of warbles on UK cattle. Amongst a myriad of toxicological effects, the systemic types of dithio-phosphate can chelate copper and open up the blood brain barrier; thereby disturbing the overall crucial balance of metals in the brain."

The application of the insecticide 'wash' onto the necks of cattle enabled the toxic chemicals to penetrate into their heads and seep into their brains. The effects were clearly extremely unpleasant for the cattle, as demonstrated by the behaviour that earned the label 'mad cow disease'. The subsequent 'outbreak' of BSE in the UK due to the high concentration of phosmet, resulted in the slaughter of millions of cattle. The incidence of BSE in countries that did not use such a high concentration of phosmet was lower than in the UK, as Mark Purdey explains,

> "The few other European countries who instigated warble fly campaigns (e.g.; France, Switzerland, Ireland, etc) used lower doses of insecticide, and, not surprisingly, developed proportionately fewer cases of BSE as a result."

Unsurprisingly, Mark Purdey's research was not widely publicised, but of greater concern are the actions taken by the authorities to discredit his research work; as he also explains in his book,

> "Despite publication in a variety of scientific journals, the authorities and their key advisors are ignoring these findings and are doing their utmost to marginalise those of us who are trying to pursue this line of research."

Unfortunately, the medical establishment invariably fails to associate toxic chemicals with the outbreak of any 'disease', except in rare circumstances, in which the link is too obvious to be ignored.

One of the likely reasons for the failure of the UK establishment to associate toxic insecticides with BSE is because of the potential consequences. The revelation that it was the high concentration of a recommended toxic insecticide wash that had caused the problem and resulted in the unnecessary slaughter of millions of cattle, would have had serious ramifications, as Mark Purdey explains,

> "If, however, it was officially verified that phosmet was a cause of BSE, compensation claims worth billions would be filed, not only against the British government but also the insecticide manufacturers."

The connection between BSE, a disease of the nervous system, and neurotoxic chemicals offers a far more compelling explanation than that of an allegedly infectious 'misfolded' protein. Although misfolded proteins have been found in connection with neurodegenerative diseases, this fact does not 'prove' that they are the cause. It is far more likely that proteins become misfolded as the result of exposures to toxins, especially neurotoxins.

Unfortunately, whilst the 'germ theory' remains firmly embedded within the medical establishment doctrines about disease, the real role of proteins within the body will not be properly studied and will remain poorly understood.

Another cattle disease that is similar to both bovine TB and BSE and also based on the 'germ theory' dogma, is foot and mouth disease (FMD), which is regarded as viral, highly infectious and sometimes fatal. The previously cited article about reservoirs of infection states that,

> "...Foot-and-mouth disease virus (FMDV) is maintained in unvaccinated cattle populations..."

However, in his book entitled *Universal Immunization, Medical Miracle or Masterful Mirage*, Dr Raymond Obomsawin PhD recounts details from his interview with Dr Archie Kalokerinos MD, who, at the time, was Chief Medical Officer at the Aboriginal Health Clinic in Australia,

> "He related an experience wherein cattle feeding on grass grown on re-mineralized soil, were grazing literally nose to nose--at the fence line--with another herd infected with hoof and mouth disease. Without the benefit of any specific protective measures including vaccines, the uninfected herd manifested total immunity."

Although not a 'laboratory experiment', this observation from the real world provides empirical evidence that FMD cannot be infectious. Furthermore, the fact that the uninfected herd were also unvaccinated supports the assertion that vaccination does not confer immunity to disease; it can, and clearly does, confer ill-health.

Myxomatosis

The OIE definition of myxomatosis refers to,

> "...an important disease of rabbits caused by a poxvirus called the *Myxoma virus* (MV)."

Myxomatosis is not classified as zoonotic; which means that it is not a disease of concern for human health. It is, however, an extremely unusual animal disease for two reasons, the first of which is that it is claimed to only affect rabbits and hares. The second reason is that its degree of virulence is claimed to be dependent upon the species of rabbit 'infected' by the virus; as the OIE states,

> "MV causes a very mild disease in its original host native to South America, but in some species of rabbits and hares, especially the European rabbits it causes a severe disease with high mortality."

It would seem that the *Myxoma virus* is highly specialised; yet, inexplicably, it is claimed that MV has a completely 'normal' mode of transmission. According to the OIE,

> "Spread mainly occurs through fleas and mosquitoes which ingest the virus while biting infected animals and then transmit the disease to other susceptible animals."

This statement suggests that transmission of the 'virus' is synonymous with transmission of 'disease', but this cannot be the case if animals must be 'susceptible' before succumbing to the disease. Unfortunately, the OIE does not explain what constitutes 'susceptibility'; but their statement indicates that the onset of disease requires other factors in addition to an alleged 'infection' with a virus.

It is claimed that a number of biting insects are carriers of the *Myxoma virus*, but that mosquitoes are the principal vectors. The two species of mosquito associated with the transmission of myxomatosis are *Aedes* and *Anopheles*, both of which are also associated with the transmission of many human diseases. *Aedes* is said to transmit diseases such as yellow fever; *Anopheles* is said to be the main vector of malaria. Yet these mosquitoes are claimed to only transmit the *Myxoma virus* to rabbits, despite the fact that they bite humans and a variety of animals.

It is reported that the *Myxoma virus* was introduced into the rabbit population of Australia in the mid-20th century as a method of 'biological control'. However, the refutation of the 'germ theory' means that myxomatosis cannot be caused by a virus; which raises questions about the Australian experience and about the real causes of this disease. These questions prompted the authors of this book to conduct a more in-depth investigation of the subject, the results of which are revealed in this discussion.

The establishment reports state that myxomatosis was first recognised in 1896 as the result of the work of Giuseppe Sanarelli, an Italian microbiologist, who is said to have imported a colony of domestic European rabbits from Brazil to Uruguay for research purposes; but all the rabbits died suddenly from a virulent 'infectious disease' that acquired the label 'myxomatosis'. Although claimed to be a viral disease, the actual 'virus' could not have been observed prior to the invention of the electron microscope in the 1930s.

The rabbit problem in Australia is reported to have begun after the inadvertent release of some European rabbits in 1859. The result of this incident was that rabbit numbers rapidly increased to such an unprecedented level that they very quickly became a significant pest, especially for Australian farmers and landowners. The prior 'discovery' that myxomatosis was a fatal disease of European rabbits led to the notion that the introduction of the 'disease' into the rabbit population might be an effective method of reducing their numbers.

The first attempt to introduce myxomatosis was conducted in 1926; it is reported to have been unsuccessful. Further attempts were made during the 1930s, but, although curtailed by the advent of WWII, they are also reported to have been unsuccessful. However, efforts to reduce the rabbit population by infecting them with myxomatosis were resumed in 1949 under a research programme headed by the Australian Commonwealth Scientific and Industrial Research Organisation (CSIRO).

Professor Frank Fenner, an Australian virologist, is regarded as the key scientist in myxomatosis research. He joined the CSIRO team in early 1951 after the first 'outbreak' of the disease; as he recounts in his book entitled *Nature, Nurture and Chance*,

"Several field trials failed, but in the Christmas-New Year period of 1950-51 the disease escaped from one of the four trial sites in the Murray valley and spread all over the Murray-Darling basin, killing millions of rabbits."

This episode is claimed to have virtually eradicated the rabbit population and is regarded as the first 'successful' introduction of myxomatosis; Professor Fenner states that it was this 'outbreak' that inspired him to study the virology of the disease. He adds an extremely interesting comment that,

"The climatic conditions at the time of the outbreak of myxomatosis in the Murray-Darling Basin had been such that there was also an outbreak of encephalitis in that region..."

The simultaneous outbreak of human encephalitis and myxomatosis generated an understandable level of concern that these diseases were somehow related; it was even suggested that the *Myxoma virus* may have been responsible for the cases of encephalitis. These fears were alleviated after it had been reported that Professor Fenner and two of his colleagues had remained unaffected after being inoculated with the virus. Although neither disease is caused by a virus, their concurrence is nevertheless significant; it will be shown that they have causes in common.

The CSIRO myxomatosis programme involved a number of field studies conducted by Professor Fenner and his team of researchers over the course of a number of years. This research is documented in a series of seven papers entitled *Studies in the Epidemiology of Infectious Myxomatosis of Rabbits*. The second paper of this series refers to the CSIRO experiments conducted during 1950, and contains some interesting information about the procedures used to 'infect' the rabbits with the 'virus'; the paper states,

"All rabbits caught were inoculated subcutaneously with 1.0ml of a glycerolated liver-lung extract from a diseased rabbit..."

This means therefore, that rabbits were inoculated with 'extract of diseased rabbit'.

This second paper also refers to the role of mosquitoes in the spread of 'infection', and states that the relevant species are *Anopheles* and *Culex*, but not *Aedes*. On the basis of the idea that they are the vectors of MV, the researchers collected mosquitoes in order to extract the 'virus'. The process of obtaining 'virus' from mosquitoes is quite revealing; it is described in the paper under the sub-heading *Recovery of virus from mosquitoes*, which states that the researchers caught 168 female *Culex* mosquitoes that were,

"...ground up in a mortar and pestle and taken up in 5ml normal saline. Of this suspension 0.5ml was inoculated subcutaneously into the right flank of a laboratory rabbit."

In other words, in these experiments, rabbits were inoculated with 'extract of ground mosquito', rather than 'extract of diseased rabbit'.

The third paper in the series documents another process of obtaining 'virus' from mosquitoes; the process is described in this paper under the sub-heading *Recovery of virus from mosquitoes* which states that the mosquitoes were,

"...quickly cooled and then ground with alundum in a cold mortar and pestle in batches of about fifty insects, taken up in 2ml of saline containing 10% horse serum, 2,000 units of penicillin per ml and 20,000 units of streptomycin per ml. After centrifugation a proportion of the supernatant material was ampouled and stored in a dry ice cabinet. The rest was inoculated intradermally in the rabbit..."

The results of the entire series of field studies display a varying degree of 'virulence' of the disease introduced into the rabbit population. The researchers also report that they had observed many rabbits with scar tissue, which they interpreted to indicate that some rabbits had been able to recover from the disease; this means that the disease cannot be inherently fatal.

The most significant aspect of these field study experiments is that 'outbreaks' of the disease, other than the one that occurred in 1950/51, were all reported to have been at a greatly reduced 'virulence'; none of them had the same devastating effect on rabbits. The researchers claim that the reason for the reduced mortality was that the rabbits had developed 'resistance' and had become 'immune' to the disease. But this claim is unfounded, because myxomatosis 'outbreaks' continue to occur in Australia.

The Australian field studies were not the only efforts to introduce myxomatosis to control rabbits. An article entitled *Failure of Myxomatosis on Skokholm Island*, published in 1955 in the journal *Nature*, details three separate attempts to introduce myxomatosis and states,

"In each attempt the marked rabbits (inoculated with the virus) appeared to have died within the usual period of less than fourteen days; but there was little or no spread to uninoculated rabbits."

The failure of any spread of disease on these occasions is claimed to be because the virus can only 'infect' a healthy animal through a scratch, cut or insect bite. However, this raises a fundamental question about the allegedly successful spread of the disease in 1950/51 that is claimed to have killed millions of rabbits.

It is clear that the many efforts to introduce an 'infectious disease' of rabbits produced inconsistent results that are inexplicable from the perspective of the 'germ theory'. These variable results are, however, more than adequately explicable from the perspective of toxic chemicals.

The phenomenal surge in rabbit numbers after 1859 had encouraged Australian farmers and landholders to utilise a variety of poisons in their attempts to exterminate the rabbit 'pest'; they had therefore used poisons for almost a century before the myxomatosis programme began. An article entitled *The Balance of Nature Upset in Australia* on the Rewilding Australia website, refers to some of the poisons used for 'pest control' during the 19th century; they include strychnine, arsenic, cyanide and phosphorous baits. Lead arsenate is also documented to have been used as a pesticide, but, although not used to poison rabbits, this highly toxic substance is a persistent environmental contaminant.

The impression from most establishment reports about myxomatosis is that the rabbit 'problem' was not successfully tackled until the field studies of the 1950s. However, this would seem to be a false impression, as the

19th century about shepherds who suffered from the effects of the toxic sheep dip; but shepherds were not the only people exposed to the hazards of arsenic. In addition to shepherds and woolsorters, anyone who handled wool from sheep dipped in arsenic-based compounds would have been affected by this highly toxic substance. The rise of 'bacteriology' in the latter part of the 19th century ensured, however, that little, if any, attention was paid to a toxicological investigation of the disease.

Although a significant contributory factor, arsenic is not the only toxic substance that can account for the poisoning of grazing animals. As will be further discussed in the next chapter, certain industries have released a wide variety of toxic substances into the environment; many of these contaminants are eminently capable of causing serious harm to the health of animals, including livestock.

One industry in particular that has been associated with anthrax 'outbreaks' is tanning; the WHO document states that,

"...the main enzootic livestock areas traditionally lay 'downstream' from tanneries and the implication has been that watercourses have carried contaminated tannery effluent..."

The use of the word 'contaminated' is intended to indicate the existence of anthrax spores from 'infected' animals; the alleged 'contamination' of hides with anthrax spores is the reason that tannery workers were vaccinated against the disease. The real contamination would be from the use of toxic chemicals by the tanning industry; these toxins included arsenic, as the *Arsenic and Old Wool* article states,

"White arsenic was further used as a preservative of hides, skins and furs."

Mining is another industry associated with the release of toxic substances that contaminate the environment. Tin mining, for example, is particularly hazardous because tin ore is usually found in association with sulphur and arsenic. Interestingly, tin mining was one of the industries in 19th century Yorkshire, the English county in which woolsorters' disease arose.

It is clear therefore, that exposure to highly toxic substances, especially arsenic used in sheep dip, provides a more compelling explanation for woolsorters' disease in humans; and that the contamination of grazing land with toxic industrial effluent and toxins released from mining provides a more compelling explanation for the animal disease known as anthrax.

Vivisection

The Oxford Concise Medical Dictionary defines vivisection as,

"a surgical operation on a living animal for experimental purposes."

According to the NAVS (National Anti-Vivisection Society) web page entitled *Areas of Science that Use Animals*,

"The scope of animal use in science today includes virtually every field of investigation."

The scientific fields that utilise vivisection are categorised by NAVS under the general headings of research, testing and education.

Investigations classified as 'testing' include experiments that are conducted to ascertain the 'safety' of chemical ingredients used in manufactured products, many of which are everyday items used by millions of people around the world. The widespread use of chemicals is discussed in the next chapter; however, testing their safety clearly relies on the idea that it is only the dose that makes a substance toxic; an idea that has been shown to be false.

The category of 'education' is self-explanatory and mainly involves the dissection of animals in classrooms.

The category of 'research' covers a range of fields of study, as described by the NAVS web page entitled *Animals Used in Research*,

> "Animals are used in basic and biomedical research, behavioural research, military research, agricultural research, veterinary research and drug development and testing."

The types of research pertinent to this discussion mainly involve biomedical research, drug development and drug testing, all of which can be combined under the general heading of 'medical research'. However, some of the arguments used, whether to support or object to animal experimentation in medical research, are applicable to other types of research and to safety testing.

The main justification for vivisection within medical research is that it is indispensable; it is claimed to be vital for the study of disease and for the development of effective drugs and vaccines to combat them. This argument is expressed by Dr Hans Selye MD in his book entitled *The Stress of Life*,

> "Yet, few antivivisectionists would consider it more ethical to stop medical research altogether and thereby expose countless human beings to unnecessary suffering."

This argument is encapsulated within the phrase 'it's the bunny or your baby'.

However, nothing could be further from the truth. Although well-intentioned, this is a fallacious argument; no bunny has to be sacrificed in order to save babies.

Dr Selye, whose important study of the role of 'stress' is discussed in chapter ten, was trained under the orthodox medical system that retains the belief in a number of flawed theories about diseases and their causes. In addition to the idea that 'germs' are the causes of 'infectious diseases', is the idea that 'genes' are relevant causal factors for a number of 'non-infectious diseases'. But both of these ideas are erroneous; neither 'germs' nor 'genes' are the causes of disease.

A wide variety of animal experiments have been conducted to investigate both 'infectious' and 'non-infectious' diseases over the course of many decades. Yet, there have been no significant reductions in morbidity or mortality; in fact, the statistics demonstrate that these problems are worsening. As indicated in the discussion about iatrogenesis, drugs and vaccines do not offer solutions to health problems; instead they exacerbate ill-health.

Anti-vivisection organisations such as NAVS correctly argue for medical research without animal experiments; it is clearly unethical to inflict suffering on animals during experiments designed to relieve human

189

suffering. However, concentrating solely on the cruelty of animal experiments misses the core issue, which is that the theories on which most medical research is based are fundamentally flawed.

Unfortunately, there is an almost complete lack of recognition of the full extent of the flaws within the teachings of the medical establishment system; and also, to a certain extent, within those of the 'alternative health community'. Although many physicians have recognised some of the problems, very few have recognised them all.

However, although they support the idea that medical research is necessary, anti-vivisection organisations raise a number of valid objections to the use of animals for research purposes. The main objections are that animals suffer during the experiments and that they have an unnatural life in the laboratory environment.

Another objection is that animals used in research are almost always killed at some stage of the experiment; to counter this objection, medical researchers often use the euphemism 'sacrificed' so that animal deaths are represented as a scientific necessity rather than cruelty. The reality is that, whether it occurs before, during or afterwards, the overwhelming majority of animals are killed so that researchers can examine them and determine the effects of the 'experiment' they have conducted.

It is probably true to say that medical researchers perform their work under the impression that they are conducting 'medical science' and that it has a genuine and meaningful purpose; as expressed by Dr Selye, who refers to,

"...one of the noblest and most human aspirations of man, the desire to understand himself."

Although the dissection of dead animals can permit an understanding of the physiological effects of 'disease', it cannot generate an understanding of disease processes within a living body, whether human or animal. Furthermore, no experimentation conducted on living, or dead, animals can take 'man' to a better understanding of 'himself'.

Despite the belief that laboratory experimentation is an essential aspect of research, there are many limitations to the experiments conducted in the name of 'medical science', one of which is, as discussed in chapter three, the failure to appreciate that the procedures used in the preparation of specimens for microscopy can directly affect the specimens, whether they are tissues, cells, disease molecules, bacteria or the particles called 'viruses'.

This limitation was acknowledged by Dr Harold Hillman, who stressed that many of the 'structures' observed under microscopes are, in reality, artefacts that have been produced by the preparation procedures such as fixation, for example. An October 2011 article entitled *Optimization of fixation methods for observation of bacterial cell morphology and surface ultrastructures by atomic force microscopy* discusses fixatives and fixation methods and makes the extremely interesting point that,

"The effects of different fixation methods on bacterial morphology were rarely studied, and thus research gaps still remained in this issue."

It should be noted that fixatives often contain toxic chemicals such as formaldehyde, which will inevitably affect living specimens, especially pleomorphic bacteria.

Although this may not seem to be relevant to a discussion about vivisection, it serves to highlight the existence of research gaps and limitations within medical research. The NAVS web page entitled *Animals Used in Research* recognises the existence of certain limitations and states,

> "Limitations of animal models are well documented, and reproducibility issues with animal experiments remain an ongoing issue for the scientific community."

Reproducibility is considered to be an essential feature of scientific experimentation.

The existence of 'research gaps' is also recognised on the NAVS web page, which states that,

> "...a large gap remains between experimental findings with animal experiments in the lab and the intended application of this information in the clinic."

This 'gap' is immensely significant; it completely undermines the fundamental belief that animal experiments are vital to the furtherance of an understanding of human disease, and to the development of suitable 'treatments'.

The existence of these limitations and research gaps demonstrates that conclusions drawn from laboratory-based animal experiments are, at best, highly questionable, even from the perspective of the medical establishment. In reality, these gaps and limitations expose a poor level of understanding about 'disease'; a situation that has been acknowledged by published 'peer-reviewed' study articles, as demonstrated by the numerous articles quoted throughout this book. Many of the cited articles admit that certain key aspects of the science relevant to the subject of the study are 'unknown', 'poorly understood' or even 'rarely studied'.

Nevertheless, the 'information' about diseases published by health organisations such as the WHO, CDC, NIH, NHS etc, implies that the 'medical establishment' is fully cognisant of all aspects of all diseases, including their causes and the appropriate methods with which to manage and treat them; the discussions in this book demonstrate otherwise.

Another limitation to the use of animal experimentation in the study of disease is that only certain effects can be observed and objectively measured; as explained by the authors of *Chemical Exposures* who state that,

> "...rats, mice and other animals are unable to tell researchers if they have headaches, feel depressed or anxious or are nauseated."

These, and many other relevant but non-measurable effects, remain unknown to researchers.

The existence of non-measurable effects is significant for animal experiments conducted to determine the 'safe dose' of chemicals. Animals cannot express many of the effects they experience; therefore, researchers cannot know all of the effects produced by any chemical.

As the discussions in this book demonstrate, the environment in the real world is very different from that of the sanitised laboratory, in which the conditions are strictly controlled and animals are usually only exposed to single substances. In the real world, people as well as all other living organisms, are exposed to multiple substances simultaneously and in varying combinations, none of which has been thoroughly tested to determine the full range of their effects.

Although most remain untested, a small percentage of substances have been tested more thoroughly than others, and an even smaller percentage of substances have been tested in a few limited combinations. The results from these tests have, however, demonstrated the existence of synergistic interactions between some substances. One substance in particular that reacts synergistically with certain others is mercury; as explained in the book entitled *Uninformed Consent*, in which the authors quote the words of Dr Boyd Haley PhD who states,

> "...the determination of safe body levels of mercury by using animal data, where the animals have not been exposed to other heavy metals, is no longer justified. Mercury is far more toxic to individuals when other heavy metals are present."

Medical research experiments that are intended to ascertain the safety of a drug suffer from the same limitations as those for chemical testing. The ingredients of pharmaceuticals are chemicals, which interact with a variety of other chemicals and many of these interactions may be synergistic. The lack of testing of all possible combinations of all substances means however, that there is a major knowledge gap, with respect to all of the effects that may be produced by interactions between the many hundreds of thousands of chemicals that now pervade the environment.

Animal research experiments are also conducted to determine the efficacy of a drug and its ability to alleviate a particular disease; but the limited knowledge about the effects of the drugs on animals means that their effects on humans remain unknown, until the drug reaches the human testing phase of clinical trials. It is claimed to be unethical to experiment on humans; however, clinical trials cannot be regarded in any other way than as human experiments. In the case of drug trials, people should not be poisoned in the mistaken belief that they are testing 'medicine'.

Another justification for the use of animals is that they are 'lesser beings', and therefore different from, humans; yet vivisection is justified on the basis that animals are sufficiently similar to humans to qualify as 'suitable models' for the study of human disease. This is a blatant contradiction.

One of the most significant objections to animal experimentation is that animals are not suitable models for studying human diseases. Each type of animal is physiologically different from all other types of animal, as well as being different from humans; this point is explained by Dr Russell Blaylock in *Health and Nutrition Secrets*,

> "Many animals have physiological and biochemical systems quite different than humans..."

These physiological and biochemical differences mean that conclusions drawn from animal experiments cannot be reliably extrapolated as if they are meaningful for human disease studies. Nevertheless, although the results are recognised to be 'approximations', medical research studies contain conclusions that are claimed to assist the development of knowledge about diseases and the appropriate measures with which to 'treat' them.

The problem with vivisection in medical research is described by Dr Moneim Fadali MD, who is firm in his condemnation of the practice, and is quoted by Hans Ruesch in his book entitled *1000 Doctors (And Many More) Against Vivisection*, to have stated that,

"Animal model systems differ from their human counterparts. Conclusions drawn from animal research, when applied to human beings, are likely to delay progress, mislead, and do harm to the patient. Vivisection, or animal experimentation, should be abolished."

There is a fundamental error in the assumption that an artificial environment created in a laboratory can simulate the environment within a living organism; this point is also discussed by Hans Ruesch who also quotes bacteriologist Rene Dubos from his own book entitled *Mirage of Health*,

"The experimenter does not produce nature in the laboratory."

It may be argued that researchers recognise this fact; nevertheless, they believe that the laboratory provides a sufficient approximation of nature and that this enables them to produce adequate experimental 'evidence' that can be reliably extrapolated and applied to the human body. These are erroneous beliefs and assumptions.

Nevertheless, in the belief that it is more ethical to experiment on animals than on humans, researchers use many types of animals; rats and mice are the most common, although others include cats, dogs, frogs, rabbits, hamsters, guinea pigs and monkeys. It may be assumed that the preference for rats and mice is because they are suitable approximations for the study of human disease; but this is not the case. Rodents are used because they are cheap, small and easy to handle, as Dr Selye admits,

"Rodents also have the advantage of being small, inexpensive and singularly resistant to infections which make them especially suitable for large-scale experimentation."

Dr Selye is by no means the only physician to acknowledge that rodents are used for these reasons; but that does not make them suitable or even approximate animal models. Furthermore, the reference to rodents being 'singularly resistant to infections' indicates that from the perspective of 'germs', the rodent response differs from the human response; a situation that raises serious questions about the relevance of any rodent-based research for the study of human 'infectious diseases'.

In fact, rodents possess a number of significant physiological differences from humans, one of which is that humans have a gall bladder, but rats do not; this means that rats digest fats differently from humans. Another difference is that rodents manufacture Vitamin B in their appendix, whereas humans do so in their liver. Another difference is that humans do not manufacture vitamin C but rodents do. A further difference is that rats and mice cannot vomit, which means that they process and expel toxins from their bodies differently from humans. These differences clearly raise even more questions about the suitability of any member of the rodent

Chapter Six

Poisoning The Planet: Science Gone Awry

"We live on a planet that has become the repository for the products, emissions and wastes of modern industry."

Joe Thornton

The discussions in the previous chapters have demonstrated that the medical establishment theories about 'disease' are flawed; that medicines do not cure disease; that vaccines do not prevent disease; and that 'germs' do not cause disease.

It is argued throughout this book that 'science' is a process and that existing scientific theories ought to remain open to reassessment and revision, and even be abandoned should new evidence be discovered that refutes their assertions; the evidence is primary. A theory is essentially an attempt to explain a phenomenon; however, each phenomenon may contain a number of different aspects, some or all of which may have been proven to be 'true' and shown to be supported by empirical evidence. Whilst the theory, as an interpretation of the phenomenon, may remain open to debate, aspects that have been demonstrated to be 'true' cannot remain subject to debate.

It is widely believed that scientific theories are highly technical and beyond the ability of the general public to understand; this attitude generates the recommendation that the public must therefore 'trust the experts'. However, statements made by certain 'experts' can often be at variance with statements made by equally qualified 'experts'; these contrasting and often conflicting views are a source of much confusion for people.

Unfortunately, it is increasingly common for experts who challenge the establishment view about a particular topic to be vilified by the mainstream media, and even denied the opportunity to present and explain their theories. This means that the general public will not be fully informed about all aspects of the topic in question, but instead will receive biased information, especially if the mainstream media is their only source of 'information'. This does not necessarily mean, however, that the establishment view is correct. The reasons for such obfuscation as well as the problems with the mainstream media and the vested interests behind the promulgation of biased 'scientific evidence' are discussed in more detail in chapter nine.

The 'environment' has become one of the dominant issues of public concern; unfortunately, discussions about this topic focus almost exclusively on 'climate change' rather than environmental pollution. Although it is widely acknowledged that the environment of the planet at the beginning of the 21st century is polluted, there are many differing opinions about the extent of the pollution, the nature of the pollutants and the appropriate measures required to address the problem.

One aspect that is inadequately covered in discussions about the environment is the extent to which pollution contributes to ill-health. Although the medical establishment theories about disease are flawed, they do recognise, albeit to a limited extent, that certain 'toxins' are environmental pollutants that contribute to certain diseases; this means that they recognise the existence of an association between the health of the environment and the health of the people who inhabit that environment. This association is recognised by the WHO and discussed in their March 2016 report entitled *Preventing disease through healthy environments*, which will be referred to in this and later chapters as the *Healthy environments* report, the purpose of which is to recommend appropriate policy measures for implementation by all WHO Member States. These policies are claimed to be able to improve public health through interventions in the environment, as outlined in the *Preface* that states,

> "Our evolving knowledge about environment-health interactions will support the design of more effective public health strategies and interventions, directed at eliminating health hazards and reducing corresponding risks to health."

Unfortunately, knowledge about 'environment-health interactions' will never be complete whilst the medical establishment remains committed to flawed theories about the nature of the hazards that threaten public health and the appropriate measures with which to address them. No policies, strategies or interventions that are based on flawed theories can effectively improve public health.

The *Healthy environments* report claims that environmental hazards significantly impact both morbidity and mortality; the severity of the problem is stated to be that approximately 23% of all deaths and approximately 22% of the global burden of disease are attributable to 'the environment'. It is stated that, in the context of the report, the definition of 'environmental risks to health' refers to,

> "all the physical, chemical and biological factors external to a person..."

The category of 'biological factors' refers to bacteria, viruses, fungi and parasites; in other words, 'germs', all of which are claimed to be more easily 'transmitted' as the result of certain environmental conditions. However, 'germs' are not the causes of disease, which means that they are not environmental risks to health.

A far more significant factor that contributes to and exacerbates the problem of environmental pollution is the plethora of substances used to eradicate the 'germs' erroneously claimed to pose health risks. The 'interventions' used for this purpose are invariably toxic; they therefore increase the risks to health; they do not reduce them. It is important in the context of this discussion to reiterate that a 'poison' is defined as,

"any substance that irritates, damages or impairs activity of the body's tissues".

It should be noted that irritation, damaged tissues and impaired activity are some of the many symptoms attributable to 'disease'. It is also important to reiterate the point that the toxic substances employed to combat 'germs' or other 'pests' are not specific to their target; they have the ability to adversely affect all living organisms exposed to them.

The category of 'physical factors' is not clearly defined by the WHO; however, the *Heathy environments* report refers to built environments and infrastructure and their association with matters such as sanitation and the supply of clean water; unclean water and poor sanitation certainly pose risks to health. Unfortunately, however, the WHO claims that the risks they pose are because they provide breeding grounds for 'germs', which are the sources of 'infection' and the causes of a variety of infectious diseases. The inappropriate measures that have been introduced to address unclean water and poor sanitation are discussed later in this chapter and in chapter eight.

The report also refers to building materials as 'physical factors' that can pose risks to health; one of the toxic substances specifically mentioned is asbestos, which is acknowledged to be a causal factor for some forms of cancer, especially mesothelioma.

The report correctly recognises that 'chemical factors' pose risks to health, and acknowledges that certain chemicals have been associated with certain diseases, especially cancers, but substantially understates the extent to which toxic chemicals contribute to environmental pollution and human illness. According to the *Healthy environments* report, the solutions to the problems caused by 'chemical factors' should include,

"...safer, more judicious use and management of toxic substances at home and in the workplace."

This solution is woefully inadequate; the mere 'management' of toxic substances in the home and the workplace will not solve the fundamental problem, which is that, as Joe Thornton succinctly describes in the quote that opens this chapter, the planet 'has become the repository for the products, emissions and wastes of modern industry'.

The only genuine solution to a problem is one that will address the root cause.

The issue is not, however, simply a matter of the injudicious use of chemicals or the failure to create and enforce effective regulations; it is far deeper, as will be further discussed in this chapter and in chapter nine.

One of the main problems with respect to toxic chemicals, is that they have been produced and used on the basis of the belief that they are safe, because it is only the dose that makes a substance a poison. This erroneous belief has had profound consequences for the health of the environment and inevitably for the health of all living organisms that inhabit that environment; in other words, for all life on Earth. However, although significant, chemicals are not the only environmental pollutants; others include electromagnetic radiation, both ionising and non-ionising, as will be discussed in this chapter.

Despite the recognition that there is an association between certain toxic chemicals and illness, a large proportion of diseases are attributed to either 'germs' or 'genes'; which means that toxicological testing is rarely used as a diagnostic tool for determining the causes of disease. The main reason that toxicology is not used for this purpose is the general denial that toxic chemicals are related in any significant degree to illness. This denial is based on two factors, one of which is the belief in the Paracelsus fallacy relating to the dose. The other factor is that it is extremely difficult to demonstrate a direct link between exposure to a single chemical and a resulting illness in the real-world environment because people are always exposed to multiple chemicals.

This difficulty is exploited by industry and used to support the denial that their products cause illness; a pertinent example is the tobacco industry's denial over the course of many decades that smoking contributed to cancer. Eventually, however, sufficient evidence accumulated to dispel the doubts and to establish a clear link between smoking and an increased risk of lung cancer.

One reason that it is virtually impossible to demonstrate a direct link between a specific chemical and a specific 'disease' is that, in reality, there are no separate and distinct disease entities with distinct causes. Another is that illness rarely has a single cause; it is almost always the result of a complex mix of factors. These topics are discussed in greater detail in chapter ten.

The failure to recognise the full extent to which toxic chemicals contribute to environmental pollution is the result of a combination of factors, one of which is that only a tiny proportion of all manufactured chemicals are tested for their safety. Another is that the testing procedures are not comprehensive; only a limited range of effects are evaluated. Furthermore, testing procedures are mainly limited to investigations of the effects from individual substances or, very rarely, to the possible effects from a few combinations of substances.

The most significant aspect of the problem is that no tests are ever conducted to assess the safety, or otherwise, of the myriad combinations of the thousands of chemicals to which people can be exposed on a daily basis in the real world. One of the reasons that comprehensive testing is not conducted is explained by Peter Montague of the Environmental Research Foundation in his May 1999 article entitled *The Waning Days of Risk Assessment*, in which he states that,

"Science has no way to analyze the effects of multiple exposures..."

Effects produced by exposures to multiple substances within a complex living human body cannot be analysed and tested in laboratory experiments that only examine tissues, cells, molecules and other fragments extracted from a living organism. The inability of 'science' to test these effects on an intact living human organism means that assurances of 'safety' cannot be relied upon.

The difficulties in establishing an association between exposures to multiple environmental pollutants and a specific disease are also discussed in a 2003 article entitled *Environmental pollution and the global burden of disease*. This article, which is published in the *British Medical Bulletin*, states that,

> "Long latency times, the effects of cumulative exposures, and multiple exposures to different pollutants which might act synergistically all create difficulties in unravelling associations between environmental pollution and health."

These 'difficulties' are obviously beneficial for polluting industries and enable them to avoid taking responsibility for their contributions to the degradation of the environment and the resulting ill-health suffered by the public.

The article claims that the major sources of 'environmental pollution' are unsafe water, poor sanitation and poor hygiene; but, in the 21st century, these conditions are largely the result of environmental pollution not their source. It was demonstrated in chapter two that the implementation of a number of sanitary measures in the 19th century substantially contributed to improved health, but these measures did not completely eradicate all illness; which means that other factors must also have been involved. The majority of 21st century pollutants differ from those of the 19th century and, to a certain extent, these differences are reflected in the different types of 'disease' with which people now suffer.

Unfortunately, the flawed understanding about the nature and causes of diseases means that the medical establishment refers to diseases as either 'infectious' or 'non-infectious' as indicated by the *Healthy environments* report, which states that,

> "The last decade has seen a shift away from infectious, parasitic and nutritional disease to NCDs..."

Strangely, however, and in contrast to this statement, is a claim made in an October 2014 article entitled *Global rise in human infectious disease outbreaks*, published by the *Journal of the Royal Society Interface*, which states that,

> "Zoonotic disease outbreaks are increasing globally in both total number and richness..."

The Royal Society is as much a part of the 'establishment' as the WHO, which makes these contrasting statements a matter of concern; they also raise the question of how such contradictions can be justified when one of the main objectives of the 'establishment' is to achieve a 'consensus' view with respect to their theories.

It is abundantly clear that, whatever the label applied to the conditions with which they suffer, increasing numbers of people around the world are experiencing worsening health; but the medical establishment is unable to effectively 'treat' these problems and help people recover their health.

One of the 'physical factors' referred to in the *Healthy environments* report requires further discussion because it is regarded as the major 'environmental problem' of the 21st century. This factor is 'climate change', which the report claims to be an emerging risk that needs to be tackled urgently. The relevance of 'climate change' to health is claimed to be that certain factors that relate to infectious diseases are 'climate sensitive'; this claim is, however, highly problematic.

The topic of 'climate change' is a controversial one; mainly due to the ideas of the scientific establishment about the causes of changes in the climate. The main claims are that unprecedented levels of atmospheric carbon dioxide have adversely affected the climate and that human activity is largely to blame for this situation; but these claims are unfounded. This is not to deny that the climate changes; that is an irrefutable fact. Climate change is a natural phenomenon that has occurred throughout the existence of the planet. The point of dispute is that it has never been proven that the level of atmospheric carbon dioxide is the driving force behind changes in the climate, or that human activity is the most significant contributory factor to the total volume of carbon dioxide in the atmosphere.

Although carbon dioxide is regarded as a greenhouse gas, it is by no means the most abundant greenhouse gas in the atmosphere; it is, however, the only gas that has been accused since the 1980s of causing 'global warming', a label that was altered to 'climate change' when global temperature readings ceased to support the notion that the planet was experiencing unprecedented 'warming'.

It is an acknowledged scientific fact that 'human emissions' form only a small fraction of the total volume of atmospheric carbon dioxide, which itself forms only a small percentage of the total volume of 'greenhouse gases'. Nevertheless, it is claimed that the contribution from 'human emissions' creates a 'dangerous' level of carbon dioxide; a claim that is refuted by palaeoclimatologist Professor Robert M Carter PhD, who states in his book entitled *Climate: The Counter Consensus* that,

> "Though we know little about the transient effect of human emissions, there is little reason to suspect that the effect is dangerous."

Carbon dioxide is not the 'dangerous' villain it is purported to be; on the contrary, Professor Carter states that increases in atmospheric carbon dioxide have been shown to be beneficial and explains that,

> "Increasing atmospheric carbon dioxide both enhances plant growth and aids the efficiency of water use."

Professor Carter is by no means alone in his recognition that atmospheric carbon dioxide is beneficial for plant growth; as demonstrated by a 2009 fact sheet entitled *Carbon Dioxide in Greenhouses* produced by OMAFRA (Ontario Ministry of Agriculture, Food and Rural Affairs), which states that,

> "The benefits of carbon dioxide supplementation on plant growth and production within the greenhouse environment have been well understood for years."

Carbon dioxide is essential for photosynthesis, which is a vital aspect of plant growth. This means that carbon dioxide is vital for life on planet Earth as many living organisms depend on plants for their food, either directly or indirectly; high levels of atmospheric carbon dioxide benefits plant growth and therefore increases the food supply.

Unfortunately, whilst the attention of the public is focused on the idea that carbon dioxide is 'bad' and the primary cause of 'climate change', the far more important and serious issue of environmental pollution is ignored. The portrayal of carbon dioxide as the 'villain' of environmental pollution has become a diversionary tactic to avoid sufficient media attention to expose the real villains, which are the plethora of toxic substances that pollute the environment.

It is often claimed that people who 'deny' climate change are funded by the oil industry to help promote their cause; the discussions in this chapter will demonstrate that the oil industry is a major polluter of the environment; this claim cannot therefore be applied to the authors of this book.

The very real and urgent problem that faces humanity is environmental pollution caused by the products, emissions and wastes of a wide variety of industries, as this chapter will demonstrate.

It must be emphasised that this discussion should not be interpreted as a polemic against 'industry' expressed from a 'Luddite' perspective, in which all industry is viewed as 'bad'. It is, however, a critique of the direction taken by many industries in respect of the processes and materials they create and utilise, as well as the irresponsible discharge of toxic industrial wastes. The sentiment of the authors of this book is described in Ralph Nader's book entitled *In Pursuit of Justice* in which he quotes the words of conservationist David Brower, who states that,

"We're not blindly opposed to progress, we're opposed to blind progress."

There is no easily discernible point in history when efforts to understand the world and how it functions developed into efforts to control and dominate the world and its resources; the process seems to have undergone a slow but insidious progression. Activities that began as the utilisation of resources for everyday life, somehow developed into a full-scale exploitation of resources by certain groups of people in the belief that they had an inalienable right to exploit those resources, without regard or responsibility for the consequences of their actions.

In addition to the exploitation of natural resources by industry in general, the chemical industry in particular has created a wide variety of new substances that could never have developed naturally; this makes it difficult, if not impossible, for them to degrade naturally. Dr Barry Commoner PhD expresses this point in his book entitled *Making Peace With the Planet*,

"Organic compounds incapable of enzymatic degradation are not produced in living things."

In this context, 'organic' means carbon-based. Enzymatic degradation is the process by which matter is broken down into its individual chemical components. If the matter is organic, these chemical components are reabsorbed into the environment where they are 'recycled' by various organisms, including bacteria. The ever-growing volume of non-organic compounds that do not biodegrade naturally is a key factor in the ever-growing level of environmental pollution.

It is no understatement to assert that science has been largely, although not completely, corrupted by those who seek to control and exploit the world's resources for their own narrow benefits, rather than to understand the importance of the maintenance of natural resources to ensure the perpetuation of life on Earth. Warnings about the dire consequences of the arrogant attitude of those who seek to control and exploit nature, have been expressed by many concerned people from various walks of life over a long period of time. One of those warnings was articulated over half a century ago by Rachel Carson in her book entitled *Silent Spring*,

> "As man proceeds towards his announced goal of the conquest of nature, he has written a depressing record of destruction, directed not only against the earth he inhabits but against the life that shares it with him."

Although her book is primarily a discussion about the dangers of toxic pesticides, Rachel Carson's words are equally applicable to various disciplines in which mankind seeks the 'conquest of nature', particularly by the manufacture of unnatural and dangerous chemicals and the generation of EM radiation. Peter Montague refers in his previously cited 1999 article to the level of awareness of the problem that existed in the 1970s,

> "Technical mastery of natural forces was leading not to safety and well being, but to a careless and accelerating dispersal of dangerous poisons into the biosphere with consequences impossible to predict."

Sadly, the situation has yet to change for the better in the intervening decades; in most instances the situation has substantially worsened. One major example is that with the development of nuclear weapons, mankind has taken the desire for control to its ultimate limit and created the ability to completely destroy the entire world; an event in which no one could ever be the winner.

This is also articulated by Peter Montague in his article, in which he states that,

> "During the late 1960s it slowly became clear that many modern technologies had far surpassed human understanding, giving rise to by-products that were dangerous, long-lived and completely unanticipated."

It is impossible in a single chapter to enumerate and detail all the ways in which the world has been, and continues to be, polluted and poisoned. Such a chapter would not only be long and cumbersome, but it would also be thoroughly depressing. The aim of this book is to inform, not to depress, and so this chapter focuses on providing information about pollutants and toxins, some of which are discussed in detail, for the purpose of demonstrating their widespread nature in everyday life and to assist people to avoid, or at least minimise, exposure to them.

The fact that people survive and are able to live despite constant exposures to a barrage of toxic substances is a testament to the body's self-regulating and self-healing mechanisms. However, whilst it is essential to bear in mind throughout this chapter that the human body is amazingly resilient, it must also be recognised that there are limits to the body's ability to withstand increasing levels of toxic intake; these limits are manifested in the serious nature of the diseases with which increasing numbers of people around the world now suffer.

This situation can be changed, but only when people have a genuine understanding of the real causes of illness, so that they can make informed decisions about matters that affect their health. However, informed decisions can only be made when people are in possession of all the relevant information about the 'poisons' to which they are exposed and can therefore avoid; providing this information is the core purpose of this chapter.

Natural Poisons

The medical establishment claims that some diseases have an ancient origin. The basis for such claims is that archaeological excavations have occasionally uncovered skeletal remains that are believed to exhibit certain pathologies indicative of certain diseases.

Although this book argues that there are no distinct 'disease entities', it is not disputed that 'diseased conditions' have existed throughout human history. Unfortunately, the ancient origin of 'disease' is frequently used as an argument against the idea that 'chemicals' can be responsible for causing disease, on the basis that the chemical industry is a relatively recent phenomenon; this is however a misleading argument.

The Earth is comprised of many different materials, some of which occur naturally in their elemental form, others occur only within compounds and are never found in nature in their elemental form. Many of these elements and compounds are beneficial for life; without these essential substances the rich variety of life-forms that exist on the planet would never have been able to develop and thrive over the course of Earth's history.

There are, however, a number of natural substances that are inherently harmful to living organisms; some of them are harmful in their elemental form but only occur in nature within a harmless compound. Others are harmful in the form in which they occur in nature, but remain deep within subterranean layers, where they are relatively harmless unless disturbed by events that precipitate their release.

Certain natural phenomena can precipitate the release of harmful substances into the environment; volcanic eruptions, for example, discharge huge volumes of minerals and gases from deep within the bowels of the earth. Volcanic eruptions do not directly cause disease, but they do introduce toxic substances into the atmosphere; it is these toxic materials that are able to spread to populated areas and cause widespread illness and death. Other natural phenomena can also contribute to increased levels of environmental pollution; the discussion in chapter four about the Black Death demonstrated that comet debris contains many toxic materials that are capable of polluting the Earth's environment and causing devastating illness and death. Hazardous materials are also released into the environment from natural processes, for example, the breakdown of radioactive materials such as uranium into their decay by-products; the health hazards from exposure to ionising radiation are discussed in more detail later in this chapter.

These natural phenomena clearly have an ancient origin; by comparison, human-generated pollution of the planet as the result of the exploitation of Earth's resources is an extremely recent phenomenon in geological terms.

Human activities have however, augmented the level of 'natural' hazardous materials in the environment; the oldest of these activities include the extraction of natural resources by mining and quarrying, both of which have origins that date back many millennia. Some of the minerals that have been discovered to be useful for human activities occur in nature within an ore, which means that the elemental mineral requires extraction from that ore; this led to the development of smelting processes, of which there are a few different types. However, mining, quarrying and smelting are all hazardous occupations; they involve substantial exposures to some highly toxic substances.

Prior to the commencement of these activities there was no knowledge about their potential hazards; nor, it would seem, were any investigations conducted to test the possibility that they may be associated with any hazards or adverse health effects. However, effects would have been noticed by those who were engaged in such activities, but their health problems may not have been directly associated with their occupations. Although men who worked in the mines, quarries and smelting works would have been exposed to the greatest levels of hazardous materials, they were not the only people to be affected. People who lived in the vicinity of these works would also have been exposed to toxic wastes and by-products released into the environment and into local sources of water.

These topics are discussed in more detail in the ensuing sections that discuss four naturally-occurring but highly toxic substances, namely, lead, mercury, arsenic and uranium. The reasons for choosing these four elements are because they are extremely toxic and because they have all been used in a variety of applications, some of which can only be described as wholly inappropriate.

Lead

The establishment definition of lead refers to,

"a soft bluish-grey metallic element that forms several poisonous compounds."

Lead usually exists in nature within an ore and in conjunction with other metals including zinc, silver and copper. The ore is mined then smelted to separate and extract the different metals. It is reported that both lead mining and smelting have long histories that date back more than three millennia. It is also reported that lead has been recognised as toxic for at least two millennia, as recorded by Sheldon Rampton and John Stauber in their book entitled *Trust Us We're Experts*,

"... lead has been a known poison since antiquity. During the first century AD, lead miners strapped animal bladders over their mouths as a way to avoid inhaling it."

The Romans were known to have used lead in their water pipes, which suggests that they may not have been fully aware of its dangers. The ancient

Greeks, however, were aware of the problem, as explained by Dr Herbert Needleman MD, in his 2004 article entitled *Lead Poisoning*,

"Warnings of lead's poisonous properties extend at least as far back as the second century BC, when Nikander, a Greek physician, described the colic and paralysis that followed lead ingestion. The early victims of lead toxicity were mainly lead workers and wine drinkers."

It is unsurprising that lead workers were early victims of lead's toxicity; lead miners are likely to have been the first to experience the adverse health effects from their exposures in the mines. The inclusion of wine drinkers as victims of lead poisoning is, however, rather more surprising; but is explained by Dr Needleman who states that lead was used in wine-making due to its 'sweet flavour' that would counteract the astringency of the tannic acid in the grapes.

The use of lead in wine-making ceased many centuries ago; but its ability to add sweetness and colour made it a useful ingredient of foodstuffs in more recent eras. In England during the 18th and 19th centuries, for example, lead was used as a red dye for children's sweets; its sweetness again masking its dangers. It would seem that English physicians were not aware of the work of Nikander or the dangers of lead, because colic and paralysis were rarely ascribed to lead poisoning.

Lead was eventually recognised to be toxic and one product in particular was manufactured to specifically take advantage of this property; the insecticide lead arsenate. This chemical compound was first used at the end of the 19th century in America as a method of destroying the gypsy moth, which is not native to the US but, in its leaf-eating caterpillar stage, had become a severe nuisance, particularly to fruit growers. It was claimed that lead arsenate had 'low phytotoxicity', which was believed to mean that it would not harm the plants even though it would poison and kill the caterpillars. Based on this claim, lead arsenate became a popular insecticide and was used on a variety of crops, including rubber and coffee, as well as fruit trees.

Lead arsenate was also available in other countries; it is reported to have been used in Canada and Australia, as well as some parts of Europe and some African countries. The claim that lead arsenate had 'low phytotoxicity' was clearly false; both lead and arsenic are highly toxic substances. This means that the insect targets of the insecticide were not the only victims of poisoning; orchard and plantation workers would also have been exposed to these poisons. Furthermore, insecticide spraying after the development of the fruit is likely to have left chemical residues on the crops, thus poisoning anyone who ate them. Residues would also have settled on the ground and contaminated the soil in which the trees and other crops were grown.

Lead arsenate does degrade, albeit very slowly, into its constituent elements, lead and arsenic; however, lead and arsenic are both persistent poisons, which means that any land previously used as orchards and plantations, on which lead arsenate had been used, will remain contaminated for a long time, even though the pesticide is no longer used.

One of the more recent and better-known applications of lead is as a motor fuel additive as it had been found to have a number of 'useful' properties, one of which is that it boosts the performance of the fuel. Lead was also found to have 'useful' properties for paints, one of which was the ability to hasten the drying process; lead was used as a paint additive for many decades.

Dr Needleman demonstrated that a clear association existed between exposure to lead and serious health hazards; his efforts over the course of many years finally resulted in the removal of lead from the manufacture of most motor fuels and most paints. He had discovered that children in particular suffered as the result of exposures to lead; many of the adverse health effects they experienced were cognitive issues, including behavioural issues and developmental problems as well as lowered IQ. The serious impact of lead poisoning has been found to occur at very low levels of exposure. Former neurosurgeon Dr Russell Blaylock MD discusses in *Health and Nutrition Secrets* the neurological dangers to children from lead exposure,

> "Several studies have shown that lead-intoxicated children experience intellectual difficulties, as well as problems with hyper-irritability and violent outbursts."

The WHO has also recognised this problem and states in the August 2018 fact sheet entitled *Lead poisoning and health* that,

> "Lead is a cumulative toxicant that affects multiple body systems and is particularly harmful to young children."

Although lead had been known to be toxic 'since antiquity', the decision to add it to motor fuel clearly ignored this fact, but the dangers from inhaling leaded fumes soon became apparent, as Dr Needleman explains,

> "When tetraethyl lead (TEL) was first produced for use as a motor fuel additive in 1925, workers at all three operating plants began to die."

These tragedies should certainly have alerted the people in charge of the operating plants to the fact that there was a serious health hazard associated with the inhalation of tetraethyl lead; but these deaths seem to have been ignored and leaded motor fuel remained in use for many decades after 1925.

Leaded fuel has been phased out of use since the mid-1970s, but, although most vehicles now use unleaded fuel, some very old vehicles in certain parts of the world still use leaded fuel. Furthermore, certain types of aviation fuel also contain lead; although it is reported that these leaded fuels will be replaced by unleaded versions in the near future. However, the stability of lead and its persistence means that the environment remains contaminated from lead emissions by leaded vehicle fuels over the course of many decades.

It is not only the atmosphere that has been contaminated; people who inhaled toxic exhaust fumes also absorbed a certain level of lead into their bodies. This means that many people also remain contaminated with lead, which takes time to be eliminated depending on which part of the body absorbed the largest level of lead. Blood lead levels are said to decrease over a comparatively short period of some months, whereas lead in bone can take years or even decades to be excreted.

The use of lead as an ingredient of paint has also been mostly, although not entirely, discontinued; some industrial paints still contain lead. Although lead is no longer an ingredient of paints used for home decorating, leaded paints had been widely used for decades in a variety of buildings, including homes, offices and industrial premises. Unless and until those layers of leaded paint have been completely and carefully removed, the hazards to health remain, even if the leaded paint is hidden beneath many subsequent layers of unleaded paint.

There is a phenomenon known as 'sick building syndrome' that is poorly understood; however, the presence of leaded paint on the walls and doors etc, could be considered as a potential and very credible contributory factor to this phenomenon. The symptoms ascribed to this condition include headaches, dizziness, runny nose and itchy watery eyes, all of which can be caused by low level but frequent exposures to lead.

The detrimental health effects from lead are numerous, depending on the degree of exposure; the most disturbing are the effects on the nervous system, some of which are explained by Dr Needleman in more detail,

> "Lead poisoning in adults can affect the peripheral and central nervous systems, the kidneys, and blood pressure. Classical descriptions of occupational toxicity depict peripheral neuropathy with wrist or foot drop.... Patients with high blood lead levels may present with severe intractable colic, motor clumsiness, clouded consciousness, weakness and paralysis. Lead has adverse effects on both male and female reproduction."

Lead poisoning is clearly capable of producing a large number of adverse health effects, one of which is paralysis, as described by Nikander more than 2,000 years ago. The establishment definition also refers to paralysis as one of the symptoms that can result from lead poisoning. This would tend to suggest that, in the 20th century, some cases of paralysis caused by lead poisoning may have been misdiagnosed and labelled as 'polio'.

Lead is one of the few chemicals specifically mentioned by the *Healthy environments* report; its dangers are also recognised in the WHO fact sheet that states,

> "There is no known level of lead exposure that is considered safe."

Mercury

The establishment definition of mercury refers to,

> "a silvery metallic element that is liquid at room temperature."

Mercury is widely regarded as one of the most toxic naturally-occurring substances on Earth. It is rarely found in its pure metallic form in nature, but usually occurs in the form of an ore called mercury sulphide, which is also known as cinnabar.

Mercury is an unusual metal because, as the definition states, in its pure metallic form at normal ambient temperatures it is liquid; a quality that gave rise to its alternative name quicksilver. This toxic metal does solidify, although this will only occur at temperatures below -38°C.

It is reported that mercury has been mined for more than two thousand years, and that it was used by the ancient Greeks in ointments and by the ancient Egyptians in cosmetics, which tends to suggest that neither of these civilisations knew about its severe toxicity. It should be clear that a long history of use does not 'prove' that a substance is safe; this is particularly pertinent with respect to mercury.

The apparent ignorance about mercury's toxicity continued into the 14th century, when it came into use as a treatment for leprosy, and the 16th century, when its use was extended to the treatment of syphilis. The recognition by the medical establishment that mercury is highly toxic has been an extremely slow process that only seems to have begun in the early 20th century; the establishment definition of mercury states the consequences of that realisation,

"Its toxicity has caused a decline in the use of its compounds in medicine during this century..."

Chapter two revealed that mercury continues to be used in the manufacture of vaccines and, although it is claimed to be 'filtered out', this claim has been shown to be unfounded, because 'trace amounts' always remain.

Mercury is utilised in the extraction of precious metals, such as gold and silver, due to its ability to dissolve metals from their ores; this further demonstrates that mining is a particularly hazardous occupation. In *Health and Nutrition Secrets* Dr Russell Blaylock states unequivocally that mercury is neurotoxic and explains how this property affected cinnabar mine workers,

"After years of working in mines, workers would often suffer from crippling neurological and mental disorders."

Mercury is released into the environment from a number of sources, some of which may be natural but others are the direct result of human activities. These activities include: mining and smelting; discharges from coal-fired power plants; and other industrial processes. Dr Blaylock indicates the scale of the release of mercury into the atmosphere,

"It has been estimated that as much as 5,000 tons of mercury are released into the atmosphere every year from burning coal and natural gas and refining petroleum products."

The dangers posed by exposure to mercury in the atmosphere far exceed those allegedly posed by carbon dioxide; yet the scientific community continues to promulgate fear through the mainstream media about 'climate change' caused by human emissions of carbon dioxide, whilst ignoring the far greater dangers posed by industrial emissions of mercury.

Despite the medical establishment denial of the dangers posed by the 'trace amounts' of mercury in vaccines, they admit to the existence of adverse health effects from small exposures to mercury; as indicated by the March 2017 WHO fact sheet entitled *Mercury and health*, that states,

"Exposure to mercury – even in small amounts – may cause serious health problems..."

The WHO claims that adverse health effects are only caused by methylmercury and that ethylmercury, the form used in vaccines, does not pose risks to health; this claim is however, unfounded.

Children's Health, which was previously cited in chapter two but deserves repetition,

"Mercury is a highly toxic element; there is no known safe level of exposure."

It is clear that mercury is finally being recognised as the highly toxic and extremely dangerous substance that it is; unfortunately, recognition of this fact has been an exceedingly slow process and has cost untold numbers of people and children their health and even their lives.

Arsenic

The establishment definition of arsenic refers to,

"...a poisonous greyish metallic element..."

Arsenic occurs naturally in conjunction with a number of other metals, such as gold, copper, zinc and lead; it is therefore a common by-product of mining and of smelting processes used to extract these other metals. Furthermore, like lead and mercury, arsenic is a persistent pollutant.

As indicated by the definition, arsenic is recognised as poisonous; a property that made it useful for a number of applications, particularly insecticides; some reports indicate that arsenic-based insecticides were first used in China in the 10th century. According to an article entitled *The Global Problem of Lead Arsenate Pesticides* on the website of the LEAD Group,

"Arsenical insecticides have been used in agriculture for centuries."

Arsenic is also used in rodenticides and remains an ingredient of many 21st century rat poisons.

Arsenic is also carcinogenic; it has been classified by the IARC as a class 1 human carcinogen, which makes it a plausible causal factor, or certainly a significant contributory factor, for many of the earliest reported cases of cancer; a point that has also been expressed by Rachel Carson in *Silent Spring*,

"The association between arsenic and cancer in man and animals is historic."

Arsenic is another of the chemicals specifically referred to as toxic by the WHO in the *Healthy environments* report. As discussed in chapter four, arsenic was a main ingredient of insecticidal sheep dips, which, although intended to only kill the insect pest, was shown to have also had a detrimental impact on the health of sheep and sheep farmers, as well as anyone who handled sheep dip or worked with fleeces treated with the toxic dip.

In his book entitled *The Arsenic Century*, James C Whorton PhD pays particular attention to the situation in 19th century Britain, where arsenic became ubiquitous,

"Arsenic lurked at every turn in the Victorian world..."

During this period, there was a substantial increase in mining throughout many parts of Britain. As mentioned above, arsenic is a common by-product of mining and smelting processes, which therefore generated an abundant supply of arsenic. Its abundance made arsenic readily available and cheap, all of which encouraged its use for a variety of applications; a situation that resulted in many sources of exposures for the population of Britain, as explained by Dr Whorton,

> "...people took it in with fruits and vegetables, swallowed it with wine, inhaled it from cigarettes, absorbed it from cosmetics and imbibed it even from the pint glass."

Anyone who is familiar with the works of Charles Dickens will be aware that, in 19th century Britain, the diet of the poor consisted mainly of bread and beer, both of which could be contaminated with arsenic. The reason that bread was contaminated, was that some farmers used an arsenic-based insecticide solution to soak their wheat seeds to prevent infestations with various 'pests'. The majority of people, especially the poor, were also exposed to arsenic released from the coal in their fires.

In common with other persistent toxins, the serious adverse health effects of arsenic are often the result of cumulative exposures, as acknowledged by the February 2018 WHO fact sheet entitled *Arsenic* that states,

> "Long-term exposure to arsenic from drinking-water and food can cause cancer and skin lesions. It has also been associated with cardiovascular disease and diabetes."

It is therefore unsurprising that people in 19th century Britain suffered ill-health, some of which can be ascribed to arsenic poisoning. However, they did not fare a great deal better if they could afford the services of a physician, because, as discussed, arsenic was an ingredient of many 'medicines' of the period. In another similarity with mercury, knowledge of arsenic's toxicity did not preclude its use in 'treatments' for a variety of conditions; compounds based on arsenic had been prescribed for many centuries, dating back to the time of Hippocrates.

Some of the conditions for which arsenic was used as a treatment during the 19th century include rheumatism, worms and morning sickness. Prescribing a poison as a 'cure' for morning sickness demonstrates an abysmally low level of knowledge about health, or the potential for serious harm to a developing baby from a poison ingested by the expectant mother. The treatment of morning sickness with arsenic-based 'medicines' is likely to have been a significant contributory factor for infant mortality and maternal death in childbirth, both of which existed at high levels at that period of time.

Arsenic was also promoted as a 'cure' for asthma. It is reported that Charles Darwin used an arsenic-based treatment for his eczema, a condition that often appears in conjunction with asthma; however, neither asthma nor eczema can be cured by arsenic, except permanently when the patient dies as the result of arsenic poisoning.

Ingestion of arsenic can produce a rather violent reaction, which often includes vomiting; it is this strong reaction that was believed to demonstrate the allegedly 'therapeutic' nature of this poison. During the 19th century, it was believed by many physicians that a person became ill due to an imbalance in their body; an idea that dates back to the time of Hippocrates. The reason for using arsenic to redress an 'imbalance' was that it would 'shock' the body back into balance and therefore back to health.

A dose of a poisonous substance that was large enough to cause a violent reaction could also result in death; it is not surprising therefore, that this kind of treatment was often referred to as 'heroic medicine'. Presumably only strong 'heroes' were able to survive being poisoned in the name of healthcare. Dr Whorton also refers to the extensive use of arsenic-based treatments and states,

"...arsenic was also a component of an array of medicines, being frequently prescribed by physicians and almost as liberally purveyed by quacks."

It is interesting to note that 'physicians' seemed to be more liberal in prescribing arsenic-based 'medicines' for their patients than 'quacks'. However, as demonstrated throughout this book, the human body cannot be poisoned back to health.

One arsenic-based 'medicine' is the substance called arsphenamine, which is also known as Salvarsan and as compound 606. Salvarsan is significant for a few reasons, one of which is that it replaced mercury ointments in the treatment of syphilis. Another is that Salvarsan is considered to have been the first 'effective' treatment for syphilis, which suggests that, despite its use over the course of a number of centuries, mercury had not been as effective as it is often claimed to have been.

The third reason that Salvarsan is significant is because this 'medicine' is regarded as heralding the beginning of the era of 'chemotherapeutic' drugs. The use of arsenic as 'medicine' must be regarded as yet another of the tragic errors of 'medical science'.

Patients were not the only victims of arsenic poisoning; medical students and the physicians who taught medicine during the 19th century also suffered, but their exposures were due to a specific aspect of medical training, which is the study of anatomy, as Dr Whorton explains,

"Not even professors of medicine were secure from the poison, the cadavers they and their pupils dissected in anatomical studies being oft-times preserved from decomposition with arsenic."

The ability of arsenic to 'preserve' specimens led to its introduction and use as an embalming fluid, although it was largely replaced by formaldehyde, which was discovered in the late 19th century; formaldehyde did not however, entirely replace arsenic as the embalming fluid of choice until the early 20th century. The main problem arising from the use of arsenic in applications such as medicines, pesticides and embalming fluid, is due to its persistence in the environment; which means that, long after this toxin has ceased to be used, it continues to pose serious hazards to health.

The seriousness of the problem caused by the widespread use of arsenic during the 19th century, led John Gay to write an article in 1859 for the *Medical Times and Gazette*; this article, which is quoted by Dr Whorton in his book, includes the question,

"How long will money-hunters be allowed, in the pursuit of their game, to vitiate the necessaries of life with the deadliest poisons?"

This plea remains pertinent more than a century and a half later; it has yet to be fully recognised as applicable to all toxic substances and acted upon!

Uranium

In common with the three previous elements, uranium is a naturally-occurring toxic substance; however, unlike lead, mercury and arsenic, uranium is radioactive. Ionising radiation, the type emitted by radioactive substances such as uranium, is discussed in more detail later in this chapter.

Interestingly, there is no establishment definition of uranium, nor has the WHO produced a fact sheet on the topic. Fortunately, the IPPNW (International Physicians for the Prevention of Nuclear War) has produced a fact sheet entitled *Health Effects of Uranium Mining*, which states that,

"Uranium is highly toxic and attacks the inner organs..."

Uranium is found in nature within an ore, which is also known as pitchblende. This ore is, however, more dangerous than elemental uranium, because it also contains various uranium decay by-products, or daughter isotopes as they are also called, many of which are more radioactive than pure uranium.

There are a number of isotopes of the naturally-occurring form of uranium and these range from U-233 to U-238, each of which has a different half-life that ranges from 69 years for U-233 to four and a half billion years for U-238. As well as being the most persistent, U-238 is also the most abundant uranium isotope found in nature.

Uranium decays by emitting alpha and beta particles, a process that results in the production of a long series of decay by-products and ultimately ends in the formation of the stable element lead. One of the decay by-products of uranium is radium, the highly radioactive and dangerous substance that was discovered by Marie Curie. Unfortunately, she was unaware of its dangers and failed to protect herself; a situation that contributed to the development of her cancer and to her early death. Radium also has many radioactive isotopes, the most stable one of which is radium-226 that has a half-life of approximately 1600 years.

Radium decays to radon gas, which has a very short half-life of approximately 4 days. Radon gas is, however, highly radioactive, dangerous and a recognised carcinogen; it is also invisible and undetectable by taste or smell. Radon gas is known to be released in areas rich in uranium deposits and a contributory factor for cancers in areas where uranium has been mined.

It is highly likely therefore, that exposures to uranium, radium and radon gas would have been significant contributory factors to cancers in the ancient past.

Uranium was discovered in 1789 and first mined in the US in 1871, although its radioactivity was not discovered until 1896 from the work of Henri Becquerel, after whom one of the units for measuring radioactivity was named.

It is clear that uranium miners would have been subjected to high levels of exposure to this dangerous substance. Unfortunately for miners, protective measures were not implemented until long after the discovery of the hazards associated with uranium mining, as Dr Rosalie Bertell PhD explains in her book entitled *No Immediate Danger*,

"The danger of uranium mining had been known for a hundred years before 1945, yet it took until 1967, with many unnecessary miner deaths from lung cancer, to legislate regulations for mine ventilation and subsequent reduction of airborne radioactive particles and gas in the mines."

Dr Bertell also explains that commercial mining for uranium began in the US in 1949; this increased activity was mainly stimulated by demands from the Manhattan Project for increased volumes of the raw materials necessary to assist their continuing development of nuclear weapons.

Whilst other factors, especially smoking, are known to contribute to an increased risk of developing lung cancer, uranium miners were shown to experience a greatly enhanced risk, as Dr Ernest Sternglass PhD describes in his book entitled *Secret Fallout*,

"...it has long been known that uranium miners have ten times the normal rate of lung cancers because of their breathing of radioactive gas in the mines."

Earth Works is a non-profit organisation concerned with a number of environmental problems, including the dangers from uranium mining; a 2011 report entitled *Nuclear Power's Other Tragedy*, available from the website, states that,

"Mining not only exposes uranium to the atmosphere, where it becomes reactive, but releases other radioactive elements such as thorium and radium and toxic heavy metals including arsenic, selenium, mercury and cadmium."

These radioactive elements and toxic heavy metals clearly increase the level of environmental contamination in the vicinity of the mines. The IPPNW fact sheet also refers to the serious hazards associated with uranium mining,

"Lung cancer, leukemia, stomach cancer and birth defects are the diseases most often to be found as a result of uranium mining."

On the CDC website is a page that refers to an ongoing series of studies of the health of uranium miners. Although called a 'worker health study', it is an investigation of the mortality of uranium miners who worked underground to determine if their mortality exceeded the 'normal' level in the general population from various diseases. The study was begun in 1950 due to,

"...concerns that uranium mining causes cancer."

It is reported within the results of the study that, unsurprisingly, uranium miners experienced far greater mortality than the general population from these diseases. The studies finally resulted in legislation in 1990 when the Radiation Exposure Compensation Act was passed.

Unfortunately, the hazards due to uranium mining remain long after the extraction processes have ceased and the mines have become inactive. A fact sheet available from the website of the organisation, Clean Up The Mines (cleanupthemines.org), provides information about the hazards of uranium mining, and exposes the existence of many thousands of abandoned uranium mines (AUMs) in the US, as well as the dangers they pose,

"AUMs remain dangerously radioactive for hundreds of thousands of years."

It is clear that decisions taken for short term goals without due regard for the long-term consequences have generated serious health hazards, particularly when they involve substances that are known to be toxic and highly dangerous.

Manufactured Poisons & Applications

The preceding discussions have shown that human activities during the last few millennia have been responsible for the discharge of various materials into the environment. Although toxic and persistent, these materials have all been 'natural'.

More recently, the quality of the environment has undergone significant and dramatic changes that began during the era of scientific advancement in the 16th and 17th centuries and continued with the era of industrialisation in the 18th and 19th centuries.

It must be emphasised that environmental pollution is not caused by 'industrialisation' per se; it is caused by the nature of the materials used and produced by industry. The vast majority of these materials are entirely man-made and inherently toxic. It is for this reason that most environmental pollution can be directly attributed to 'manufactured poisons' and the applications in which they have been employed.

It is often claimed that the changes brought about by the combination of science and industry represent advances in 'civilisation', and that these innovations have generated improved standards of living. This claim is unfounded; the major beneficiaries of industrialisation have been industrialists, many of whom became extremely wealthy. The 'ordinary people', by comparison, were not so fortunate; large numbers of them merely exchanged a life of poverty and deprivation from subsistence farming in rural areas, to poverty and deprivation from factory employment in urban areas. The changed living and working conditions they endured cannot be described as representing an improvement to their living standards.

Previous chapters have described some of the appalling living conditions that had existed over the course of many centuries in various European countries, some of which became centres of 'industrialisation'. The working conditions, especially in factories, were no better. People were made to work long hours, adults were usually expected to work for a minimum of 12 and even up to 16 hours per day for 6 days per week; children would also work in the factories because they were a cheap source of labour. The conditions in the factories were appalling and often dangerous; as well as the hazards they faced from the machines they operated, people were also exposed to a variety of hazardous and invariably toxic substances.

Industrialisation together with science and technology are promoted as necessary for 'development' that leads to better standards of living for the whole population; it is also claimed to lead to better health for everyone, but this is not borne out by the evidence that shows the incidence of chronic diseases in 'developed' countries to be continuing to increase, not decrease. Chronic diseases, also known as NCDs, are often referred to as 'diseases of affluence', but this term is an oxymoron. Affluence is usually associated with better health, but clearly is not the case. A number of the most significant ubiquitous; it is an ingredient of a significant proportion of chemical compounds used in a wide variety of everyday products.

It is widely recognised that many thousands of chemicals have never been tested for their safety, or their health effects. However, many of the chemicals that have been tested and shown to induce adverse health effects nevertheless remain in use. Chlorine is a particularly appropriate example; one of its main uses is in the treatment of water in order to kill 'germs', as will be discussed later in this chapter. Joe Thornton explains the adverse health effects associated with exposure to organochlorines,

> "Several hundred compounds have now been tested, and virtually all organochlorines examined to date cause one or more of a wide variety of adverse effects on essential biological processes, including development, reproduction, brain function and immunity."

The TSCA was originally passed in 1976 in order to regulate chemicals; as the title of the act suggests, it was intended to control 'toxic substances'; but it has clearly failed to do so. The Act has since been amended; the June 2016 amended legislation effectively requires the EPA to clear their 'backlog' and test all remaining untested chemicals that have nevertheless been approved for use.

However, even if the EPA conducted all the required tests, this would still fail to ensure the integrity of the environment or to safeguard public health, because the testing procedures are inadequate. The reason they are inadequate is because they are based on flawed theories, including the theory related to 'risk assessment'.

Peter Montague's hope that the days of inadequate 'risk assessment' were waning unfortunately has yet to be fulfilled. This flawed method remains firmly entrenched within chemical safety testing procedures, as demonstrated by the IPCS (International Programme on Chemical Safety), a WHO programme, the functions of which are explained on the WHO web page entitled *Methods for chemicals assessment,*

> "IPCS work in the field of methodology aims to promote the development, harmonization and use of generally acceptable, scientifically sound methodologies for the evaluation of risks to human health from exposure to chemicals."

There are many problems with this approach, not least of which is the idea that any level of 'risk' to human health from exposure to chemicals should be deemed acceptable. In his article entitled *Making Good Decisions,* Peter Montague refers to risk assessment as 'inherently misleading' and states that,

> "Risk assessment pretends to determine 'safe' levels of exposure to poisons, but in fact it cannot do any such thing."

He expands on this point in his previously cited 1999 article about risk assessment, in which he states that,

> "Science, as a way of knowing, has strict limits..."

He elaborates on this point and further states that,

> "...risk assessment is not a science, it is an art, combining data gathered by scientific methods with a large dose of judgement."

One of the main tenets of 'science' is that results should be reproducible, but judgement is clearly not reproducible; a situation that raises serious questions about the 'scientifically sound methodologies' that the IPCS claims to use to evaluate 'risks' to human health.

Existing regulatory systems, as discussed further in chapter nine, increasingly favour industry over the consumer; they allow the swift release of products onto the market but involve many difficulties for the removal of products after the discovery of any adverse effects. This situation is described by Dr Devra Davis in *The Secret History of the War on Cancer*,

> "It can take 3 weeks to approve a new chemical and 30 years to remove an old one."

There are many examples to illustrate this situation; a pertinent one is DDT, an organochlorine that was first introduced onto the market in 1938 when it was hailed as a 'miracle' pesticide. As well as being sprayed on crops, it was also sprayed on people of all ages to destroy any insect 'pests' they may have been carrying.

It must be noted that the DDT used for spraying people was in the form of a powder that was claimed to be less easily absorbed into the skin and therefore less hazardous; but this does not mean it was 'safe'. The DDT used for spraying crops was an oil-based product that was said to be more easily absorbed, which made it more hazardous. Although people were sprayed with DDT powder many were also exposed to the oil-based DDT used for crop-spraying, as Joe Thornton explains,

> "Once oil-soluble organochlorines are released into the environment, however, they accumulate in the fatty tissues of living things, a process called bioaccumulation."

The PR campaign that promoted DDT as 'good for you' ensured that the public remained completely oblivious of its dangers. But some scientists, especially those studying the natural world, began to notice a serious level of decline in certain animal populations, especially birds. One bird species in particular that experienced a dramatic decline in numbers was the bald eagle, the iconic symbol of the US. Concerns about these changes were raised mainly, but not solely, by Rachel Carson and recorded in *Silent Spring*, in which she demonstrated clear links between the introduction of heavy pesticide spraying and a number of adverse conditions observed in many wildlife species.

Nevertheless, it was almost a decade after the publication of the book that DDT was finally banned, although it was only banned in certain countries. The delay and the failure to implement a worldwide ban provides just another example of the power of industry to obstruct efforts to remove a lucrative product, despite the fact that it has been proven to be an environmental hazard.

Unfortunately, the proverbial genie had already been let out of the bottle. In common with most other organochlorines, DDT is persistent and had been steadily released into the environment over the course of a period of more than 30 years prior to the ban. Of particular concern is that DDT is being re-introduced to help 'fight' a war against mosquitoes in many of the much larger than 'pests' is not a relevant criterion for determining the effects of toxic pesticides; as has been discussed, some chemicals produce serious effects in very low concentrations. The important point is that the effects of organophosphate exposure can be devastating, as Dr Blaylock explains,

"Heavy exposures can cause rapid death from respiratory paralysis."

But even if exposure is not 'heavy', there are many other potentially serious adverse effects, as Dr Blaylock continues,

"In fact, low-concentration exposure can produce lasting neurological problems, such as memory defects, impaired vigilance and a reduced ability to concentrate."

One very serious concern is that organophosphate-based chemicals are ingredients of treatments to combat head lice and therefore mainly used for children. The hazards associated with organophosphates indicate that the head of a growing child should be the very last place that these neurotoxic chemicals ought to be applied.

Another effect of organophosphate exposure is that it can induce the chelation of copper from the body; this can result in copper deficiency, which is also associated with neurological problems.

It is clear that pesticides can produce many adverse health effects.

The reason that this discussion has focused on chemicals used for 'pest control' is to demonstrate that many chemicals are manufactured for the specific purpose of acting as a poison in order to kill 'pests'. Yet none of these chemicals only affects the intended 'target'; they can all adversely affect a far greater variety of living organisms than they are intended to attack, incapacitate or kill; the other species harmed by the use of pesticides are far too numerous to mention.

However, the public's attention is invariably diverted away from the dangers of toxic chemicals and towards various scapegoats; usually 'germs' and 'viruses' in particular. This tactic of blaming 'germs' instead of toxins was used to great effect in the 2016 'outbreak' of the so-called 'Zika virus', which was alleged to have been the cause of microcephaly and other birth defects.

It is claimed that the Zika 'virus' is transmitted by mosquitoes; a claim that resulted in the launch of an intensive pesticide spraying campaign in the name of 'protecting' people from the 'virus'. Yet the endocrine-disrupting chemicals used in many of the pesticides deployed against mosquitoes are significant contributory factors to the onset of birth defects, as will be discussed in the next chapter.

Although pesticides are produced for their ability to 'poison', they are not the only chemicals in widespread use that have the ability to adversely affect living organisms. Previous discussions have exposed the dangers associated with antibiotics. One of the major problems is the fundamental belief that 'poisons' offer solutions to many of the problems that face humanity; in reality, it is the plethora of manufactured chemical poisons that pose some of the greatest threats to human health.

There are clearly far too many chemicals to discuss any of them in depth;

however, petrochemicals are one group that does require further discussion for a number of reasons, one of which is that they have been shown to be directly associated with adverse health effects. Petroleum refining and the manufacture of petrochemicals are associated with chemicals called aromatic hydrocarbons, of which there are many types, but all of them are associated with varying degrees of toxicity.

There are six basic petrochemicals, two of which are benzene and toluene; the former is a proven carcinogen, the latter a known neurotoxin. Yet, according to the ACS (American Chemical Society) web page entitled *Organic Chemistry*,

"Petroleum is also the raw material for many chemical products including pharmaceuticals..."

Chlorine is also important for the manufacture of pharmaceuticals. On the website of the American Chemistry Council is a page entitled *Chlorine Chemistry: Providing Pharmaceuticals That Keep You and Your Family Healthy*, which states that chlorine remains 'present' in many medicines.

The discussion about modern medicine in chapter one referred to the toxic nature of the wastes of the pharmaceutical industry; these wastes include dioxins, as Joe Thornton explains,

"Dioxins have even been identified at low levels in wastes from the synthesis of pharmaceuticals, presumably because chlorinated benzenes and phenols are common feedstocks for drug synthesis."

The use of highly toxic substances as feedstocks for pharmaceuticals means that it is entirely unsurprising that 'medicines' have been demonstrated to adversely affect health.

Pharmaceuticals are not the only applications in which petrochemicals are used. The petrochemical industry claims that the six basic petrochemicals, namely benzene, toluene, ethylene, propylene, butadiene and xylene, are used to make petrochemical derivatives and, according to the AFPM (American Fuel & Petrochemical Manufacturers) web page entitled *Petrochemicals*,

"The most basic petrochemicals are considered the building blocks for organic chemistry."

Although originally the term 'organic' was used in reference to living organisms, it has been extended to include all carbon-based chemicals, whether natural or synthetically manufactured. Organic chemistry in the 21st century predominantly involves the creation of entirely new synthetic chemical compounds; according to the ACS web page entitled *Organic Chemistry*,

"The range of applications of organic compounds is enormous and also includes, but is not limited to, pharmaceuticals, petrochemicals, food, explosives, paints and cosmetics."

The use of synthetic chemicals in foods is discussed later in this chapter.

The range of products made using organic chemistry is clearly immense, as the AFPM website states,

"Most, if not all, finished goods depend on organic chemicals."

This therefore means that virtually all industrial manufacturing depends upon petrochemicals and therefore the oil industry.

This reliance on petroleum highlights another popular theory, which is that the supply of 'oil' is finite; however, as will be discussed in chapter nine, this theory, which is also referred to as 'peak oil', is false. Furthermore, as also discussed in chapter nine, oil is not a 'fossil fuel', but that does not mean it should continue to be used. Petrochemicals are inherently toxic and therefore inherently harmful to the environment and to all living organisms.

One group of materials that are widely used in the manufacture of a vast proportion of everyday products are plastics. There are many types of plastic, but they are all said to fall into one of two categories; they are either thermoplastics, such as nylon, PVC and polythene, or thermosets, such as epoxy resin and urea formaldehyde.

Plastics are used extensively in the manufacture of electrical and electronic equipment; this means that plastics are central to the technology industry. A large proportion of plastics are manufactured from materials derived from petrochemicals and some plastics are derived from chlorine; PVC (polyvinyl chloride), for example, is produced using both.

As mentioned in the previous section, rare earth elements are also central to modern technology; they are used in many items of electronic equipment, such as computers, tablets and mobile phone devices. Rare Earth Technology is part of the American Chemistry Council, Inc; on their website is an article entitled *What Are Rare Earths?* that states,

"Rare earths are a series of chemical elements found in the Earth's crust that are vital to many modern technologies..."

A September 2016 article entitled *Effects of rare earth elements on the environment and human health: A literature review* states that one of the major industrial uses of rare earth elements (REE), or (RE),

"...is in the production of catalysts for the cracking of crude petroleum."

REEs are clearly vital for the oil industry; however, the article also states that,

"There are many environmental and health issues associated with the production, processing and utilization of REEs."

In common with most other resources that are developed for their usefulness, REEs have been poorly studied or tested for their toxicity, as indicated by a March 2013 article entitled *Toxicological Evaluations of Rare Earths and Their Health Impacts to Workers: A Literature Review* that states,

"Although some RE have been used for superconductors, plastic magnets and ceramics, few toxicological data are available in comparison with other heavy metals."

The article focuses on occupational health hazards, which are significant for people who are involved in the extraction of rare earth elements because,

"Generally, most RE deposits contain radioactive materials..."

The article summarises the problem and states that,

"...there are many environmental issues associated with RE production."

These environmental issues include water pollution and the destruction of farmland, both of which are associated with significant adverse health effects for the people living in the vicinity of such facilities.

It is clear that chemicals have been exploited by many industries; this includes the military that has taken advantage of the nature of certain chemicals, such as sulphur and saltpetre (potassium nitrate), for example, that were used in the manufacture of explosives. The chemical industry has also directly assisted the military; for example, with the production of chlorine gas for use as a chemical weapon during WWI. Although weapons of the 21st century involve highly advanced forms of technology, many chemicals are still utilised by the military.

One surprising area in which the chemical industry has cooperated with the military is in the field of intelligence; there is ample evidence that many intelligence agencies have employed a variety of chemicals for use in certain applications. In their book entitled *Acid Dreams*, authors Martin A Lee and Bruce Shlain explain that, in both America and Germany, scientists have experimented with chemicals to ascertain their usefulness during interrogation and for more nefarious purposes, such as 'mind control',

> "The navy became interested in mescaline as an interrogation agent when American investigators learned of mind control experiments carried out by Nazi doctors at the Dachau concentration camp during World War II."

After WWII, many German scientists were taken to the US under Operation Paperclip in order to assist the Americans in a variety of programmes, the best-known of which is the American space programme; but these programmes also included the development and testing of chemicals for their potential use as 'truth drugs'. In 1942, William Donovan of the OSS (Office of Strategic Services), the precursor of the CIA, requested that a group of prestigious scientists undertake some top-secret research. In *Acid Dreams*, the authors state that the purpose of this mission,

> "...was to develop a speech-inducing drug for use in intelligence interrogations."

The research extended beyond the field of interrogation; it moved into the fields of behaviour modification and mind control under a number of different projects, the best known of which is Operation MKULTRA. In his book entitled *Operation Mind Control*, author Walter Bowart includes a copy of a document that lists the drugs used by the CIA in their many human experiment programmes that were designed to investigate the ability to influence, interrogate and control people. The list comprises 139 substances that include heroin, cannabis, cocaine, quinine, strychnine and morphine.

Although often referred to as a separate entity from the 'chemical industry' as a whole, the pharmaceutical industry is, in reality, an integral part of the chemical industry. It should not be surprising therefore, that a number of pharmaceutical drugs were included amongst the substances tested in those experiments. The 'medicines' listed include epinephrine, insulin, novocaine and chloral hydrate.

The participants in these experiments were often military personnel and invariably volunteers, although they were generally kept ignorant of the nature of the substances they were 'testing' on the basis of the claim that it was a matter of 'national security'.

Legislation was introduced in the US to regulate the use of illegal drugs by the general public in the 1960s; it would seem, however, that the military and CIA programmes were exempted from these restrictions, as the authors of *Acid Dreams* explain,

> "The CIA and the military were not inhibited by the new drug laws enacted during the early 1960s."

It would seem that they were not accountable under any other regulations either, as the authors continue,

> "The FDA simply ignored all studies that were classified for reasons of national security, and CIA and military investigators were given free rein to conduct their covert experimentation."

One of the many substances tested by the military, in their search for substances that could assist them to extract information and control subjects, was LSD (lysergic acid diethylamide). These experiments were conducted despite the claim that human experimentation is widely accepted as unethical. Nevertheless, as the authors state in *Acid Dreams*,

> "By the mid-1960s nearly fifteen hundred military personnel had served as guinea pigs in LSD experiments conducted by the US Army Chemical Corps."

However, LSD proved to be ineffective for intelligence gathering purposes, therefore it was decided to test a number of other drugs, one of which was heroin. This drug did prove useful, mainly because it is highly addictive; which meant that it allowed experimenters to 'control' their subjects by either providing or withholding the drug. The consequences of the change from LSD to heroin are described by Walter Bowart,

> "Simultaneously, as the LSD supply dried up, large supplies of heroin mysteriously became available. It was strong heroin, imported from the Golden Triangle in Southeast Asia (largely under CIA control)."

Clearly, 'mind control experiments' and 'the drugs trade' are huge subjects that are outside the intended scope of this book; they are, however, topics about which a great deal has been written; in addition to the books referred to above is *The Politics of Heroin* by Professor Alfred W McCoy. One of the reasons for referring to these topics in a discussion about the chemical industry, is to demonstrate that many human experiments have been conducted that were not intended to determine the safety, or potential health effects of chemicals.

It is clear that chemicals significantly contribute to pollution of the environment; which means that they significantly affect the health of the people who inhabit that environment; these effects are almost invariably detrimental.

One of the main priorities of huge corporations is to make profits for their shareholders; their efforts to maximise profits often involve minimising costs, especially when these costs are deemed unnecessary to the goods they produce and sell. The costs that would be considered 'unnecessary' will inevitably include those involved in processes to safely dispose of their toxic wastes, because, as Peter Montague indicates in his 1999 article,

> "In the short run, corporations that dump their toxic wastes into a river, or bury

them in the ground, make much more money than corporations that sequester and detoxify their wastes at great expense."

Dr Barry Commoner expands on this point in *Making Peace With the Planet*,

"The arithmetic is deadly: if the chemical industry were required to eliminate toxic discharges into the environment, the cost would render the industry grossly unprofitable."

These statements demonstrate the inherently dangerous nature of most of the substances manufactured by the chemical industry; many of these synthetic substances are used as ingredients in a wide variety of products and applications in everyday use.

Ionising Radiation

The 'natural' substances of which the Earth is comprised include radioactive materials, such as uranium and its decay products; these materials together with cosmic radiation from the sun and stars are collectively referred to as 'natural background radiation'. This type of radiation is known as 'ionising'; non-ionising radiation is discussed in the next section.

Scientists estimate that the Earth is approximately four and a half billion years old and that the first 'life-forms' emerged approximately three and a half billion years ago; natural background radiation therefore substantially pre-dates the existence of all living organisms. However, on the basis that living organisms have always co-existed with this 'background radiation', it is assumed that there is a 'safe' level of ionising radiation; but this is a mistaken assumption.

The NIRS (Nuclear Information & Resource Service) summarises the energy of ionising radiation on a web page entitled *Radiation*,

"Ionizing radiation can actually break molecular bonds causing unpredictable chemical reactions."

The NIRS fact sheet entitled *No Such Thing as a Safe Dose of Radiation* cites the work and words of a number of reputable scientists, one of whom is Dr Karl Z Morgan PhD, an American physicist who stated in 1978 that,

"There is no safe level of exposure and there is no dose of radiation so low that the risk of a malignancy is zero."

The term 'natural background radiation' has recently been redefined and expanded; as Dr Rosalie Bertell PhD explains in *No Immediate Danger*,

"Thorium, uranium, radium, radon gas and its radioactive daughter products are officially called 'natural background radiation' in nuclear jargon, even though they have been removed from their relatively harmless natural state deep in the earth."

Dr Bertell's use of the word 'relatively' indicates that, whilst they remained undisturbed deep within the earth, these naturally radioactive substances had a minimal impact on the environmental level of ionising radiation. This point is also made by the NIRS in their fact sheet entitled *Radiation Basics* that states,

"These substances were, with few exceptions, geologically isolated from the environment under layers of shale and quartz before human beings dug them up by the ton and contaminated the biosphere."

"Beginning in April of 1945 and continuing through July of 1947, eighteen men, women and even children, scattered in quiet hospital wards across the country, were injected with plutonium."

Unlike uranium, plutonium is not a naturally-occurring substance; it is only created within a nuclear reactor; however, like uranium, plutonium is radioactive and dangerous. There are a number of different isotopes of plutonium, one of which, plutonium-244, has a half-life of more than 80 million years.

Further investigations led Eileen Welsome to discover that the eighteen cases she had initially uncovered represented only a small fraction of the total number of people used as 'guinea pigs' for radiation experiments, as she explains,

"It turned out that thousands of human radiation studies had been conducted during the Cold War. Almost without exception the subjects were the poor, the powerless and the sick..."

Further investigations reveal that civilians were not the only people used as 'test subjects' for radiation experiments. In their 1982 book entitled *Killing Our Own*, journalists Harvey Wasserman and Norman Solomon report their detailed investigations into many cases of US military personnel who had been exposed to radiation as the result of their duties that included 'clean-up' operations in Nagasaki and Hiroshima. These military personnel were also required to be in attendance in the vicinity of many nuclear bomb test detonations, especially the Nevada Test Site and the Marshall Islands in the Pacific Ocean. The authors describe some of the effects these men and women endured,

"Some developed terminal illnesses affecting bone marrow and blood production – the kind of biological problems long associated with radiation exposure."

These illnesses included certain types of cancer, as well as a number of debilitating conditions,

"Others found that at unusually early ages they were plagued by heart attacks, severe lung difficulties, pain in their bones or joints, chronic fatigue and odd skin disorders."

Although certain effects, particularly vomiting, were experienced immediately after their exposures, more serious effects developed years later; a situation that presented difficulties for the attempts to 'prove' that these illnesses had been the direct result of radiation exposure. Some veterans had realised that their exposure to radiation was the only possible cause of their severe health issues, but their requests for assistance from the VA (US Department of Veterans Affairs) were denied. They were told that radiation could not have caused their illness and that they had only been exposed to levels of radiation that were 'low' and below the level that had been proven to be 'safe'. The authors state that the veterans were,

"...consistently ignored and denied at every turn by the very institutions responsible for causing their problems."

One of the problems was that the 'authorities' had only considered the possibility of external exposures, for which dosimeter badges had sometimes been distributed to enable radiation levels to be monitored. However, and far more importantly, many veterans had also been exposed to internal radiation in the course of their duties. The source of their internal exposure was mainly from the inhalation of radiation-contaminated air; but those assigned clean-up duties in Hiroshima and Nagasaki would have also had internal exposures from the radiation-contaminated foods and drinks they consumed. The fact that radiation is undetectable by the senses meant that they were completely oblivious to the hazards they faced, until they began to experience a deterioration in their health and the onset of some very serious health problems. Radionuclides, when ingested, are known to cause serious damage to the soft tissues of which the body's organs are comprised; certain radionuclides cause damage to other parts of the body; strontium-90 for example, is known to damage bone.

The Nuremberg trials held after WWII resulted in a set of ethical guidelines for research experimentation that involved human participation; these guidelines, published in 1947, are referred to as the Nuremberg Code. One of the major principles of this Code is the requirement for informed consent; which means that all participants must be made fully aware of the nature of the experiment and provide their consent prior to participation. In the research for her book, Eileen Welsome discovered that the Nuremberg Code had frequently been flouted in the radiation experiments; a fact that had remained a secret for decades,

"The vastness of the human experimentation became clear only in 1994..."

The information was revealed in 1994 in a US GAO (General Accounting Office) Report entitled *Human Experimentation: An Overview on Cold War Programs*. The report includes the comment that,

"GAO discussed federal experimentation on humans for national security purposes..."

The report further states that,

"The tests and experiments involved radiological, chemical and biological research and were conducted to support weapon development programs..."

The period under review includes the years between 1940 and 1974; human experimentation conducted after 1947 would therefore have been subject to the Nuremberg Code; however, amongst its findings, the report states that,

"In some cases, basic safeguards to protect people were either not in place or not followed. For example, some tests and experiments were conducted in secret; others involved the use of people without their knowledge or consent or their full knowledge of the risks involved."

During their participation in the Manhattan Project bomb test experiments, many servicemen and servicewomen were sent to areas that were in close proximity to the site of explosions, but rarely were they fully informed of the potential hazards they faced; as reported by the authors of *Killing Our Own*. The dangers of radiation were known by the 1940s, but the bomb development programme was deemed to have priority, and was certainly considered to be more important than concerns about the consequences from increased environmental contamination with ionising radiation. This opinion was, of course, held mostly by people within the Manhattan Project and the military establishment.

Between 1945 and 1949, the US was the only country to have developed and tested nuclear bombs; however, and inevitably, other nations began to develop nuclear capabilities and create their own weapons programmes. The Soviet Union was the first of these other nations; their first bomb was detonated in August 1949; an event that added further to the tensions of the Cold War period and intensified the 'arms race' between these two 'superpowers'.

It is reported that hundreds of nuclear bombs were detonated in the atmosphere between 1945 and 1963, after which above ground testing was prohibited under the Partial Test Ban Treaty. But radiation hazards did not dissipate when the bomb tests ceased, as Dr Bertell explains,

> "In above-ground nuclear weapon testing, there is no attempt to contain any of the fission or activation products. Everything is released into the air and onto the land."

Radioactive materials have half-lives of different duration; however, they all decay into 'daughter products', some of which can be more dangerous that the 'parent'.

There are five countries referred to as 'nuclear weapon states'; these are the US, Russia, UK, France and China. The UK tested its first bomb in 1953, France in 1960 and China in 1964. Three more countries acknowledged to possess nuclear weapons are India, North Korea and Pakistan; it is claimed that Israel also possesses nuclear weapons, but that this has not been publicly acknowledged.

Unfortunately, the Partial Ban Treaty of 1963 only prohibited atmospheric tests; it did not prohibit underground or underwater tests, both of which continued. Furthermore, the treaty was only signed and agreed to by three nations; the US, Russia and the UK; France continued atmospheric testing until 1974 and China continued until 1980.

A Comprehensive Nuclear Test Ban Treaty was proposed in 1996 but, more than two decades later, it has yet to be enacted for the simple reason that it has not been ratified by all countries; the most significant country that has not ratified this treaty is the United States.

In addition to military personnel, there is another extremely significant group of people who have also been exposed to radiation discharged from the detonation of hundreds of nuclear bombs. This group comprises the entire civilian population of the world; none of whom has ever been fully informed about the hazards to which they have been and continue to be exposed. Nor is there any evidence that this group has ever given their informed consent to being irradiated. Within this group there is however, a much smaller group of civilians who have been subjected to higher levels of radiation exposure; these are the people who lived, and still live, 'downwind' of the various detonation sites around the world.

In *Killing Our Own*, the authors provide details of the numbers of bombs detonated each year by the US between 1945 and 1980; they total 691, of which 563 are reported to have been exploded at the Nevada Test Site. Dr Bertell reports in *No Immediate Danger* that epidemiological studies have discovered an increased incidence of health problems in the Nevada area; including significant increases in the incidence of cancers. Furthermore, she explains that,

> "The civilian population downwind of the Nevada test site was never warned of the health effects which might result from their exposure."

Some of these health effects are described by the authors of *Killing Our Own*,

> "...in one small community after another, people died from diseases rarely seen there before: leukemia, lymphoma, acute thyroid damage, many forms of cancer."

Although the immediate vicinity of a bomb test receives a more concentrated 'dose', the radiation released by the explosions does not remain in that location. The course taken by radiation is determined by the prevailing weather conditions; which means that radiation can spread for hundreds or even thousands of miles, as Dr Bertell explains,

> "The Nevada nuclear tests have spread radiation poisons throughout central and eastern United States and Canada and produced in the stratosphere a layer of radioactive material which encircles the globe."

The health hazards associated with exposure to ionising radiation are acknowledged by the WHO in the April 2016 fact sheet entitled *Ionizing radiation, health effects and protective measures*,

> "Beyond certain thresholds, radiation can impair the functioning of tissues and/or organs..."

It is clear from this statement that the medical establishment still follows the notion that there is a 'safe' threshold level of exposure, despite abundant evidence to the contrary.

The Environmental Health and Safety (EHS) department of the University of Washington published a 2006 report entitled *Biological Effects of Ionizing Radiation*, which contains extracts from a 1990 FDA report of the same name. The EHS report refers to the existence of knowledge about the dangers of exposure to high levels of radiation long before the first nuclear bombs were tested and states that,

> "Early human evidence of harmful effects as a result of exposure to radiation in large amounts existed in the 1920s and 1930s, based upon the experience of early radiologists, miners exposed to airborne radioactivity underground, persons working in the radium industry and other special occupational groups."

The belief in the existence of a 'safe' dose or exposure unfortunately resulted in a serious delay to the discovery of the harm that low level exposures could cause, as the report states,

> "The long term biological significance of smaller, repeated doses of radiation, however, was not widely appreciated until relatively recently..."

The report claims that most of the existing knowledge has developed since the 1940s. It must be emphasised that small doses do not have to be repeated in order to be able to cause harm. The report discusses those most at risk from low exposures,

"...embryonic and fetal tissues are readily damaged by relatively low doses of radiation."

Dr John Gofman, who earned his PhD in nuclear and physical chemistry and later qualified as a medical doctor, had been involved with the Manhattan Project and had originally been supportive of atomic energy. In 1963 he was asked by the AEC (Atomic Energy Commission) to head a programme to study the effects of man-made radiation, the result of which was anticipated by the AEC to support the planned expansion of the use of nuclear energy for 'peaceful purposes'. The authors of *Killing Our Own* report that the study did not support the AEC, but that its conclusions led Dr Gofman and his team in 1969 to recommend,

"...a tenfold reduction in the AEC's maximum permissible radiation doses to the general public from nuclear reactors."

The result of his work led Dr Gofman to recognise that there is no safe dose of radiation; he is quoted in the NIRS fact sheet to have stated in 1990 that,

"...the safe-dose hypothesis is not merely implausible – it is disproven."

In a 1994 interview with *Synapse*, a publication of the University of California, Dr Gofman referred to his long-held criticisms of the DoE and the AEC, its predecessor. He also referred to the human body's ability to repair a certain level of radiation damage and stated that, if the biological repair mechanisms are working perfectly,

"Then a low dose of radiation might be repaired."

This does not mean that a low dose is 'safe', but that in the absence of other serious health issues, the body may be able to heal damage caused by a low level of radiation.

Dr Ernest Sternglass PhD is another decades-long critic of the nuclear establishment and their efforts to play down the dangers of ionising radiation. In *Secret Fallout*, he demonstrates that, devastating though the immediate effects of nuclear bombs are, the more insidious, long-term and disastrous effects are from radioactive 'fallout',

"By 1953, it was already known that many of the radioactive elements (called isotopes) created by an atomic explosion, once they entered the atmosphere in the form of tiny fallout particles, would contaminate food, water and air and thus find their way into the human body."

This is precisely the route by which the veterans had received their internal exposures to radioactive particles. The establishment defines radioactivity as,

"disintegration of the nuclei of certain elements, with the emission of energy in the form of alpha, beta or gamma rays."

Ionising radiation is 'energy' emitted with the power to break molecular bonds, as described at the beginning of this section. When the energy breaks molecular bonds, it can dislodge electrons from an atom. These free electrons become electrically charged and highly reactive. Although referred to as 'free radicals', these free electrons are far more dangerous and cause far more harm than 'free radicals' generated by metabolic processes.

The scientific and medical establishment have denied for many decades that low level ionising radiation is dangerous; they have continued to assert that there is a 'safe' threshold, despite substantial evidence to the contrary. This situation is, however, changing; as indicated by the WHO fact sheet that admits,

"Low doses of ionizing radiation can increase the risk of longer term effects such as cancer."

Interestingly, a definitive refutation of the claim of the existence of a 'safe' level of ionising radiation has been published by the prestigious NAS (National Academy of Scientists). A 2005 report entitled *Low Levels of Ionizing Radiation May Cause Harm* is the 7th in a series on the topic of the biological effects of ionising radiation. This report is available from the NAS website and accompanied by a Press Release statement that quotes the words of the committee chair,

"The scientific research base shows that there is no threshold of exposure below which low levels of ionizing radiation can be demonstrated to be harmless or beneficial."

In other words, the scientific establishment has finally admitted that there is no 'safe' level of exposure to ionising radiation.

It should be noted that this statement also acknowledges that no level of ionising radiation is 'beneficial'. Yet, despite this statement, which was made in 2005, the 2016 WHO fact sheet refers to 'beneficial applications' of ionising radiation in medicine; the fact sheet also indicates the immense scale of the field of nuclear medicine,

"Annually worldwide, more than 3600 million diagnostic radiology examinations are performed, 37 million nuclear medicine procedures carried out and 7.5 million radiotherapy treatments are given"

Nuclear medicine is clearly of great financial benefit to the nuclear industry, which may explain the reluctance to recognise the scientific findings of the NAS report that stated no dose of ionising radiation can be demonstrated to be harmless or beneficial.

The idea that ionising radiation could be useful in the field of 'medicine' arose from the work of Marie and Pierre Curie, who had observed that exposures to radium had caused the death of 'diseased' cells. The long-held but incorrect beliefs about 'diseases' and methods of treatment have been discussed and will be discussed in more detail in chapter ten. Nevertheless, the widespread medical belief that 'disease' must be attacked and destroyed, naturally encouraged the idea that radioactive materials may be useful in the continuing 'battle' against disease. The problems arising from the use of radiation in the treatment of cancer are discussed in chapter seven.

There are other medical applications of ionising radiation, in addition to its use for diagnostic examinations and for treatments. One of these applications is the 'sterilisation' of medical supplies; however, although this may not result in a direct exposure there are indirect hazards due to the existence of radionuclides in the working environment. In his book *In Pursuit of Justice*, consumer advocate Ralph Nader states in his 2001 essay entitled *Irradiation Craze* that,

"Between 1974 and 1989 alone, forty-five accidents and violations were recorded at US irradiation plants, including those used to sterilise medical supplies."

Another application of ionising radiation, and one that is wholly inappropriate, is food irradiation. The FDA website contains a page entitled *Food Irradiation: What You Need to Know* that claims irradiated foods do not become radioactive; it also states that food irradiation,

"...is a technology that improves the safety and extends the shelf life of foods by reducing microorganisms and insects."

This is clearly yet another application of the 'germ theory' and the obsession with killing 'germs'. According to the FDA,

"...irradiation can make food safer."

Nothing could be further from the truth. Food irradiation is not only entirely inappropriate, it is also highly dangerous. Irradiation affects foods at an absolutely fundamental level, as Ralph Nader also reports in his essay,

"We do know that irradiation destroys essential vitamins and minerals in foods..."

The detrimental effects of irradiation are reported by the Center for Food Safety (CFS) on a page entitled *About Food Irradiation* that states,

"Radiation can do strange things to food...."

A 2006 report entitled *Food Irradiation: A Gross Failure*, published by the CFS in conjunction with Food and Water Watch, refers to the many research studies that have demonstrated that the irradiation process has detrimental effects on the flavour, odour, appearance and texture of foods; these changes indicate that the foods have been dramatically altered. Furthermore, the destruction of vitamins and minerals means that these 'food products' can no longer be considered capable of providing nourishment. The result of all these alterations caused by irradiation means that the products subjected to this unnatural process cannot be regarded as 'food' suitable for human consumption.

An even more worrying discovery is that, according to the CFS web page,

"Research also shows that irradiation forms volatile toxic chemicals such as benzene and toluene..."

The serious health hazards associated with these highly toxic chemicals have been previously discussed.

The nuclear industry is clearly immense; but it is also supported by a number of extremely powerful international bodies, especially the International Atomic Energy Agency (IAEA), a UN organisation created in 1957. The objectives of the IAEA are stated to be,

"The Agency shall seek to accelerate and enlarge the contribution of atomic energy to peace, health and prosperity throughout the world."

These are indeed lofty aims; however, the reality of the situation is that 'atomic energy' is entirely unable to achieve them.

First of all, nuclear power has its origins within the military industry and the production of weapons of mass destruction. The proliferation of nuclear weapons continued to expand beyond 1957 when the IAEA was formed; the existence of thousands of nuclear weapons that have the power to destroy the world many times over cannot be called a 'peaceful' contribution to the world. It is usually claimed that these highly destructive weapons are powerful 'deterrents' against nuclear war; this argument is disingenuous, the fact that they remain in existence means that they could be used.

Secondly, atomic energy generation does not and cannot contribute to improved health. Ever since the creation and detonation of the first bomb in July 1945, the environmental level of ionising radiation has increased. But, as has been asserted by many eminently qualified scientists, there is no safe level of exposure to ionising radiation; which means that increasing levels of radiation in the environment exacerbate health problems. Furthermore, as confirmed by the NAS report, no level of radiation is beneficial.

The third claim, which is that atomic energy contributes to world prosperity, is made on the basis of the idea that atomic energy is a cheap method for generating electricity. This too is a false notion, as Dr Bertell explains,

"...no country has been able to develop a commercially viable nuclear industry. The industry is kept alive by the will of governments through taxpayer subsidies."

If the true costs were included within the price of electricity, consumers would soon realise that it is not the cheap source of power it is claimed to be; the existence of subsidies masks the real costs.

These three claims made by the IAEA about the alleged advantages of nuclear power appear to be based more on PR than science and reality. However, the consequences from the use of atomic energy to produce electricity extend far beyond its failure to be commercially viable; nuclear power plants are accompanied by many hazards that include the continual release of ionising radiation; Dr Bertell explains,

"It is not possible to operate a nuclear plant without any releases of fission fragments and activation products (also called radionuclides and radioactive chemicals)."

Many of the dangers posed by nuclear power reactors are reported by Beyond Nuclear; one of their pamphlets, entitled *Routine Radioactive Releases from US Nuclear Power Plants*, includes the following statement,

"Every nuclear power reactor dumps radioactive water, scatters radioactive particles, and disperses radioactive gases as part of its routine, everyday operation."

Furthermore, nuclear power plants only have a limited lifespan after which they are decommissioned; but this too is highly problematic because there is no safe method of disposal of radioactive materials, some of which have incredibly long half-lives that can be in the thousands, millions or even billions of years.

The hazards caused by nuclear power plants are not restricted to the discharges of radioactive materials during the course of their 'normal' operations; there have been many accidents that have exacerbated the problem of environmental contamination with ionising radiation. The three main accidents that have been reported were those that occurred in 1979 at Three Mile Island; in 1986 at Chernobyl; and in 2011 at Fukushima.

Each of these accidents should have brought the nuclear power industry to a grinding halt. But, whilst they have generated some reluctance within certain countries to proceed with the development of nuclear energy production, these accidents have not generated a sufficient level of public outrage with a demand for nuclear power to be ceased with immediate effect. The main reason for a lack of outrage is because the public is deliberately misinformed about the full extent of the dangers associated with nuclear power generation.

In addition to these 'big' accidents, there have been a number of 'small' accidents, some of which have been reported to have been 'contained'; although this does not necessarily mean that they have been made 'safe'. The total number of 'small' accidents is however, entirely unknown; their existence remains largely undisclosed, as Dr Bertell states,

"Many military accidents have gone unreported, shrouded in secrecy for 'national security' reasons."

The fundamental problem with the nuclear industry is that it is inextricably connected to the military industry; or more correctly to the military-industrial complex. In fact, many industrialists are reported to have taken a keen interest in nuclear power at a very early stage of its development, as the authors of *Killing Our Own* state,

"To astute financiers, the late 1940s signalled prospects for huge profits to be made from nuclear investments."

In their book, the authors refer to a number of large US corporations that became interested in industrial uses for nuclear power; many of these corporations remain household names.

The justification for the continuing existence of a huge nuclear arsenal is the idea that they are a deterrent against war. However, although nuclear war is an extremely frightening prospect as it has the potential to annihilate the entire world population, the very real and far more immediate danger for humanity is the continuing contamination of the environment with ionising radiation. It has been acknowledged that the greatest exposures to ionising radiation resulted from nuclear bomb tests, as indicated by the 2000 *Report of the United Nations Scientific Committee on the Effects of Atomic Radiation to the General Assembly* that states,

"The man-made contribution to the exposure of the world's population has come from the testing of nuclear weapons in the atmosphere from 1945 to 1980."

To this must be added the continual discharge of radioactive materials from nuclear power stations, as well as exposures to ionising radiation from other sources, especially radiology examinations with X-rays and radiotherapy treatments.

The idea that carbon dioxide poses the greatest threat to humanity is clearly ludicrous by comparison to the very real threat posed by ionising radiation, which has been proven by many eminent scientists to be hazardous at any level of exposure.

During 2017 however, hopes were raised that nuclear weapons might finally be banned. A July 2017 page on the website of the United Nations proclaimed *Treaty adopted on 7th July* and explained,

"By resolution 71/258, the General Assembly decided to convene in 2017 a

United Nations conference to negotiate a legally binding instrument to prohibit nuclear weapons leading towards their total elimination."

The treaty was endorsed by 122 of the 192 UN Member States. However, and most significantly, all NATO (North Atlantic Treaty Organization) countries, with the sole exception of the Netherlands, failed to participate in the conference. Although the Netherlands attended the conference, they did not endorse the treaty. Unsurprisingly, the countries that did not attend the conference included the nine countries, referred to earlier in this discussion, known to possess nuclear weapons.

The New York Times reported the result of the conference and treaty in an article entitled *A Treaty Is Reached to Ban Nuclear Arms. Now Comes the Hard Part* that states,

"Some critics of the treaty, including the United States and its close Western allies, publicly rejected the entire effort, calling it misguided and reckless..."

The article also reports that the US, Britain and France, three of the major nuclear 'powers', issued a joint statement that they,

"...do not intend to sign, ratify or ever become party to it."

It is, however, the retention of these deadly weapons that is reckless, not efforts to eliminate them.

Clearly the nations that possess nuclear arsenals refuse to acknowledge that lives are endangered by their decisions; it is no exaggeration to state that the fate of the world population rests in the hands of those who are in charge of these nations. The point they seem to fail to appreciate is that there could be no winner of such a war. They also fail to acknowledge that their actions continue to endanger the health of the entire population of the world; including those in charge of the weapons programmes; they are not 'immune' to the health hazards caused by ionising radiation.

Non-Ionising Radiation

The 'electromagnetic spectrum' is the term used to refer to the entire range of electromagnetic (EM) radiation, each type of which is described by reference to a specific range of frequencies and wavelengths.

The types of EM radiation that have the highest frequencies, shortest wavelengths and sufficient energy to break molecular bonds are referred to as 'ionising radiation', as previously discussed. All other types of EM radiation have a wide range of frequencies and wavelengths, but do not have sufficient energy to break molecular bonds; these are collectively referred to as 'non-ionising radiation', which is defined on the WHO web page entitled *Radiation, Non-ionizing* as,

"...the term given to radiation in the part of the electromagnetic spectrum where there is insufficient energy to cause ionization. It includes electric and magnetic fields, radio waves, microwaves, infrared, ultraviolet and visible radiation."

Clearly, therefore, there are many different types of 'non-ionising' radiation, but the fact that they do not cause ionisation does not mean that they are harmless.

In common with ionising radiation, non-ionising radiation, with the exception of visible light, is undetectable by the senses; as Dr Robert Becker

energy to function, as Dr Becker states in *Cross Currents,*

"The body's internal energetic control systems are subtle, and they operate with minute amounts of electromagnetic energy."

He adds that,

"A little goes a long way, and very often, more is not better."

It is clear from the growing body of evidence that 'more' EM radiation has been proven to be decidedly harmful.

Unfortunately, the situation is likely to worsen with the continuing development of new technologies; as indicated by the WHO web page entitled *Electromagnetic fields* that states,

"Electromagnetic fields of all frequencies represent one of the most common and fastest growing environmental influences about which anxiety and speculation are spreading. All populations are now exposed to varying degrees of EMF, and the levels will continue to increase as technology advances"

The reference to the spread of 'anxiety and speculation' indicates that the WHO does not accept the huge body of scientific evidence that demonstrates conclusively that artificial EMFs cause many adverse health effects. It also indicates that by ignoring the evidence the WHO is failing to fulfil its stated aim to achieve 'health' for everyone.

The powerful electromagnetic fields that radiate from the plethora of telecommunications and electrical power sources can and do disrupt the body's bio-electrical system at the cellular level. In his 2012 article entitled *The Biological Effects of Weak Electromagnetic Fields*, Dr Andrew Goldsworthy PhD summarises the situation and states that,

"...the evidence that alternating electromagnetic fields *can* have non-thermal biological effects is now overwhelming."

The studies included in the BioInitiative Report refer to a variety of non-thermal effects that can induce a wide range of symptoms, some of which may be mild, such as headaches, others may be far more serious, such as heart problems and cancers. Dr Goldsworthy explains the effects that occur at a cellular level,

"The explanation is that it is not a heating effect but mainly an electrical effect on the fine structure of the electrically-charged cell membranes upon which all living cells depend."

The magnitude of the effect will depend upon which part of the body is affected. As will be further discussed in chapter seven, the endocrine system is particularly sensitive and can be disrupted by exposure to EM radiation. All hormones are important; any disruption to their production and release, whether from chemical or electrical influences, will affect the body's ability to function properly. However, disruption to the production of melatonin can have a significant impact on a number of important functions. In his 2002 article entitled, *EMF/EMR Reduces Melatonin in Animals and People*, Dr Neil Cherry explains the range of possible effects from low levels of melatonin in the body,

"...reduced melatonin output causes many serious biological effects in humans and other mammals, including sleep disturbance, chronic fatigue, DNA damage leading to cancer, cardiac, reproductive and neurological diseases and mortality."

Melatonin is an extremely potent antioxidant; inadequate levels of this important hormone can therefore result in increased levels of metabolic free radicals that can cause damage at a cellular level. As Dr Cherry indicates, the damage from insufficient melatonin and excess free radicals can lead to cancer. The association between exposures to EM radiation and cancer is demonstrated by the IARC classification of RF and ELF as 'possible' human carcinogens; the BioInitiative Report however, states the case rather more strongly,

"There is little doubt that exposure to ELF causes childhood leukaemia."

Exposure to ELF generates elevated risks for a number of types of cancer, but most of them develop slowly over the course of a number of years. This means that the likelihood of associating a person's prior exposure to EM radiation with the later onset of cancer is fairly slim; however, exposure to EM radiation is only one of many factors that contribute to the development of cancer, as discussed in more detail in chapter seven.

In a disturbingly familiar situation, certain frequencies of 'non-ionising' radiation are utilised by the medical establishment in certain applications, most of which are based on the ability of these frequencies to produce heat in the body.

One of the first applications to be developed was 'diathermy', which is the use of radio wave frequencies for the 'treatment' of a number of different conditions, which originally included arthritis, migraine headaches and cancer. Dr Becker explains the origin of diathermy in *Cross Currents* and states that, in the late 1920s, workers at a factory that was developing an experimental radio transmitter with a high frequency began to feel ill. The most significant symptom they experienced was a raised body temperature, or fever, which the medical establishment of the period attributed to being a 'good' reaction to illness and injury. This led to the idea that heat could be induced using these radio frequency waves, which, in turn, led to the development of 'diathermy' as a method for treating various conditions of illness. Dr Becker notes that diathermy can produce a number of 'undesirable side effects', which include sweating, weakness, nausea and dizziness. Diathermy continues to be used, although for a smaller range of ailments; it is now mainly used as a method of treatment for muscle and joint conditions.

A more recent medical application that uses EM radiation as a method to induce heat is called 'hyperthermia', which is a cancer treatment that utilises certain frequencies to heat cancer cells in order to kill them. Hyperthermia refers to an elevated body temperature; hypothermia is the term that refers to a low body temperature. An ACS article entitled *Hyperthermia to Treat Cancer* states that,

"Radio waves, microwaves, ultrasound waves, and other forms of energy can be used to heat the area."

The idea on which this treatment is based is that tumours have a high water content and are therefore susceptible to high heat, however, the ACS admits that there are side effects from this treatment but claims that,

"Most side effects don't last long, but some can be serious."

Hyperthermia treatment can be applied to large or small areas of the body; when applied to a small area it is referred to as 'local hyperthermia', the side effects of which are described in the ACS article,

> "Local hyperthermia can cause pain at the site, infection, bleeding, blood clots, swelling, burns, blistering, and damage to the skin, muscles, and nerves near the treated area."

Although called 'side effects', it should be obvious that they are direct effects; they also provide a clear indication of the extent of the damage that this 'treatment' can cause.

Diathermy and hyperthermia are treatments that obviously rely on the heating effect of EM radiation frequencies; but, as demonstrated by many studies, 'heat' is not the only effect. Furthermore, and most importantly, the BioInitiative Report states unequivocally that some effects occur at levels far below that at which heating occurs, as indicated by the so-called 'side effects' listed above. Yet, as demonstrated by the WHO fact sheet, the medical establishment refuses to acknowledge the existence of these non-thermal effects; the 'attractiveness' of the technology has yet again overpowered the objective contemplation of possible adverse effects and their detrimental consequences for health.

Another example of a medical technology that uses EM radiation, although not for the 'heating effect', is MRI (Magnetic Resonance Imaging), which is described on the NHS web page entitled *MRI scan* as,

> "...a type of scan that uses strong magnetic fields and radio waves to produce detailed images of the inside of the body."

The dangers associated with X-rays and CT scans, both of which use frequencies in the ionising range of the electromagnetic spectrum, have led to the assumption that MRI scans are safer because they use frequencies in the 'non-ionising' range of the spectrum. The fact that the IARC has classified RF waves as a 'possible' carcinogen for humans should raise questions about the claim that MRI scans are 'safe'.

The Johns Hopkins Medicine Health Library web page entitled *How Does an MRI work?* states that they can be used for imaging any part of the body, including the brain and explains that,

> "The magnetic field, along with radio waves, alters the hydrogen atom's natural alignment in the body."

The radio waves are pulsed; when they are turned on, they cause the protons within the hydrogen atoms to be 'knocked out of alignment'; the protons realign when the waves are turned off. This is clearly an unnatural process; however, the UK NHS refers to it as,

> "...one of the safest medical procedures currently available."

The fact that many studies have demonstrated the adverse effects of RF waves at exposure levels that are orders of magnitude lower than those deemed 'safe', should raise serious and fundamental questions about the appropriateness of this procedure.

Although reports are occasionally published about the hazards associated with exposures to artificial EM radiation, there are a number of obstacles that impede public awareness of the full extent of the problem. Many of these obstacles have been recognised and explained in the BioInitiative Report in the *Summary for the Public*,

"The exposures are invisible, the testing meters are expensive and technically difficult to operate, the industry promotes new gadgets and generates massive advertising and lobbying campaigns that silence debate, and the reliable, non-wireless alternatives (like wired telephones and utility meters) are being discontinued against public will."

Another obstacle is that the work of scientists, who have discovered the adverse effects of exposures to EM radiation and attempt to inform the public, is discredited by other scientists who refute their findings. This problem is also explained in the BioInitiative Report *Summary*,

"Other scientific review bodies and agencies have reached different conclusions than we have by adopting standards of evidence so unreasonably high as to exclude any conclusions likely to lead to new public safety limits."

There are reasons that different scientists reach different conclusions; however, some of these reasons are not based in science nor are they based on the findings from scientific research. The BioInitiative Report lists 10 reasons, the most significant of which is a familiar obstacle to public awareness,

"Vested interests have a substantial influence on the health debate."

The main vested interests behind the censorship of information about the hazards of exposures to artificial EM radiation are, unsurprisingly, the technology and telecommunications industries. Another significant 'vested interest' with a strong influence over technology and the use of various electromagnetic frequencies, is the military industry, as explained by Dr Becker in *Cross Currents*,

"Military services of every country use all parts of the electromagnetic spectrum for communications and surveillance..."

It is important to reiterate that the problem is not 'technology' per se. The problems that exist have been caused by the type of technology that has been developed, together with the range of electromagnetic frequencies that have been used for the operation of those technologies; the effects they produce have been proven beyond doubt to be detrimental to health.

Despite the increasing volume of evidence that electromagnetic radiation in the radiofrequency range causes harm, new technologies that utilise these frequencies continue to be developed. The most significant development with respect to the current discussion is 5G, the new generation of telecommunications systems that has begun to be introduced earlier than had originally been planned. One of the most likely reasons for this early release, is to avoid the possibility that efforts to issue a moratorium until potential health hazards have been fully investigated will be successful.

The 'establishment' promotes 5G as able to facilitate faster speeds and greater capacity to meet increasing demand for access to wireless technologies; however, it should be noted that 5G will augment not replace the earlier generations of 2G, 3G and 4G. This means that 5G will involve chemicals found in association with fracking operations. The *Study* reports that,

"A list of 944 products containing 632 chemicals used during natural gas operations was compiled."

The *Study* acknowledges that this is not a complete list,

"...but represents only products and chemicals that we were able to identify, through a variety of sources, as being used by industry during natural gas operations."

The list of chemicals identified by the *Study* reveals that a significant percentage of them are highly toxic. These chemicals include arsenic, barium, benzene, cadmium, cyanide, fluoride, lead, mercury, methylene chloride, toluene, uranium, radium-226 and radium-228, which are some of the most dangerous substances known to science. Each of these 13 substances has been proven to be extremely toxic and highly dangerous; their combined toxicity is however, entirely unknown. There is no evidence that any tests have been conducted to determine the health effects from this combination, which it would be no exaggeration to describe as a highly lethal cocktail. Yet these deadly poisons, together with many hundreds of other chemicals, many of which remain undisclosed, have been pumped under the ground in order to extract oil and natural gas.

As part of their investigations, Dr Colborn and her colleagues obtained CAS (Chemical Abstract Service) numbers for 353 of the chemicals they had discovered were used in fracking operations. These CAS numbers enabled them to obtain further information, especially in respect of the adverse health effects associated with these chemicals, about which the *Study* states,

"...more than 75% of the chemicals on the list can affect the skin, eyes, and other sensory organs, the respiratory system, the gastrointestinal system and the liver."

These are not the only effects; the *Study* also discovered that,

"More than half the chemicals show effects on the brain and the nervous system."

The reported adverse health effects are those that have been shown to be associated with exposures to each individual chemical; there is no information about the health effects from exposures to any combinations of multiple chemicals.

The *Study* refers to some of the functions attributed to these chemicals to justify their use as ingredients of fracking fluids,

"Chemicals are added to increase the density and weight of the fluids in order to facilitate boring, to reduce friction, to facilitate the return of drilling detritus to the surface, to shorten drilling time, and to reduce accidents."

The reason that these processes are facilitated by some of the most toxic chemicals known to science remains unclear. Unsurprisingly though, the industry claims that fracking fluids do not pose any hazards to health, as the *Study* reports,

"Industry representatives have said there is little cause for concern because of the low concentrations of chemicals used in their operations."

This is clearly another practice that is based on the Paracelsus theory that a 'low dose' is not a 'poison'; but, as discussed, this theory is not only unproven it has been repeatedly demonstrated to be false. The *Study* confirms this stance in the statement that,

> "...pathways that could deliver chemicals in toxic concentrations at less than one part-per-million are not well studied and many of the chemicals on the list should not be ingested at any concentration."

The previous discussion about chemicals showed that no chemical has been fully tested for all possible effects; but, more specifically, no chemical has been thoroughly tested at very low exposure levels to determine its effects on the endocrine system. This means that the oil and gas industry's assertion that there is no need for concern about the low concentrations of chemicals is unfounded. Many of the scientific studies that have been conducted demonstrate that, contrary to the industry's claim, there is a genuine cause for concern.

In addition, the assertion that fracking fluids only contain low concentrations of chemicals is disingenuous; fracking operations utilise millions of gallons of fluids, therefore a low concentration is not synonymous with a low volume. A 'low concentration' within millions of gallons of liquid can translate to hundreds if not thousands of gallons of fluids containing hundreds of different toxic chemicals. Yet no tests have been performed to determine the safety of these compounds or to investigate the possible health effects.

The existence of synergistic interactions between chemicals is well-known; some chemical interactions have been shown experimentally to produce a level of toxicity that is many times greater than would be expected by their combined toxicities. The extent and nature of all possible synergistic interactions between the hundreds of chemicals used in fracking fluids is entirely unknown; they have never been studied. As previously stated, science has no method to analyse multiple substances, which means that science is unable to determine the consequences arising from the chemical compounds used in fracking products. It is important to reiterate that the health of the environment and the health of the inhabitants of that environment are inextricably interconnected.

Although some aspects of fracking operations remain unknown, certain aspects are under investigation, the most important of which are the effects on human health; there is an increasing level of awareness that fracking operations are associated with increased health problems for people living in their vicinity. Even the medical establishment has reached a limited recognition of the risks posed to health by fracking operations; as indicated by an October 2016 article entitled *Fracking Linked to Cancer-Causing Chemicals, New YSPH Study Finds* published on the website of the Yale School of Public Health (YSPH). This article reports that more than 1,000 chemicals were examined in their analysis and states that,

> "An expansive new analysis by Yale School of Public Health researchers confirms that numerous carcinogens involved in the controversial practice of hydraulic fracturing have the potential to contaminate air and water in nearby communities."

The work of Dr Colborn and her colleagues demonstrates that the as reported in the *Study*,

> "In the eastern United States, and increasingly in the West, these chemicals are being re-injected underground, creating yet another potential source of extremely toxic chemical contamination."

The idea of burying 'waste' is not new; it is a method used for the disposal of 'ordinary waste', which has resulted in the huge and ever-increasing number of landfill sites that contaminate vast areas of land in most, if not all countries around the world.

Underground burial does not and cannot solve the problem of toxic waste; it merely relocates the problem. But this method also generates a further level of environmental contamination, the consequences of which are also unknown because they have not been studied. One inevitable impact of the burial of toxic substances will be on food crops grown in contaminated soil moistened by contaminated water. When buried underground, the toxic fluid wastes will also poison the myriad of organisms that dwell in the ground and are vital to the health of the soil.

Another method for the disposal of fracking wastewater is through sewage treatment plants. Fortunately, this is not a widely-used method because these treatment plants are unable to process and detoxify liquids contaminated with highly toxic chemicals. There are serious implications that arise from the inability of sewage or water treatment plants to detoxify chemicals; these are discussed in more detail later in this chapter.

In addition to contaminating water, the chemicals used in fracking operations also contaminate the air in the immediate vicinity. Some of the chemicals involved in these operations are classified as volatile organic compounds (VOCs); which means that they can readily become airborne. Not all VOCs are inherently toxic; however, the *Study* mentions certain VOCs that are known to be used in fracking operations and are known to be toxic,

> "In most regions of the country, raw natural gas comes out of the well along with water, various liquid hydrocarbons including benzene, toluene, ethylbenzene and xylene (as a group, called BTEX) hydrogen sulphide (H_2S), and numerous other organic compounds that have to be removed from the gas."

These VOCs can mix with other compounds, including any 'natural gas' that has escaped from the wells, and with diesel exhaust. The combination of these compounds produces 'ground level ozone', the dangers of which are also explained in the *Study*,

> "One highly reactive molecule of ground level ozone can burn the deep alveolar tissue in the lungs...Chronic exposure can lead to asthma...and is particularly damaging to children..."

This is not only dangerous to humans, as the *Study* also states,

> "Ozone not only causes irreversible damage to the lungs, it is similarly damaging to conifers, aspen, forage, alfalfa and other crops..."

One of the primary components of 'natural gas' is methane, which is a highly flammable gas that contributes further to the hazards associated with hydraulic fracturing. The March 2012 Food & Water Watch report refers to a number of incidents that have occurred as the result of the escape of methane gas from nearby fracking operations. In one of these incidents, a house is reported to have exploded due to the infiltration of highly-flammable methane gas into the water supplied to the house. In another incident, the contamination of the local water supply with 'natural gas' required the intervention of the EPA, whose officials instructed the local inhabitants not to drink the contaminated water. These are not isolated incidents; as the report indicates,

"ProPublica identified more than 1,000 cases of water contamination near drilling sites documented by courts, states and local governments around the country prior to 2009."

The Food & Water Watch group condemns fracking in that it entails,

"...a legacy of air pollution, water pollution, climate pollution and public health problems."

The main health problems associated with fracking operations are due to exposures to the toxic chemicals used in these operations that contaminate the water and air. But, as with deleterious effects caused by many pollutants, the health problems from exposures to toxic fracking fluids are unlikely to be recognised by physicians who are simply not trained to detect symptoms caused by chemical poisoning. People affected by these toxic substances will most likely be prescribed a pharmaceutical drug intended to alleviate their symptoms; but no drug can effectively 'treat' health damage that has been caused by chemical poisoning.

A further consequence of hydraulic fracturing operations is one that has serious repercussions for the entire region in which they are conducted. There is a growing body of evidence that fracking operations can generate increased earthquake activity. An April 2016 article entitled *Do fracking activities cause earthquakes? Seismologists and the state of Oklahoma say yes* states that,

"University of Calgary seismologist David Eaton says in the past six years, 90 percent of earthquakes larger that magnitude three taking place in the Western Canada Sedimentary Basin can be linked to fracking or waste water disposal."

The article also states that, in David Easton's opinion,

"...the earthquakes are being caused by changes in pressure underground."

There are clearly a large number of detrimental effects due to fracking operations that together far outweigh any of the purported benefits that the industry claims are gained.

It is obvious from their report about the impacts of fracking operations on drinking water that the EPA is aware that these operations can contaminate the environment; but this raises the question of why regulations have not been able to curb the polluting activities of the oil and gas industry. The alarming answer to this question is that, in the US, fracking operations have been excluded from certain aspects of legislation designed to protect the environment. The oil and gas industry clearly have very powerful lobbyists that have been extremely successful in protecting their clients. The *Study* explains the situation,

"In tandem with federal support for increased leasing, legislative efforts have granted exclusions and exemptions for oil and gas exploration and production

that has no qualms about using the planet as their experimental laboratory.

According to the Royal Society report, geoengineering interventions fall into two categories, which are labelled carbon dioxide removal (CDR) and Solar Radiation Management (SRM).

In addition to not being the cause of climate change, carbon dioxide is not dangerous; as the earlier discussion explained, it is essential for plant growth, which makes it essential for food production and therefore for life on planet Earth, as many living organisms are dependent on plants for their food supply. CDR procedures are clearly inappropriate; however, they are not the focus of this discussion.

Of particular concern are the interventions and technologies associated with the category of SRM, the function of which, according to the report, is to,

"...reduce the net incoming short-wave (ultra-violet and visible) solar radiation received, by deflecting sunlight, or by increasing the reflectivity (albedo) of the atmosphere, clouds or the Earth's surface."

The report acknowledges that SRM strategies would not address the alleged 'problem' of atmospheric levels of carbon dioxide; they are, however, intended to mitigate the effects. In other words, SRM interventions are intended to reduce the absorption of solar radiation in order to assist the process of cooling the Earth, despite the complete absence of evidence that the planet is undergoing 'unprecedented warming'.

The interventions suggested under the category of SRM include the use of 'stratospheric aerosols'; however, the report only discusses the use of sulphur-based chemicals such as hydrogen sulphide or sulphur dioxide, both of which are claimed to be able to induce a cooling effect. Significantly the report adds the comment that, although reference is only made to the use of sulphate particles,

"This does not mean that some other type of particle may not ultimately prove to be preferable to sulphate particles."

The evidence indicates that many other types of particle have proved to be preferable to sulphur-based substances.

Another 'suggested' SRM technique refers to the introduction of materials to act as sun-shields that will reflect solar radiation; one of the proposals for this technique includes the use of,

"a superfine mesh of aluminium threads..."

The reason for selecting aluminium is because it is a highly reflective metal.

The documentary film entitled *What In The World Are They Spraying* (WITWATS) was produced in 2010. The research for this film involved the attendance of the filmmakers at the February 2009 AAAS Geoengineering Conference, one of the main speakers at which was Professor David Keith, a key scientist in the field of geoengineering and a member of the working group that authored the 2009 Royal Society report.

The documentary refers to the work of a number of researchers, including former USDA biologist Francis Mangels PhD, who have independently collected soil and water samples from a variety of locations in the US, including snow from Mount Shasta, a pristine mountain range at a significant distance from industrial activities. The samples were analysed and demonstrated to contain unusually high concentrations of certain materials, most notably aluminium, but also barium and strontium. Dr Mangels also reported that his analysis over a period of years had demonstrated that the soil pH had altered so significantly that, instead of being acidic, it had become alkaline.

The researchers referred to in the WITWATS documentary are not the only ones to have analysed soil and water samples and found many anomalous results. These discoveries cannot be dismissed as irrelevant to the strategies to be employed in geoengineering programmes; the high concentration of aluminium in water and soil samples is highly correlated with the 'suggested' use of aluminium to reflect solar radiation.

Human intervention in the climate is not, however, a recent phenomenon; there are many historic precedents, as indicated by Professor James Fleming who, in his essay entitled *The Climate Engineers*, refers to,

"...the long and checkered history of weather and climate control..."

He explains that some of the earliest 'weather manipulation' experiments were conducted during the 19th century and that these were largely attempts to induce rain or to increase rainfall. He also indicates that rainmaking experiments continued into the 20th century, although the nature of the experiments changed with the introduction of new technologies.

An August 2001 article entitled *RAF rainmakers caused 1952 flood* reports that, on August 15th 1952, the English town of Lynmouth was hit by a 'flash flood' that has been described as one of the worst to have occurred. The article reports that, according to unearthed documents, 'rainmaking experiments' had been conducted by scientists and the British RAF during the two weeks prior to the flood. Although it is officially denied that these experiments caused the flood, the close timing of these events cannot be easily dismissed as a chance 'coincidence'.

Experiments of a similar nature have also been conducted in the US, especially by certain factions within the US military during the Cold War period. The reason that 'weather manipulation' interests the military is that the ability to control the weather is considered to be a very useful tool; it can be used to disrupt the operations of the enemy. It is officially reported that weather manipulation programmes were conducted during the Vietnam War. One of these programmes, codenamed Operation Popeye, involved a number of aircraft flights that released particles of silver iodide in order to increase precipitation and therefore disrupt the movements of the enemy.

It is clear therefore from these and many other examples that 'weather modification' techniques have been utilised, particularly by the military. However, these activities were ostensibly curtailed by the UN *Convention on the Prohibition of Military or Any Other Hostile Use of Environmental Modification Techniques* (ENMOD) that came into force in 1978. According to Professor Fleming, under the ENMOD Convention, the term 'environmental modification' means,

"...any technique for changing – through the deliberate manipulation of natural processes – the dynamics, composition or structure of the Earth, including its biota, lithosphere, hydrosphere and atmosphere, or of outer space."

The ENMOD treaty should therefore preclude all activities intended to deliberately manipulate the atmosphere or alter the weather or the climate; this would include all of the activities 'suggested' by climate scientists and reported in documents such as the Royal Society report. The evidence indicates that this treaty has at the very least been circumvented, if not completely disregarded, not only by scientists but also by the military. Although it is claimed that none of the suggested geoengineering techniques has been implemented, the evidence indicates otherwise.

There are a number of factors involved in presenting the evidence to support the claim that geoengineering is an active programme; one of these factors requires a discussion about aircraft trails. The term 'contrail' is defined by the US NOAA (National Oceanic and Atmospheric Administration) as follows,

"A contrail is the condensation trail that is left behind a passing jet plane."

The NOAA explains how these trails are formed,

"Contrails form when hot humid air from jet exhaust mixes with environmental air of low vapour pressure and low temperature."

It is clear therefore, that these trails are formed under specific atmospheric conditions; the NOAA describes their duration,

"The length of time that a contrail lasts is directly proportional to the amount of humidity that is already in the atmosphere."

This means that all aircraft flying within the same atmospheric conditions at similar altitudes ought to produce 'trails' that are very similar, if not the same, in appearance. Empirical evidence obtained from direct observation of aircraft in the sky demonstrates that this is not the case; different aircraft can be seen to leave different kinds of trails, despite flying at similar altitudes and in similar atmospheric conditions.

Some of these trails bear no resemblance to the 'contrails' described by the NOAA. Many aircraft eject long white trails that remain in the sky long after the planes have disappeared from view. Each trail continues to spread in width and often merges with other trails to form a misty white blanket across large regions of the sky. It should be noted that the Royal Society report suggests that 'cloud condensation nuclei' increase the formation of clouds, which reduce solar radiation.

These long white trails that are clearly not condensation trails have become known as 'chemtrails', which is not a recognised scientific term, mainly because the mainstream scientific community denies the existence of any trails other than ordinary 'contrails'. The reason they have become known as 'chemtrails' is because they contain a variety of chemical substances, including aluminium, barium, strontium and silver, which, although ejected by aircraft into the sky, do not remain there. These substances descend to the ground where they contaminate the soil and water, as indicated by the results of soil and water analyses.

Many of these substances are hazardous to health, but their dangers are exacerbated by the use of extremely fine particles, or nanoparticles as they are more correctly called. One of the metals detected in extremely high concentrations is aluminium, which, as previously discussed, is neurotoxic. Dr Russell Blaylock explains the dangers posed by nanoparticles of aluminium in his July 2013 article entitled *Impacts of Chemtrails in Human Health. Nanoaluminum: Neurodegenerative and Neurodevelopmental Effects*,

> "It has been demonstrated in the scientific and medical literature that nanosized particles are infinitely more reactive and induce intense inflammation in a number of tissues."

In his article, Dr Blaylock expresses his concerns about the adverse health effects on the neurological system due to exposures to aluminium nanoparticles,

> "Of special concern is the effect of these nanoparticles on the brain and spinal cord, as a growing list of neurodegenerative diseases, including Alzheimer's dementia, Parkinson's disease, and Lou Gehrig's disease (ALS) are strongly related to exposure to environmental aluminium."

A 2004 study by Mark Purdey reveals health hazards associated with some of the other toxic metals that have been found in unusually high concentrations, especially silver (Ag), barium (Ba) and strontium (Sr). The study is reported in his article entitled *Elevated silver, barium and strontium in antlers, vegetation and soil sourced from CWD cluster areas: do Ag/Ba/Sr piezoelectric crystals represent the transmissible pathogenic agent in TSEs?* CWD is chronic wasting disease, which is regarded as a TSE that is only experienced by certain types of deer. The discussion in chapter five about BSE referred to the claim that a protein called a 'prion' is regarded as the cause of all TSEs, but demonstrated that this is not the case. In the abstract of his article, Mark Purdey indicates clearly that 'atmospheric spraying' was not theoretical in 2004,

> "The elevation of Ag, Ba and Sr were thought to originate from both natural geochemical and artificial pollutant sources – stemming from the common practise of aerial spraying with 'cloud seeding' Ag or Ba crystal nuclei for rain making in these drought prone areas of North America, the atmospheric spraying with Ba based aerosols for enhancing/refracting radar and radio signal communications as well as the spreading of waste Ba drilling mud from the local oil/gas well industry across pastureland."

Although CWD is alleged to be restricted to certain members of the deer family, silver, barium and strontium have known adverse health effects for many living organisms, including humans.

Allan Buckmann trained as a US Air Force weather observer and worked in this field for the military during the early 1960s; he also trained as a wildlife biologist, which enabled him to recognise wildlife health problems. In his August 2012 article entitled *Chemtrail Whistleblower Allan Buckmann: Some Thoughts on Weather Modification* he states,

> "The cloud nuclei being used are composed of metallic salts in nano form, all potentially toxic to life as we know it. We have documented accumulations of aluminium, strontium, barium and many others in the soil, the rainwater, snow and plants at levels thousands of times higher than any normal condition, and many should not be present at all."

In the article he also refers to the replacement of sulphur-based materials with those of other metals,

"The USAF and NASA say aluminium coated fibreglass (chaff) is 20 times more reflective than sulphur and the metallic particles have strong electromagnetic properties."

The use of weather modification by the US military in programmes such as Operation Popeye, indicates that any technology with a perceived usefulness for their operations is invariably incorporated into military projects and programmes. Although geoengineering is claimed to be solely for the purpose of mitigating global warming, there is evidence that the military industry has developed climate intervention technologies that are capable of altering far more than just global temperatures and for more nefarious purposes. To discuss these purposes requires reference to another controversial programme, namely HAARP (High Frequency Active Auroral Research Program), which is described by co-authors Dr Nick Begich PhD and Jeane Manning, in their book entitled *Angels Don't Play This HAARP*, as,

"...a research program designed to study the ionosphere in order to develop new weapons technology."

The authors refer to the ionosphere as a shield that protects the planet from bombardment by high energy particles and explain that,

"The transmitter or HAARP device on the ground is a phased array antenna system – a large field of antennas designed to work together in focusing radio frequency energy for manipulating the ionosphere."

The discussion about non-ionising radiation highlighted the dangers of introducing 'unnatural' frequencies into the environment of the planet; this 'environment' is not restricted to the lower atmosphere. The potential hazards that could result from experimental manipulation of the ionosphere is further explained by Dr Begich in his article entitled *Ground Based 'Star Wars'*, in which he states that,

"The ionosphere is alive with electrical activity, so much so that its processes are 'non-linear'. This means that the ionosphere is dynamic, and its reactions to experiments are unpredictable."

The unpredictable nature of their experiments has rarely stimulated the scientific community, or the military, to proceed with caution or to consider the full extent of the potential consequences of their actions prior to conducting full-scale experiments; the detonation of the first nuclear bomb is a prime example.

The poor level of understanding about the nature of the climate system is also explained by Dr Begich and Jeane Manning, who state that,

"...leading edge scientists are describing global weather as not only air pressure and thermal systems, but also as an electrical system."

One of the key drawbacks of the early 'weather manipulation' techniques was their lack of ability to control and steer the weather systems they produced; this capability is, however, provided by HAARP. The ability to steer the weather is clearly unrelated to 'global warming', 'climate change' or to 'carbon dioxide removal'; it has a far more nefarious purpose that is described by Professor Gordon MacDonald in his 1968 essay entitled *How To Wreck the Environment,*

"Among future means of obtaining national objectives by force, one possibility hinges on man's ability to control and manipulate the environment of his planet."

Although wrecking the environment is not the intended goal of programmes designed to manipulate the environment, the techniques involved certainly have the ability to do so; as Professor MacDonald states,

"When achieved, this power over his environment will provide man with a new force capable of doing great and indiscriminate harm."

The main goal of these programmes is to develop technologies that can be used to achieve 'national objectives' through the use of force or the threat of force. It is for this reason that the main 'power' in this field is wielded by the military. This is further demonstrated by Dr Rosalie Bertell, who states in her 1996 article entitled *Background on the HAARP Project* that,

"Basic to this project is control of communications, both disruption and reliability in hostile environments."

In her book entitled *Chemtrails, HAARP, and the Full Spectrum Dominance of Planet Earth,* author Elana Freeland refers to patent #4,686,605 entitled *Methods and Apparatus for Altering a Region in the Earth's Atmosphere, Ionosphere, and/or Magnetosphere.* This patent was held by Bernard Eastlund, an American physicist and advocate of weather manipulation; it is claimed by Dr Begich that this patent is the basis for HAARP, although it is officially denied. The abstract of the patent states,

"The region is excited by electron cyclotron resonance heating to thereby increase its charged particle density."

Any technologies implemented in accordance with this patent would clearly contravene the terms of the ENMOD convention.

Elana Freeland explains in her book that HAARP can be used to heat the ionosphere, which would create high-pressure areas that can be used to move the jet stream. This can significantly alter the weather at specific locations to create floods or droughts, which, as indicated by Professor MacDonald, can be used to achieve 'national objectives' by a different type of 'force' than the usual tactics employed by the military.

Documents and information about technologies developed for use by the military are invariably kept secret under the rubric of 'national security'. Occasionally, however, useful information does become available; one example is a document entitled *Weather as a Force Multiplier: Owning the Weather in 2025,* a 1996 USAF research paper. The Executive Summary at the beginning of this document includes the following statement,

"A high-risk, high-reward endeavour, weather-modification offers a dilemma not unlike the splitting of the atom. While some segments of society will always be reluctant to examine controversial issues such as weather-modification, the tremendous military capabilities that could result from this field are ignored at our peril. From enhancing friendly operations or disrupting those of the enemy via small-scale tailoring of natural weather patterns to complete dominance of global communications and counterspace control. Weather-modification offers the war fighter a wide-range of possible options to defeat or coerce an adversary."

Prior to the implementation of any large-scale programme that conducts experiments to manipulate the climate and has the potential to affect the entire population of the world, there ought to be a public debate that would raise the essential question articulated by Professor Fleming in his previously cited essay,

"Who would be given the authority to manage it?"

With his knowledge of history, he supplies a response indicating the most likely candidates,

"If, as history shows, fantasies of weather and climate control have chiefly served commercial and military interests, why should we expect the future to be different?"

It is time to expect a different future and to wrest control over the climate of the planet out of the hands of the commercial and military interests! Although the geopolitical aspect of the efforts to control all of the resources of the world are beyond the intended scope of this book, further indications of the strategies involved and the manner in which they are promoted to the general public are discussed in chapters eight and nine.

It should be clear from the weight of evidence, only some of which has been presented in this discussion, that despite the establishment claims to the contrary, geoengineering is not a 'theoretical' programme; it is an active one with additional and far more sinister purposes than the stated objective of addressing the alleged problem of 'climate change'.

Poisoned Food

Food can be 'poisoned' in a few different ways, both directly and indirectly; the deliberate poisoning of food with intent to cause harm does not, however, form any part of this discussion.

Food can be directly, although unintentionally, poisoned by toxic substances used for other purposes; the spraying of food crops with pesticides, for example. Food crops can be indirectly poisoned by natural toxic substances within the environment, such as arsenic in the soil or water, or by unnatural toxic substances that have been released into the environment, radiation fallout, for example. Important and relevant though they all are, these ways in which food can be poisoned have been discussed elsewhere.

The purpose of the following series of discussions is to reveal another way in which certain foods are directly 'poisoned'; but before embarking on a discussion with the ominous title of 'poisoned food' it is important to clarify these terms to avoid misunderstanding.

The word 'poison' refers to a substance that interferes with the body's normal functions by causing damage to cells and tissues. The extent of the damage that a poison can inflict on the body depends mainly, but not entirely, on its innate toxicity; it also depends on other factors, as will be discussed in chapter ten.

It may be assumed that the meaning of the word 'food' is universally understood and requires no further clarification; but this would be a mistaken assumption, because the word is often applied to substances that do not conform to its true meaning. The fundamental purpose of food is to supply the body with the materials necessary for normal functioning; these materials are collectively known as 'nutrients'.

In his book entitled *Excitotoxins: The Taste That Kills*, Dr Russell Blaylock explains that,

"Every second of every day thousands of chemical reactions are taking place throughout every cell and in every tissue of the body."

He expands on this point and states that,

"The primary purpose of eating is to support these chemical reactions."

Dr Blaylock indicates that the reactions he refers to are 'biochemical' in nature rather than simply 'chemical'. Chemistry and biology are separate scientific disciplines, although they converge in the field of 'biochemistry', which is defined as the study of the chemistry of living organisms, as described on the Biochemical Society website that states,

"It is a laboratory based science that brings together biology and chemistry."

Laboratory experiments conducted by biochemists primarily involve the study of processes at the cellular and molecular level and of the substances necessary to those processes. These substances include proteins, many of which are essential for the body's biochemical reactions. However, investigations that are restricted to the study of isolated substances and processes within the confines of the laboratory, cannot facilitate a full understanding of their role in the complex, interconnected, self-regulating living organism that is the human body.

The body's biochemical reactions are supported by the chemicals obtained from food; but these chemicals must be in the 'right' form in order to be metabolised and utilised by the body to power the vital processes of life; Dr Blaylock explains,

"Many of the substances absorbed from our food play a vital role in the overall metabolic process of life."

It is clear therefore, that foods must provide the range of nutrients necessary to support those metabolic processes; which means that 'nutritious foods' are key elements of a 'healthy diet'. The medical establishment however, maintains a slightly different perspective; as indicated by the October 2018 WHO fact sheet entitled *Healthy diet*, which claims that,

"A healthy diet helps to protect against malnutrition in all its forms, as well as noncommunicable diseases (NCDs)..."

This is another demonstration of the medical establishment's incomplete understanding about nutrition, because a healthy diet does not merely 'help' to protect against 'disease'. Furthermore, according to the February 2018 WHO fact sheet entitled *Malnutrition*,

"Malnutrition refers to deficiencies, excesses, or imbalances in a person's intake of energy and/or nutrients."

The topic of malnutrition is discussed in chapter eight; however, it is important to make the point for the current discussion that the word does not merely refer to a deficiency of food. The claim by the WHO that malnutrition is the result of an imbalance in a person's intake of energy is also misleading. A calorie is a unit of 'energy', it is not a unit of 'nutrition'; these terms are not synonymous. It is possible for a 'foodstuff' to provide calories but not to contain any nutrients; a substance of this nature would not support the body's vital metabolic processes and cannot therefore be correctly described as 'food'.

The *Healthy diet* fact sheet does refer to aspects of a diet that are important, such as the consumption of fruit and vegetables; it also recommends that the intake of fats, free sugars and salt should be limited. This recommendation is supported by the February 2018 WHO fact sheet entitled *Obesity and overweight*, which suggests that the food industry can also assist by,

"...reducing the fat, sugar and salt content of processed foods."

The recommendation to reduce fat, sugar and salt intake suggests that these substances form part of a healthy diet, provided they do not exceed a certain level of intake, but this too is misleading. Although the request to the food industry to reduce them would be useful, it is inadequate, because excess fat, sugar and salt content are not the only problems associated with manufactured food products, as the discussions in the following sections will demonstrate.

The body absorbs and metabolises foods in order to extract the nutrients; however, processed food products manufactured by the food industry contain various synthetic chemicals that are used in production processes to perform certain 'technological functions', as will be discussed. These synthetic chemicals do not contribute to the nutritional content of foods, but they are not harmless. Any chemical food ingredient that is not a nutrient can react with other substances within the body, but these reactions are not part of the body's normal and vital metabolic processes. Instead, the 'non-nutrient' chemicals can interfere with 'normal' processes at the cellular level; it is wholly appropriate, therefore, to describe these chemicals as 'poisons'.

The food industry is immense; it is reported to be one of the largest industries in the world. It is certainly regarded as one of the most important, mainly because it is claimed that the food industry is vital to ensure a continuing supply of food for the ever-increasing population of the world. The theory on which this claim is based is seriously flawed, as will be explained in more detail in chapter eight.

The manufacture of food is governed by a variety of laws and regulations that were created to ensure that food products meet certain criteria, which include the requirements for food to be 'safe' and fit for consumption. One of the main reasons for the original introduction of food legislation was to address the problem of food adulteration, which generally entails the addition of ingredients that make the resulting product of a lower quality than it is perceived to be. Although the adulteration of food can involve the use of toxic substances, this is not always the case; for example, in the 19th century it was a not uncommon practice to add chicory as a 'filler' ingredient to coffee. The resulting product had certainly been adulterated because it was no longer 'pure' coffee; however, chicory is not toxic, therefore the coffee had not been 'poisoned'.

Unlike most 21st century food outlets, the grocery shops of earlier periods did not sell many pre-packaged goods; instead they mainly held loose commodities that were sold in the quantities requested by customers. This situation provided opportunities for some of the more unscrupulous traders to increase their profits by adulterating their loose commodities with cheap 'filler' ingredients. Unfortunately, not all adulterations were as innocuous as the addition of chicory to coffee.

The practice of adulteration in England was first exposed in the early 19th century by Friedrich Accum, a German chemist who lived and worked in London. In 1820 he wrote a book entitled, *A Treatise on Adulterations of Food and Culinary Poisons*, the purpose of which he claimed was,

"...to put the unwary on their guard against the use of such commodities as are contaminated with substances deleterious to health."

He provides a number of examples of contaminated foods,

"Our pickles are made green by copper, our vinegar rendered sharp by sulphuric acid...."

Other examples include such delights as custard poisoned with laurel leaves, tea falsified with sloe leaves, pepper mixed with floor sweepings and sweets dyed red with lead. None of these examples are mere 'adulterations'; the foods had been contaminated by substances that were decidedly 'deleterious to health' and are clear examples of 'poisoned food'.

Another form of adulteration perpetrated by unscrupulous traders was the addition of ingredients to a food that had perished, and should therefore no longer have been available for sale. Friedrich Accum reports that an example of this form of adulteration involved the addition of either rice powder or arrowroot to bad milk, which was then sold as 'cream'. This practice was clearly intended to deceive the public about the quality of the product but the added ingredients did not poison the basic food; their purpose was to mask the fact that it was not fit for consumption.

Friedrich Accum left England in 1821 and the battle against food adulteration was temporarily suspended. It was, however, resumed in the 1850s by Thomas Wakley, a surgeon and the founder of *The Lancet*, and Dr Arthur Hill Hassall, a physician. Together these men investigated a number of foods and discovered many that had been adulterated; their findings were published in *The Lancet*. The investigations conducted by these men and other food safety campaigners, such as John Postgate, finally led to the enactment of legislation, namely the 1860 Food Adulteration Act, which was the first in a series of laws passed in England in the effort to protect the integrity of foods.

Food adulteration was not exclusive to England; the battle against the problem in America was led by Dr Harvey Washington Wiley MD, who is regarded as the foremost pioneer of the effort to protect the safety of food in the US. The result of his work and campaigning was the enactment of legislation, the 1906 Pure Food and Drug Act, which also enabled the

materials, are not the same as natural chemicals. However, this does not mean that 'natural' is synonymous with harmless; previous discussions have demonstrated that many natural substances are extremely toxic. Of particular importance is that the synthetic compounds used in the manufacture of food products are often derived from petrochemicals, which are inherently toxic to the human body and therefore totally unsuitable for human consumption.

The EFSA acknowledges, to a certain extent, that some chemicals may cause 'effects' but claims that they are not harmful,

"...unless we are exposed to them for a long time and at high levels."

The dependence on 'science', and particularly on the Paracelsus fallacy, becomes all too apparent in the additional EFSA statement that,

"Scientists help to safeguard against these harmful effects by establishing safe levels."

If a substance used in a food has the ability to cause harmful effects it is, by definition, a poison; which means that the adulteration of food with substances that are 'deleterious to health' was not abolished by the creation of food safety laws and regulations.

In his 1982 book entitled *Beating the Food Giants*, Paul Stitt, a biochemist who worked in the food industry for a number of years, discusses many aspects of food manufacturing including the use of chemicals, about which he states,

"An ever-increasing proportion of the food we eat is no longer food but is now a conglomerate of high-priced chemistry experiments designed to simulate food."

The increased reliance by the food industry on the ingenuity of chemists has resulted in the situation whereby synthetic chemicals can also be used to replace basic ingredients, as Paul Stitt explains,

"When flavors, colors, texture, indeed when the food itself is synthesized, the corporations are freed from dealing with the cost and bother of real foods like vegetables and fruit."

The activities of the food industry include the packaging and distribution of whole foods including produce, such as fruits and vegetables, that do not become ingredients of processed food products. These whole and fresh foods are not the main focus of this discussion, although it should be noted that they may be subjected to certain processes to ensure that they comply with food standards; these processes may involve the use of chemicals, especially those for the purpose of killing 'germs'.

The *Codex* report includes an extract from the *Statutes of the Codex Alimentarius Commission* that lists the purposes of the Codex food standards, the first of which is,

"protecting the health of consumers and ensuring fair practices in the food trade."

The idea that Codex food standards fulfil the purpose of protecting consumer health is supported by the claim in the *Codex* report that,

"For more than five decades Codex texts have contributed immensely to the safety and quality of the food we eat."

This claim is misleading. The scientific establishment has revised the meanings of the terms 'safety' and 'quality' to ensure that they conform to criteria set by 'risk assessment' evaluations. The discussion about chemicals earlier in this chapter referred to the 1999 article by environmentalist Peter Montague, who stated that 'risk assessment' is not a science, but involves a great deal of judgement, which is how the word 'safe' has become a relative term, rather than an absolute one.

The CAC, previously stated, is a collaboration of the FAO and WHO. The WHO web page entitled *International Food Standards (FAO/WHO Codex Alimentarius)* states that,

> "FAO and WHO work on the provision of independent international scientific advice on microbiological and chemical hazards."

As demonstrated throughout this book, the WHO, the leading health 'authority' within the medical establishment, operates from the basis of fundamentally flawed theories; particularly, the 'germ theory' and the idea that a substance is only a poison with reference to the quantity used. Nevertheless, these theories, flawed though they are, are used to determine the safety of food. With respect to 'microbiological hazards', the word safe means 'free from germs'; whereas, with respect to 'chemical hazards', the word safe means that the quantity used does not exceed the level at which an adverse effect may be observed.

It is the aim of the CAC to 'harmonise' all food standards in all countries so that they conform to those of Codex Alimentarius, because, as the *Codex* report states,

> "Food regulations in different countries are often conflicting and contradictory."

It is claimed in the *Codex* report that these differences create barriers to trade, and that harmonisation of standards would reduce or eliminate those barriers and thus enable 'fair practices' in the food trade. In reality, the harmonisation of food standards and the removal of trade barriers will mainly serve the interests of the large food manufacturers that dominate the food industry. The harmonisation of food regulations in conformity with Codex standards would not ensure the safety of food products, nor would they protect the health of consumers.

The food standards set by the CAC include a number of codes of practice that govern various aspects of food production; one of these relates to hygiene and states that,

> "In almost all cases it is required that the product shall be free from pathogenic microorganisms, toxins or other poisonous or deleterious substances in amounts that represent a hazard to health."

There are a number of joint FAO/WHO 'expert' groups that address specific aspects of the food industry; one of these groups is JEMRA (Joint FAO/WHO Expert Meetings on Microbiological Risk Assessment). This group was founded in 2000 for the stated purpose as described in the *Codex* report,

> "JEMRA aims to optimize the use of microbiological risk assessment as the scientific basis for risk management decisions that address microbiological hazards in foods."

The work of JEMRA is clearly based on the flawed idea that it is the 'microbes' that poison foods, rather than any toxic chemicals used in their manufacture.

The Codex standard that relates to food contaminants, entitled *General Standard for Contaminants and Toxins in Food and Feed* (Codex STAN 193-1995), is clearly based on the Paracelsus fallacy. This standard provides information about the recommended maximum limits (MLs) for a variety of contaminants to ensure that any exposure to them is as low as possible. The principles for setting MLs include a number of criteria, the first of which states,

> "MLs should be set only for those contaminants that present both a significant risk to public health and a known or expected problem in international trade."

This criterion demonstrates the equal status afforded to public health and international trade, as also demonstrated by the first purpose of Codex food standards listed in the CAC *Statutes* previously referred to. However, there are circumstances that create conflicts between practices that would benefit the food industry and those that would benefit consumers; in the event of such conflicts it is invariably the interests of the food industry that are given priority. Furthermore, the *Codex* report would seem to suggest that the contamination of food is a normal occurrence by the statement that,

> "Everything that finds its way into food, if not used correctly, can be dangerous."

The examples cited by the report include food additives, pesticide residues and veterinary drugs. The most significant veterinary drugs are antibiotics, the dangers of which have been discussed; however, there are potential hazards from residues of all types of veterinary drugs. Pesticides have been discussed at length, although it is important to reiterate that pesticide residues can also affect food crops used as ingredients of processed food products. Pesticide residues are governed by a separate FAO/WHO 'expert' group called JMPR (Joint Meeting on Pesticide Residues).

The measures introduced by many of the original food laws also included the requirement to provide 'honest' information about the food to prevent deceptions, such as the sale of bad milk as 'cream'; honest labelling remains a key feature within food regulations. The Codex standard that regulates food labelling is *General Standard for the Labelling of Prepackaged Foods* (Codex STAN 1-1985) which, under the heading *General Principles*, states,

> "Prepackaged food shall not be described or presented on any label or in any labelling in a manner that is false, misleading or deceptive or is likely to create an erroneous impression regarding its character in any respect."

The Codex labelling standard not only regulates the manner in which prepackaged foods must not be described on the labels, it also stipulates the ingredients that must be declared on them. There is, however, a provision that relates to ingredients that do not require a declaration on a food label; this provision states,

> "Where a compound ingredient (for which a name has been established in a Codex standard or in national legislation) constitutes less than 5% of the food, the ingredients, other than food additives which serve a technological function in the finished product, need not be declared."

It may be argued that a requirement to declare every single ingredient would result in an unwieldy label; whilst this may be true, the counter argument is far stronger. This argument maintains that the granting of exclusions for certain ingredients results in food products that can, and invariably will, contain ingredients of which the consumer is unaware. The absence of information about all ingredients of a product means that consumers can be misled about the nature of the prepackaged food products they buy; a situation that clearly contravenes the Codex standard that food labels should not be misleading.

Exclusions can also be exploited to enable food manufacturers to use substances as ingredients that, were they declared on the label, may discourage customers from purchasing the product. One example is that, under certain conditions, foods are permitted to contain ingredients made with MSG without that fact being declared on the label; MSG is discussed later in this chapter.

The Codex standards generally recognise that foods should contain nutrients, although this is another word that has been assigned a revised meaning, as indicated by the *Codex* report that states,

"Numerous experts tell us which nutrients are good for us and which are not and we need to know what is in a food in order to compose a healthy diet."

The idea that a nutrient might not be 'good for us' indicates a very poor level of understanding about nutrition. A nutrient, by definition is 'good for us'; conversely a substance that is not 'good for us' cannot be a nutrient.

The Codex standard that governs information about nutrients to be declared on food labels is entitled *Guidelines on Nutrition Labelling* (CAC/GL 2-1985), the purpose of this information includes,

"...providing the consumer with information about a food so that a wise choice of food can be made..."

Consumers can only make a 'wise choice' if they have all of the necessary information to do so. Unfortunately, the medical establishment, which includes the WHO, does not understand nutrition, and is therefore unable to provide all of the required information so that consumers can be 'well-informed' and able to make 'wise choices' about their food purchases. Instead, they promulgate confusing and misleading information, as indicated by the *Guidelines on Nutrition Labelling* that incorrectly defines a nutrient as,

"...any substance normally consumed as a constituent of food..."

The guideline expands on this basic statement with reference to three categories of 'substances' that they refer to as 'nutrients'. The first category refers to any substance that 'provides energy'; however, energy is not a measure of nutrition. The second refers to substances that are needed for the maintenance of life. The third refers to substances a deficiency of which would produce adverse effects. It should be clear that the second and third categories are interconnected and represent the real meaning of 'nutrient'.

Although it is clear that the CAC recognises nutrients as important for the maintenance of life, it limits the ability to make claims about the relationship between food and health; as demonstrated by the Codex standard entitled *Guidelines for Use of Nutrition Claims* (CAC/GL 23-1997)

that defines a nutrition claim as,

"...any representation which states, suggests or implies that a food has particular nutritional properties..."

This statement is anomalous. The sole purpose of food is to provide the body with nutrients; therefore, nutrition claims can be made about all foods, which, by definition, have nutritional properties. It would seem, however, that the purpose of this standard is to refute claims that certain foods have specific health benefits, but this too is misleading. Unfortunately, the problem is exacerbated by the limited information permitted by the guidelines with respect to 'nutrition claims' and 'nutrients',

"The only nutrition claims permitted shall be those relating to energy, protein, carbohydrate and fat and components thereof, fibre, sodium and vitamins and minerals for which Nutrient Reference Values (NRVs) have been laid down in the Codex *Guidelines for Nutrition Labelling*."

A genuinely healthy diet will include a variety of foods that each contain various nutrients, including vitamins and minerals. Food labels that claim to provide 'nutritional information' list carbohydrates, fats, proteins and other permitted 'nutrients' in the food; but this does not provide consumers with useful information about the real nutritional value of the product. Nutrition is discussed in detail in chapter ten, but there are two important points with reference to this discussion; these are: that nutrients should not be evaluated individually; and that processing and storage reduce the nutritional content of foods.

Different countries are likely to have different regulations that govern the information provided on food labels, but the increasingly 'international' nature of the food industry means that manufactured food products will usually contain the information referred to in this discussion.

In addition to 'nutritional' information, labels are required to provide details of the product's ingredients; the Codex labelling standard Codex STAN 1-1985 defines an ingredient as,

"...any substance, including a food additive, used in the manufacture or preparation of a food and present in the final product although possibly in a modified form."

The standard states that certain foods and ingredients must be declared on the label, especially those, such as peanuts, that have been identified to cause hypersensitivity; 'peanut allergies' are discussed in chapter seven.

It is a recognised phenomenon that food product labels often contain a list of unfamiliar and often unpronounceable ingredients; these are almost invariably chemical compounds used as food additives to perform specific 'technological functions'. It is claimed that consumers are able to make 'wise choices' about food products based on information provided on the label, but the increasing use of synthetic chemicals means that only people with an extensive knowledge of chemistry are in a position to decipher the labels and understand the ingredients of the food products they buy.

It is clear that the food industry does not serve the interests of consumers; this can be demonstrated by a number of factors, which are: the failure to understand the real purpose of food; the poor level of knowledge about nutrition; the utilisation of synthetic chemicals; and the prioritisation of trade and profits. The food industry is clearly aided and abetted by the international 'expert' groups responsible for the creation of the food regulations that govern the production of processed food products.

People are encouraged to believe that these manufactured food products fulfil the function of food and provide them with all the nutrients their bodies require; but this is not the case; the emphasis on calories also adds to the confusion.

People are also encouraged to believe that these products are entirely 'safe'; but this is another mistaken belief. Most, if not all, manufactured food products contain a variety of chemical 'additives' that not only adulterate the foods, but also poison them; a situation that is summarised succinctly by Paul Stitt, who stated in his 1982 book that,

> "Processed foods are terrible things for your body for two reasons – they are stripped of their nutrient value in the refining process, and they are poisoned with sugar and other harmful additives."

This situation has not improved in the intervening decades since the 1980s, as the following discussions about a variety of food additives will demonstrate.

Food Additives

The EFSA web page entitled *Food Additives* provides an overview of the purpose of these substances in manufactured food products,

> "Food additives are substances added intentionally to foodstuffs to perform certain technological functions, for example to colour, to sweeten or to help preserve foods."

The Codex standard that governs food additives is the *General Standard for Food Additives Codex STAN 192-1995* (GSFA), which is clearly intended to be regarded as the definitive guidance for all food manufacturers, as indicated by the statement that,

> "The *General Standard for Food Additives* (GSFA) should be the single authoritative reference point for food additives."

The intended 'authority' of this standard, which will be referred to as the *GSFA*, is further demonstrated by the statement that,

> "Only the food additives listed herein are recognized as suitable for use in foods in conformance with the provisions of this Standard."

Although originally adopted in 1995, the *GSFA* has been regularly revised; it is the 2016 version that is used as the source of references cited in the following discussions. The term 'food additive' is defined in the *GSFA* as follows,

> "Food additive means any substance not normally consumed as a food by itself and not normally used as a typical ingredient of the food, whether or not it has nutritive value..."

The efforts of the 19th century food safety campaigners generated legislation that was claimed to prevent food adulteration. However, the permission granted for the use of substances that are 'not normally consumed as food' means that the *GSFA* provides official approval for the

One of the main problems arising from the procedures used to determine 'safe use levels' is that, as for virtually all chemicals, safety testing procedures are conducted almost entirely on each individual substance. Although studies may be conducted to test some combinations of food additives, these are generally limited in range, and are mostly conducted after the substances have been introduced into the foods additives market and incorporated into food products to be consumed by the public.

None of the assessments involves an evaluation of the effects of varying combinations of the thousands of chemical food additives used in all manufactured processed food products; nor do they evaluate the effects of exposures to the mix of chemical food additives in combination with chemicals used in other products. More importantly, the tests that are conducted are based on the assumption that humans are alike and will therefore all react in exactly the same way to food additives; this is, however, yet another mistaken assumption.

Although some chemicals are known to interact synergistically, this is a poorly tested phenomenon. The failure to test all combinations of all chemicals used as food additives means that any synergies that do occur remain unidentified; assurances of 'safety' cannot be relied upon. Furthermore, many of the chemicals used to create food additives are derived from petrochemicals; which means that they are inherently toxic and consequently entirely unsuitable for use in food products intended for human consumption.

It is important to note that JECFA does not conduct studies; at their meetings, the Committee assesses various studies, published papers and other relevant documentation made available to them, from which they make their evaluations about the substances under review. These evaluations are incorporated into the relevant Codex standard; they are also published as reports and made available on the website of the WHO as part of their Technical series. This means that the Committee should be aware of the latest results from scientific studies that have investigated food additives. However, some food additives continue to be permitted for use by JECFA, despite the fact that published scientific studies have demonstrated the existence of adverse health effects that have occurred due to the consumption of these substances.

The role of JECFA has been expanded to also include risk assessments and safety evaluations of contaminants, natural toxins and residues of veterinary drugs in animal products. The results of these evaluations are incorporated into Codex Standard STAN 193-1995, as discussed in the previous section. The FAO website provides an overview of the expanded role of JECFA under the heading *Chemical risks and JECFA*,

> "The Committee has also developed principles for safety assessment of chemicals in foods that are consistent with current thinking on risk assessment and take account of developments in toxicology and other relevant sciences."

The purpose of the November 2016 meeting of JECFA in Rome was to evaluate six 'contaminants' in foods, one of which is a group of substances called 'aflatoxins'; which are described in the report from that meeting as,

"...one of the most potent mutagenic and carcinogenic substances known..."

Aflatoxins are said to be produced by two types of the *Aspergillus* fungus. There are a few crops that are reported to be particularly susceptible to aflatoxins; they include corn, peanuts and cotton, all three of which are acknowledged to receive some of the heaviest applications of pesticides, herbicides and fungicides. A heavy application of fungicide should, however, prevent the growth of any fungus; which raises the question of what is the real source of these 'potent' toxins that are claimed to be produced by the *Aspergillus* fungus.

The fact that these crops become 'toxic' in the presence of toxic pesticides should not be surprising; there is no need to invoke the existence of a so-called 'toxic fungus' to be able to explain the consequences of the application of toxic chemicals onto these crops. The discussion in chapter three demonstrated that most fungi, if not all of them, are harmless and that many of them are, in fact, beneficial. An important point to note is that an association has been identified between 'aflatoxin exposure' and liver cancer. As will be further discussed in chapter seven, cancer is mostly associated with, although not exclusively caused by, exposures to toxic substances; it should be emphasised that the liver is the body's main detoxification organ.

The reason for referring to aflatoxins in a discussion about food additives is to demonstrate the errors of the medical establishment, especially the adherence to the 'germ theory' in order to blame 'germs' for problems that are, in reality, caused by toxic chemicals. Their failure to properly acknowledge the role of toxic chemicals continues to influence regulations that claim to ensure the 'safety' of food. The WHO permits the use of toxic chemicals to kill 'germs', but claims that these toxic substances do not pose human health risks provided that they are used at the appropriate 'dose'.

The efforts to achieve a global harmonisation of food regulations have resulted in a certain level of success, although regional differences remain and these are discussed in an April 2013 article entitled *Review of the regulation and safety assessment of food substances in various countries and jurisdictions*. The countries and jurisdictions included in the review were Argentina, Australia, Brazil, Canada, China, the European Union, Japan, Mexico, New Zealand and the United States. The 'food substances' considered by the review article include,

"...direct food additives, food ingredients, flavouring agents, food enzymes and/or processing aids, food contact materials, novel foods, and nanoscale materials for food applications."

All of these 'food substances', with the sole exception of any real food ingredients, can be regarded as falling under the generic label of 'food additives' for the purposes of this discussion and the ensuing sections that discuss a few significant types of additive. The article recognises the existence of variations in the different regulatory frameworks that govern the approval of food additives within each country, but also recognises that there were similarities,

"...including the use of positive lists of approved substances."

The reference in the article to 'approved substances', and to JECFA evaluations of the safety of food additives, is a clear indication that the *GSFA* is increasingly recognised by the scientific community as the authoritative guidance for food additives.

There is, however, one aspect of US food regulations that is unique. This is the ability to categorise substances as GRAS (generally recognised as safe); a category that was created by the Food Additives Amendment of 1958 to enable commonly-used food ingredients to be exempted from the usual FDA approval process. However, this legislation inadvertently created a loophole, which has been exploited by some food manufacturers to claim GRAS status for new chemicals that are not common food ingredients. The consequence of this loophole was exposed by the NRDC (Natural Resources Defense Council) in an April 2014 report entitled *Generally Recognized as Secret: Chemicals Added to Food in the United States*. On a web page with the same title, the NRDC states that,

"The exemption allows manufacturers to make safety determinations that the uses of their newest chemicals in food are safe without notifying the FDA."

This means that manufacturers can claim an exemption under GRAS for certain chemicals; this situation parallels that of fracking companies that are permitted to make a claim of 'proprietary information' for the chemical products they use in their operations, as previously discussed. The problem is not merely that food manufacturers fail to notify the FDA; the salient point is that the public remains ignorant about the inclusion of these chemicals in the food products they buy, as explained by the NRDC in the *Conclusion* to their report,

"A chemical additive cannot be 'generally recognized as safe' if its identity, chemical composition and safety determination are not publicly disclosed."

In view of the efforts towards the harmonisation of standards and the increasingly global nature of the food industry, the question arises therefore, as to whether harmonisation will eliminate the GRAS category in the US or whether 'GRAS' will become the 'authoritative guideline' for all other countries; at the time of writing, this question had yet to be resolved.

It is clear that the standards and regulations that govern the manufacture of food products and their permissible ingredients do not preserve the purity, safety or nutritional content of food. On the contrary, the regulations that claim to protect the integrity of food, in reality, permit the use of a variety of chemical compounds under the label 'food additives', none of which has been proven to be absolutely safe to consume.

Furthermore, additives are used in multiple combinations in a wide variety of manufactured, processed food products; but there is no evidence that these combinations of food additives have ever been tested to determine their safety, or to assess any adverse health effects that may arise from their consumption.

The WHO acknowledges that there are some risks posed by some chemicals, as demonstrated on their web pages relating to the topic of *Food Safety* that include a page entitled *Chemical risks*, which states,

"Chemicals can end up in food either intentionally added for a technological purpose (e.g. food additives), or through environmental pollution of the air, water and soil."

This is a clear acknowledgement that 'chemicals' can be defined as environmental pollutants; although it is highly unlikely that the WHO intended this statement to be a confirmation that the chemicals used as food additives are toxic and therefore environmental pollutants; nevertheless, this is the case, as the ensuing discussions will demonstrate.

It should be noted that food additives are used to serve 'technological functions' and that most of them are purely cosmetic; this is particularly the case with respect to the use of chemicals to add colour to foods.

Food Colouring

The visual appeal of a food is important; it depends, at least to a certain extent, upon the food's colour. In order to make them visually appealing, food manufacturers must therefore create products that present foods in the colours with which they are normally associated.

Unfortunately, most natural foods, especially fruits and vegetables, lose some of their brightness of colour when they undergo any form of processing, including home cooking. The loss of colour is, however, more pronounced when foods undergo manufacturing processes, but the food industry compensates for this problem in a number of ways, one of which is through the use of 'food colourings', the purpose of which is explained by First Steps Nutrition Trust on the web page entitled *Additives*, which states that,

> "They are used solely as cosmetic additives to boost the consumer appeal of products, for example by adding brightness lost in processing or storage, mimicking the colour profile of healthier ingredients such as fruits and vegetables, or overcoming colour variations that occur in natural products."

The use of certain natural materials to add colour to foods has a long history. Saffron, the name given to the dried stigmas of the plant *Crocus Sativus*, is a spice known for its ability to impart a yellow colour to food. However, saffron contains nutrients; which means that it is a 'food' as well as a food colouring agent.

By comparison, the synthetic chemical compounds used to impart colour to processed food products are entirely different substances. As previously discussed, Friedrich Accum's investigations discovered that chemicals had been used to enhance the colour of certain foods; for example, copper was used to dye pickles green and lead was used to dye sweets red. Although 'natural', copper and lead are both highly toxic and should not have been added to foods.

The rise of the chemical industry, and particularly the petrochemical industry, resulted in the manufacture of chemical compounds that were found to be useful as dyes. In 2010, CSPI (Center for Science in the Public Interest) published a report entitled *Food Dyes: A Rainbow of Risks*, which explains,

> "Dyes are complex organic chemicals that were originally derived from coal tar, but now from petroleum."

These dyes were initially created for the textile industry, but were inexplicably deemed useful for the food industry; although it should be noted that petrochemical-derived compounds were also deemed useful for the pharmaceutical industry. However, petrochemicals are inherently toxic; which means that, like copper and lead, they are entirely unsuitable substances to be added to food.

Despite the efforts of the CAC to ensure that the *GSFA* is the sole 'authority' with respect to food additives, there are still some variations within different countries. The CSPI is based in the US; their report therefore focuses on the situation in that country, where the consumption of food dyes is reported to have increased five-fold since the mid-20th century. However, certain food dyes that are permitted in the US have been withdrawn from use in other countries, and some have even been banned.

As discussed in the previous section, the *GSFA* states that the use of food additives is justified when there is an advantage; the CSPI report describes some of those 'advantages', which are clearly of the kind that benefit the food industry rather than the consumer,

> "Companies like using them because they are cheaper, more stable, and brighter than most natural colourings."

These advantages do not ensure that chemical dyes are 'safe' for use in foods. Further confirmation that these dyes are neither safe nor suitable for consumption is provided in the report, which states that,

> "It is worth noting that dyes are not pure chemicals, but may contain upwards of 10 percent impurities that are in the chemicals from which dyes are made or develop in the manufacturing process."

These impurities are 'permitted' by the FDA with the proviso that they do not exceed a specified concentration; however, these contaminants may include some highly dangerous substances, such as benzene, lead, mercury and arsenic, to name just a few. Nevertheless, chemical dyes are used to brightly colour a wide variety of 'food products', many of which are intended to appeal to and be consumed by children.

Despite the claim that food colouring additives have been assessed and shown to be 'safe', a wealth of scientific evidence shows this not to be the case. This evidence, which has accumulated since the 1970s, demonstrates the existence of a clear association between adverse health effects and the consumption of food dyes. These adverse effects, which are more pronounced in children, are mainly behavioural; as indicated by a January 2016 CSPI article entitled *Fact Sheet: The Science Linking Food Dyes with Impacts on Children's Behavior* that states,

> "Over the past 40 years, many double-blind studies have concluded that food dyes and other ingredients can impair behavior in some children."

The UK establishment also acknowledges that there is at least a potential problem associated with the consumption of chemical food dyes. A September 2007 University of Southampton news release entitled *Major study indicates a link between hyperactivity in children and certain food additives* states that,

> "A study by researchers at the University of Southampton has shown evidence of increased levels of hyperactivity in young children consuming mixtures of some

artificial food colours and the preservative sodium benzoate."

The food colours include tartrazine, quinoline yellow and allura red, all of which are commonly found in drinks, confectionery and bakery goods, as well as a number of other 'food products', and all of which are derived from petrochemicals.

The food dye coding systems vary according to country or region; the EU food additive numbering system classifies tartrazine as E102, quinoline yellow as E104 and allura red as E129. In the US, tartrazine is classified as FD&C Yellow 5 and allura red as FD&C Red 40. Quinoline yellow is not recognised by the US dye codes, but is claimed to be 'structurally equivalent' to FD&C Yellow 10, which is approved for use in the US in medicines and cosmetics, although it is not approved for use in foods.

The inherent toxicity of these food dyes can be demonstrated by the example of allura red. This dye is a derivative of naphthalene, which is an aromatic hydrocarbon that is used in insecticides and pest repellents; it is also commonly used in mothballs. It should be obvious that these applications indicate that naphthalene is toxic; evidence of its toxicity is shown by the classification of naphthalene as a Group C carcinogen; which means that it is regarded as a 'possible' cause of cancer; it is clearly not 'safe'.

The significance of the Southampton University study results was that adverse health effects were discovered to be caused by the combination of certain chemical food dyes and a certain chemical preservative. This finding demonstrates that chemical reactions can occur between different types of food additives and indicates the existence of chemical synergies that can produce a more intense adverse reaction.

These results demonstrate the consequences of safety testing procedures that only investigate individual food additive compounds, and therefore fail to study the effects of the many combinations of chemical additives that are commonly used in food products. This point is further demonstrated by the CSPI *Food Dyes* report that discusses nine food dyes, three of which account for approximately 90 per cent of all food dyes used in the US; the report refers to the studies that had been conducted to determine their safety and states that,

> "...virtually all the studies tested individual dyes, whereas many foods and diets contain mixtures of dyes (and other ingredients) that might lead to additive or synergistic effects."

Although referred to as food dyes, these chemical compounds are also used in other products, as explained in the 2016 CSPI report entitled *Seeing Red: Time for Action on Food Dyes*, which states that,

> "Most of the dyes used in food are also permitted to be used in other products such as cosmetics, personal-care products like mouthwash, shampoo and toothpaste; over-the-counter medications; dietary supplements; and prescription drugs."

The safety studies that only test individual food dyes, and only consider exposures from their use in food, clearly fail to take account of multiple exposures to chemical dyes in all of the other products in which they are used, especially personal care products used on a daily basis; personal care

development of a new branch of the food additives industry that was dedicated to the creation of 'flavourings'. The scientists in the 'flavourings industry' are referred to as 'flavourists' or as 'flavour chemists' and their work is primarily conducted in laboratories. According to the *Review*, the flavourings industry constitutes the largest sector of the huge global food additives industry. The flavourings produced by this industry perform a variety of functions; as indicated by the *Review*, which states that they are used,

> "...in order to alter the taste profile of the basic ingredients of the product, to flavour tasteless base materials, to mask 'off-notes', to boost flavour after food processing, to enhance flavours present, or for reasons of economy, as flavourings are generally cheaper than flavourful base ingredients."

In common with food colourings, food flavourings are also claimed to be 'safe'; as demonstrated by the EFSA web page entitled *Flavourings* which states that,

> "Flavourings have a long history of safe use in a wide variety of foods..."

The word 'safe' is again used in its revised context as a relative term; in other words, flavourings are 'safe' on the proviso that they meet certain conditions, as demonstrated by the further EFSA comment that,

> "They are used in comparatively small amounts so that consumer exposure is relatively low."

The use of a 'small amount' of a flavouring does not render it 'safe' for consumption; the need to ensure a low level of 'consumer exposure' clearly indicates that these substances pose a potential, if not a genuine health hazard if used in larger amounts. Another reason for using a 'small amount' of a flavouring substance is explained in the *Review*,

> "Flavourings can be potent and may be needed in very small quantities..."

Some natural flavourings, such as spices, are also potent and only needed in small quantities, but this is due to the intensity of their flavour, not to the possibility that they pose a potential health hazard if consumer exposure is not kept to a low level. It should be clear that spices and chemical flavourings are fundamentally different; unprocessed spices that contain nutrients are foods, whereas all chemical flavourings are devoid of nutrients and are therefore not foods.

Although flavourings are a type of food additive, and therefore governed by the *GSFA*, they are also governed by a Codex standard that is specific to flavourings. This standard, reference number *CAC/GL 66-2008*, is entitled *Guidelines for the Use of Flavourings*; its purpose is stated to be to provide,

> "...principles for the safe use of the components of flavourings..."

The 'safety' of these flavourings, as with all food additives, is based on evaluations conducted by JECFA that have determined that these compounds,

> "...present no safety concern at estimated levels of intake..."

However, a significant property that chemical flavourings have in common with chemical food dyes is the basic type of chemicals from which many of them are derived; as the *Review* explains,

"Petrochemicals are the most common source materials for flavourings in the category 'flavouring substances'..."

Unlike food dyes, food flavourings were not originally created for use in another type of industry; however, the 'flavourings industry' supplies chemical compounds to industries other than the food industry; the *Review* explains,

"Most companies that supply flavourings to the food and drink industry also supply fragrances for use in non-comestible products like perfumes, cosmetics, toiletries and household cleaning products."

A number of 'non-comestible' products are discussed in more detail later in this chapter.

It is a known phenomenon that there is a close association between the sense of taste and the sense of smell; many natural materials that impart flavour to foods also impart a distinctive aroma. It is therefore unsurprising that certain materials, including fruits and other parts of plants, are used as fragrances for non-food products; 'lemon', for example, is a common fragrance of household products as well as a common flavouring for food products. The flavourings industry utilises this close association between flavour and aroma to produce chemical compounds that can be used to fulfil both functions, as the *Review* explains,

"Both flavourings and fragrances are often referred to as 'aroma chemicals' with many of the same raw materials and similar production processes."

These chemical compounds can be used in various combinations to create a wide variety of flavours, as the *Review* indicates,

"For example, a popular strawberry flavouring may contain approximately 30 flavouring substances plus a flavouring preparation."

Due to their chemical nature, it is highly likely that none of these 30 flavouring substances has been extracted from a real strawberry.

The continuing growth of the flavourings industry means that new flavouring compounds are continually being developed; however, it should be noted that some flavouring compounds have also been withdrawn from the market after they have been found to be associated with adverse health effects. Although the exact number is unknown, it is estimated that there are in excess of 2,500 flavouring compounds currently in use by the food and other industries. These substances are categorised by the Codex *Flavourings* standard under four headings,

"Flavourings may consist of flavouring substances, natural flavouring complexes, thermal process flavourings or smoke flavourings..."

The first category of flavouring substances is further subdivided by the standard into two more categories, which are labelled, 'natural' and 'synthetic'. Synthetic flavouring substances are defined as,

"...flavouring substances formed by chemical synthesis."

Flavourings produced by chemical synthesis may be 'chemically identical' to natural flavouring substances, but that does not make them identical. The difference between them can be illustrated by an example provided in the *Review*, which refers to the extraction of vanillin and states,

"Synthesised vanillin is chemically identical to vanilla extracted using physical, enzymatic and microbiological processes, but cannot be labelled as 'natural'."

Clearly, a synthesised flavouring cannot be labelled as 'natural', but this highlights the fact that they are different and that the difference is more fundamental than their chemical structure; foods are far more complex than a conglomeration of chemicals.

Food 'flavourings' are not comprised entirely of synthetic chemicals; some of them are compounds that have been derived from natural plant materials that have a particular flavour or aroma component. It is the work of 'flavour chemists' to extract the required 'components' from these plants or other sources and create 'natural flavouring substances', which are defined by the Codex *Flavourings* standard as,

> "...flavouring substances obtained by physical processes that may result in unavoidable but unintentional changes in the chemical structure of the components of the flavouring..."

It should be clear that changes in the chemical structure of a substance, including natural substances, can significantly affect its properties and functions. Furthermore, some of the processes involved in the extraction of a 'flavour component' have some unpleasant consequences, one of which is described in the *Review*,

> "The extraction of flavourings often requires the use of solvents which may leave a residue in the food or drink when the flavour is added."

Solvents are used solely to assist the extraction processes, they are not added directly to foods; however, it is clear that solvent residues can remain in the flavouring compounds, which means that they may be transferred to the food. The presence of residues in foods is acknowledged on the web page entitled *Extraction solvents*, that refers to these solvents,

> "...which are removed but which may result in the unintentional, but technically unavoidable, presence of residues or derivatives in the foodstuff or food ingredient."

One of the solvents used in some extraction processes is methanol, a hazardous chemical that is discussed in more detail later in this chapter. Another of the solvents used in extraction processes is propylene glycol, which is a main ingredient of antifreeze. Although classified in the US as GRAS, propylene glycol is associated with certain 'side effects', which is a clear indication that it cannot be regarded as 'safe' in the true meaning of the word.

Flavourings, as indicated by Action on Additives, are also used in 'non-food' products, including 'medicines'. The purpose of flavourings in medicines, especially in liquid medicines intended for children, is to mask their unpleasant and often bitter taste and to therefore make them palatable. However, the pleasant taste imparted by 'flavourings' also masks the reason that these drugs have an unpleasant flavour, which is because they are manufactured from a variety of chemical compounds, many of which are derived from petrochemicals.

The Codex guideline clearly acknowledges that there is at least a potential health 'risk' from the consumption of 'flavouring' compounds but only refers to the management of this risk and to the establishment of,

"... risk management measures to reduce the risk to human health from such flavouring substances..."

As repeatedly discussed, safety testing is virtually always conducted on individual chemicals or, very occasionally, on a limited combination of chemicals. But, no matter how rigorous the testing protocols may have been, they are unable to evaluate the full extent of the 'risks' to health because they do not test all possible interactions between all combinations of all the different food additives used by the food industry.

There are clearly some serious health concerns for people who consume significant quantities of highly processed food products that contain a variety of flavourings as well as other food additives. Although the regulatory bodies such as the CAC claim that their calculations incorporate sufficient safety margins to cover all consumption habits, the *Review* indicates that these evaluations may not be adequate,

"There remains debate over the safety of a number of flavouring compounds and whether methods to assess intakes are sufficiently robust"

A page entitled *Flavourings-related lung disease* on the NIOSH section of the CDC website, discusses food flavourings that have been found to be associated with respiratory problems for the workers in factories that utilise or produce these compounds. The web page refers to these flavouring chemicals as 'very volatile', which is the reason that they are easily inhaled and cause respiratory problems. One of the flavourings discussed on the page is diacetyl, a compound that imparts a buttery flavour to foods. The factory where the respiratory problems had been identified was one that used diacetyl in the manufacture of microwaveable popcorn, although NIOSH claims that the studies,

"...were not able to definitely determine if diacetyl exposure contributed to lung disease..."

Nevertheless, the discussion on the NIOSH web page about the problems due to the various flavourings includes a particularly significant comment,

"Given the complexity of flavourings mixtures, and the lack of health data for many of the component materials..."

This statement is a clear acknowledgement that 'flavourings' are produced from complex combinations of compounds, as indicated by the previously cited example that 30 different flavouring substances are used to produce one particular strawberry flavour. It is also clear that the lack of health data means that many of the 'component materials' have not been adequately tested to determine their health effects, if at all. Nevertheless, diacetyl has been classified by the FDA as GRAS. Diacetyl is not the only flavouring ingredient that is capable of producing harm; the NIOSH web page also states that,

"...the flavourings industry has estimated that over a thousand flavouring ingredients have the potential to be respiratory hazards due to possible volatility and irritant properties..."

These properties indicate that there are at least a thousand flavouring substances that can be regarded as toxic and therefore capable of causing harm to health, but respiratory problems are not the only adverse health effects they may cause. Flavourings that are produced from petrochemicals must all be regarded as inherently toxic and therefore totally unsuitable for use in foods.

Monosodium Glutamate (MSG)

Monosodium glutamate (MSG) is more correctly described as a 'flavour enhancer' rather than a 'food flavouring' as it possesses no actual flavour of its own. Dr Russell Blaylock explains in *Health and Nutrition Secrets* that,

"Monosodium glutamate is the sodium salt of glutamic acid, a form of glutamate..."

He adds the statement that,

"Glutamic acid is an amino acid that occurs naturally in many foods."

The creation of MSG is attributed to Professor Kikunae Ikeda, a Japanese chemist who discovered that foods which contained a type of kelp used extensively in Japanese cuisine had a more intense flavour. In 1908, he isolated the chemical that seemed to produce the intensified flavour and developed a process for its manufacture. The process by which MSG is manufactured has since changed; according to the FDA web page entitled *Questions and Answers on Monosodium Glutamate (MSG)*,

"Today, instead of extracting and crystallizing MSG from seaweed broth, MSG is produced by the fermentation of starch, sugar beets, sugar cane or molasses."

Since the initial introduction of MSG into the food industry in the US in the late 1940s, its production and use have rapidly expanded to the extent that this substance is a common food additive in a wide variety of manufactured food products. On the basis that no recorded adverse events had been associated with MSG, the FDA classified it as 'GRAS' when that category was first established in 1958. Another justification for this classification is that the chemical structure of MSG is claimed to be identical to that of naturally occurring glutamic acid; as explained on the FDA Q&A web page,

"The glutamate in MSG is chemically indistinguishable from glutamate present in food proteins."

As demonstrated in the previous discussion, the fact that two substances are regarded as 'chemically indistinguishable' does not mean that they are identical; particularly if one substance is naturally occurring and the other has been synthesised in a chemist's laboratory. This point is discussed in an article entitled *On the Subject of Manufactured vs Natural Glutamic Acid* by Truth in Labeling, an organisation that was founded by Dr Adrienne Samuels MD and her husband. The article, which is published on their website, states that,

"Central to their argument is the lie that the processed free glutamic acid used in processed food is identical to the glutamic acid found in unprocessed, unadulterated food and in the human body."

The reason that the natural unprocessed glutamic acid found in foods is not identical to the processed glutamic acid is explained by Dr Blaylock,

"In nature, it is bound by peptide linkages, which are broken down solely during the digestive process, thereby preventing the sudden surges that are associated with the pure, processed additive MSG."

The 'safety' of MSG is the subject of an ongoing controversy, which began in the late 1950s after animal experiments revealed that MSG could cause the destruction of nerve cells in mice. In the late 1960s, Dr John Olney MD repeated the animal experiments, the results of which not only revealed the same nerve damage, they also revealed that damage had occurred in cells within the hypothalamus. Although he reported his findings to the FDA, no action was taken to withdraw MSG from the market.

As mentioned in the Truth in Labeling article, glutamic acid is also found in the body; more specifically, this amino acid is a neurotransmitter that is found in the brain and spinal cord. Under normal circumstances, glutamic acid is carefully regulated by the body's self-protective mechanisms, one of which is the blood-brain barrier, a boundary that protects most areas of the brain and, as Dr Blaylock explains,

"...prevents most harmful substances in the blood from entering the interior of the brain."

The blood-brain barrier does permit the passage of certain substances, including amino acids, although the passage of any substance across this barrier is usually carefully controlled. It should be noted, however, that some toxic substances, including some pharmaceutical drugs, are able to breach the blood-brain barrier.

The level of glutamic acid from a diet of unprocessed foods that do not contain MSG is clearly regulated by a number of different mechanisms in the body. However, the consumption of processed MSG-laden food products can result in these normal protective mechanisms being overpowered; this, in turn, can lead to a build-up of high levels of glutamate in the blood, as Dr Blaylock explains,

"By artificially adding very high concentrations of free glutamate to food, blood glutamate levels in most people are far higher than were ever intended..."

The consumption of MSG-laden food products can increase the amount of glutamate in the blood to the extent that it reaches a level that Dr Blaylock refers to as critical. At this stage, the body's normal protective mechanisms will be unable to function properly and the concentration of glutamate will become toxic to neurons and cause them to become 'excited'. Glutamate is not the only substance capable of causing harm to neurons; aspartate, which is discussed later in this chapter, acts in a similar manner. In *Excitotoxins: The Taste That Kills*, Dr Blaylock explains the effects caused by critical levels of these substances,

"When neurons are exposed to these substances, they become very excited and fire their impulses very rapidly until they reach a state of extreme exhaustion."

Unfortunately, exhaustion is not the only type of harm that can be caused; Dr Blaylock continues,

"Several hours later these neurons suddenly die, as if the cells were excited to death."

These are serious effects that demonstrate the harmful nature of MSG.

Another significant difference between manufactured MSG and natural glutamic acid is that the latter is comprised of a single amino acid, whereas

mistaken assumption. One of the reasons this is a mistaken assumption is because the impact of chemical food preservatives on the nutritional content of the food products to which they have been added, is virtually unknown. This aspect of food preservation has not been studied, as indicated by a 1992 article entitled *Nutritional aspects of food preservatives* that states,

"Surprisingly, there is quite a lack of scientific knowledge in this field."

Nevertheless, despite an almost complete lack of knowledge about their impact on the nutritional value of foods, different chemical substances are used to perform at least one of three different functions that are claimed to preserve foods. These functions are: to prevent microbial growth; to prevent or delay oxidation; and to inhibit the natural ripening process.

The first function of 'food preservatives' clearly owes its origin to the 'germ theory' and the erroneous belief that microorganisms, especially bacteria, are 'dangerous'; as indicated by the EUFIC (European Food Information Council) web page entitled *Preservatives to keep foods longer – and safer*, which states that,

"The primary reason for using preservatives is to make foods safer by eliminating the influence of biological factors."

These 'biological factors' include yeasts and moulds as well as bacteria. The discussion in chapter three explained that bacteria are saprobes, or 'natural decomposers'; which means that they break down dead and decaying matter into its constituent elements for reabsorption into the environment; this is 'natural recycling'. The erroneous idea that bacteria, rather than natural processes, are the cause of food decay has resulted in the creation of an entire range of chemical food additives intended to 'attack' them; as explained on the EUFIC web page,

"To delay the spoiling of foodstuffs by micro-organisms, anti-microbial substances are used which inhibit, delay or prevent the growth and proliferation of bacteria, yeasts and moulds."

Antimicrobial substances that are intended to poison bacteria, yeasts and moulds do not make food 'safer'; instead, these poisons make foods less safe.

A similarly erroneous idea about the effect of bacteria on food is shown by the claim that bacteria cause 'food poisoning', which has been renamed and is now referred to as 'food-borne disease'. The original label was, however, far more apt as it described the real cause of the problem. Worryingly, 'food-borne disease' is said to have become a significant health problem; as indicated by the June 2019 WHO fact sheet entitled *Food safety*, which states that,

"An estimated 600 million – almost 1 in 10 people in the world – fall ill after eating contaminated food and 420,000 die every year..."

The WHO attributes the causes of food contamination to a number of factors,

"Unsafe food containing harmful bacteria, viruses, parasites or chemical substances causes more than 200 diseases – ranging from diarrhoea to cancers."

It should be clear that bacteria, viruses and parasites can be eliminated from this list of causes. The remaining factor, namely 'chemical substances', are the only ones relevant to 'food-borne disease'. The fact sheet provides some examples of 'chemical substances' that include POPs (persistent organic pollutants), such as dioxins, and heavy metals, such as lead, cadmium and mercury. There are, however, many thousands of chemicals that are eminently capable of causing severe health problems if consumed.

Despite the recognition that chemical substances are relevant contributory factors, the medical establishment nevertheless retains its focus on 'germs' as the major causes of 'food-borne disease', one example of which is botulism. Although it is not a common condition, botulism is said to be caused by toxins produced by a bacterium called *Clostridium botulinum*. These bacterial 'toxins' are claimed to be neurotoxic; the symptoms they are said to cause can include respiratory problems and paralysis. There is no explanation of how a bacterium is able to produce these symptoms; however, there are many neurotoxic chemicals that have been proven to cause such symptoms; organophosphate pesticides for example, as previously discussed.

Some of the other substances that have the ability to induce symptoms that may be diagnosed as a 'food-borne disease' include the chemical compounds used as 'food preservatives'. The EUFIC web page about *Preservatives* refers to a group of compounds and states,

"Benzoic acid and its calcium, sodium or potassium salts (E210-213) are used as antibacterials and antifungals in foods such as pickled cucumbers, low sugar jams and jellies, dressings, condiments."

The EUFIC page also refers to the fact that, prior to their use, these chemicals would have undergone safety assessments by the EFSA and JECFA; previous discussions have shown that these evaluations do not ensure that chemicals are absolutely safe, but only relatively safe when used below the maximum permitted level in a food.

It is claimed that benzoic acid occurs naturally in many plant and animal species and that it can be produced by microorganisms. Yet it is also claimed that benzoic acid and its salts have antimicrobial properties; this anomaly is not explained. One of the methods by which benzoic acid is commercially produced involves the oxidation of toluene, a highly toxic petrochemical that has been classified as a Group 1 carcinogen. Sodium benzoate is the benzoic acid salt that was demonstrated by the Southampton University study to cause adverse health effects when consumed in combination with certain food colourings; it has been shown to release benzene when used in soft drinks and other beverages that also contain ascorbic acid.

Other preservatives that are claimed to prevent bacterial growth include sodium nitrate and sodium nitrite, both of which are commonly used in meats; they also act as colour fixatives to enhance the bright red colour of processed meats and meat products such as bacon, ham, sausages and hot dogs. But these chemical preservatives have long been known to be toxic, as Dr Blaylock explains in *Health and Nutrition Secrets*,

"For decades, food scientists and cancer specialists have known that nitrates and nitrites were converted in the human stomach into powerful cancer-causing substances called nitrosamines."

The second function of preservatives is to prevent oxidation, which is a normal process that results from exposure of foods to oxygen in the atmosphere and causes discolouration; oxidation is the process that turns apples brown when they are cut open. This discolouration can be prevented or delayed through the use of antioxidants; but 'antioxidants' are not all the same. In common with most food additives, the antioxidants used by the food industry are generally synthetic chemical compounds that are very different from the antioxidants that occur naturally in plant foods.

The third function of preservatives is to inhibit the ripening process, which is claimed to enable the shelf-life of food products to be significantly prolonged. One method used for this purpose is sterilisation, which destroys enzymatic activity. However, enzymes are extremely important; they act as catalysts for many of the body's biochemical reactions. They are also essential for the processes of digestion, as they assist the break-down of the component materials of foods and the absorption of nutrients.

Foods can be sterilised by a few different methods, some of which involve chemicals; sulphur dioxide for example, is used in some wines and in some dried fruits. Despite the claim that food preservatives make food 'safer', the EUFIC web page acknowledges that both sulphite compounds and benzoic salts are associated with asthma, although it is claimed that asthma is only 'triggered' in people who already suffer from this condition; asthma is discussed in chapter seven.

Two other chemicals used to inhibit the natural ripening processes are BHA (butylated hydroxyanisole) and BHT (butylated hydroxytoluene), which are used in a large range of products that include margarines, salad dressings, cereals, preserved meat, beer and baked goods. The benefits of these chemicals to the food industry is explained by Paul Stitt,

"Preservatives like BHT, BHA and EDTA keep food fresh for months, enabling them to be manufactured more cheaply in huge centralized factories and shipped long distances, or stockpiled until the price goes up."

The use of chemicals to inhibit ripening does not, however, keep food genuinely fresh.

The FDA has classified both BHA and BHT as GRAS, however, the 14th Report on Carcinogens published in 2016, described BHA as,

"Reasonably anticipated to be a human carcinogen."

BHT is not claimed to be carcinogenic, but it has been associated with adverse effects in the liver, which is indicative of its inherent toxicity.

It is clear that all of the chemicals used for the purpose of preserving foods are toxic by nature; their function is to destroy enzymatic activity and impede natural processes. The disruption to these processes means that the nutritional content of any real food ingredients can be adversely affected by chemical preservatives to the extent that the food may no longer be able to fulfil its basic function.

The use of preservatives to prolong the shelf-life of foods may be beneficial to food producers, but it is far from beneficial for consumers. The inherently toxic nature of their chemical ingredients does not make food products safer; on the contrary, chemical preservatives poison foods and therefore, make them far less safe.

Salt

In chemistry, according to the Oxford Dictionary, a 'salt' is defined as,

"any compound formed by the reaction of an acid with a base."

More commonly, 'salt' refers to the chemical compound, sodium chloride.

Salt has been used for millennia as a food preservative; the mechanism of action by which salt achieves preservation involves osmosis and the withdrawal of water from the cells, which inevitably causes dehydration. It is for this reason that salt is claimed to have antimicrobial properties.

This mechanism of action means that salt also causes the cells of all living organisms, including humans, to become dehydrated. This is demonstrated by the fact that highly-salted foods generate thirst, which is the body's mechanism for indicating a need for rehydration. Unfortunately, thirst is all too often addressed by the consumption of liquid in the form of processed soft drinks. But these beverages are a poor choice of liquid with which to quench thirst; not only do they fail to adequately rehydrate the body, but they increase the intake of toxins as they contain a number of food additives, especially sugars or sweeteners, which are discussed in the next sections.

There are a few different types of salt, the most common of which is referred to as 'table salt'; a highly processed product. The basic materials required for the manufacture of 'table salt' can be sourced from salt crystals or rock salt, which is then subjected to a number of processes. The first process involves the removal of all other substances, including other minerals, to leave the basic compound of sodium chloride. This compound is then subjected to two further processes, the first of which involves bleaching in order to whiten it. The second process involves the addition of aluminium, which is said to act as an anti-caking agent. It should be noted that bleach and aluminium are both hazardous substances.

Salt is also used as a 'flavour enhancer'; the food industry's enthusiasm to use salt for this purpose is indicated by an IoM (Institute of Medicine) 2010 Report entitled *Strategies to Reduce Sodium Intake in the United States* that states,

"Added salt improves the sensory properties of virtually every food that humans consume, and it is cheap."

The October 2018 WHO *Healthy diet* fact sheet recommends people to reduce their intake of salt and states,

"Keeping salt intake to less than 5g per day (equivalent to sodium intake of less than 2g per day) helps to prevent hypertension, and reduces the risk of heart disease and stroke in the adult population."

Although the WHO recommends a reduced salt intake and the IoM recommends a reduced sodium intake, the discussion about hypertension in chapter one demonstrated that heart problems are more likely to occur due to an imbalance between sodium and potassium at the cellular level, and not to the absolute level of sodium as the result of the consumption of salt.

There is, however, a great deal of confusing information about the consumption of salt; the central theme of most debates on the topic is that it is only the highly-processed form of salt that is unhealthy. The proponents of this idea claim that there are other types of salt that retain their original mineral content and are therefore nutritionally beneficial. But this idea is misleading.

Sodium and chloride are essential mineral nutrients; they are both required for the body's bioelectrical system and chloride combines in the stomach with hydrogen to form hydrochloric acid, which is essential for proper digestion. However, like all nutrients, it is essential that sodium and chloride are in the correct 'form' for absorption into and utilisation by the body. But whether other minerals are present or not, the compound called 'salt' does not contain the correct forms of sodium or chloride for the body; as indicated by Herbert Shelton in *Natural Hygiene Man's Pristine Way of Life*,

"How can salt be a food when it passes through the body unchanged, being ejected from all of the ejector organs in the same state in which it is taken into the stomach?"

Dr Henry Bieler MD, who studied the effects of salt on the body and particularly on the endocrine system, explains in *Food Is Your Best Medicine* that,

"Salt (sodium chloride) is frequently used to excess on foods because it stimulates the adrenal glands, but it is really a highly corrosive drug – a former embalming fluid which cannot be used in the body economy."

Its former usefulness as an embalming fluid is a clear demonstration that the main effect of salt in the body is to destroy enzymatic activity and cause dehydration; it is also clear that the body does not recognise salt as an essential nutrient.

It may be argued that some animals can absorb minerals directly from salt; however, as explained in chapter five, animals have different bodily systems, many of which are not directly comparable with the systems of the human body. For example, elephants are said to obtain minerals from 'salt-licks', but this does not mean that humans can do likewise; elephants can consume and digest whole acacia trees, including the bark and the leaves, humans are clearly unable to do likewise.

Herbert Shelton also explains that salt has been used as an emetic; in other words, salt can be used to induce vomiting. It is claimed by the medical establishment that this effect is only produced by the ingestion of a large amount of salt; the influence of the Paracelsus fallacy is again apparent. However, as Dr Bieler and Herbert Shelton have explained, salt is rejected by the body whatever the amount ingested; a larger 'dose' only causes a more pronounced effect.

The human digestive system absorbs its required nutrients from a diet that includes plants, fruits and vegetables, all of which provide a wide variety of minerals, including sodium and chloride.

Sugar

Sugar is the collective name for a particular group of carbohydrates; these include glucose, which is produced by the body, and fructose, which is found predominantly in fruits, although also in some vegetables. Glucose and fructose are monosaccharides that have identical chemical formulae. Other sugars include lactose, which is found in milk, and sucrose, which is found in both sugar cane and sugar beet. Lactose and sucrose are disaccharides that have identical chemical formulae, although these differ from the formulae of glucose and fructose.

It is often claimed that all sugars are the same; however, nothing could be further from the truth.

Sugar cane is a plant of the grass family that is indigenous to Asia and only grows in a tropical climate; the initial discovery that this plant produced a sweet-tasting juice is reported to have occurred many millennia ago. It is also reported that India was the first country to develop a method to process the liquid sap of the sugar cane and to produce sugar crystals.

The introduction of sugar to other parts of the world is reported to have begun with the planting of sugar cane in Brazil by the Portuguese. The popularity of sugar in Europe encouraged the expansion of sugar production and led to the establishment of many sugar cane plantations throughout South America and the Caribbean. The discovery that beets were also able to produce a sweet-tasting substance occurred in the 18th century; sugar beets only grow in a temperate climate.

The basic ingredient for the manufactured products generically referred to as 'sugar' is the juice extracted mainly from cane sugar, although beet sugar may also be used. However, the extracted juice, which contains sucrose, is subjected to many processes before it is transformed into 'refined sugar'. William Dufty describes this form of 'sugar' in his book entitled *Sugar Blues*,

> "Refined sucrose, $C_{12}H_{22}O_{11}$, produced by multiple chemical processing of the juice of the sugar cane or beet and removal of all fiber and protein, which amount to 90% of the natural plant."

The fact that these refining processes remove the nutrients means that the resulting product cannot be described as a 'food'. Refined sugar is often described as providing 'empty calories'; but this is not the only problem. The consumption of this highly processed form of sugar is also associated with certain adverse effects that make it harmful to the human body, as William Dufty explains,

> "In addition, sugar is worse than nothing because it drains and leaches the body of precious vitamins and minerals through the demand its digestion, detoxification and elimination make upon one's entire system."

Glucose is an entirely different type of sugar; it is produced by the body as the result of the consumption of many types of food, as William Dufty explains,

> "Many of our principal foods are converted into *glucose* in our bodies. Glucose is always present in our bloodstream, and it is often called blood sugar."

Under normal circumstances, glucose is carefully controlled by the body; it plays an important role in many aspects of metabolism. However, the consumption of refined sugars disrupts the body's regulatory mechanisms and interferes with the production of insulin; this disruption can result in diabetes, which is discussed in chapter seven.

Fructose, which is the type of sugar that occurs naturally in many different fruits and some vegetables, is also manufactured commercially and used to sweeten food products and drinks. Manufactured fructose is not the same as natural fructose; one of the main differences is that they are metabolised differently in the body. Whole foods, such as fruits, contain other elements, such as fibre, that enable the body to metabolise the fructose content slowly and release the sugar into the bloodstream in a controlled manner. Refined fructose, by comparison, does not contain those other elements and the body is unable to regulate the release of the sugar into the bloodstream.

In common with salt, a great deal of misleading information is reported about sugar, including its role in the human diet and its effects. The adverse health effects associated with the consumption of refined sugar are, albeit to a limited extent, recognised by the medical establishment, as indicated by the October 2018 WHO *Healthy diet* fact sheet that recommends,

"Limiting intake of free sugars to less than 10% of total energy intake..."

The reference to 'energy intake' is a clear indication of the erroneous notion about the importance of 'calories' as the criteria by which nutrition should be measured. The WHO explains the meaning of the term 'free sugars' in the March 2015 Press release entitled *WHO calls on countries to reduce sugars intake among adults and children*,

"Free sugars refer to monosaccharides (such as glucose, fructose) and disaccharides (such as sucrose or table sugar) added to foods and drinks by the manufacturer, cook or consumer..."

Although this press release refers to glucose and fructose as 'free sugars' that need to be limited in the diet, this is misleading; it is also somewhat confusing because the WHO appears to clarify their statement by the comment that,

"The WHO guideline does not refer to the sugars in fresh fruits and vegetables..."

The reason that the guidelines do not apply to the natural sugars found in whole foods, such as fresh fruits and vegetables, is because, as the WHO acknowledges,

"...there is no reported evidence of adverse effects of consuming these sugars."

The WHO therefore makes the point very clearly that the consumption of whole fruits and vegetables does not cause the health problems associated with the consumption of refined sugars. This is one point on which the WHO has not erred. Nevertheless, their recommendation that the intake of sugar should be 'limited' is inadequate, because processed refined sugars are not foods and do not, therefore, form part of a healthy diet.

In addition to being a common food 'ingredient', processed sugar is also used as a 'food preservative'. The reason it is useful as a preservative is because refined sugar has a similar effect on cells as salt; in other words, refined sugar draws water from cells through osmosis. It is for this reason that refined sugar is also claimed to have 'antimicrobial properties' and to therefore be able to 'protect' foods.

Sugar and salt are two of the most common food additives; although one is sweet and the other savoury, they are frequently used in the same food products and often on the basis that they perform similar 'technological functions'. They are both considered to be preservatives and flavour enhancers; but neither of them can be accurately described as a food.

Although all forms of sugar are perceived to be food, this is misleading; refined sugar is associated with many adverse health effects, which are listed on a page entitled *141 Reasons Sugar Ruins Your Health* on the website of Dr Nancy Appleton PhD; the list includes,

"Sugar interferes with the body's absorption of calcium and magnesium;

Sugar can cause tooth decay;

Sugar can lead to obesity;

Sugar can cause arthritis;

Sugar can cause asthma;

Sugar can contribute to osteoporosis;

Sugar can cause toxemia during pregnancy;

Sugar can cause free radicals and oxidative stress;

Sugar upsets the mineral relationships in the body."

These are nine very good reasons to completely avoid refined sugar. One of the most significant effects is the production of free radicals, which is at the heart of virtually all health problems, as discussed more fully in chapter ten.

Another adverse health effect, and one to which Dr Appleton does not refer, is that sugar is associated with tuberculosis, although it is not claimed to be the cause. In his book, William Dufty states that the number of deaths from tuberculosis increased in Britain during the 1700s, a period during which the consumption of sugar also increased. He further states that,

"In 1910, when Japan acquired a source of cheap and abundant sugar in Formosa, the incidence of tuberculosis rose dramatically."

It is officially recognised that there is an association between diabetes mellitus and tuberculosis; as indicated by a December 2009 article entitled *Tuberculosis and diabetes mellitus: convergence of two epidemics*, which states that,

"There is growing evidence that diabetes mellitus is an important risk factor for tuberculosis..."

Whilst the medical establishment continues to adhere to the 'germ theory' and the mistaken idea that TB is caused by a bacterium, they will never solve this problem, or that of diabetes, both of which are related to nutrition as well as other factors. The article also reports that ancient Indian writings record certain conditions that display similar symptoms to those of diabetes; this will be further discussed in chapter eight, as TB and diabetes are both major health problems in India.

It is clear that the natural sugars found in fresh foods are nutrients that the body is perfectly able to metabolise and convert into materials necessary for normal functioning. Unnatural sugars, such as those that have been refined by manufacturing processes, are not metabolised by the body; in fact, they have been shown to be deleterious to the body. These refined sugars are appropriately described by William Dufty as,

"...the sweetest poison of all."

Artificial Sweeteners

The recommendation by the WHO to reduce the intake of 'free sugars', in other words, processed refined sugars, is mainly based on the idea that sugar is high in calories and therefore contributes to obesity and overweight, which are 'risk factors' for heart disease.

The discussion in the previous section shows that the health problems associated with refined sugars is not related to the number of calories they contain. Unfortunately, the emphasis on the calorific value of foods encouraged the food industry to develop substances that provide sweetness but contain few, if any, calories. Foods that contain these sweeteners are often labelled 'sugar-free' or 'low calorie'.

However, the replacement of sugars with artificial sweeteners, whether as an additive to hot drinks, such as tea and coffee, or as additives in the manufacture of processed food products and drinks, is not an appropriate solution.

Although it may be assumed that foods and drinks with a reduced sugar content are lower in calories and therefore a 'healthy option', this would be a mistaken assumption for a number of reasons, not least of which is that these foods and drinks are invariably processed food products, which means they inevitably contain a number of additives.

The main reason is that artificial sweeteners are mostly, if not entirely, synthetic chemical compounds that are detrimental to health; they are not a suitable replacement for refined sugars, as two examples will demonstrate.

Saccharin

Saccharin is the name given to the chemical compound benzoic sulphimide, a coal tar derivative that is used by the food industry to sweeten both foods and drinks. It is claimed to be approximately 300-400 times sweeter than sugar and cheaper to produce.

The discovery that benzoic sulphimide had a sweet flavour is reported to have arisen accidentally as the result of laboratory experiments with coal tar derivatives conducted in 1879 by Constantin Fahlberg, a chemist who was working at the Johns Hopkins University. This discovery led to the development of a product that was introduced into the market and sold to the public as a 'low calorie' sweetener called saccharin.

In the early 20th century, Dr Harvey Wiley mounted a challenge to the use of saccharin during his relentless campaign against food adulteration. In 1908 he claimed that, as a coal-tar derivative, saccharin was not a 'food'; he also claimed that it was not fit for human consumption and proposed that it should be banned. Although his claims were correct, saccharin was not banned; the results of a number of experiments were claimed to demonstrate that small amounts were not harmful; saccharin was classified by the FDA as GRAS in 1959.

However, animal feeding studies were later conducted to assess the effects of saccharin consumption on rats. These experiments revealed that saccharin was a potential carcinogen; a revelation that led to its removal from the status of GRAS in 1972 and to its listing as a carcinogen in 1981. It has subsequently been revealed that rats have a different bodily mechanism and that it was this mechanism that accounted for the development of bladder tumours. As this mechanism does not exist in humans, it has been claimed that saccharin cannot cause human cancer. This new discovery has led to the removal of saccharin from the list of carcinogens in 2000 and to its approval for use, as indicated by the FDA website on a page entitled *Additional Information about High-Intensity Sweeteners Permitted for Use on Food in the United States* that states,

"Saccharin is approved for use in food as a non-nutritive sweetener."

Furthermore, the FDA refers to saccharin as 'safe for human consumption'.

Chapter five discussed the evidence that animals are not suitable models for humans, which was clearly demonstrated by the difference between rats and humans; however, that does not provide evidence that saccharin is therefore 'safe' for humans. It is a coal-tar derivative, which means that it is inherently toxic and should not be consumed.

Its toxicity is demonstrated by the fact that saccharin is known to be associated with a number of 'side effects'; these include headaches, breathing difficulties, diarrhoea, and skin problems. As previously discussed, all 'side effects' are, in reality, direct effects; these 'effects', which result from the consumption of saccharin, indicate that it cannot be considered 'safe' for consumption.

Aspartame

Aspartame is a highly popular and widely used artificial sweetener that is said to be 200 times sweeter than sugar; it is a complex chemical compound that is described as 'a methyl ester of the aspartic acid/phenylalanine dipeptide'. The EFSA published its assessment of aspartame in 2013, and states, on the web page entitled *Aspartame*, that,

"The opinion concludes that aspartame and its breakdown products are safe for general population (including infants, children and pregnant women)."

Unfortunately, however, nothing could be further from the truth.

The discussion about MSG revealed that glutamate and aspartate have a number of common characteristics; they are both naturally-occurring amino acids and are both neurotransmitters, which, under normal circumstances, are carefully controlled by the body's protective mechanisms.

Aspartame is a manufactured food additive product; it is used by the food industry to sweeten foods and drinks. The effects of aspartame are comparable to those of MSG, because it increases the body's level of the amino acid, in this case aspartate, and leads to circumstances that are no longer 'normal'. Under these circumstances, the body's normal protective mechanisms become overwhelmed and processed aspartate, like processed glutamate, becomes neurotoxic.

In *Death by Modern Medicine,* Dr Carolyn Dean refers to the research conducted by Dr Betty Martini, who has revealed that the dangers from aspartame are a direct result of its chemical composition,

> "Aspartame in molecular chemistry is composed of one molecule of aspartic acid, one molecule of methanol (free methyl alcohol) and one molecule of phenylalanine. Consider that this means 33% free methyl alcohol, a severe metabolism poison"

Dr Blaylock has also investigated the health hazards caused by aspartame and explains in *Health and Nutrition Secrets* how these hazards occur,

> "Both phenylalanine and aspartic acid are normally found in the nervous system, but at higher concentrations both are neurotoxic."

It is for this reason that the establishment claim that aspartame is 'safe' is erroneous. Dr Blaylock further explains why aspartame is not safe for consumption,

> "...the metabolic breakdown of aspartame yields about a dozen toxic compounds, some of which have been associated with cancer induction and alteration of brain function."

In common with aspartame's other components, methanol occurs naturally; however, there are natural mechanisms that prevent it from being toxic, as Dr Martini explains,

> "Methanol occurs naturally in all plants, fruits and vegetables, but – in nature – it is tied to the fibre pectin and is accompanied by its antidote, ethanol, in greater quantities that prevents the methanol being metabolized and it passes safely through the body's system without causing any harm."

This demonstrates another similarity with glutamate, which, in nature, is bound to peptide linkages; this also indicates the errors that are made by the assumption that manufactured chemicals are identical to their natural counterparts; clearly, this is not the case. The 'natural' form of methanol is processed differently by the body; methanol, or methyl alcohol, is described by Dr Blaylock as a 'powerful toxin'; he adds that,

> "When methyl alcohol is consumed, it is converted in the cells to formaldehyde and formic acid, both potent toxins."

Foods and drinks that contain aspartame are claimed to be a healthier option because they do not contain sugar; this too is clearly not the case. Unfortunately, soft drinks in aluminium cans pose an additional hazard; as Dr Blaylock explains,

> "So, in the case of diet drinks in aluminium cans, the very brain-toxic aluminium fluoride compound co-exists with multiple toxins found in aspartame, thus creating the most powerful government-approved toxic soup imaginable."

The health hazards associated with aspartame consumption include birth defects and mental retardation; it is also associated with a number of diseases, including multiple sclerosis. Birth defects and autoimmune diseases are discussed in chapter seven.

The dangers associated with aspartame led Dr Blaylock to conclude that,

> "This particularly nasty substance should have never even been approved for human use."

Genetically Engineered Food

Genetic engineering (GE), also referred to as genetic modification (GM), is a technology that is claimed to be vital for the ability to produce the ever-increasing volume of food necessary to feed the ever-growing population of the world; this technology is, however, highly controversial, as are many of the claims associated with it.

A May 2016 report entitled *Genetically Engineered Crops: Experiences and Prospects* was produced as the result of a study conducted by the US National Academies of Sciences, Engineering and Medicine. This report, which will be referred to as the *NASEM report*, defined the term 'genetic engineering' as,

> "a process by which humans introduce or change DNA, RNA, or proteins in an organism to express a new trait or change the expression of an existing trait."

Although the terms 'genetic engineering' and 'genetic modification' are often used interchangeably, they are not regarded as identical techniques. It is claimed that genetic engineering was first developed in the 1970s and that genetic modification, or manipulation, is a much older practice that is said to refer to the processes by which plants and animals have been 'domesticated'. The latter claim is, however, grossly misleading; genetic modification techniques do not resemble traditional breeding methods, as will be demonstrated.

The focus of this book is primarily on matters pertaining to health; however, in some instances, as with the current topic, a more wide-ranging discussion is necessary to provide a fuller understanding of the topic and the issues involved. The important additional issues for inclusion in the current discussion involve the origins of the technology and the ideas from which it has been developed, as well as the real purpose it is intended to serve, which is not the elimination of hunger, as claimed. The existence of world hunger and its causes are discussed further in chapter eight.

Author F. William Engdahl has investigated the history of the ideas behind the development of GE technology and recorded his findings in his book entitled *Seeds of Destruction*, which is one of the sources for this discussion and will be referred to as *Seeds*. In the introduction to *Seeds*, William Engdahl explains the wider context in which this subject needs to be contemplated,

> "In actual fact, the story of GMO is that of the evolution of power in the hands of an elite determined at all costs to bring the entire world under their sway."

In addition, he ascribes the idea that a certain faction exerts control over the production of food to a statement that is attributed to Henry Kissinger,

> "Control the food, and you control the people."

The idea that groups of people exert control over certain aspects of everyday life may seem incredible, but the evidence provided by the discussions in both this chapter and chapter nine will demonstrate otherwise.

In his investigation of its history, William Engdahl explains that the origin of genetic engineering lies in 'eugenics'. Although it is beyond the intended scope of this discussion to explore the subject in detail, it must be noted that eugenics did not originate in Germany in the 1930s as is commonly believed. Instead, it began in Britain and was readily adopted in America, which became the two foremost countries to develop eugenics programmes. The term 'eugenics' was coined in 1883 by Francis Galton, a British polymath and scientist, who was a major proponent of eugenics and who encouraged the implementation of eugenics programmes in Britain and the US. The purpose of these programmes was to develop methods with which to 'improve the breed of man'; some of the methods used by the programmes' scientists included the sterilisation of people who were deemed to be 'defective'.

Outrageous though these programmes were, it can be seen that the underlying idea of 'eugenics' has similarities with the underlying idea of genetic engineering as defined in the *NASEM report*. The purpose of manipulating genes is to alter the expression of existing traits or characteristics of organisms, which can be plant or animal in origin. The development of GE techniques resulted in the creation, in 1974, of a genetically modified mouse; in 1994, a tomato was the first genetically modified food to become commercially available, although it was not commercially successful.

The techniques of genetic engineering are different from those used in eugenics programmes, but they are both the result of the claim by certain groups of people that they have the 'right' to use 'science' to create all kinds of experiments, including those that can manipulate nature and alter the characteristics of living organisms.

The remainder of this discussion will focus on the genetic engineering of food.

William Engdahl explains in *Seeds* that GE technology was developed as the result of decades of prior agribusiness research that has its roots in the 'Green Revolution', the purpose which he also explains,

> "The heart of its strategy was to introduce 'modern' agriculture methods to increase crop yields and, so went the argument, thereby to reduce hunger and lessen the threat of a potential communist subversion of hungry unruly nations."

The threat of 'communist subversion' has not been relevant since the end of the Cold War; nevertheless, this same 'strategy' provides the essential aspects of the main argument that is used to promote genetic engineering; in other words, to increase crop yield and thereby reduce world hunger.

Although referred to as 'green', this revolution was not 'environmentally friendly'; it has proven to be the complete opposite because it involved the widespread use of large quantities of chemicals, as indicated in *Seeds*,

> "As one analyst put it, in effect, the Green Revolution was merely a chemical revolution."

Some of the major problems faced by farmers involve 'pests', whether of the insect or plant variety; another major concern for them is crop yield. The 'solutions' to these concerns of the farmers, to whom the 'Green Revolution' was promoted and sold, were found within the laboratories of the rapidly expanding chemical industry.

Nitrogen had long been used as a component of explosive weapons; TNT (trinitrotoluene) for example, was developed in 1863. Many of the weapons employed during WWII also utilised nitrogen in its nitrate form as a main component of the explosive material for bombs and shells. The US had produced a substantial quantity of nitrates for their weapons, but were left with a large stock of the material at the end of that conflict.

Plants require a variety of nutrients, one of which is nitrogen; however, plants cannot absorb atmospheric nitrogen, they can only absorb nitrates that are present in the soil. It was soon recognised that the stock of nitrates that was surplus to the requirements of the military could be made useful for agricultural purposes, as it would provide the basic material for nitrate fertilisers, which, together with pesticides and herbicides formed the core components of the 'Green Revolution'. These 'modern agricultural methods' provided a substantial boost to the output and profits of the chemical industry as the 'Green Revolution' was gradually introduced during the 1950s and 1960s into many countries, the first of which was Mexico.

At the beginning of the 1980s, genetic engineering technologies were in the early stages of development in the US and solely restricted to laboratory experimentation; at that time, there were mixed opinions within the scientific community about the introduction of plants created through GE technology, as explained in *Seeds*,

> "In 1984, no serious scientific consensus existed within America's research laboratories on the dangers of releasing genetically modified plants into a natural environment."

Nevertheless, in 1991, a mere seven years later, GM plants were experimentally introduced into Argentina whose population essentially became the first human 'guinea pigs' on whom this technology was tested. However, no substantial or long-term safety trials had been conducted prior to the release of this completely novel technology into the real-world environment. The reason that the industry failed to conduct substantial safety trials is explained by Jeffrey Smith in his book entitled *Genetic Roulette*, in which he quotes the US FDA 1992 policy on GM foods,

> "The agency is not aware of any information that foods derived by these new methods differ from any other foods in any meaningful or uniform way."

This policy effectively claims that GM crops are the same as traditionally-grown crops; its purpose was to provide assurances to the general public that foods produced by this new technology were entirely 'safe'. Although the FDA was in agreement with the industry about the alleged 'safety' of GM foods, there was a difference of opinion on the matter of which organisation should bear the responsibility for those assurances of safety. In *Genetic Roulette*, Jeffrey Smith quotes the FDA as being of the opinion that,

> "Ultimately it is the food producer who is responsible for assuring safety."

He also quotes the industry opinion on the matter, which, according to Philip Angell of Monsanto, was that,

> "Assuring its safety is the job of the FDA."

The denial of responsibility by both the biotech industry and the FDA is egregious.

The claim that GE crops and non-GE crops are not meaningfully different led to the creation of the term 'substantial equivalence'. This is, however, a false notion; there are significant differences between GE crops and non-GE crops, as will be demonstrated.

The failure to conduct thorough, long-term safety trials to determine whether this entirely novel method of creating food was absolutely safe prior to release into the real-world environment, has had serious consequences. Despite the claims that GE foods are 'safe', they have been proven to be otherwise, but the evidence of their health hazards is mostly, although not entirely, suppressed by the biotech industry.

In 2012, Earth Open Source produced a report entitled *GMO Myths and Truths: An evidence-based examination of the claims made for the safety and efficacy of genetically modified crops*, the Executive Summary of which states,

> "Genetically modified (GM) crops are promoted on the basis of a range of far-reaching claims from the GM crop industry and its supporters."

As indicated by its title, the report demonstrates that these claims are 'myths' rather than 'truths'. This report, which will be referred to as the *GMO Myths* report, is divided into seven sections, each of which contains a group of related 'myths' that are countered by 'truths', all of which are supported by evidence. Section seven refers to a number of myths grouped under the general heading *Feed the World*; the first myth of this group refers to the industry claim that,

> "GM crops are needed to feed the world's growing population."

This myth is countered by the statement that,

> "GM crops are irrelevant to feeding the world."

The theory that existing methods of food production are inadequate to feed the growing population of the world is based on an idea that is attributed to Thomas Malthus, a 19th century English economist, who claimed that food production increases at a different and much slower rate than that of population growth. It was believed that this discrepancy between the growth rates of food and population numbers meant that there must be a maximum world population 'carrying capacity', beyond which it would be impossible to produce sufficient food to feed everyone.

The *GMO Myths* report states that world hunger is not caused by an inadequate level of food production; a topic that is discussed in more detail in chapter eight. The viewpoint expressed in the *GMO Myths* report concurs with that of the Union of Concerned Scientists (UCS), who, in 2009, produced a report entitled *Failure to Yield: Evaluating the Performance of Genetically Engineered Crops*, the Executive Summary of which states,

> "Driven by economic and political forces, food prices soared to record highs in 2007 and 2008, causing hardships around the world. Although a global food shortage was not a factor then or now – worldwide food production continues to exceed demand – those recent price spikes and localized scarcity, together with rising populations in many countries and individuals' rising aspirations, have brought renewed attention to the need to increase food production in the coming decades."

The existence of hunger is not in dispute; the reality of this tragic situation is demonstrated by a September 2017 WFP news release entitled *World Hunger Again On The Rise, Driven By Conflict And Climate Change, New UN Report Says*. The number of people living in hunger is estimated to be approximately 815 million.

Conflict is certainly relevant to the creation of conditions that can give rise to hunger; but it is not one of its direct causes. The *GMO Myths* report claims that hunger is,

"...a problem of distribution and poverty, which GM cannot solve."

These factors are certainly relevant, but they are not the only causes of hunger.

It should be clear from previous discussions that 'climate change' cannot be regarded as the cause of any of the world's problems, including hunger; nevertheless, it is implicated as a causal factor of problems associated with agriculture. Section six of the *GMO Myths* report refers to the claim that,

"GM will deliver climate-ready crops."

Farmers have used traditional breeding methods to improve tolerance to a variety of conditions for millennia; these methods are able to improve crop tolerance to extreme weather conditions such as floods and drought, neither of which is caused by or is specific to 'climate change'. The biotech industry, on the other hand, believes that only GE technology can address these environmental stresses. An example of the industry efforts to control the situation can be seen in US Patent number 7851676 entitled *Stress tolerant plants and methods thereof*; although there are six individuals listed as the inventors, the assignee, or owner, is Monsanto Technology LLC. The first claim of this patent refers to,

"A method of generating a transgenic plant with enhanced tolerance to environmental stress..."

The *GMO Myths* report explains that,

"Tolerance to extreme weather conditions involves complex, subtly regulated traits that genetic engineering is incapable of conferring on plants."

According to the *GMO Myths* report, one of the reasons that GE technology is irrelevant to 'feeding the world' is because it is unable to achieve the increased crop yields it is claimed to produce. This point is confirmed by the UCS report, which was produced as the result of a detailed evaluation of GE crops,

"This report is the first to evaluate in detail the overall, or aggregate, yield effect of GE after more than 20 years of research and 13 years of commercialization in the United States. Based on that record, we conclude that GE has done little to increase overall crop yields."

In the conclusion to the report it is acknowledged that there have been overall increases in crop yields, but that these increases were largely achieved by methods other than those that involved GE technology,

"Most of the gains are due to traditional breeding and improvements of other agricultural practices."

The fact that traditional breeding methods outperform GE technology methods is discussed in section one of the *GMO Myths* report, the first 'myth' of which claims that GE technology is an extension of natural

315

breeding techniques. This myth is refuted by the 'truth' that,

"...GM is a laboratory-based technique that is completely different from natural breeding."

Throughout a large part of human history, people have grown food and developed methods for 'breeding' crops and for creating hybrid varieties; these processes were, and still are, 'natural'. These methods enable different varieties of the same crop to be cross-bred, the result of which is intended to encourage certain beneficial traits, such as drought resistance, for example. If successful, the improved traits will be emphasised in the new seeds and successive generations of the plants and crops.

Genetic engineering is not an extension of natural breeding; GE techniques involve the insertion of genetic material into a plant cell. This is a completely unnatural process that bears no resemblance to traditional cross-breeding methods and techniques. The *GMO Myths* report explains the GE process to highlight the difference between this technology and natural breeding,

"The genetic engineering and associated tissue culture processes are imprecise and highly mutagenic, leading to unpredictable changes in the DNA, proteins and biochemical composition of the resulting GM crop..."

Another myth that is exposed by the *GMO Myths* report is that GM crops reduce the use of pesticides and herbicides; this myth is countered by the truth that GM crops increase their use because,

"Herbicide-tolerant crops have been developed by agrochemical firms specifically to depend upon agrochemicals and have extended the market for these chemicals."

In 2003 the Institute of Science in Society prepared a Report entitled *The Case for a GM-Free Sustainable World*. This report, which is authored by a number of independent scientists, discusses many of the problems and issues with GM crops including the use of toxic herbicides, which they have been developed to tolerate. These herbicides include glufosinate ammonium and glyphosate, about which the report states,

"Both are systemic metabolic poisons expected to have a wide range of harmful effects and these have been confirmed."

It should be noted that glyphosate has been classified by the IARC as a 'probable' human carcinogen.

On the website of the Center for Food Safety is a September 2014 article entitled *Debunking Popular Myths about GE Crops Portrayed in the Media*. Included in this article is a reference to the myth that GE crops use chemicals of lower toxicity, but more worryingly, is the statement that,

"...next generation GE crops will further increase pesticide usage of even stronger, more toxic herbicides..."

The reason for the perceived need to use stronger pesticides is that many of the 'pest' plants, on which the toxic herbicides have been used, have developed resistance, especially to glyphosate. The biotech industry's 'solutions' to this problem, as indicated by the article, include the introduction and use of stronger pesticides and the development of a new generation of GE crops.

One particularly toxic pesticide, which was approved by the EPA in 2014 for use with GE crops, is a product that contains a blend of glyphosate and 2,4-D (2,4-Dichlorophenoxyacetic acid). 2,4-D is not a new pesticide; it was one of the ingredients of Agent Orange, the highly toxic chemical that is best known for its use as a defoliant during the Vietnam war. The Beyond Pesticides fact sheet about 2,4-D states that the health hazards with which this toxic substance has been linked include cancer, endocrine disruption and neurotoxicity.

Another of the industry claims exposed in the *GMO Myths* report is that GM crops are safe to eat; however, the truth is that,

"Studies show that GM foods can be toxic or allergenic."

It is impossible to tell the story of GMOs without referring to Dr Arpad Pusztai PhD, a biochemist who formerly worked at the Rowett Research Institute in Scotland and who, initially, was a supporter of GE technology and believed it would help to improve crop yield. In the mid-1990s, he conducted rat-feeding studies with genetically modified potatoes; however, the results of his experiments caused him to be concerned because they demonstrated a range of adverse effects.

In 1998, a programme was aired on British TV that contained an interview with Dr Pusztai in which he openly discussed his research and the results he had obtained; he is also reported to have stated that he would not eat GM foods. Although he had received prior approval from the Rowett Institute for this interview, the programme caused a furore; it had exposed the existence of health hazards as a direct result of the consumption of GM foods, which was in direct contradiction to the biotech industry's claims of safety. Shortly afterwards, Dr Pusztai was suspended from the Institute and vilified in the press on the basis that his work had not been published or 'peer-reviewed'. This situation was rectified in 1999 by the publication of his study article in *The Lancet*; a reputable journal that was, nevertheless also attacked and subjected to severe criticism by the pro-GM community. The study article is entitled *Effect of diets containing genetically modified potatoes expressing Galanthus nivalis lectin on rat small intestine*; it is available from the website of *The Lancet*.

The unfounded claims levelled against Dr Pusztai and his work were clearly intended to discredit him, despite the fact that he was considered to be an authority in his field of research and that, at that time, his study was considered by many to have been the most thorough research that had been conducted on a GM food. It is clear that his study results needed to be suppressed as they posed a serious challenge to the biotech industry and contradicted the claim that GM foods were safe.

In his 2009 article entitled *GMO Scandal: The Long Term Effects of Genetically Modified Foods on Humans* published on the website of the Center for Research on Globalisation, William Engdahl reports the continuing suppression of study results other than those that have been approved by the industry. He states that,

"The only research which is permitted to be published in reputable scientific peer-reviewed journals are studies which have been pre-approved by Monsanto

317

and the other industry GMO firms."

In 2011 Dr Vandana Shiva PhD, Debbie Barker and Caroline Lockhart of Navdanya, co-authored a report entitled *The GMO Emperor Has No Clothes*, which discusses the problems with GMOs. This report, which will be referred to as the *GMO Emperor* report, refers to information obtained by a group, comprised of CRIIGEN (the Committee of Independent Research and Information on Genetic Engineering) and two French universities, about Monsanto's 2002 rat feeding trials. The information discovered by the group was that the rats had suffered organ damage after being fed three varieties of approved GE corn. The *GMO Emperor* report cites the words of Dr Gilles Eric Seralini PhD, a molecular biologist, who refers to this information about the effects on the rats and states that it,

"...clearly underlines adverse impacts on kidneys and liver, the dietary detoxification organs, as well as different levels of damage to the heart, adrenal glands, spleen and haematopoietic systems."

Although, as discussed, animals are not suitable models for humans, these results demonstrate the existence of serious harm to rats and indicate the potential for harm to humans; it is therefore inappropriate for the industry to claim that GM foods are safe. These adverse impacts cannot be dismissed as irrelevant; they are systemic and not merely due to a different mechanism in one organ, as was the case with saccharin.

One of the theories on which genetic engineering is based claims that each gene codes for a single protein that expresses a specific trait or characteristic. On the basis of this theory, it was assumed that, as the human body contained approximately 100,000 proteins, it would contain an equal number of protein-coding genes. It was also believed that this assumption would be verified by the Human Genome Project.

However, to the amazement of many scientists, the results from this Project have revealed that the human genome only contains approximately 20,000 protein-coding genes; far fewer than had been expected. This discovery has completely undermined the theory that one gene codes for one protein; a theory that is central to genetic engineering. The implication of this discovery is explained by Dr Barry Commoner, a former senior scientist at the Centre for the Biology of Natural Systems at Queens College, who states, in his 2002 article entitled *Unraveling the DNA Myth: The spurious foundation of genetic engineering*, that,

"The fact that one gene can give rise to multiple proteins ... destroys the theoretical foundation of a multibillion-dollar industry, the genetic engineering of food crops."

The problem with GE technology extends beyond the discovery that genes can code for multiple proteins; it is exacerbated by the fact that the genes inserted into a plant cell have been taken from another species, often a bacterium; a situation that has absolutely no precedent in nature. Dr Commoner expands on this point in his article and states,

"In genetic engineering it is assumed, without adequate experimental proof, that a bacterial gene for an insecticidal protein, for example, transferred to a corn plant, will provide precisely that protein and nothing else."

The techniques involved in genetic engineering are claimed to be precise and the results predictable; the *GMO Myths* report, however, states that the processes are crude, imprecise and unpredictable and that GM technology,

"...is based on a naïve and outdated understanding of how genes work."

Dr Commoner expands further on the failure of GE processes to be either precise or predictable and indicates the potentially serious consequences,

"Yet in that alien genetic environment, alternative splicing of the bacterial gene might give rise to multiple variants of the intended protein – or even to proteins bearing little structural relationship to the original one, with unpredictable effects on ecosystems and human health."

On the basis that many proteins play important and even critical roles in the body, GE technology is clearly another example of a misplaced intervention in natural processes that has proven to cause a range of adverse consequences, some of which are entirely unpredictable. Molecular geneticist, Dr Michael Antoniou PhD, is quoted by Jeffrey Smith in his book, to have stated that,

"If the kind of detrimental effects seen in animals fed GM food were observed in a clinical setting, the use of the product would have been halted..."

In addition to the modification of seeds, genetic engineering is also used to create various enzymes and proteins that are included in the ingredients of many processed food products, although not always labelled as such. For example, two of the amino acids that comprise aspartame, namely aspartic acid and phenylalanine, are produced using processes that involve genetically modified bacteria.

Another 'myth' is the industry claim that GM foods are more nutritious. The *GMO Myths* report refutes this claim with specific reference to certain GM rice varieties that,

"...had unintended major nutritional disturbances compared with non-GM counterparts, although they were grown side-by-side in the same conditions."

The fundamental purpose of eating is to supply the body with nutrients; the disturbances to the nutritional content of GM foods by comparison with non-GM foods further demonstrates that they are not 'substantially equivalent'.

There is clear evidence that GM foods are not 'safe' and that, in reality, they are harmful. Herbicides are, by definition, toxic; their purpose is to kill unwanted plant 'pests' whilst sparing the crops that have been genetically engineered to be resistant to them. Although Dr Pusztai claimed that pesticides were not the cause of the adverse health effects he observed, the fact that GM crops are liberally sprayed with these toxic chemicals means that they will inevitably contain residues that are harmful to human health.

One of the most widely-used herbicides is glyphosate, which is the main active ingredient in a popular product called Roundup. In his 2010 article entitled *Study Shows Monsanto Roundup Herbicide Link to Birth Defects*, William Engdahl states,

"Roundup in far lower concentrations than used in agriculture is linked to birth defects."

The study to which he refers is reported in an article entitled *Glyphosate-*

based herbicides produce teratogenic effects on vertebrates by impairing retinoic acid signalling, on the website of the American Chemical Society. The study was initiated due to,

"Reports of neural defects and craniofacial malformations from regions where glyphosate-based herbicides (GBH) are used..."

The study investigated the effects of glyphosate on animal embryos; the abnormalities, including teratogenic effects, that were discovered bore a striking similarity to the malformations observed in human babies, as the article explains,

"The direct effect of glyphosate on early mechanisms of morphogenesis in vertebrate embryos opens concerns about the clinical findings from human offspring in populations exposed to GBH in agricultural fields."

Glyphosate is not the only chemical that has been associated with birth defects.

Many animal feeding studies involving GM foods have demonstrated a variety of adverse effects that have involved various organs, mainly the liver and kidneys, and many different systems, such as the bloodstream and digestive system and particularly the endocrine system, which is the reason for birth defects.

The failure to conduct long-term safety testing trials of GM foods prior to their release into the market has been exposed by the launch of a new long-term study. This study is reported in a November 2014 article entitled *Largest international study into safety of GM food launched by Russian NGO*. The article states that the study was to begin in 2015 and to be a 3-year experiment to investigate the long-term health effects of GM foods. It is reported that the researchers plan to use GM maize developed by Monsanto and that the purpose of the study is to answer the question about the safety of GM food. This is clearly a question that should have been both asked and satisfactorily answered long before any GM crops were allowed to be introduced into the real-world environment. However, the control by the biotech industry over the publication of the results of GM food studies, if they are unfavourable, raises questions over the information this study will be able to reveal.

Furthermore, the term 'substantial equivalence' was deliberately created not only to generate the impression that GE foods were no different from non-GE foods, but to also avoid conducting expensive safety trials. This is revealed by the *GMO Emperor* report that quotes a 1999 article entitled *Beyond 'substantial equivalence'*, which refers to substantial equivalence as,

"...a pseudo-scientific concept... It is, moreover, inherently anti-scientific because it was created primarily to provide an excuse for not requiring biochemical or toxicological tests."

It is clear, therefore, that the real purpose behind the introduction of GE 'technology' is largely related to the ability to control the food supply; some of the mechanisms through which this control is being established involves the use of patents, as the *GMO Emperor* report states,

"GMOs are intimately linked to seed patents. In fact, patenting of seeds is the real reason why industry is promoting GMOs."

The report expands on this point to show that the acquisition of seed patents does not conform to the normal procedures of competition within the same industry,

> "The giant seed corporations are not competing with each other. They are competing with peasants and farmers over the control of the seed supply."

One of the essential elements of traditional breeding methods involves the collection of seeds, either for planting to produce the next crop or for developing new varieties or new tolerances. But this practice is being eroded by the biotech industry that denies farmers the 'right' to collect seeds because GM seeds do not 'belong' to them; farmers are therefore forced to purchase seeds annually from the giant biotech corporations that seek to control agriculture, as the *GMO Emperor* report states,

> "Monopolies over seeds are being established through patents, mergers and cross licensing arrangements."

This situation makes farming far more expensive for the people, but hugely lucrative for the corporations, as the report continues,

> "Patents provide royalties for the patent holder and corporate monopolies."

The problem is not merely one of profiteering by the industry, it has far-reaching consequences, as the report indicates,

> "The combination of patents, genetic contamination and the spread of monocultures means that society is rapidly losing its seed freedom and food freedom."

Despite the claim by establishment scientists that genetic engineering technology is specific, precise, predictable and safe, it has been demonstrated in this discussion to be unspecific, imprecise, unpredictable and unsafe. Dr Barry Commoner stated in 2002 that,

> "The genetically engineered crops now being grown represent a massive uncontrolled experiment whose outcome is inherently unpredictable. The results could be catastrophic."

There is a growing awareness about the problems associated with GM foods, but it has led to calls for them to be labelled; these efforts, although well-meaning, are misplaced, they will ultimately result in the elimination of choice, as the *GMO Emperor* report states,

> "GMOs contaminate non-GE crops. Contamination is inevitable, since cross-pollination is inevitable, within the same species or with close relatives."

The only genuine solution to the problem of GE technology is an immediate and outright ban; it is the only course of action that can genuinely ensure the continuing availability of wholesome foods for the entire world population; not only for present generations, but for all future generations.

Poisoned Water

Water is an essential component of the cells of living organisms, including humans.

Although not categorised as a nutrient, water plays a vital role in all of the body's biochemical processes, as Herbert Shelton explains in *Natural*

Hygiene: Man's Pristine Way of Life,

> "Indeed, all the chemico-vital processes or changes that take place in the living body require the presence of water and a deficiency of it soon manifests itself in disturbances of these operations."

Water is lost from the body through natural functions, such as excretion and sweating, and therefore needs to be replaced to avoid dehydration, which can have serious health consequences. Although it is essential that lost fluids are replaced, there are differing opinions about the quantity of water that should be consumed each day; this important topic is discussed in chapter ten. It is the quality of drinking-water that is the focus of the discussion in this section.

The importance of providing good quality water for all purposes is recognised by the February 2018 WHO fact sheet entitled *Drinking-water* that states,

> "Safe and readily available water is important for public health, whether it is used for drinking, domestic use, food production or recreational purposes."

According to the USGS (US Geological Society) web page entitled *How Much Water is There on Earth?* an estimated 71 per cent of the Earth's surface is covered by water, of which approximately 96.5 per cent is sea-water. Of the remaining 3.5 per cent that is fresh water, more than two-thirds is locked in ice, glaciers and permanent snow. This means that only about 1 per cent of the total volume of water on the planet is in the form of liquid freshwater, most of which is located in groundwater and therefore below the surface; this leaves only a comparatively tiny volume located in surface waters, such as rivers and lakes. Yet this precious resource in all its locations has been, and continues to be, 'poisoned'.

It must be noted that, as with 'poisoned food', the deliberate poisoning of water with intent to cause harm forms no part of this discussion.

The WHO *Guidelines for Drinking Water Quality* report, originally published in 2011, was updated in 2017; this fourth edition of the report incorporates additional material, including the SDGs (Sustainable Development Goals) that relate to water. The UN 2030 Agenda and a number of the SDGs are discussed in greater detail in chapter eight; it should be noted for the purposes of this discussion that SDG 6.1 aims to,

> "By 2030, achieve universal and equitable access to safe and affordable drinking water for all."

The WHO report, which will be referred to as the *Water Guidelines* report, states that,

> "The primary goal of the Guidelines is to protect public health associated with drinking-water quality."

It would seem from the stated objectives of the UN and WHO that their policies will ensure that water made available for human consumption will be safe. Unfortunately, the word 'safe' is used in the same context in these reports as it is used in the Codex Alimentarius food guidelines; in other words, 'safe' is a relative term, as demonstrated by the *Water Guidelines* report that states,

> "Every effort should be made to achieve drinking water that is as safe as

practicable."

Efforts to make water 'safe' ought to involve the removal of all hazardous materials prior to the water being made available for human consumption. However, 'as safe as practicable' does not mean that all hazards have been removed; as the *Water Guidelines* report indicates, the purpose of the recommended strategies is to,

"...ensure the safety of drinking-water supplies through the control of hazardous constituents of water."

Unfortunately, their rigid adherence to the 'germ theory' means that, according to the medical establishment, the main 'hazardous constituents of water' are microbes; as indicated by the report that refers to,

"microbial hazards, which continue to be the primary concern in both developing and developed countries."

The main strategies to address these microbial hazards in order to make water 'safe' are discussed in the next section.

It is recognised that sanitation, hygiene and water are closely related issues; this is demonstrated by SDG 6.2, the aim of which is to,

"By 2030, achieve access to adequate and equitable sanitation and hygiene for all..."

It was shown in chapter two that the introduction of sanitary measures played a significant role in achieving improved public health, although this is often erroneously attributed to vaccination programmes. It is clear that insanitary conditions can adversely affect water quality, but the WHO nevertheless promotes the erroneous idea that 'germs' are the major cause of health problems. The WHO web page entitled *Water-related diseases* lists a number of diseases claimed to be caused by 'germs' and transmissible through water; one of these diseases is cholera, which is discussed in chapter eight. Surprisingly, this list also includes malnutrition; the WHO claims the nature of the relationship between water and malnutrition to be that,

"Nutritional status is compromised where people are exposed to high levels of infection due to unsafe and insufficient water supply and inadequate sanitation."

Unsafe water does not cause 'infections'; however, inadequate sanitation measures can clearly lead to the contamination of water, which, if consumed, would certainly be detrimental to health. The real relationships between malnutrition, insanitary living conditions and illness are also discussed in chapter eight.

The erroneous belief that 'microbes' pose the main threat to water quality means that an inadequate level of attention is paid to the real sources of water pollution. Although the phrase 'dangerous contaminants' refers to 'microbes', nevertheless, the WHO *Drinking-water* fact sheet does refer to genuine contaminants in the statement that,

"Inadequate management of urban, industrial and agricultural wastewater means the drinking-water of hundreds of millions of people is dangerously contaminated or chemically polluted."

The recognition that industrial wastes and chemicals are major sources of water pollution is demonstrated by the aim of SDG 6.3, which is to,

"By 2030, improve water quality by reducing pollution, eliminating dumping and minimizing release of hazardous chemicals and materials…"

Although the *Water Guidelines* report refers to the contamination of water by chemicals, it downplays their importance as pollutants in the statement that,

"There are many chemicals that may occur in drinking-water; however, only a few are of immediate health concern in any given circumstance."

The main justification for making such a statement is that the chemicals occur in amounts that are considered to be too low to cause any 'risks' to health; the erroneous nature of the theory on which this justification is based has been discussed.

Previous discussions have also demonstrated that chemicals are inadequately tested for their safety, and that the tests that have been conducted fail to investigate effects from exposures to the multiple combinations of chemicals to which people are exposed, including those that may occur in drinking water.

The claim that water is 'safe' because it is contaminated by only a few chemicals 'of concern' is therefore unfounded as it is not supported by evidence. More importantly, there is a large body of evidence that demonstrates many of the chemicals that pollute water are of significant concern with respect to human health.

There are many chemicals that pollute water and most of them are produced and discharged by a variety of different industries, as will be discussed. There are, however, two chemicals that are intentionally added to water, although for different purposes, which require particular attention.

Water Chlorination

One of the main ways in which drinking-water is poisoned is, paradoxically, the process by which water is claimed to be made 'safe', namely disinfection, about which the *Water Guidelines* report states,

"Disinfection is of unquestionable importance in the supply of safe drinking-water."

Nothing could be further from the truth. Disinfection is inherently toxic; its sole purpose is to kill germs, as the report states,

"The destruction of pathogenic microorganisms is essential and very commonly involves the use of reactive chemical agents such as chlorine."

Chlorine has been discussed at some length earlier in the chapter; however, its use as a water 'disinfectant' requires further examination.

One of the earliest applications of chlorine involved textile bleaching. Another application arose from the discovery by French scientists that chlorine compounds would not only reduce the 'odours of putrefaction' that permeated the streets of France in the early 19th century, they would also delay putrefaction; these chemicals therefore became useful for industries that produced noxious putrefaction odours; abattoirs, for example.

Although chlorine compounds may have succeeded in masking odours from decomposed organic material and waste matter, they did not eliminate the cause of the problem. The discussion about preservatives demonstrated that decomposition is a normal process and that delaying this process does not 'solve' the problem. The use of chlorine compounds to mask 'noxious odours' merely exacerbated the hazards to health.

The emergence and dominance of the 'germ theory' in the late 19th century encouraged the notion that 'germs' needed to be destroyed. The belief that diseases were transmitted through water stimulated scientists to believe that chlorine would be a useful ally in the battle against the 'germs' found in water; the addition of chlorine compounds to water supplies for disinfection purposes began in the early 20th century. At the time it was believed that, when added to water, chlorine would dissipate and leave no residue; this was, however, a mistaken belief, but the mistake was not discovered until the 1970s.

The reality is that, as discussed, chlorine-based compounds react with organic matter to produce toxic organochlorines that are persistent; which means that they remain present throughout the water system.

One of the major problems resulting from the use of chlorine for 'disinfection' is the production of DBPs (disinfection by-products), which are explained by Joe Thornton in *Pandora's Poison*,

> "The myriad by-products formed in the disinfection of drinking water with chlorine also find their way to people mainly though tap water – by drinking, absorption through the skin, or inhalation during a hot shower or bath."

The DBPs formed as the result of water chlorination include a group called THMs (trihalomethanes), a common type of which is chloroform, a toxic substance that has been classified by the IARC as 'possibly carcinogenic'.

The EPA web page entitled *National Primary Drinking Water Regulations* contains a table that lists various water pollutants, one of which is labelled TTHMs (total trihalomethanes). Within the table is a heading labelled 'Potential Health Effects from Long-Term Exposure Above the MCL'; the entry in this table for TTHMs lists,

> "Liver, kidney or central nervous system problems; increased risk of cancer."

MCL means 'maximum contaminant level'. The claim that health problems only occur when exposures exceed the MCL is unfounded. The serious nature of the effects produced in the body's important detoxification organs and the CNS is a clear indication of the severe toxicity of TTHMs. It should be clear that toxic substances always cause harm; the size of the 'dose' only determines the degree of harm they cause.

The EPA recognises that DBPs generate risks to health, but water disinfection is nevertheless claimed to be essential due to the perceived need to destroy germs. This paradox, which claims that toxic substances can be used to make water 'safe', creates a challenge for the water industry, as the EPA explains in a document entitled *Introduction To The Public Water System Supervision Program*,

> "A major challenge for water suppliers is how to balance the risks from microbial pathogens and disinfection byproducts."

The health risks from DBPs are deemed 'acceptable' because it is believed that many 'infectious diseases' are associated with water and inadequate sanitation, as indicated by the February 2018 WHO fact sheet entitled *Sanitation* that states,

"Poor sanitation is linked to transmission of diseases such as cholera, diarrhoea, dysentery, hepatitis A, typhoid and polio."

It should be clear that the addition of toxic chemicals to faecally-contaminated water does not remove the faecal matter, even though it may delay or even halt the processes of decomposition. The use of chlorine-based compounds, or any other toxic chemicals, to 'disinfect' water clearly does not make it 'safe'; this fact is acknowledged, albeit to a limited extent, by the *Water Guidelines* report that states,

"Chemical disinfection of a drinking-water supply that is faecally contaminated will reduce the overall risk of disease, but may not necessarily render the supply safe."

Faecally-contaminated water will certainly induce illness; faeces are waste matter that, if ingested, will be rejected by the body through vomiting or diarrhoea, or both, but these are natural processes, not 'diseases'.

The reason that the WHO claims water is not necessarily made 'safe' is due, in part, to the idea that some 'pathogens' are resistant to some disinfectants; the erroneous nature of this idea has been discussed. The real reason that water is not made 'safe' by disinfection is because the chemicals used are toxic; they clearly cause the water to become 'poisoned'.

Water Fluoridation

Fluorine and chlorine are two of a group of five closely-related chemical elements called halogens. The closeness of the relationship between them means that fluorine and chlorine have many properties in common, the most significant of which are that they are both corrosive, reactive and toxic, and that neither of them occurs in nature in their elemental gaseous form. However, unlike water chlorination, water fluoridation is not practised in all countries; only a small percentage of the world population receives artificially fluoridated water, although there are efforts to expand this practice.

Fluorine and chlorine are both claimed to have 'antibacterial' properties, but water fluoridation is used to serve a different purpose. The addition of fluoride to water supplies is based on the claim that it helps to reduce tooth decay, but this is yet another false claim.

Water fluoridation was first introduced in 1945 in the North American city of Grand Rapids, Michigan, where the inhabitants were the subjects of the initial human trial. The purpose of the experiment was to study the effects of fluoride on children's teeth and to compare the results with the condition of children's teeth in Muskegon, Michigan, where water was not fluoridated. This experiment is claimed to have shown that water fluoridation improves children's dental health; these results have been used to justify the introduction of water fluoridation into most parts of the US, where, according to the CDC web page entitled *Water Fluoridation Data & Statistics*,

"In 2014, 74.4% of the U.S. population on public water systems, or a total of 211,393,167 people, had access to fluoridated water."

Although fluoride is claimed to be beneficial, it is also recognised to be harmful; as indicated by the WHO web page entitled *Inadequate or excess fluoride*, which claims that fluoride has both beneficial and negative effects but that,

"The ranges of intakes producing these opposing effects are not far apart."

The claim that fluoride produces beneficial effects is, however, totally unfounded; fluoride only produces negative effects on teeth and on health.

The history of fluoride and its industrial applications is recounted by Christopher Bryson in his book entitled *The Fluoride Deception*. In particular he relates that, in the 1930s in Denmark, Dr Kaj Roholm MD discovered that workers who processed cryolite to extract aluminium suffered from multiple crippling ailments that mainly occurred in their bones, but also affected their central nervous systems. Cryolite is sodium hexafluoroaluminate, a major component of which is fluoride. Dr Roholm concluded from his investigations that the cryolite workers' health problems were caused by their exposure to fluoride; he called their condition 'fluorine intoxication'.

Christopher Bryson explains that the theory that fluoride was beneficial for teeth was first posited, although without any supportive evidence, as early as the 19th century. He also refers to a 1925 rat-feeding study, the results of which refuted the theory; this study demonstrated that fluoride weakened teeth, not strengthened them. Christopher Bryson reports that Dr Roholm made the same discovery,

"The workers' teeth he studied were bad, and the worst teeth had the most fluoride in them."

Aluminium is one of the most abundant elements in the Earth, but, like many other elements, it only occurs within an ore, from which it must be extracted. Although originally extracted from cryolite, aluminium is now mainly extracted from bauxite. The reason for this change is due to the depletion of cryolite deposits. The extraction of aluminium from bauxite still utilises cryolite, which, although now a manufactured substance, inevitably contains fluoride; aluminium extraction processes therefore still produce fluoride as a by-product.

Another industry that produces a significant volume of fluoride as a by-product is the phosphate fertiliser industry; the rock phosphate used as feedstock for the production of fertiliser contains a concentration of fluoride that ranges between 2 to 4 per cent.

The wastes discharged by the phosphate fertiliser industry originally caused a significant level of environmental damage; as discussed in a May 2003 article entitled, *The Phosphate Fertilizer Industry: An Environmental Overview*, in which the author, Michael Connett of the Fluoride Action Network (FAN), states,

"In the past when the industry let these gases escape, vegetation became scorched, crops destroyed, and cattle crippled."

The article reports that the damage caused by the toxic emissions of the phosphate fertiliser industry during the 1950s and 1960s was so severe that local communities pressured the industry to implement measures to reduce them. The action taken by the industry involved the installation of pollution capture devices, called 'wet scrubbers'.

The processes that convert phosphate rock to fertiliser produce wastes in the form of toxic silicofluorides. Although fluoride was useful for a number of industrial processes, the presence of silica in the wastes was a serious obstacle to their sale because the costs involved in removing silica rendered it uneconomical. But the toxicity of fluoride presented the industry with another difficulty, the disposal of the wastes captured by the 'scrubbers'; Dr Russell Blaylock explains,

> "Because of its intense corrosive ability and extreme toxicity, disposal of fluoride had, up until that time, been a very expensive and controversial proposition."

Fortunately for the industry, this difficulty was solved by the suggestion that these silicofluorides, which include fluorosilicic acid, could be utilised for water fluoridation, as explained on the FAN web page entitled *Fluoridation Chemicals*,

> "Until recently, all fluoridation chemicals were obtained from the wet scrubbing systems of the phosphate fertilizer industry in Florida."

The current source of fluoridation chemicals used in the US is reported on the FAN web page to be China, where regulations are reputed to be more lax. However, although Chinese industry is said to be poorly regulated, the fluoridation chemicals obtained from the wastes of the US phosphate fertiliser industry can also be contaminated by toxic materials, such as arsenic. Another common contaminant is uranium, which occurs naturally, although in varying concentrations, within phosphate rock.

The existence of 'regulations' does not ensure 'safety'; this is demonstrated by the fact that the EPA supported the use of toxic wastes from the phosphate fertiliser industry as the appropriate material to use in water fluoridation. The position of the EPA is made clear on the FAN web page about *Fluoridation Chemicals* that provides an extract from, and a link to a copy of, a letter written in 1983 by a senior EPA official; the letter states,

> "In regards to the use of fluosilicic acid as a source of fluoride for fluoridation, this Agency regards such use as an ideal environmental solution to a long-standing problem."

Fluosilicic acid is another name for fluorosilicic acid.

That the EPA would consider the use of toxic waste by-products to be an 'ideal' solution to an environmental problem is outrageous; the purpose of the EPA, as indicated by its name, is to protect the environment, not permit it to be poisoned.

The proposal to add fluoride to the US water system was opposed by many scientists and doctors who were aware of fluoride's toxicity; this opposition was originally endorsed by the ADA (American Dental Association), as indicated by Dr Blaylock, who quotes from the 1944 journal, in which the ADA referred to fluoride and concluded that,

> "...the potential for harm outweighed those for good."

The ADA has, however, reversed their position since 1944; the ADA web page entitled *Fluoride in Water* claims that water fluoridation,

> "...is safe and effective in preventing tooth decay..."

The promulgation of this claim by the ADA means that dentists are misinformed by the organisation responsible for their education; a situation that mirrors that of medical practitioners who are similarly misinformed by the organisation responsible for their education. The problems with dentistry are further discussed later in this chapter; the problems with medical education are discussed in chapter nine.

The idea that water fluoridation would help to prevent tooth decay was also a boon for the sugar industry, as it deflected attention away from evidence that showed sugar to be one of the main causes of tooth decay. Although the correct solution is to avoid sugar, the 'germ theory' was yet again invoked as it was claimed that bacteria were the cause of dental caries and that fluoride, which was toxic to bacteria, would assist in solving that problem. But fluoride is highly toxic, as Dr Blaylock explains,

> "It is essential to remember that fluoride is so reactive it can eat through steel, glass, iron, aluminium and most other substances: it joins mercury as being one of the most poisonous substances on earth."

Its inherently toxic nature is demonstrated by some of the main industrial applications of fluoride, which Dr George Waldbott MD discusses in his 1978 book entitled *Fluoridation: The Great Dilemma*,

> "Commercially, their only outlets were insecticides and rodenticides."

One fluoride-based pesticide is compound 1080 (sodium fluoroacetate), which is extensively used to control 'pests' such as rodents; this toxic compound was mentioned in the discussion about myxomatosis in chapter five.

Despite its highly toxic nature, fluoride has another, more surprising, industrial application; Dr Waldbott explains,

> "Simultaneously, the pharmaceutical industry discovered that fluorine reinforces the action of many molecules."

The result of this 'discovery' is that an estimated 20 to 30 per cent, of pharmaceutical drugs contain organofluorine compounds; their perceived mechanism of action includes certain functions, one of which is to slow the speed of drug metabolism; this function is also claimed to improve the drug's bioavailability. Some of the drugs that contain fluorinated compounds include: anti-cancer agents, antidepressants, anti-inflammatory agents and anaesthetics.

The FAN web page entitled *Sources of Fluoride* contains a section about *Pharmaceuticals*, which states that consumption of most of the drugs that contain fluorinated compounds will not increase exposure to fluoride. It is claimed that these drugs do not increase the intake of fluoride due to the tight bond between the fluorine and carbon atoms; this bond is said to resist metabolic processes that would release the fluoride ion.

However, the body will recognise pharmaceuticals that contain fluoridated compounds as toxic and attempt to expel them, but if these natural elimination processes are impeded, the body burden of toxins will increase, which will exacerbate health problems, not resolve them.

In common with many toxic chemicals, fluoride is widely used in many applications; although some have been discussed, Christopher Bryson provides a number of examples,

"We are exposed to fluorine chemicals from often-unrecognized sources, such as agricultural pesticides, stain-resistant carpets, fluorinated drugs, and such wrapping as microwavable popcorn bags and hamburger wrappers, in addition to industrial air pollution and the fumes and dust inhaled by many workers inside their factories."

One major difference between fluoride and chloride is that the latter is required by the body, whereas there is no evidence that fluoride plays any role in the body's biochemical processes. Although the WHO *Water Guidelines* report acknowledges that there is no recognised role for fluoride within the human body, it is tempered by the statement that,

"Fluoride may be an essential element for humans; however, essentiality has not been demonstrated unequivocally."

In his April 2012 article entitled *Fluoride and Biochemistry*, Dr Paul Connett PhD discusses the lack of evidence that fluoride plays any role in the human body and states,

"...there are no known biochemical processes that need the presence of the fluoride ion to function properly."

The article also states that some of the first opponents to water fluoridation were biochemists, who used fluoride for experimental purposes because it was known to act as a poison. In his article, Dr Connett quotes the words of biochemist Dr James Sumner, who stated in the 1950s that,

"Everybody knows fluorine and fluorides are very poisonous substances and we use them in enzyme chemistry to poison enzymes, those vital agents in the body."

Dr Sumner won a Nobel Prize in 1946 for his work on enzyme chemistry.

In his August 2012 article entitled *Fluoride is not an Essential Element* Michael Connett states categorically that,

"It is now known that fluoride is not a nutrient."

Despite the efforts of the WHO to suggest that fluoride 'may be' an essential element for the human body, the *Water Guidelines* report recognises fluoride to be a water contaminant of a similarly toxic nature to arsenic; as indicated in the reference to,

"...key chemicals responsible for large-scale health effects through drinking-water exposure (e.g. arsenic, fluoride, lead, nitrate, selenium and uranium) ..."

This recognition of fluoride's toxicity is in direct contradiction to the idea that fluoride is capable of protecting teeth from decay or is able to confer any 'beneficial' effects.

The idea that a tiny amount of fluoride is beneficial owes its existence to the Paracelsus fallacy, and is the basis for the reduction in 2015 of the concentration of fluoride added to the US water supply; it is claimed that the previous level had been 'too high'.

It should be clear that fluoride is toxic and should not be added to the water supply in any concentration; fluoride is, in fact, a major source of 'poisoned' water.

More Water Poisons

The *Water Guidelines* report states that,

"Access to safe drinking-water is essential to health, a basic human right and a component of effective policy for health protection."

Although access to water is a major problem for many people in certain regions of the world, the more fundamental problem, which affects everyone, is water quality.

The previous two sections have shown that, in countries where water is accessible through public water systems, the quality of the water delivered to people has almost invariably been compromised by 'treatment' with chlorine-based disinfectants to destroy 'germs'; in certain areas, fluoride 'treatments' exacerbate the problem and further compromise water quality. Other discussions in this chapter have indicated that most bodies of fresh water have become 'contaminated'; but, contrary to the information promulgated by the medical establishment, 'germs' are not contaminants.

The most significant factors that contribute to water pollution are toxic industrial wastes; a problem that is recognised by the EPA web page entitled *Industrial Wastewater*, which states that,

"Wastewater discharges from industrial and commercial sources may contain pollutants at levels that could affect the quality of receiving waters or interfere with publicly owned treatment works (POTWs) that receive those discharges."

The EPA has created a programme called NPDES (National Pollutant Discharge Elimination System) to 'control' the discharge of industrial wastes into local waterways by setting 'discharge limits' for each type of industry. This approach is clearly based on the idea that low levels of toxins are 'safe'; but it fails to recognise that multiple industrial discharges into the same body of water are extremely likely to exceed the limits deemed to be 'safe'. The EPA recognises that different industrial operations produce different volumes of wastes of varying degrees of toxicity and sets industry-specific guidelines. Two industries specifically referred to by the EPA are mining and oil and gas extraction, both of which have been discussed and shown to be significant sources of water pollution.

AFOs (Animal Feeding Operations) are another group of industrial operations that pollute the environment, especially local sources of water. A 2015 Food and Water Watch report entitled *Factory Farm Nation* refers to the huge growth in the US of large factory farms, also called CAFOs (Concentrated Animal Feeding Operations), and states that they,

"...produce millions of gallons of manure that can spill into waterways from leaking storage lagoons or fields where manure is over-applied to soil."

Although manure is often regarded as a good source of fertiliser for the soil, the wastes from CAFOs invariably contain a variety of contaminants, which include large volumes of antibiotics that are routinely used to 'treat' animals; the report states that,

"...most industrial livestock facilities treat the animals with low levels of antibiotics to try to prevent illness and compensate for stressful conditions."

Previous discussions have demonstrated that antibiotics are unable to prevent 'infections', or any other illness; they are, however, eminently capable of causing ill-health for animals as well as humans. In *Seeds of Destruction*, William Engdahl refers to the repeal by the EPA of a rule that had formerly held corporate livestock owners liable for pollution caused by animal wastes; he adds that,

> "The EPA also dropped a requirement that would have forced facilities to monitor groundwater for potential contamination by animal waste, which often seeped into the earth, leaving communities vulnerable to potentially dangerous drinking water supplies."

This is clearly another example of the failure of the EPA to protect the environment.

The chemical industry also contributes substantially to water pollution, both directly, via wastes produced from the manufacture of chemicals, and indirectly, via wastes produced by other industries that utilise chemicals in the manufacture of their own products, many of which are used on a daily basis. The use and disposal of products by the general public also contribute to environmental pollution, including water pollution. These direct and indirect sources are acknowledged by the *Water Guidelines* report that states,

> "Chemicals from industrial sources can reach drinking-water directly from discharges or indirectly from diffuse sources arising from the use and disposal of material and products containing the chemicals."

One group of chemicals that are of particular concern are POPs (persistent organic pollutants), which are discussed on the EPA web page entitled *Persistent Organic Pollutants: A Global Issue, A Global Response* that states,

> "Many POPs were widely used during the boom in industrial production after World War II when thousands of synthetic chemicals were introduced into commercial use."

Nevertheless, the EPA acknowledges that,

> "These same chemicals, however, have had unforeseen effects on human health and the environment."

To call the effects 'unforeseen' is disingenuous; had these chemicals been thoroughly tested prior to their introduction into commercial use, their nature as both toxic and persistent would have been discovered. This is not, however, a problem that only affects the US; POPs are indeed a 'global issue', their use is global and their effects are global.

A group of twelve POPs are referred to as the 'dirty dozen' due to their particularly toxic and persistent properties; this group includes pesticides such as aldrin, chlordane, dieldrin and heptachlor. It should be noted that all of the 'dirty dozen' are organochlorines, although they are not all pesticides. Another member of this group is TCDD, the most toxic member of the dioxin family. The persistence of dioxins in the human body is revealed by the October 2016 WHO fact sheet entitled *Dioxins and their effects on human health*, which states that,

> "Their half-life in the body is estimated to be 7 to 11 years."

Pesticides, whether used to kill insects, plants or animals, are recognised to be toxic and capable of contaminating sources of fresh water. However, pesticides, and particularly insecticides, are deemed to be necessary, as discussed in the *Water Guidelines* report,

"The diseases spread by vectors are significant causes of morbidity and mortality. It is therefore important to achieve an appropriate balance between the intake of the pesticides from drinking-water and the control of disease-carrying insects."

The most common 'vectors' are mosquitoes, which live near and breed in water; this means that mosquito-killing insecticides will be applied into or around bodies of water in which these insects are found. But insecticides are not specific to mosquitoes; they will poison all organisms, including people, that live in or rely on, the bodies of fresh water to which insecticides are applied. Yet again, the 'germ theory' provides the justification for the use of toxic chemicals to 'control' vectors that are claimed to transmit pathogenic microorganisms. The October 2017 WHO fact sheet entitled *Vector-borne diseases* claims that,

"The growth of urban slums, lacking reliable piped water or adequate solid waste management can render large populations in towns and cities at risk of viral diseases spread by mosquitoes."

The *Water Guidelines* report claims that the most significant type of virus that causes such diseases are enteric viruses, which,

"...infect the human gastrointestinal tract and are predominantly transmitted by the faecal-oral route."

Previous discussions have demonstrated that no diseases, including diarrhoea and similar gastrointestinal problems, are caused by viruses, nor are they caused by any other so-called 'germ'. Faeces, whether human or animal, are waste materials that the human body will recognise as 'toxic' and attempt to reject as quickly as possible, often producing diarrhoea and vomiting, both of which are natural mechanisms; the ingestion of water contaminated by toxic insecticides will also produce these symptoms.

Another significant member of the 'dirty dozen' is dichloro-diphenyl-trichloroethane, more commonly known as DDT. The EPA web page about POPs describes DDT as both 'controversial' and 'effective'; it also refers to the health and environmental damage caused by this toxic pesticide, which was documented by Rachel Carson in her seminal book *Silent Spring*. Although listed as a member of the 'dirty dozen' and banned in many countries, DDT remains one of the main tools used in the battle against mosquitoes in malaria-endemic regions of the world. As previously discussed, the ban on the use of DDT was not universally applied; DDT remained in use in certain countries, where it continued to contribute to health problems.

The WHO web page entitled *Persistent organic pollutants (POPs)* recognises that 'low level exposures' can lead to health problems that include increased cancer risk, increased birth defects and neurobehavioural impairment. The page also states that,

"POPs bio-magnify throughout the food chain and bio-accumulate in organisms."

The 'organisms' highest on the food chain, which include humans who consume animal-based foods, will therefore suffer the greatest accumulation of POPs; yet food production often involves the use of a variety of chemicals, including POPs. As discussed, the 'Green Revolution' promoted the idea that agricultural practices should increase the use of synthetic chemicals. Although nitrate is a soil nutrient, synthetic nitrate fertilisers are not 'natural'; they are pollutants that often leach from the soil and contaminate water sources, as explained by a Soil Association report entitled *Just Say N₂O: From manufactured fertiliser to biologically-fixed nitrogen* that states,

> "Nitrate leaching can lead to eutrophication and acidification in fresh waters, estuaries and coastal zones..."

There are far too many water-contaminating chemicals to discuss them all; the *Water Guidelines* report lists more than 100 substances under the sub-heading *Chemical contaminants in drinking water*. It should be noted that this list includes: aluminium, arsenic, asbestos, barium, benzene, cadmium, cyanide, fluoride, formaldehyde, lead, mercury, toluene and uranium; these are some of the most toxic and dangerous substances known to science and none of them should be present in water that has been deemed to be 'safe' for drinking.

Radioactive materials, such as uranium and its decay products, clearly present extremely serious health hazards, as the *Water Guidelines* report acknowledges,

> "Drinking-water may contain radioactive substances ('radionuclides') that could present a risk to human health."

Despite recognition of the health risk, the report continues with the statement that,

> "These risks are normally small compared with the risks from microorganisms and chemicals that may be present in drinking-water."

This is grossly misleading; the 'risk' from microorganisms is zero, as has been discussed. There are certainly health risks from ingesting chemicals. The discussion about ionising radiation demonstrated that there is no 'safe' level of exposure; the risks from ingesting water contaminated with radionuclides cannot be regarded as small.

The health hazards due to 'medicines' have been discussed, especially in the section about iatrogenesis; however, pharmaceuticals also pose a direct threat to water; as Dr Carolyn Dean states in *Death by Modern Medicine*,

> "One astounding fact about our overuse of medications is that every body of water tested contains measurable drug residues."

In addition, she states that,

> "Following that abuse are the tons of drugs and drug metabolites that are flushed down our toilets making their way around the world and ending up in our drinking water."

The 'astounding fact' that water is contaminated by huge volumes of pharmaceutical drugs is supported by the findings of a US Geological Survey study discussed by the NRDC in their December 2009 White Paper entitled *Dosed Without Prescription: Preventing Pharmaceutical Contamination of our Nation's Drinking Water*. In this paper, the NRDC reports that the Survey team,

> "...found organic wastewater contaminants and pharmaceuticals in 80 percent

of sampled sites – including antibiotics, hypertensive and cholesterol-lowering drugs, antidepressants, analgesics, steroids, caffeine and reproductive hormones."

This situation is not unique to the US; it will exist in every country in which pharmaceutical drugs are consumed. Another significant source of water pollution by pharmaceutical drugs involves the operations of the pharmaceutical industry itself, as the NRDC White Paper states,

"The amount and variety of waste created during the manufacture of pharmaceuticals dwarfs the amount of the actual finished product."

The ever-greater variety of chemicals that continue to be developed, used and discharged into the environment continue to exacerbate water pollution, as indicated by the EPA on a web page entitled *Contaminants of Emerging Concern including Pharmaceuticals and Personal Care Products* that states,

"Contaminants of emerging concern (CECs), including pharmaceuticals and personal care products (PPCPs), are increasingly being detected at low levels in surface water..."

This situation had been anticipated by Rachel Carson who wrote in *Silent Spring* that,

"Ever since chemists began to manufacture substances that nature never invented, the problems of water purification have become complex and the danger to users of water has increased."

It is, however, a situation that has substantially worsened due to the thousands of new chemicals that have been produced and introduced onto the market since the 1960s. The refusal to acknowledge that it is not 'germs' but toxic chemicals that pose the greatest threat to human health, permits the chemical industry to continue polluting and contaminating the environment, including vital sources of fresh water.

Water purification can no longer be described as merely 'complex'; it is widely recognised that most water treatment plants are unable to remove the vast majority of chemicals; which means that 'treated' water remains chemically-polluted. Nevertheless, this 'treated' water may be returned to the water system. A November 2013 article entitled *Only Half of Drugs Removed by Sewage Treatment* refers to a report, which revealed that the 'treatment' of effluent subsequently discharged into the Great Lakes had failed to remove six chemicals, which were,

"...an herbicide, an anti-seizure drug, two antibiotic drugs, an antibacterial drug and an anti-inflammatory drug."

The concentration of these chemicals is reported to have been 'low', but that does not mean that they pose no threat; as repeatedly stated, low doses of toxic substances are not 'safe'.

Although regulatory agencies set a 'safety limit' for the concentration of each chemical, these are often breached, as indicated by an August 2016 press release entitled *Unsafe levels of toxic chemicals found in drinking water for six million Americans*. This press release, issued by the Harvard School of Public Health states that,

"Levels of a widely used class of industrial chemicals linked with cancer and other health problems – polyfluoroalkyl and perfluoroalkyl substances (PFASs) – exceed federally recommended safety levels in public drinking water supplies."

Clearly, the existence of regulations does not guarantee that they will be implemented. However, even if fully complied with, regulations that limit the amount of each chemical discharged by each industry will not solve the problem, because industrial wastes contain multiple chemicals in varying combinations, none of which has ever been tested for the level at which they can be deemed 'safe'.

Furthermore, the failure to test all combinations of all chemicals means that by-products of chemical interactions are entirely incapable of detection; their effects remain unknown and unknowable. Peter Montague's comment in his 1999 article about risk assessment, which was quoted at the beginning of the chapter, deserves repetition,

"Science has no way to analyze the effects of multiple exposures..."

Rachel Carson made a similar comment with specific reference to organic chemicals; she states that,

"The chemist who guards water purity has no routine tests for these organic pollutants and no way to remove them."

The degree to which drinking water is contaminated by toxic substances will depend on where people live; however, water is a vital resource for everyone wherever they live. Water is essential for all forms of life on planet Earth; it is far too important a resource to be contaminated, polluted and poisoned.

Poisoned Bodies

Previous discussions have shown that 'poisons' can be absorbed into the body through ingestion, injection and inhalation; there is, however, a further pathway through which poisons can be absorbed into the body. Although the skin has been referred to as an organ of elimination, the process operates in both directions; in other words, the skin can absorb toxic substances as well as eliminate them.

The IPCS (International Programme on Chemical Safety) is a collaboration between the WHO, ILO (International Labour Organisation) and UNEP (United Nations Environmental Programme) that, in 2006, produced a report entitled *Dermal Absorption*; a term that is used to describe,

"...the transport of chemicals from the outer surface of the skin both into the skin and into the systemic circulation."

The skin is the body's largest organ; it has three layers. The outermost layer, called the epidermis, acts as a waterproof barrier that can nevertheless permit the transport of substances into other layers and into the systemic circulation; which enables toxic chemicals to enter the bloodstream.

Although the report claims that skin permeability is variable, Dr Samuel Epstein MD states in his book entitled *Toxic Beauty* that the skin is 'highly permeable'; he also explains that toxic substances absorbed into the body through the skin can be more harmful than if they had been ingested. The reason for this is because the digestive system carries ingested substances into the liver where they can be processed and detoxified by enzymes. But these enzymatic processes are bypassed when toxic substances are absorbed through the skin. It should be noted that these enzymatic processes are also bypassed when toxic substances are injected into the body, whether injections are administered intradermally, intramuscularly or subcutaneously.

In 2014 the IPCS published a further report entitled *Dermal Exposure*, which recognises that health hazards can arise from skin exposures to toxic substances and states,

> "Diseases resulting from dermal exposure (and consequently absorption) may have a significant impact on human health."

Specific chemicals do not cause specific 'diseases' per se; as will be discussed in chapter ten. However, the report recognises that chemicals can cause various degrees of damage and states that,

> "Dermal exposure can lead to local damage to the skin and/or systemic effects after crossing the skin barrier..."

The report also recognises the variety of products in which chemicals can be found,

> "Dermal exposure has been identified as an important exposure route, as people are exposed to a variety of substances and products either directly or indirectly while at work, in the home or in public facilities."

The report claims that 'skin diseases' are the second most frequent type of occupational health problem; it also claims that the second highest incidence of occupational health problems occurs in manufacturing workers. Although there is a huge variety of chemical-based products utilised for industrial purposes, some types are more common.

One group of widely-used products are organic solvents, which have a number of applications that range from degreasing agents to ingredients of paints, varnishes, adhesives and glues. The chemical ingredients of solvents can include benzene, formaldehyde and toluene, all of which have been discussed and shown to be highly toxic and even carcinogenic. Solvents also contain chemicals that are volatile, which means that they can be inhaled and cause respiratory problems, as discussed in the section about fracking. Some of the solvent chemicals are lipophilic; which means that they dissolve in fats or oils and, if they cross the skin barrier, the report states that they,

> "...may become systemically available in considerable amounts."

The highly toxic nature of some of these chemicals means that 'considerable amounts' can lead to extremely serious health problems.

NIOSH (National Institute for Occupational Safety and Health) is part of the CDC and responsible, as its name implies, for health and safety in the workplace. The NIOSH section of the CDC website includes a page entitled *Skin Exposures and Effects* which recognises that,

> "Dermal exposure to hazardous agents can result in a variety of occupational diseases and disorders, including occupational skin diseases (OSD) and systemic toxicity."

Contact dermatitis, which is said to be a type of eczema, is claimed to be one of the most common skin diseases, the symptoms of which can include irritation, dryness and inflammation. It is incorrect to refer to these symptoms as a 'disease' when they are recognised to have resulted from exposures to hazardous substances; eczema is discussed further in chapter seven.

The toxic ingredients of industrial products can result in far greater health hazards than irritation, dryness and inflammation of the skin; as recognised by the reference to systemic toxicity. However, other than a passing reference to 'skin cancer', NIOSH fails to discuss the full extent of the potential adverse health consequences that can result from the absorption of highly toxic chemicals into the bloodstream; chapter seven discusses cancer and many of its causes.

The *Dermal Exposure* report acknowledges that exposure to toxic substances is not limited to occupational environments, although non-occupational exposures involve different products; the report states that,

> "...people can be dermally exposed to chemicals in a variety of chemical classes through use of a diverse range of consumer products. Most relevant types of products include personal care products and cosmetics, textiles (including shoes) and household products..."

A number of consumer products and their toxic ingredients are discussed in the ensuing sections; however, in common with all other chemicals, the determination of their 'safe use' in consumer products is based on risk assessment, as indicated by the *Dermal Absorption* report that states,

> "Risk assessments are usually performed to determine the extent to which exposure to a particular substance is acceptable and therefore the extent to which the substance is safe to use."

The claim that risk assessments ensure that people are never exposed to harmful 'doses' of any toxic substance has been repeatedly shown to be unfounded, as Dr Epstein asserts in *Toxic Beauty*,

> "The poison is only in the dose, they tell us, and claim (falsely) that the doses to which we are exposed are too low to be harmful."

Surprisingly, however, the *Dermal Absorption* report makes a significant admission, which is that,

> "For many chemicals, there is no information on dermal absorption."

This means that the medical establishment has a poor level of knowledge about the full extent of the potential health effects from the absorption of chemicals through the skin. Despite this paucity of knowledge, the 'safe' level of a substance used in consumer products is determined by reference to the NOAEL established through experimentation that, in the vast majority of cases, only investigates each substance individually. This is acknowledged by a 2012 EU report entitled *Toxicity and Assessment of Chemical Mixtures*, which states that,

> "The EU Chemicals legislation, in common with the situation in other parts of the world, is based predominantly on assessments carried out on individual substances."

Although legislation and regulations in many countries are based on assessments of individual substances, the EU report recognises that, in the real world, people are exposed to multiple chemicals in many different combinations in the reference to,

> "...the almost infinite number of possible combinations of chemicals to which humans and environmental species are exposed..."

Most people probably assume that consumer products that are intended for use on the skin, or are likely to make direct contact with the skin, have been proven safe to use on the skin; this is yet another mistaken assumption. One of the main obstacles to a greater awareness of this problem is the lack of information about the ingredients provided on a product's label. In Dr Epstein's book entitled *The Politics of Cancer Revisited* is an Appendix entitled *Shopper Beware* in which he states,

> "Consumers have an inalienable right to know what ingredients are in products they use daily..."

This problem is not one that can be solved by demanding that manufacturers provide better information on product labels and include all of their chemical ingredients. The fundamental problem is that toxic chemicals are used in the manufacture of consumer products intended for use on the skin or are likely to make contact with the skin.

However, people do not have to use these products; in addition to the 'right' articulated by Dr Epstein, is an even more basic 'right', which is the right not to be poisoned, which means that people can choose to purchase non-toxic products; or even create their own.

Surprisingly the EPA has provided some suggested solutions, which are available on the web page entitled *Household Hazardous Waste (HHW)*,

> "When shopping for items such as multipurpose household cleaners, toilet cleaners, laundry detergent, dish soap, dishwashing machine pods and gels, bug sprays and insect pest control, consider shopping for environmentally friendly, natural products or search online for simple recipes you can use to create your own."

Solutions to these and many other problems discussed in this book are explored further in chapter ten.

Household Products

The term 'household products' applies to a wide range of goods, from large electrical appliances to small consumable items. Although a range of different materials are used in the manufacture of these products, some materials are common to a substantial proportion of them; metals and plastics, for example.

The first synthetic plastic was developed in the early 20th century; the intervening century has, however, seen a phenomenal increase in their manufacture and use, the result of which is that plastics have become ubiquitous. Plastics are entirely synthetic materials that are mostly, although not exclusively, made from petrochemicals; they are used in a wide range of applications that extend from insulation for electrical wiring to baby toys; from hard plastics for device casings to soft plastics for food wrapping.

The main advantage of plastics is said to be their stability, a quality that ensures their durability; unfortunately, their durability is also their main disadvantage, because synthetic plastics are incapable of natural degradation, they are virtually indestructible and have become highly persistent environmental pollutants.

There are many types of plastic; one of the most widely used is PVC (polyvinyl chloride), a product of both the petrochemical and chlor-alkali industries. Like all plastics, PVC is durable; it is also an extremely effective insulating material, which makes it ideal for use as protective covering for electrical wiring.

Plastics have many applications, some of which require them to be solid and strong, others of which require them to be soft and flexible. For the latter type of application, plastics are required to undergo further treatment with chemicals called plasticisers. One of the most common group of plasticiser chemicals are members of the family of phthalates, which are also petrochemicals. Although they are mainly used as plasticisers, phthalates also perform other 'functions' and can be found in a wide variety of consumer products, as indicated by the FDA web page entitled *Phthalates* that states,

> "Phthalates are a group of chemicals used in hundreds of products such as toys, vinyl flooring and wall covering, detergents, lubricating oils, food packaging, pharmaceuticals, blood bags and tubing, and personal care products such as nail polish, hair sprays, aftershave lotions, soaps, shampoos, perfumes and other fragrance preparations."

The plastics industry unsurprisingly claims that phthalates are 'safe'; for example, according to a PVC industry promotion website,

> "Plasticised PVC has been used for over 50 years without a single known case of it having caused any ill-health..."

The FDA's position on the safety of phthalates, by comparison, is rather vague,

> "It's not clear what effect, if any, phthalates have on human health."

These comments are disingenuous; there is ample evidence that demonstrates phthalates produce many adverse effects. A 2008 article entitled *Environmental phthalate exposure in relation to reproductive outcomes and other health endpoints in humans* indicates that phthalates, like all other chemicals, have not been thoroughly tested; as the article states,

> "Though the number of phthalates is large, many have not been examined in humans."

The article refutes the claim that there are no adverse human health effects from exposures to phthalates and states that,

> "...evidence for significant impacts on human health is mounting."

These health impacts are a matter of serious concern, particularly as the FDA indicates that the medical establishment utilises plastics containing phthalates in blood bags and tubing. Phthalates are also used in pharmaceuticals, in which their main function is to act as excipients in drugs. According to the page entitled *Pharmaceutical Excipients* on the American Pharmaceutical Review website,

> "Generally, an excipient has no medicinal properties. Its standard purpose is to

streamline the manufacture of the drug product and ultimately facilitate physiological absorption of the drug."

The PVC industry website contains a page entitled *PVC: The most widely used polymer in medical applications* that lists some of the applications, which include: inhalation masks, catheters and cannulae, and surgical and examination gloves. All of these applications utilise softened plastics, which means they contain plasticisers; and they all make direct contact with the skin or body of medical staff and patients.

The FDA also lists food packaging as one of the uses of phthalates, one of the most common of which is called DEHP (di-2-ethylexyl phthalate). Phthalates have been increasingly recognised as endocrine disrupting chemicals and, in some instances, have been replaced. One of the main chemicals introduced to replace DEHP is a substance called DEHA (di-2-ethylhexyl adipate); however, in *The Politics of Cancer Revisited*, Dr Epstein states that,

> "Cling film contains carcinogens such as di-2-ethylhexyl phthalate (DEHP) and di-2-ethylhexyl adipate (DEHA), which will migrate into foods, especially fatty foods."

The recognition that DEHA is also carcinogenic raises serious questions over its suitability as a replacement chemical for DEHP; it is clearly not 'safer'. Although not a member of the family of phthalates, adipates are similarly derived from petrochemicals. Dr Theo Colborn also refers to the leaching of phthalates on the page entitled *Phthalates* on the Our Stolen Future website,

> "Now they are ubiquitous, not just in the products in which they are intentionally used, but also as contaminants in just about anything."

In their March 2012 *Phthalates Action Plan*, the EPA claims that phthalate exposures have been associated with adverse health effects, but have not been proven to directly cause ill-health problems; nevertheless, they state,

> "EPA is concerned about phthalates because of their toxicity and the evidence of pervasive human and environmental exposure to them."

Furthermore, the EPA's TEACH (Toxicity and Exposure Assessment for Children's Health) programme has produced a document about phthalates that discusses some of the adverse effects reported by animal experiments and states,

> "Exposure to phthalates has been reported to result in increased incidence of developmental abnormalities such as cleft palate and skeletal malformations, and increased fetal death in experimental animal studies."

Children are clearly vulnerable to toxic chemicals; however, pregnant women are particularly vulnerable to endocrine disrupting chemicals, which can have devastating effects on the developing baby; the endocrine system and its importance is discussed further in chapter seven.

Another group of plastics that have been the subject of health concerns are polycarbonate plastics; the reason for this concern is because they often contain a chemical called bisphenol A, also known as BPA. Plastics that contain BPA have been used for food containers and baby bottles, as well as for the resin used in the inner lining of tins. Although BPA is widely recognised as an endocrine disrupting chemical, the FDA refers to it as,

"...safe at the current levels occurring in foods."

This statement suggests that at other levels BPA may not be 'safe'; which demonstrates the reliance on the Paracelsus fallacy to permit the continuing manufacture and use of products that nevertheless can and do cause adverse health effects. In contrast to the view of the FDA, is that expressed by the ECHA (European Chemicals Agency) on the web page entitled *MSC unanimously agrees that Bisphenol A is an endocrine disruptor*; the title is self-explanatory. MSC refers to the Member State Committee of the ECHA.

Despite the position taken by the FDA, there has been a considerable degree of publicity in the US about the hazards of BPA and this has led to its removal from some plastic products. However, although plastic bottles may be promoted as 'BPA-free', the chemicals used to replace it have not necessarily proven to be a safer option. A March 2011 article entitled *Most Plastic Products Release Estrogenic Chemicals: A Potential Health Problem That Can Be Solved* states that,

"Almost all commercially available plastic products we sampled – independent of the type of resin, product, or retail source – leached chemicals having reliably detectable EA, including those advertised as BPA free."

EA means oestrogenic activity, (estrogenic is the American spelling). One of the chemicals introduced to replace BPA is called BHPF (fluorene-9-bisphenol), but this is also associated with endocrine disruption; as indicated by a March 2017 article entitled *Fluorene-9-bisphenol is anti-oestrogenic and may cause adverse pregnancy outcomes in mice*; the title is self-explanatory.

In addition to the materials with which many types of household goods and containers are manufactured, are the chemicals that comprise the ingredients of consumables, such as cleaning products for example. Every year the chemical industry produces large quantities of chemicals, unknown numbers of which are contained in a profusion of products that have a multitude of purposes within the home. It may be assumed that, because these products are intended for use within the home, they have been thoroughly tested for their safety; unfortunately, yet again, nothing could be further from the truth.

Fortunately, public awareness about the toxic ingredients of many everyday household products is growing, as Dr Epstein explains,

"In the last few years consumers have discovered that some of the chemicals in household products whose safety was taken for granted are hazardous."

One particular group of household products that contain hazardous chemicals are 'cleaning products', which include a myriad of polishes, creams, liquids, sprays, lotions and potions to brighten, whiten, sparkle, gleam and otherwise clean everything in the home, as well as an array of 'fresheners' to disperse those 'unwanted odours'. These products promise to make the chore of cleaning easy, but this ease is achieved through the use of some extremely powerful, but highly toxic chemicals. The extent of this problem is succinctly explained by the Organic Consumers Association in an article entitled *How Toxic Are Your Household Cleaning Supplies?*

"In fact, some cleaners are among the most toxic products found in the home." This article, which will be referred to as the OCA article, states that,

"In 2000, cleaning products were responsible for nearly 10% of all toxic exposures reported to US Poison Control Centers, accounting for 206,636 calls."

The article reports that more than half of these calls related to children younger than six years old. The adverse effects from exposure to the chemicals in cleaning products can vary from mild irritation to chronic health problems, including cancer. Clearly, some chemicals are more dangerous than others; however, cleaning chemicals are rarely harmless. The OCA article quotes Philip Dickey of the Washington Toxics Coalition, who states that,

"The most acutely dangerous cleaning products are corrosive drain cleaners, oven cleaners, and acidic toilet bowl cleaners."

The article also confirms that combinations of products can significantly add to the dangers of the various toxic chemicals contained in each different product,

"Combining products that contain chlorine and ammonia or ammonia and lye (in some oven cleaners) produces chloramines gases, while chlorine combined with acids (commonly used in toilet bowl cleaners) forms toxic chlorine gas."

Chlorine is a common ingredient of bleach, which, together with ammonia are the two chemicals most often used as cleaning agents. In 1999, the *NEJM* (New England Journal of Medicine) published an article entitled *Severe Lung Injury after Exposure to Chloramine Gas from Household Cleaners*, which also refers to the production of chloramine gas from the combination of ammonia and chlorine and explains the effects,

"When inhaled, chloramines react with the moisture of the respiratory tract to release ammonia (NH_3), hydrochloric acid (HCl) and oxygen free radicals."

It should be noted that chloramines are also used as secondary water disinfectants on the basis of the claim that they are longer lasting; however, chloramines are not a 'safer' option for water disinfection. Chloramines can also generate toxic by-products, a significant one of which is a chemical called NDMA (N-Nitroso-dimethylamine) that is described in the March 2014 EPA Technical Fact Sheet as a group B2 carcinogen; which means it is a 'probable' human carcinogen. The fact sheet states that,

"NDMA is also an unintended by-product of the chlorination of wastewater and drinking water at treatment plants that use chloramines for disinfection."

Exposures to the toxic chemicals used in cleaning products arise not only from direct contact with the skin but also from inhalation because many of these chemicals are volatile as Dr Epstein explains,

"That means they become gaseous at room temperature or are sprayed from an aerosol can or hand pump and this takes the form of microscopic particles that are easily inhaled."

The inhalation of volatile toxic chemicals means that they are absorbed into the respiratory system where they can cause serious damage to the lungs.

Another chemical of concern, and one that is also associated with cleaning products, is called 1,4-dioxane, which, despite its similar name, is not a

343

member of the family of dioxins; it is, however, classified as a 'probable' carcinogen. The Environmental Working Group (EWG) refers to it as a by-product and states that it has been found in products such as liquid laundry detergents, as indicated on the EWG web page entitled *Cleaning Supplies and Your Health*,

"Common cleaning ingredients can be laced with the carcinogenic impurity 1,4-dioxane..."

Some chemicals used as ingredients of household products have been withdrawn from use when they were discovered to be particularly hazardous; but their replacements have often been discovered to be similarly toxic, or in some cases more so. It is common for the new formulation to be promoted as 'new and improved', but the new ingredients may only have a different mechanism of action. It should be clear that 'new and improved' does not necessarily mean 'safer'.

In addition to the chemicals that perform the task of 'cleaning' are the increasing array of chemicals used in order to impart 'fragrance'; these chemicals include, amongst others, the ubiquitous family of phthalates. Some of the adverse effects caused by 'fragrance' chemicals are discussed in the OCA article,

"Fragrances added to many cleaners, most notably laundry detergents and fabric softeners, may cause acute effects, such as respiratory irritation, headache, sneezing and watery eyes in sensitive individuals or allergy and asthma sufferers."

Although 'sensitive individuals' are more likely to suffer acute symptoms, 'non-sensitive' people will also be affected by these toxic chemicals; chapter seven discusses sensitivity to chemicals.

The OCA article also refers to the use of 'trade secrets' to prevent disclosure of fragrance chemicals, the consequences of which are that these ingredients are not listed on the product label. The customer is only provided with limited information, which may state that the product contains 'fragrance', 'perfume', or sometimes 'parfum'; however, 'fragrance' chemicals are not restricted to household cleaning products; they are widely used in cosmetics and personal care products, which are discussed in the next section.

It is clear that one of the main problems for consumers is the lack of information they are provided about all of the chemical ingredients of the products they purchase. This dearth of information is not restricted to fragrance chemicals, as Dr Epstein explains,

"Some leading household products do not disclose to the consumer that they contain carcinogens...neurotoxins, such as formaldehyde..."

The toxic chemical ingredients of cleaning products do not necessarily remain in the home; they often enter the water or sewage systems; but as discussed, most water treatment plants are unable to remove most toxic chemicals. It is therefore not only their use, but their disposal that makes household products significant contributors to environmental pollution. The page entitled *Household Hazardous Waste (HHW)* on the EPA website refers to the 'improper disposal' of hazardous substances and states that this includes pouring the chemicals into toilets and drains, because,

> "...improper disposal of these wastes can pollute the environment and pose a threat to human health."

This point is not disputed; however, the EPA fails to recognise or mention the far more important and fundamental problem, which is that industries are permitted to manufacture and sell products that contain extremely hazardous chemicals that threaten not only the environment, but also human health; both of which the EPA claims to protect.

The foregoing clearly represents only a very small selection of the household products that are used on a regular, if not daily basis; but they highlight the problem that, by using these products, people are regularly exposed to highly toxic and often dangerous chemicals that can and do adversely affect their health.

Cosmetics and Personal Care Products

The use of 'cosmetics' has a long history that, in some parts of the world, spans many millennia. However, a long history is not proof that a practice is inherently safe, particularly as some of the substances used in cosmetics applied to the face have been decidedly toxic. For example, during the period between the 15th and 18th centuries, it was a custom for some European women to apply white lead to their faces and either cinnabar or red lead to their cheeks; cinnabar is mercury sulphide. Another example is the ancient Eastern practice of applying 'kohl' around the eyes; although different substances have been and still are used, the traditional source of kohl was stibnite, which is the primary ore of antimony, a toxic metalloid.

The application of toxic materials to any part of the body is hazardous to health due to the skin's permeability; the application of neurotoxic substances, such as mercury and lead, to the face poses even greater hazards to health due to the close proximity of the brain and other vital organs in the head and neck.

The rise of the chemical industry during the 19th and 20th centuries stimulated the replacement of natural materials with synthetic chemical compounds in an ever-wider variety of applications, and this inevitably extended to the use of chemicals in cosmetics, as Dr Epstein explains in *Toxic Beauty*,

> "During the Roaring Twenties chemists further expanded the cosmetics industry with their laboratory discoveries."

All statements attributed to Dr Epstein in this discussion are from *Toxic Beauty*, unless otherwise stated.

The chemicals developed for use by the cosmetics industry in the early 20th century were treated in the same manner as those developed for other industrial purposes; in other words, these chemicals were not subjected to rigorous safety testing procedures prior to their release onto the market, despite the fact that they were intended for use in cosmetics products and that many of them would be applied to the face. The enthusiasm of the cosmetics industry to exploit the market and sell a wide range of new products seems to have outweighed any concerns about potential adverse health effects; as Dr Epstein states,

> "Synthetics captured the imagination of manufacturers, and their advantages helped blind the industry to any consideration of the unknown impact these synthetic ingredients would have on health."

It was not just the industry that was blinded; Dr Epstein explains that, in the early 1930s, certain eyelash and eyebrow colourants were manufactured from aniline dyes, which are toxic coal-tar derivatives, and that these products literally blinded some of the women who used them.

It would appear that the situation has changed in the intervening decades as the cosmetics and personal care products industry now asserts that the chemical ingredients used in their products undergo rigorous safety testing to ensure that they are 'safe'. However, the procedures employed for testing the safety of the chemical ingredients of these products are the same as those employed for all other applications of chemicals; their purpose is to determine a 'safe level of use' for each individual ingredient.

In addition to conducting tests of individual ingredients, the industry states that they also assess the 'safety' of the combination of ingredients in each product, as indicated by a page entitled *Science & Safety Information*, on the website of Cosmetics Info, that states,

> "All ingredients are evaluated in the final product to confirm that their actual use is within the safe range for both consumers and the environment."

The claim that the use of chemicals falls within a 'safe range' means that there must also be an 'unsafe range' of these chemicals and that therefore they are not absolutely safe. It is clear that the Paracelsus fallacy is again the basis for the safety testing procedures and product evaluations that apply to cosmetics and personal care products. The idea that there can be a 'safe' dose of a toxic chemical or of a combination of toxic chemicals within a single product ignores the situation in the real world, in which exposures are always to multiple combinations of substances in multiple products.

Despite assurances by the industry that their products have been tested and proven to be 'safe' for their intended use, the *Dermal Exposure* report acknowledges that direct skin contact is a recognised source of exposure to chemicals and that cosmetics and personal care products are relevant to such exposures. The report also admits that these products,

> "...can damage the skin's function and eventually contribute to the risk of ill-health."

Although promoted as enhancers of beauty, the reason that these products can damage the skin is due to the toxic nature of their chemical ingredients, and the harsh manufacturing processes they undergo, some of which are described by Dr Devra Davis in *The Secret History of the War on Cancer*,

> "To make some of the chemicals that are widely used in personal care products, toxic materials like ethylene oxide and propylene oxide are placed in oversize pressure reactors and pushed to react with oils or with amines, while they cook for a day."

It should be noted that propylene oxide has been categorised as reasonably anticipated to be a human carcinogen and that the EPA lists ethylene oxide as a Group B1 'probable' human carcinogen.

346

Some of the chemical ingredients of cosmetics and personal care products are used for purposes that are more akin to the 'technological functions' performed by food additives; for example, one of the additional purposes is 'preservation'. In common with all other preservative chemicals, those used in cosmetics and personal care products are claimed to possess 'antimicrobial' properties; which means that, by definition, they must be toxic. The chemicals most commonly used for this purpose belong to a group referred to as parabens, of which there are many different types. Dr Epstein refers to parabens and states that they are,

> "...the most common of all ingredients in cosmetics and personal-care products. They are also widely used in foods and pharmaceuticals."

He adds that,

> "Numerous studies over the last decade have shown that parabens pose weakly estrogen-like effects."

Although described as 'weak' these effects cannot be dismissed as irrelevant, as the discussion about the endocrine system in chapter seven will demonstrate. However, the FDA promulgates a different view of these chemicals and states on their web page entitled *Parabens in Cosmetics* that,

> "At this time, we do not have information showing that parabens as they are used in cosmetics have an effect on human health."

This statement is disingenuous in the light of Dr Epstein's reference in his 2009 book to the numerous studies that have shown parabens to demonstrate effects on the endocrine system. But further studies have been conducted since 2009 and they continue to demonstrate that parabens can cause adverse effects. One study is reported in a September 2010 article entitled *Toxic effects of the easily avoidable phthalates and parabens* that refers to the use of parabens in anti-perspirants and states that,

> "Their estrogenicity and tissue presence are a cause for concern regarding breast cancer."

As the article indicates, phthalates are another group of toxic chemicals used in many cosmetics and personal care products, including soaps, shampoos and perfumes. Dr Epstein explains that their function in these products is,

> "...to increase their flexibility and to stabilise fragrances."

The phthalates used in cosmetics and personal care products include diethyl phthalate (DEP), dibutyl phthalate (DBP) and di(2-ethylhexyl) phthalate (DEHP), all of which are categorised on the TEDX website as endocrine disrupters; additionally, the IARC has classified DEHP as a Group 2B 'possible' human carcinogen. Furthermore, the EU has banned the use of DBP and DEHP due to concerns about their adverse health effects.

In addition to products such as perfumes that are intended to deliver 'fragrance', many cosmetics and personal care products also contain 'fragrances', which are mostly chemical in nature, as Dr Epstein explains,

> "The chemicals that give perfumes and fragrances their aromas are manufactured in one of three ways: chemical synthesis from petrochemicals; chemical modification of isolates from natural sources; or direct extraction from

natural sources."

He adds that,

"In various combinations, perfumes and fragrances use at least 5,000 different ingredients, and about 95 percent of these are synthetic."

Although some are obtained from 'natural sources', the processes to which these substances are subjected may substantially alter their nature to the extent that they may no longer bear any resemblance to their original state. These changes can significantly alter the way these processed chemicals function or even the way they react with other chemicals.

Another toxic chemical extensively used in cosmetics and personal-care products is formaldehyde, which, as discussed, is claimed by the medical establishment and vaccine manufacturers to be endogenously produced. This claim is refuted, however, by the re-classification of formaldehyde by the IARC in 2006 to Group 1 status; which means that it is a proven human carcinogen. In addition to the direct use of formaldehyde, certain personal care products, including some intended to be used on babies and small children, contain chemicals that Dr Epstein refers to as 'formaldehyde releasers', which he describes as some of the many 'hidden carcinogens' in these products.

Triclosan is another preservative chemical claimed to have 'antibacterial' properties. It was originally introduced in the 1970s and initially only used in hospitals and health-care facilities, but was subsequently introduced into a wide range of consumer products, especially 'antibacterial' soaps and handwashes. Triclosan is, however, an organochlorine and therefore not 'safe', as Dr Epstein explains,

"Triclosan interacts with free chlorine in tap water and degrades under sunlight to produce chloroform."

Furthermore, in addition to the production of chloroform, which is categorised as a 'probable' human carcinogen, triclosan poses other health hazards, as Dr Epstein continues,

"It also produces a class of persistent, highly toxic, carcinogenic chemicals known as dioxins..."

Although triclosan is not a pesticide, the organisation Beyond Pesticides has led a campaign to remove it from the market; their web page entitled *Triclosan* refers to,

"...the mounting scientific evidence documenting adverse health effects, including impacts to the thyroid hormone..."

One of the results of the campaign has been that some manufacturers have voluntarily removed triclosan from their products. Another major result has been that in September 2016 the FDA issued a rule, which establishes that,

"...over-the-counter (OTC) consumer antiseptic wash products containing certain active ingredients can no longer be marketed."

The ingredients referred to include triclosan and triclocarban, amongst others; the reason for this rule is claimed to be because they are no better than soap and water for 'preventing the spread of germs'. However, the FDA also admits that,

"In fact, some data suggests that antibacterial ingredients may do more harm than good over the long-term."

It should be noted that the EU also removed their approval of triclosan in 2016.

Although the removal of any toxic chemical is a 'victory' against the use of 'poisons' in consumer products, it must be remembered that thousands of chemicals remain on the market and that most of them have not been fully tested for their safety, if at all, despite their use as ingredients of products that are used on a daily basis by millions of people around the world.

Many cosmetics and personal care products also contain chemicals that act as emulsifiers and foaming agents; these functions are important for liquid products such as shampoos, bodywashes and bubble baths, amongst others. One chemical commonly used for these purposes is DEA (diethanolamine), which is acknowledged by the EPA to cause adverse effects,

"Acute inhalation exposure to diethanolamine in humans may result in irritation of the nose and throat, and dermal exposure may result in irritation of the skin."

Adverse health effects are not restricted to mere irritation; the IARC classified DEA in 2013 as a Group 2B carcinogen, in other words, it is 'possibly' carcinogenic to humans. Dr Epstein refers to DEA as one of three detergents that are 'common penetration enhancers', because they,

"...facilitate the absorption of other ingredients through the skin by damaging the skin to increase its permeability."

It should be clear that substances known to damage the skin should not be ingredients of products intended for use on the skin.

There is a variant of DEA called cocamide DEA that is promoted as being naturally derived from coconut oil; which suggests it is a 'natural' ingredient, but this is not the case. The coconut oil from which the chemical has been derived is certainly natural; but this natural substance is then subjected to chemical processes that substantially alter its nature, as indicated by the IARC classification of cocamide DEA in 2013 as a Group 2B 'possible' human carcinogen.

Other chemicals of concern that are used in cosmetics and personal care products, as well as in household products, include sodium lauryl sulphate (SLS) and sodium lauryl ether sulphate (SLES); the latter may also be referred to as sodium laureth sulphate. The purpose of these chemicals is to act as surfactants, which means that they break the surface tension of the liquid to produce a greater interaction between the products and the surfaces to which they are applied. These may be inanimate surfaces, such as kitchen worktops, or they may be living surfaces, such as human skin. Dr Epstein explains that SLS and other harsh detergents are also penetration enhancers that, like DEA, damage the skin and increase its permeability, which enables toxic chemicals to be absorbed into the body and systemic circulation. He adds that these harsh detergents,

"...are invariably contaminated with high concentrations of the volatile and carcinogenic ethylene dioxide and 1,4 dioxane..."

In addition to their everyday use by the general public at home, cosmetics and personal care products are employed in a number of occupational settings; for example, many different types of products are used on a daily basis by beauticians and hairdressers. Another major consumer of cosmetics is the entertainment industry, in which many people, especially actors, are regularly exposed to 'make-up' applied to the face. It should be noted that the people who apply these products to actors are also exposed, although to a lesser extent, to the chemical ingredients of these products.

Regulatory bodies claim that responsibility for the safety of cosmetics and personal care products rests with the manufacturers. The industry claims that their products are thoroughly tested and proven to be 'safe' prior to their release onto the market. Despite these claims, however, every year some products are recalled for various reasons, which include the detection of toxic substances known to cause health hazards. Some of the detected toxic materials include lead, mercury and antimony. An April 2017 article entitled *Number of cosmetic product recalls spikes 63% in 2016* was published on the Cosmetics Business website; the article states that,

"Using the European Commission's rapid alert system for product notification (RAPEX), SGS released its 2016 RAPEX Recalls report presenting the number of recalls by country and product category."

The SGS report states that during 2016, 124 cosmetics and other chemical products were recalled, which, although not a large number, nevertheless indicates that products claimed to be safe' have subsequently been discovered to be 'unsafe'. The report shows that the products with the greatest number of recalls are in the category of bodywashes and cleansers. The Cosmetics Business article adds that,

"Certain ingredients were highlighted in the report as being 'frequently implicated substances'."

These 'frequently implicated' substances are reported to include parabens, phthalates and formaldehyde, all of which have been shown in this discussion to be toxic and hazardous to health; which raises the question of why these hazardous chemicals continue to be permitted in consumer products.

Two other chemicals common to a number of the products recalled are methylisothiazolinone (MIT) and methylchloroisothiazolinone (CMIT); these are both preservative chemicals that are claimed to possess 'antibacterial' properties. The main hazard associated with their use is reported to be 'contact dermatitis', which is a clear indication that they are skin irritants. This situation raises serious concerns about the rationale behind the continued use of known skin irritants in products intended for use on the skin.

It is clear that most cosmetics and personal care products contain a wide variety of chemical ingredients, many of which are toxic and known to cause adverse health effects; however, although there is increasing pressure by concerned groups for all product ingredients to be fully listed on labels, this will not solve the problem; as Dr Epstein states,

"...product labelling per se is still inadequate to protect consumer health..."

Consumer health can only be protected by the rejection of products that contain toxic ingredients. The recommendation by the EPA that people should find ways to source non-toxic alternatives for household products should be extended to apply to cosmetics and personal care products. Safer alternatives are being produced and are becoming more readily available, as will be discussed in chapter ten.

Clothes

It is disquieting to contemplate that the ordinary, everyday activity of wearing clothes could be a source of exposure to toxic chemicals; nevertheless, that is the case, as acknowledged by the *Dermal Exposure* report, which, as previously cited, includes textiles and shoes in the list of 'relevant products'.

Although the production of textiles has a long history, especially in countries such as India, the modern textile industry has its origins in the Industrial Revolution; it was one of the first to benefit from the mechanisation processes developed during that period of vast industrial expansion. The textile industry also benefited from the creation of petrochemicals, some of which were the basic ingredients used in the manufacture of synthetic fibres, the first of which was nylon that began commercial production in 1939.

The manufacture and use of synthetic fibres have increased phenomenally since the mid-20th century; according to the Statista website, the worldwide production of synthetic fibres was 5,000 tons in 1940; by 2015, the volume is reported to have increased to 62.9 million tons. Synthetic fibres are claimed to possess certain advantageous qualities, particularly durability, for which they are increasingly developed and used in preference to natural fibres. It is claimed that clothes manufactured using synthetic fibres are 'safe'; but this is another unfounded claim, as Dr Brian Clement PhD and Dr Anna Maria Clement PhD explain in their book entitled *Killer Clothes*,

> "Synthetic-fiber clothing is worn with an illusion of safety but hides invisible chemical and other dangers that clothing manufacturers and much of the world's health-care industry ignores, or attempts to rationalize away."

Clothing made from synthetic fibres is also discussed by Nicholas Ashford and Dr Claudia Miller in *Chemical Exposures*, in which they refer to some of the serious health effects that can be produced,

> "Synthetic fabrics have been implicated in elevated blood pressure, increased heart rate, arrhythmias, and angina."

This statement indicates that these conditions have causes other than those claimed by the medical establishment; cardiovascular diseases are discussed in more detail in chapter seven.

Fortunately, there is an increasing level of awareness of the adverse impacts on the environment due to the manufacture of clothing. Greenpeace, for example, produced two reports in 2012 about the use of toxic chemicals in the textile and clothing industries. The October 2012 report, entitled *Toxic Threads: The Big Fashion Stitch-Up*, indicates the phenomenal output of the industry,

> "Around 80 billion garments are produced worldwide, the equivalent of just over 11 garments a year for every person on the planet."

The manufacture of clothing is not only a source of environmental pollution, it also poses hazards to human health, especially as the vast majority of the 80 billion garments produced each year are manufactured utilising processes that involve a huge number of chemicals, as indicated by a January 2008 article entitled *The A-Z of Eco Fashion* that states,

"...at least 8,000 chemicals are used to turn raw materials into clothes..."

The article adds that,

"Many of these cause irreversible damage to people and the environment."

The durability of synthetic fabrics is a contributory factor to one of the world's major environmental problems; non-biodegradable waste. The article cites the example of polyester and states that it is,

"Non-biodegradable, it will be around for another 200 years or so."

The use of synthetic chemicals in the manufacture of textiles and clothing is not restricted to the creation of durable fabrics; clothes are increasingly subjected to a number of additional processes, for example 'finishes' that are claimed to impart properties labelled as 'easy care', 'water repellent', and 'wrinkle free', to name just a few. Although seemingly useful, these properties are accomplished solely through the use of chemicals, many of which are far from benign, as indicated in the *Eco Fashion* article that states,

"The bleaching, dyeing, sizing and finishing of textiles all result in large quantities of effluent often containing highly toxic heavy metals that pollute the soil and water and damage aquatic life."

Heavy metals are by no means the only toxic substances in textile industry effluent; for example, toxic organochlorines are formed as the result of chlorine-based chemicals, such as sodium hypochlorite, that are used to bleach textiles.

One of the additional processes applied to some fabrics, especially those used for clothing manufactured for babies and small children, involve their treatment with 'flame-retardant' chemicals, but these do not prevent fires, as explained in *Killer Clothes*,

"These chemicals delay ignition of products exposed to flames but don't stop fires, and at low temperature combustion, they release high levels of brominated dioxins, which are toxic substances."

Some of the chemicals that have been used as flame retardants are called PBDEs (polybrominated diphenyl ethers), which are discussed on the EPA web page entitled *Polybrominated Diphenyl Ethers (PBDEs)* that states,

"EPA is concerned that certain PBDE congeners are persistent, bioaccumulative, and toxic to both humans and the environment. The critical endpoint of concern for human health is neurobehavioral effects."

The term 'congener' refers to related chemicals.

Neurobehavioural effects are not the only issue of concern; there is evidence that PBDEs produce a range of effects, some of which can occur at exposure levels below those claimed to have been proven to be 'safe'. A September 2003 EWG article entitled *Mother's Milk: Health Risks of PBDEs* refers to animal research studies that have,

"...linked PBDE exposure to an array of adverse health effects including thyroid hormone disruption, permanent learning and memory impairment, behavioural changes, hearing deficits, delayed puberty onset, decreased sperm count, fetal malformations and, possibly, cancer."

A few different PBDE compounds have been produced and used, although in many countries most have now been banned or voluntarily removed from use by the manufacturers due to their toxic nature. Nevertheless, these chemicals continue to pose health hazards and to be a source of environmental pollution due to their persistent nature; PBDEs are now widely recognised as being 'POPs'.

The concerns about PBDEs has led to the introduction of a variety of other flame-retardant chemicals to replace them; unfortunately, most of these other chemicals have also been discovered to be toxic. Some of the chemicals introduced to replace PBDEs are chlorinated compounds; which means that they will inevitably produce highly toxic carcinogenic dioxins when subjected to combustion. A 2013 article entitled *PBDEs and Their Replacements: Does the Benefit Justify the Harm* concludes that,

"Flame-retardant chemicals can pose a potentially greater hazard to health and environment than the risk of the fires they are supposed to prevent."

Flame-retardant chemicals are also used in home furnishing fabrics; however, although there is less direct skin contact with furniture than with clothes, these treated fabrics are nevertheless another source of exposure to toxic chemicals.

As discussed, certain groups of chemicals have multiple applications; it is therefore unsurprising to discover that some of the chemical ingredients of consumer products have applications in the processes used to produce textiles and clothing; for example, finishes such as dyeing and printing. The *Dermal Exposure* report refers to some of these processes and states,

"Of toxicological interest are, in particular, those chemicals that are involved in the dyeing and printing processes, optical brighteners and chemical finishes."

The chemicals involved in dye printing include some members of the family of phthalates, as explained in *Killer Clothes*,

"...the pigments in printing must be bound to the fabric with a polymer, and the most commonly used plasticizers are a family of phthalates."

The subtitle of the October 2012 Greenpeace report is: *How big brands are making consumers accomplices in the toxic water cycle*; this report found that phthalates can leak from printed images and states that,

"Phthalates in plastisol formulations are not tightly bound to the plastic and can therefore be released from the product over time."

Although the main purpose of the Greenpeace report is to highlight the pollution of water with toxic chemicals, the release of phthalates from clothing is another source of dermal exposure to these poisons.

Azo dyes are widely used as textile dyes; however, they are another group of synthetic chemicals that are not permanently bound to fabrics; they are also toxic, as the Greenpeace report states,

"Certain azo dyes can break down under reductive conditions to release aromatic amines."

Aromatic amines are toxic and some have been proven to be carcinogenic.

The November 2012 Greenpeace report is entitled *Toxic Threads: Putting Pollution on Parade*; its purpose is to expose the pollution produced by the textile industry in China. The report refers to the fact that some clothing manufacturers, including many brand names, source their textile manufacturing from China and states that,

> "The textile industry is built upon the use of a large number of chemicals, and China is now the largest consumer of textile chemicals, with 42% of global consumption."

The report focuses on pollution caused by the discharge of toxic chemical wastes into the environment; but this is not the sole issue of concern. The major issue from a human health perspective is that the manufacture of clothes utilises processes that involve many different toxic chemicals that can seep out of the clothing fabric. These chemicals can be absorbed into the skin, which enables them to pass into systemic circulation and therefore poison the bloodstream.

The emphasis by the report on the situation in China creates the impression that it is Chinese industry that is the source of the problem due to their bad manufacturing practices; but this impression is misleading. The textile industry in China does utilise toxic chemicals in the manufacture of textiles and clothing and therefore does pollute the environment; however, the pollution it produces is the direct result of the use of toxic chemicals; a practice that is not exclusive to China. Most, if not all manufacturing processes that utilise toxic chemicals will inevitably discharge toxic wastes, pollute the environment and generate human health hazards; the clothing industry is no exception.

The clothing manufacturers that source their textiles from China have generally made that decision for commercial reasons, which include lower costs and less restrictive or even absent regulatory oversight; the relocation of industries to countries in Asia and other parts of the world is discussed further in chapter eight.

Formaldehyde is another chemical of concern that is utilised by the textile industry; some of its uses include finishes that are claimed to impart properties such as anti-cling, anti-static, waterproof, perspiration-proof and moth-proof, amongst others. Although known to be highly toxic, formaldehyde is claimed to be useful, because, as explained in *Killer Clothes*,

> "...it's a simple molecule that can connect individual fibers and enable them to hold their shape after repeated cleanings."

It is claimed that formaldehyde helps to prevent colours from 'running'; which is the reason for its use in dyes and printing inks. The focus of the Greenpeace report on pollution levels in China overlooks the fact that formaldehyde is commonly used in clothing, wherever it is manufactured; an issue that is recognised in *Killer Clothes*,

> "When it comes to the presence of formaldehyde in clothing, no country in the world bans its use in textiles..."

It has been discovered that formaldehyde is another chemical that does not remain tightly bound. The ubiquitous nature of formaldehyde together with its ability to leak from fabrics, inks and dyes provide many sources of exposure to this carcinogenic chemical that can be absorbed, especially by inhalation, into the body. Some of the symptoms known to result from the inhalation of formaldehyde include severe coughing, bronchitis, asthma, chest pain, wheezing, and inflammation of the windpipe, bronchi and even lungs. These adverse effects can occur due to exposure to concentrations of formaldehyde that are lower than those deemed to be 'safe'.

Another treatment to which some textiles are subjected involves the use of 'antibacterial' substances on the basis of the claim that bacteria are the cause of 'unpleasant body odours'; this is yet another unfounded claim. The substances utilised for this purpose in clothing are mainly triclosan, triclocarban and silver, the first two of which have been discussed. Although a natural metal, silver is claimed to be toxic to bacterial cells; however, according to a 1994 article entitled *Antibacterial Silver*,

"...its toxicity to human cells is considerably lower than to bacteria."

A 'considerably lower' level of toxicity is not synonymous with 'non-toxic' nor does it mean that silver is 'safe' for humans; it should be noted that silver is not considered to be an essential component of the human body. In addition to its use as an antibacterial, silver is also claimed to 'kill' viruses; an entirely unfounded claim as the particles called 'viruses' are not living entities.

Although nanotechnology is still in its infancy, the silver incorporated into clothing for 'antibacterial' purposes is increasingly in the form of nanoparticles. The EU website contains a number of pages that discuss nanotechnologies and nanoparticles, one of which, entitled *What are potential harmful effects of nanoparticles*, states that,

"Nanoparticles can have the same dimensions as biological molecules such as proteins."

The page also refers to inflammation that can be induced by nanoparticles and claims that,

"Nanoparticles may cross cell membranes."

As demonstrated throughout this book, the medical establishment does not possess a comprehensive knowledge of the functions of the human body, especially at the cellular level. Dr Harold Hillman has extensively documented that most procedures and preparation materials used in the investigation of cells significantly alter their nature. He also states that these procedures generate cell 'artefacts', even though the medical establishment regards them as natural components of cells.

The medical establishment's poor level of understanding about the human body in the state of health or disease means that the full extent of the potential consequences from the use of silver nanoparticles is entirely unknown. These knowledge gaps with respect to nanoparticles are recognised, albeit to a limited extent, by the EU web page which acknowledges that,

"There remain many unknown details about the interaction of nanoparticles and biological systems..."

Another 'finish', which is mainly applied to outer layers of clothing, is one intended to provide 'protection' from insects, for which the toxic chemical most frequently used is permethrin. The use of insecticides in clothing originates from the military and is based on the idea that insecticide-treated clothing will protect people who wear them from insect-borne diseases, especially malaria. The use of insecticides has however been expanded to include civilian clothing, as reported in *Killer Clothes*,

"The practice of intentionally adding toxins to fabrics as an insect repellent is now commonplace throughout both the military and civilian clothing industries worldwide."

The development of permethrin was based on the discovery that chrysanthemums contain compounds called pyrethrins, which appear to act as natural insect repellents. Permethrin is, however, a synthetic derivative of pyrethrin and, although considered to be of low toxicity, the Beyond Pesticides fact sheet entitled *Permethrin* states that,

"Permethrin can be irritating to both the eyes and the skin."

Although clothes treated with permethrin are not generally worn next to the skin, that does not mean there will be no exposure to this irritant.

There are many different chemicals used in the manufacture of clothes and, although some are claimed to be tightly bound to fabrics or printed images, this has been shown not to be the case. The 'leaking' of any chemicals out of clothing will result in dermal exposure and can also result in dermal absorption of substances into the skin or even into the bloodstream and the whole bodily system.

In addition to the chemicals used in the manufacture of clothes are those used as ingredients of clothes-cleaning products; especially laundry detergents and fabric softeners, as discussed. Residues of some laundry products are intended to remain in the clothes; this particularly applies to their 'fragrance' chemicals, as also discussed.

However, although the combination of chemicals in domestic laundry cleaning products may cause concern, dry cleaning is not a safer option as it also involves the use of a variety of chemicals, many of which are equally, if not more, toxic. One of the most significant groups of chemicals used are solvents, some of which are known to 'off-gas' from the fabric and pose hazards to the respiratory system. The most common chemical used as a dry-cleaning solvent is perchloroethylene, also referred to as 'perc', which is described by Joe Thornton in *Pandora's Poison*,

"Perchloroethylene is a particular problem, because its use as a solvent in thousands of small dry cleaning shops means that it pollutes the homes and workplaces of millions of people at short range."

Perc is toxic; it is known to severely affect the respiratory system and cause a wide range of adverse health effects. This volatile chemical poses a clear health hazard, not only to people who wear dry-cleaned clothes but also to the people who operate the dry-cleaning machinery and are therefore exposed to this toxic solvent on a daily basis.

It is evident that clothes can contain a rich variety of toxic chemicals; it is also evident that there is little public awareness of this problem; the reason for the existence of this situation is suggested in *Killer Clothes*,

> "Clothing manufacturers and even many toxicologists choose to believe that absorbing tiny amounts of toxic chemicals from individual items of clothing cannot be harmful to you."

This is yet another application of the Paracelsus fallacy that is of benefit to clothing manufacturers but has detrimental consequences for the people who wear the clothes.

As discussed, some chemicals interact synergistically, which can raise their individual toxicities by orders of magnitude, but these synergies are rarely recognised and even more rarely are they tested; as indicated in *Killer Clothes*,

> "Those synergistic processes constitute the 'black hole' of ignorance within the fields of toxicology and preventive medicine."

There is indeed an immense 'black hole of ignorance' with respect to the full potential for harm caused by exposures to the thousands of toxic chemicals used in the manufacture of clothes that are intended to be worn next to or close to the skin.

Another detrimental feature of synthetic fibres is one that is not directly related to the use of toxic chemicals; this is the fact that, unlike their natural counterparts, most synthetic fibres do not allow the skin to 'breathe', as discussed in *Killer Clothes*,

> "Human-made petrochemical fibers restrict and suffocate the skin, our largest and most sensitive body organ, making it unable to breathe properly..."

It may be suggested that the solution to this problem would be to source clothes made from 'natural' fibres, such as cotton, wool, flax, hemp and silk. However, even natural fibres may be 'poisoned' in a number of ways, one of which may result from 'treatments' applied to their source. For example, as previously discussed, sheep are dipped in order to 'treat' their fleeces with toxic insecticides, residues of which may remain throughout the manufacturing processes that produce woollen garments. Similar problems occur with cotton, one of the main issues with which is that it is increasingly grown as a GM crop that is 'treated' with large volumes of pesticides, residues of which can remain within cotton fabric used in the manufacture of clothes.

The solution to this problem first requires knowledge of its existence. Although 'toxic clothes' may not be easily or entirely avoidable, knowledge of the extent of the problem enables people to make informed decisions and choices in order to at least reduce, if not entirely eliminate their exposures to the 'poisons' in their clothes. Solutions to this problem are discussed in chapter ten.

Dentistry

The establishment definition of dentistry refers to,

> "the study, management, and treatment of diseases and conditions affecting the mouth, jaws, teeth and their supporting tissues."

Despite the claim that dentistry involves the study and treatment of diseases specific to the area surrounding the mouth, it is not classified as a branch of 'medicine'; nevertheless, dentistry utilises some of the same flawed theories and practices as the medical establishment, especially the 'germ theory' and the use of toxic substances as 'treatments', on the basis that they are 'safe' if used at the right dose.

In their book entitled *Uninformed Consent*, dentist Hal Huggins DDS MS and physician Dr Thomas Levy MD explain that dentists are largely oblivious to the toxic nature of the substances that they use, often on a daily basis,

> "Most dentists are entirely unaware of either the contents of the dental materials they implant or the potential consequences of those materials after they get into your body."

Dentists are obviously aware of some of the hazards involved in their work, particularly the dangers from exposure to X-rays. However, like their colleagues in the medical establishment, dentists ought to be fully aware of the toxic nature of all of the substances they use, especially mercury and fluoride, both of which have been acknowledged by the WHO to be toxic. Although mercury and fluoride have been discussed elsewhere in this chapter, they require further examination in respect of their use in dentistry; they are not, however, the only toxic substances used by dentists.

The main application for which mercury is used in dentistry is dental amalgam, as explained in *Uninformed Consent*,

> "Called 'silver fillings' due to their initial shiny appearance, amalgam is made from powders of copper, tin, silver and zinc mixed with approximately 50% liquid elemental mercury."

Despite the increasing acknowledgement of mercury's toxicity, the medical establishment continues to claim that it is 'safe' for use in the mouth; this is demonstrated by the EPA web page entitled *Mercury in Dental Amalgam* that states,

> "Amalgam is one of the most commonly used tooth fillings, and is considered to be a safe, sound and effective treatment for tooth decay."

The EPA page contains a link to an FDA web page entitled *About Dental Amalgams*, which, under the heading *'Potential Risks'*, explains some of the risks associated with amalgam, about which it states,

> "It releases low levels of mercury in the form of a vapour that can be inhaled and absorbed by the lungs. High levels of mercury vapour exposure are associated with adverse effects in the brain and the kidneys."

This statement would seem to contradict the EPA's claim that amalgams are 'safe'; however, the position of the FDA seems to be self-contradictory as the same web page contains the statement that,

> "The weight of credible scientific evidence reviewed by FDA does not establish an association between dental amalgam use and adverse health effects in the general population."

These contradictory statements made by the FDA and EPA are seemingly 'resolved' by the idea that it is only high levels of exposure to mercury that are problematic and by the claim that amalgams do not represent high exposure levels. There is, however, a significant volume of credible scientific evidence that establishes a clear association between adverse health problems and exposures to very low levels of mercury. One surprising source of this evidence is the WHO in a 2005 policy paper entitled *Mercury in Health Care* that states,

"Recent studies suggest that mercury may have no threshold below which some adverse effects do not occur."

Other sources state unequivocally that there is no safe level of exposure to mercury.

Corroboration of the assertion that mercury is an extremely hazardous material is demonstrated by the fact that dental amalgam is treated in dental surgeries as 'hazardous waste' that requires special procedures to be followed to ensure its safe removal and safe disposal. It is therefore disingenuous for dentists to claim ignorance about the hazards associated with either mercury or amalgam.

Nevertheless, amalgam fillings continue to be used on the basis of the claim that amalgam is a stable compound within which mercury is 'inert' and therefore 'harmless'. But this claim is refuted by the EPA statement referred to above, which states that one of the 'risks' associated with amalgams is the release of mercury vapour that can be absorbed into the lungs. This point is further substantiated in *Uninformed Consent*, in which it is stated that released mercury vapour can be detected,

"After implantation in your teeth, and for an indefinite period of time, silver mercury fillings outgas readily detectable amounts of mercury vapor."

The EPA statement also referred to the ability of mercury vapour to cause adverse effects in the brain and kidneys. The effects in the brain should not be surprising on the basis of mercury's known neurotoxicity. The kidneys are organs of detoxification, therefore effects in these organs are indicative of systemic poisoning. Furthermore, the 'normal' levels of mercury released from amalgam fillings are increased in the presence of dental work that utilises other metals, for example gold or nickel crowns.

In *Uninformed Consent*, Hal Huggins relates an incident that demonstrates the effects of dental amalgams on health. A young patient of his, who had previously had amalgam fillings placed in her teeth, had been diagnosed with leukaemia. Her treatment consisted of the removal of her amalgam fillings, after which her health improved. Her physician declared that her leukaemia was 'in remission' but refused to consider that the removal of her fillings had been relevant to her recovery. At her next visit to Hal Huggins, he replaced the amalgam fillings in her teeth, after which her leukaemia returned. In her next visit, he removed the fillings and she again recovered her health.

As will be discussed in chapter seven, cancer is rarely, if ever, caused by a single factor, but this example, even though 'anecdotal', is a clear demonstration that amalgam fillings can have a significant adverse impact on health, and that their removal can result in a significant improvement to health.

It must be emphasised that amalgam fillings should only be removed by dentists who are aware of and follow the correct procedures; there are potentially serious adverse effects that can result if these procedures are not followed.

In *Death by Modern Medicine*, Dr Carolyn Dean provides an interesting summary of the origin of the use of mercury in dentistry in America,

"Around the 1830s, dentistry was an unregulated service. Free market medical men, barbers, and blacksmiths elbowed each other for patients. They found that mercury amalgams fitted much more easily than hot lead, and were much cheaper than gold. Since mercury fillings, technically, were outside the body, most lay dentists were not concerned about potential toxicity. Medical-dentists who were concerned tried to warn the public but the initial rush for cheap fillings drowned them out. The lay dentists and the pro-amalgam dentists became so powerful they eventually formed their own dental association in 1859, the American Dental Association (ADA). The ADA continued to promote and support the use of mercury amalgams as a safe dental product."

The choice of lead for fillings is yet another example of the inappropriate use of highly toxic materials. However, despite Dr Dean's reference to 'medical-dentists' who, even in the 19th century, were aware of its toxicity, mercury continued to be used in some 'medicines' in the 20th century and is still used in the 21st century in certain antiseptic substances, as well as certain vaccines and amalgam fillings.

The March 2017 WHO fact sheet entitled *Mercury and health* claims that an outright ban of amalgam fillings would be 'problematic' for the dental sector; this is disingenuous because these fillings are extremely detrimental to human health, which ought to be the priority of the WHO. Nevertheless, the WHO recommends that the use of amalgam dental fillings should be 'phased out' and that cost-effective alternatives should be developed.

Another hazardous material used in dentistry is nickel, which is a component of crowns, bridges, braces and partial dentures; its dangers are explained in *Uninformed Consent*,

"Nickel is one of the most durable yet most carcinogenic metals on this planet."

The authors explain that many dentists are under the impression that stainless steel, which is also used in dental products, is 'safe'; they also explain that this is a mistaken impression because stainless steel contains nickel. Some of the alloys used for dental products, such as crowns and bridges for example, are compounds that, in addition to nickel, can contain substances such as beryllium, cobalt and chromium, all of which are toxic. As has been discussed, some metals interact synergistically; for example, cobalt can enhance the carcinogenicity of nickel; the mixture of cobalt and nickel in an alloy used for dental products can only be described as entirely inappropriate.

Metals are not the only toxic ingredients used in the manufacture of dental products; dentures for example, may be made from acrylic, which is another toxic material that has been associated with adverse health effects, as reported in *Chemical Exposures*,

"Acrylic dentures may provoke headache, joint pain, fatigue and rashes."

As previously discussed, the body is not solely biochemical in nature, it is also bioelectrical; therefore, dental products and fillings made from certain metals are able to interfere with and disrupt the body's bioelectrical functions; as discussed by the authors of *Uninformed Consent*,

"Fillings are like little tiny batteries. They have an electrical charge."

Adverse effects can also result from the electrical charges produced by fillings; these effects can include an increased release of mercury from amalgams, especially in the presence of other metals; the authors explain that,

"This is due to the electric current generated by the presence of dissimilar metals being present in an electrolyte such as saliva."

The electric current generated in the mouth can alter 'normal' bioelectrical activity and, in the same way that chemicals can poison the brain, this 'abnormal' electrical activity can adversely affect the brain and effectively 'poison' it, as they state,

"Fillings are pushing very high electrical charges into the brain relative to what the brain normally operates on..."

Fluoride is yet another highly toxic substance used in dentistry. It is widely promoted as beneficial for 'dental health' when applied directly onto the teeth, which is the justification for the addition of fluoride to products such as toothpastes and mouthwashes. This is demonstrated by the WHO September 2018 fact sheet entitled *Oral health* which includes the following statement quoted as a 'fact',

"Dental caries can be largely prevented by maintaining a constant low level of fluoride in the oral cavity."

This claim is based on the idea that fluoride protects and strengthens weak teeth by replacing lost minerals; but as the previous discussion about water fluoridation demonstrated, fluoride weakens teeth by causing a condition called dental fluorosis. Nevertheless, the medical establishment continues to promote the use of fluoridated toothpastes, as indicated by the UK NHS web page entitled *Fluoride* that states,

"Brushing your teeth thoroughly with fluoride toothpaste is one of the most effective ways of preventing tooth decay."

This web page also recommends that mouthwashes should not be used after brushing the teeth with fluoridated toothpastes as this will wash the fluoride away. These statements clearly raise questions about the rationale behind the alleged benefits of water fluoridation, because water that is ingested does not remain in the mouth to 'coat' the teeth.

As previously discussed, the overwhelming weight of evidence demonstrates that not only does fluoride confer no benefits for dental health, it is highly toxic and extremely dangerous; as indicated by Christopher Bryson in *The Fluoride Deception*,

"Fluoride is so potent a chemical that it's also a grave environmental hazard and a potential workplace poison."

This potent poison cannot strengthen teeth by replacing lost minerals; it can only cause damage to the teeth and to the whole body when ingested.

The cause of weakened or decayed teeth is claimed to be bacterial acids that attack teeth when sugary foods and drinks are consumed; this is yet another fallacy generated by the rigid adherence to the 'germ theory'. There is however, no need to invoke the existence of 'germs' to explain tooth decay, one of the causes of which is explained by Dr George Waldbott in

Fluoridation: The Great Dilemma,
"It is now well established that consumption of sugar and other refined carbohydrates associated with civilisation has been primarily responsible for the recent dramatic increase in caries."

One of the major causes of tooth decay is clearly the consumption of refined sugars in various forms, including processed food products that contain high levels of sugars, and particularly confectionery that is frequently given to small children as 'treats'; but these so-called treats are detrimental to health in a number of ways.

The problem of tooth decay caused by a high consumption of refined sugar products clearly cannot be solved by the application of toxic fluoride 'treatments'. Problems can only be solved by the removal of their cause; the problem of tooth decay therefore can only be 'solved' by the elimination from the diet of all forms of refined sugars. As previously discussed, many other health benefits can be achieved by the elimination of this 'sweet poison' from the diet.

It is clear that many dental products, processes and 'treatments' involve the use of some highly toxic materials that are significant contributors to the 'poisoning' of the body.

In Summary

The discussions in this chapter have explored the myriad ways in which people are 'poisoned' on a daily basis. However, as stated at the outset, the purpose of this chapter has been to inform, not depress; for it is only by possessing all of the required information that people are able to make informed decisions.

It is clear from the discussions in this chapter that toxic substances are ubiquitous; they are used in a wide variety of applications that impact virtually every aspect of life in the 21st century.

The medical establishment recognises that some substances are toxic, but downplays their significance in the causation of 'disease' in order to maintain the false narrative that 'germs' pose far greater hazards to human health. As discussed at the beginning of this chapter, the WHO recognises that the health of the environment affects the health of the people who inhabit that environment; but this too is downplayed in favour of another false narrative, which claims that atmospheric carbon dioxide is the cause of climate change and that this is the most important environmental issue of the 21st century.

The close relationship between the health of the environment and the health of the human inhabitants of the environment means that it is extremely important to pay attention to activities that pollute the environment. The most important environmental problem is due to pollution, contamination and degradation, which are almost entirely due to the sum total of all industrial activities, but mainly to those that involve: the extraction of resources; the development, use and disposal of toxic chemicals; the development of nuclear weapons and power; and the development of technologies that utilise unnatural electromagnetic radiation.

These activities are mostly, although not entirely, conducted without due consideration for their consequences, their impact on the environment or their impact on human health. Furthermore, despite assurances that industrial activities and their products are all 'safe', this chapter has demonstrated otherwise.

The essence of this problem is articulated by Dr Paul Craig Roberts in his March 2015 article entitled *The Oceans Are Dying* in which he states that,

> "While the powerful capitalists use the environment for themselves as a cost-free dumping ground, the accumulating costs threaten everyone's life."

The claim that 'industry' is largely responsible for environmental problems and human illness is often regarded as 'Luddite' and usually criticised as representing a view that is 'anti-progress', 'anti-science' and 'anti-development'. This point is encapsulated by medical writer Martin J Walker, whose words are quoted by Dr Samuel Epstein in *The Politics of Cancer*,

> "The dissident who questions the chemical companies, the industrial food companies, and inevitably the state, is branded as irrational, anti-science and anti-technology and hence as a subversive standing in the way of progress."

This type of criticism falls within the logical fallacy referred to as the 'ad hominem attack', the sole purpose of which is to vilify the person rather than discuss their work; this form of attack always fails to address the issues raised.

Each section within this chapter has provided at least some of the available evidence that refutes the establishment claims about each of the topics under discussion; furthermore, the discussions have demonstrated the contribution of each industrial activity to human illness and environmental degradation.

Many scientists claim to be able to understand the laws of nature; but this is sheer hubris; as this book demonstrates, there are vast gaps in 'scientific knowledge'. Dr George Waldbott MD recognised the disingenuous nature of such claims in *Fluoridation: The Great Dilemma*,

> "We assume that the laws of nature are universal and constant. Man, however, does not always understand nature's laws; his interpretations are imperfect, and today's wisdom is often merely tomorrow's folly."

The discussions in the next chapter provide yet more examples of the 'knowledge gaps' that exist within 'modern medicine' as well as the poor level of understanding of the medical establishment about the major 'diseases' that are said to afflict millions of people around the world.

It has been shown that manufacturers are held responsible for the safety of their products; it has also been shown that the basis of their claims about 'safety' rely on the idea that a 'safe dose' of each individual substance can be determined by reference to testing procedures conducted within a laboratory. The laboratory setting is, however, completely divorced from the real-world environment, in which the everyday experiences of most people involve exposures to a wide variety of multiple toxic substances in combinations that have never been tested for their safety, nor have they been evaluated for their effects on human health.

Under the existing 'system', adverse health effects are generally discovered as the result of epidemiological studies, which, although conducted in the real world, are unable to determine a single specific effect that results from a single activity or exposure to a single substance. For example, after many years of epidemiological studies, smoking was finally linked to lung cancer, however, this illness is clearly not inevitable as some smokers never contract lung cancer; which means that other factors must be involved. Ill-health is always the result of multiple influences. This means that there is rarely a single causal factor for any of the conditions of ill-health that are incorrectly referred to as 'diseases'; these points are discussed in detail in chapter ten.

It is abundantly clear that the human body is amazingly resilient, as demonstrated by the ability to withstand exposures to many different toxins. However, as stated at the beginning of this chapter, there is a limit to the ability of the human body to function properly under a constant barrage of toxic substances and unnatural electromagnetic radiation.

It is possible to reduce exposures to these hazards and even to eliminate some of them entirely; but it requires knowledge of their existence and the applications in which they are used, which is the main purpose of this chapter.

The final comment in this chapter is reserved for Rachel Carson, who wrote one of the major exposés of the 20th century in which she alerted the world to the dangers posed by the vast array of toxic chemicals applied for a wide variety of purposes. In *Silent Spring*, she also provided a lasting message that is as relevant in the early 21st century as it was in the mid-20th century,

> "The choice, after all, is ours to make. If, having endured much, we have at last asserted our 'right to know', and if, knowing, we have concluded that we are being asked to take senseless and frightening risks, then we should no longer accept the counsel of those who tell us that we must fill our world with poisonous chemicals..."

Chapter Seven

'Non-Infectious' Diseases: More Medical Misconceptions

"Each of these recurrent exposures, no matter how slight,
contributes to the progressive build-up of chemicals in our
bodies and so to cumulative poisoning."

Rachel Carson

The WHO is the authoritative body of the medical establishment responsible for providing information about matters pertaining to health. This includes the identification of diseases, which is provided by the ICD (International Classification of Diseases); this is described by the ICD information sheet on the WHO website as,

"...the global health information standard for mortality and morbidity statistics."

The information sheet also states that,

"The ICD defines the universe of diseases, disorders, injuries and other related health conditions."

The ICD lists all 'known' diseases and conditions, each of which is sub-divided according to certain criteria and each individual element within each category of disease is allocated a unique ICD code. However, the purpose of the ICD is not solely to enable the monitoring of health trends and the compilation of statistics; it is also described as,

"...the diagnostic classification standard for all clinical and research purposes."

It is clear therefore, that the ICD is intended to be the definitive guide to 'disease' for the entire medical establishment.

The ICD lists many thousands of different 'diseases', but they are all categorised as either 'infectious' or 'non-infectious'. Previous discussions have, however, exposed the fatally flawed nature of the theories pertaining to 'infectious diseases'; they have also demonstrated that the explanations offered by the medical establishment about these diseases contain many anomalies, inconsistencies and contradictions and present a number of aspects that remain poorly understood.

The flawed nature of the medical establishment's theories and explanations about 'infectious diseases' inevitably raises questions about the veracity of their theories and explanations about 'non-infectious diseases', which are usually referred to as 'noncommunicable diseases' or NCDs.

A number of the most significant NCDs are discussed in this chapter, in which it will be shown that the information promulgated by the medical establishment about them contain many anomalies, inconsistencies and contradictions. The discussions will also demonstrate that, for the vast majority, if not all, of these diseases, the medical establishment has a poor level of understanding about their nature, as well as their causes and the mechanisms of action involved.

It is claimed that NCDs are responsible for the majority of all deaths worldwide; the June 2018 WHO fact sheet entitled *Noncommunicable diseases* states that,

"Noncommunicable diseases (NCDs) kill 41 million people each year, equivalent to 71% of all deaths globally."

According to the fact sheet, CVDs (cardiovascular diseases) are the most serious group of diseases and cause 17.9 million deaths each year. Cancer is the second most serious group and accounts for 9.0 million deaths; respiratory diseases, the third group, is said to account for 3.9 million deaths; diabetes, the fourth most serious, is said to account for 1.6 million deaths. The fact sheet adds that,

"These 4 groups of diseases account for over 80% of all premature NCD deaths."

The term 'premature' refers to deaths that occur in people younger than 70.

The 2013 WHO report entitled *Global Action Plan for the Prevention and Control of Noncommunicable Diseases 2013-2020*, which will be referred to as the *Global Action Plan* report, states that,

"NCDs are now well-studied and understood..."

The level of confidence expressed in this statement is, however, unfounded; whilst NCDs may be 'well-studied' they cannot be described as 'understood', as the discussions in this chapter will demonstrate.

Unlike 'infectious diseases', there is no core 'theory' on which NCDs are based; however, the fact sheet describes some of the features these diseases are claimed to share,

"Noncommunicable diseases (NCDs), also known as chronic diseases, tend to be of long duration and are the result of a combination of genetic, physiological, environmental and behavioural factors."

Although 'genetic factors' are claimed to contribute to the onset of many NCDs, this is another medical misconception, as a number of the discussions in this chapter will demonstrate.

The role of 'environmental factors' in NCDs is only referred to by a general comment in the fact sheet that,

"These diseases are driven by forces that include rapid unplanned urbanization, globalization of unhealthy lifestyles and population ageing."

The previously cited *Healthy Environments* report does acknowledge that 'environmental factors' contribute to ill-health, although that recognition does not extend to all of the food, water and environmental pollutants discussed in chapter six.

The references in the fact sheet to 'behavioural factors' and 'unhealthy lifestyles' are linked in the claim that there are four 'risk factors' with which all NCDs are associated,

> "Tobacco use, physical inactivity, the harmful use of alcohol and unhealthy diets all increase the risk of dying from a NCD."

This statement is not entirely incorrect, because smoking has been proven to be harmful to health; nevertheless, it is misleading with respect to risks posed by 'physical inactivity', about which the fact sheet states,

> "1.6 million deaths annually can be attributed to insufficient physical activity."

This is misleading; insufficient physical activity alone does not cause death.

Whilst one school of thought suggests that a moderate level of alcohol consumption is harmless and another suggests it may be beneficial, it should be noted that alcohol can harm the body, especially the liver and brain. Furthermore, alcoholic beverages may contain additives that, although permitted, are toxic; as discussed in chapter six, sulphur dioxide is used as a preservative in some wines and beers.

An unhealthy diet is certainly one of the main factors that contribute to ill-health, as will be discussed in chapter ten; but the fact sheet only makes a specific reference to one aspect of an unhealthy diet, namely, an excess intake of salt/sodium. The discussions in the previous chapter about 'poisoned food' indicate that an appropriate explanation of an 'unhealthy diet' ought to include reference to the wide range of processed 'food products' that contain toxic chemical additives, and therefore fail to fulfil the fundamental purpose of food to provide nutrients. The reason for this omission may relate to the involvement of the WHO with the CAC, which regards food additives created from synthetic chemicals as 'safe' when used at the appropriate 'level'.

In addition to the four behavioural risk factors, the fact sheet refers to four 'metabolic' risk factors, which are stated to be raised blood pressure, overweight/obesity, hyperglycaemia and hyperlipidaemia. These factors are said to increase the risk of developing cardiovascular diseases, which are discussed in the next section.

It is claimed that overweight and obesity are the result of an intake of calories in excess of those expended, and that physical activity should therefore be increased to reduce these excess calories and solve the problem; but this is yet another medical misconception. One of the main factors that contributes to obesity is a diet that consists almost entirely of processed 'food products' that are high in non-nutrients but contain few, if any, essential nutrients; a situation that cannot be solved through an increased level of physical activity. Problems can only be resolved when their root causes have been identified and addressed.

By definition, NCDs are not 'communicable'; which means that they are not transmissible between people; nevertheless, the *Global Action Plan* report claims that,

"The role of infectious agents in the pathogenesis of noncommunicable diseases, either on their own or in combination with genetic and environmental influences, has been increasingly recognized in recent years."

The claim that 'infectious agents' play a role in the pathogenesis of NCDs indicates that the medical establishment has completely redefined the term 'noncommunicable'; this claim is, however, unfounded, 'germs' play no role in the development of any disease.

Two 'noncommunicable diseases' in which the WHO claims 'infectious agents' play a direct causal role, are cervical cancer and hepatitis, both of which are said to be caused by 'viruses'. The discussion about cervical cancer in chapter two demonstrated that this condition is not caused by a virus. The discussions in chapter three demonstrated that 'viruses' cannot be the cause of 'hepatitis', which is a health problem that involves damage to the liver, the body's main detoxification organ. Hepatitis is discussed further in chapter eight; however, it should be noted that this condition is indicative of toxins that have adversely affected the liver; as demonstrated by the recognised association between alcoholism and 'liver disease'.

Another factor that is claimed to be associated with NCDs is poverty; the fact sheet states,

"NCDs disproportionately affect people in low- and middle-income countries where more than three quarters of global NCD deaths – 32 million – occur."

This is misleading because the majority of the world population lives in low- or middle-income countries. It is also erroneous because NCDs are claimed to be 'diseases of affluence', which means they should be mainly, if not solely, experienced by people in high income countries. According to a November 2018 article entitled *The macroeconomic burden of noncommunicable diseases in the United States: Estimates and projections* states that,

"In the United States, NCDs account for 89% of all deaths..."

This is clearly a far higher burden than the global average of 71 per cent quoted in the WHO NCD fact sheet; it is also higher the 'more than three quarters' experienced in low- and middle-income countries; yet the US is claimed to be a high-income country. As the discussion about iatrogenesis in chapter one revealed, the US has the most expensive healthcare system, yet Americans are some of the least healthy people by comparison to the populations of other 'high-income' countries; the article states that,

"...the United States has extraordinarily high health expenditures, but does not attain the best health outcomes."

The reasons for this apparent paradox are explained throughout this book. It is perfectly clear, however, that neither high income status nor high health expenditures equate to better health for people.

The reason that NCDs are claimed to be linked to poverty is expressed in the NCD fact sheet to be that,

"Vulnerable and socially disadvantaged people get sicker and die sooner than people of higher social positions..."

The fact sheet also claims that poor people have 'limited access to health services'. This problem is also discussed in the *Global Action Plan* report, which states, under the heading *Universal Health Coverage*, that,

"All people should have access, without discrimination, to rationally determined sets of the needed promotive, preventive, curative and rehabilitative basic health services and essential safe, affordable, effective and quality medicines."

The health services referred to as 'needed' are clearly those that are provided by the medical establishment system, which has been shown to be based on flawed theories of disease causation. Furthermore, as previous discussions have also demonstrated, pharmaceutical drug treatments are not 'curative' and vaccines are not 'preventive'; it has been shown that, contrary to the claims made by the medical establishment, these 'interventions' cause harm and exacerbate ill-health.

The increased efforts to 'harmonise' all aspects of life under a 'global' system are represented by a number of UN programmes. One of the most significant recent programmes of this type is the 2030 Agenda that contains 17 Goals, each of which contains a number of different 'targets' and all of which are to be achieved by the year 2030. The core aim of SDG 3 is to,

"Ensure healthy lives and promote well-being for all at all ages."

A number of the 2030 Agenda goals are discussed in more detail in chapter eight; however, one of the targets of Goal 3 specifically refers to NCDs and states the aim to,

"By 2030, reduce by one third premature mortality from non-communicable diseases through prevention and treatment and promote mental health and well-being."

The ability to create solutions to any problem first requires a full understanding of the nature of the problem; the problems of 'disease' are no exception. However, as the discussions in this chapter will demonstrate, the medical establishment does not possess a full understanding of the nature of non-communicable diseases, and even admits to possessing a poor level of understanding about the mechanisms involved in most, if not all of them. The topic of 'mental health' has been discussed in chapter one with reference to psychiatric medications, and will be further discussed in chapter ten.

In common with other chapters, the 'establishment definition' of each disease has been taken from the 2007 edition of the Oxford Concise Medical Dictionary, unless otherwise indicated.

Cardiovascular Diseases

Cardiovascular diseases (CVDs) are those that affect the cardiovascular system, which is defined by the establishment as,

"the heart together with two networks of blood vessels..."

The definition expands on this description and states that,

"The cardiovascular system effects the circulation of blood around the body, which brings about transport of nutrients and oxygen to the tissues and the removal of waste products."

The May 2017 WHO fact sheet entitled *Cardiovascular diseases* states that CVDs are the leading cause of death and were responsible for 31 per cent of worldwide mortality in 2015. The two CVDs of greatest significance are coronary heart disease and cerebrovascular disease; coronary heart disease is described in the fact sheet as,

"disease of the blood vessels supplying the heart muscle."

Cerebrovascular disease is described as,

"disease of the blood vessels supplying the brain."

It is clear that any influence that impairs the cardiovascular system will affect the circulation of the blood and the body's two most vital organs; Dr Russell Blaylock explains in *Health and Nutrition Secrets* that,

"Of all the organs, the brain and the heart are most vulnerable to impaired circulatory function."

Heart attacks and strokes are the two most common CVD 'events', the risk factors for these events are claimed to be the same as those for all NCDs; namely tobacco use, unhealthy diet, physical inactivity and harmful use of alcohol. The fact sheet adds that,

"The effects of behavioural risk factors may show up in individuals as raised blood pressure, raised blood glucose, raised blood lipids, and overweight and obesity."

The WHO recommends that these 'risk factors' are addressed, although further measures may be required for people with underlying conditions,

"In addition, drug treatment of diabetes, hypertension and high blood lipids may be necessary to reduce cardiovascular risk and prevent heart attacks and strokes."

The WHO also recommends people with established disease to be treated with 'medicines', the most common of which are aspirin, beta-blockers, angiotensin-converting inhibitors and statins.

The fact sheet refers to the importance of addressing all NCDs; a concern that resulted in the creation of the *Global Action Plan* report that contains nine 'targets', two of which relate specifically to CVDs. One of these targets aims to reduce the incidence of raised blood pressure by 25 per cent, on the basis of the claim that,

"Raised blood pressure is the leading risk factor for cardiovascular disease."

Raised blood pressure is defined as a reading that exceeds the specific range deemed appropriate to the person's age group. The discussion about hypertension in chapter one discussed the results of the SPRINT study and the likelihood that the range of blood pressure readings regarded as 'normal' may be further reduced. The other target of the *Global Action Plan* report aims to ensure that at least half of all 'eligible people' receive drug treatments in order to prevent heart attacks and strokes. It is clear that the intention is to substantially increase the number of people deemed 'eligible' for drug treatments. However, although this will result in an immense boost to the sales and profits of the pharmaceutical industry, it will not achieve the intended aims of addressing CVDs; pharmaceutical drugs can neither prevent nor alleviate disease.

The fact sheet claims that, in addition to the four 'behavioural' risk factors, there are other 'determinants' that affect CVDs; these are the same determinants that are said to apply to all NCDs; namely, globalization, urbanization and population ageing. The WHO clearly recognises that multiple factors affect health and cause illness, but does not refer to the plethora of toxic substances that permeate and pollute food, water and the environment as the result of industrial activities. The fact sheet refers to another group of factors and states that,

"Other determinants of CVDs include poverty, stress and hereditary factors."

Poverty is discussed in more detail in chapter eight; stress and 'ageing' are discussed in more detail in chapter ten.

The establishment view that hereditary factors can cause cardiovascular diseases is illustrated by a February 2017 article entitled *Sudden death warning over faulty heart gene*, which states that,

"Research has helped to discover many of the faulty genes that cause inherited heart conditions."

This is another medical misconception; genes do not control the functions of the body nor do they cause diseased conditions; on the contrary, genes are themselves controlled by other factors that turn them on or off. These 'other factors' are discussed by Dr Robert Hedaya MD in his 4-part article series entitled *Nutrition and Depression*; it is the second article of the series that is of particular interest for the purposes of this discussion. In this second article, which is subtitled *Nutrition, Methylation and Depression*, Dr Hedaya refers to research findings within the field of epigenetics that have demonstrated that genes,

"...are turned on or off by one's environment, one's diet, by stress or by one's experience..."

Dr Hedaya is not alone in expressing the view that genes are not controlling influences, but are themselves controlled by other factors. Dr Bruce Lipton PhD has also undertaken important research on the function of genes and the environmental influences that affect and control the fate of cells, as will also be discussed in chapter ten.

Furthermore, as previously mentioned, the body is bioelectrical in nature as well as biochemical; the two main organs that function electrically are the brain and the heart, as demonstrated by the fact that their electrical activity can be measured by EEG and ECG machines, respectively. Therefore, any influence that disrupts the body's bioelectrical system can disrupt the normal functioning of these two vital organs. The BioInitiative Report 2012 refers to evidence that exposures to ELF-EMF (extremely low frequency electromagnetic fields) and RFR (radiofrequency radiation) have been linked to some cardiovascular effects. Although this finding should not be surprising, a more significant finding is that the mechanism that connects EMF exposures to CVDs is oxidative stress. Within the BioInitiative Report is the statement that,

"...oxidative stress is gaining more and more ground as being the initial mechanism of action of EMFs..."

There is a large and growing body of scientific evidence that recognises oxidative stress to be a key mechanism for many diseases, including CVDs;

as the discussions in this chapter will demonstrate.

Oxidative stress is the result of an excess generation of free radicals, which are atoms or molecules that have one or more unpaired electrons; these radicals are unstable and highly reactive, which is the reason that they cause damage to the body's cells and tissues. There are different types of free radicals, most of which are formed by reactions involving oxygen and are referred to as ROS (reactive oxygen species). They can, however, be formed by reactions involving other elements, for example, those involving nitrogen are referred to as RNS (reactive nitrogen species). The web page entitled *Free Radicals and Reactive Oxygen* states that 'radicals' are formed during 'normal biochemical reactions', but that,

> "...when generated in excess or not appropriately controlled, radicals can wreak havoc on a broad range of macromolecules."

A 2004 article entitled *Reactive oxygen species, vascular oxidative stress, and redox signaling in hypertension: what is the clinical significance?* states that under 'normal conditions' there is a balance between oxidant formation and elimination; but that,

> "...an imbalance between prooxidants and antioxidants results in oxidative stress..."

A 2008 article entitled *Free Radicals, Antioxidants in Disease and Health* states that some studies,

> "...have provided precious evidence supporting the role of oxidative stress in a number of CVDs..."

A 2012 article entitled *Drug-Induced Oxidative Stress and Toxicity* states that, for some drugs,

> "...there is evidence of elevation in cellular ROS in response to drug exposure, and evidence implicates ROS and oxidative stress in toxicity..."

The discussion about statins in chapter one referred to the medical misconception about cholesterol and the idea that LDL cholesterol is 'bad'; whereas the real problem is the presence of oxidised cholesterol, both LDL and HDL; as Dr Blaylock explains,

> "Free radicals in the blood oxidize the cholesterol-carrying lipoproteins called LDL and HDL."

The highly reactive nature of these free radicals means that they can cause damage in the circulatory system; Dr Blaylock further explains,

> "Once oxidised, they can damage blood vessel walls which leads to atherosclerosis and all of its related complications including heart attacks, strokes and peripheral vascular disease."

Another substance that has been demonstrated to contribute to cardiovascular disease is refined sugar. One of the reasons that refined sugar is harmful is because it increases metabolism, which in turn increases oxidation and the generation of free radicals, as Dr Blaylock states,

> "It is also well known that overfeeding, especially of high-energy foods like sugars and carbohydrates dramatically increase metabolism and hence free radical generation."

He explains that a high intake of sugar results in 'glycation', which is a chemical reaction between sugar molecules and proteins, and that, when glycolated, proteins are more easily oxidised. This provides an explanation for the association between diabetes and cardiovascular problems, as indicated by the suggestion in the fact sheet that the treatment of diabetes may prevent heart attacks and strokes.

It should be clear that pharmaceutical drugs can neither treat not prevent CVDs, or any of the health conditions that relate to the cardiovascular system. One of the most effective solutions to the problem of oxidative stress is an increased intake of antioxidants. A 1996 article entitled *Randomised controlled trial of Vitamin E in patients with coronary disease: Cambridge Heart Antioxidant Study (CHAOS)* concluded that,

"...alpha-tocopherol treatment substantially reduces the rate of non-fatal MI..."

MI is myocardial infarction, which is defined by the establishment as,

"death of a segment of heart muscle..."

Oxidative stress clearly plays a contributory role in the onset of CVDs; equally clear is that the resolution of cardiovascular problems will require the removal of influences that generate high levels of free radicals; one of those influences are pharmaceutical drugs that are known to be toxic, not curative.

It is increasingly recognised that toxic substances exert their harmful effects through the generation of free radicals that lead to oxidative stress and result in free radical damage at the cellular level. It is for this reason that attention needs to be paid to the foods consumed to ensure that the diet contains a variety of food-based antioxidants; the importance of diet is discussed in more detail in chapter ten.

Multiple Chemical Sensitivity

Multiple Chemical Sensitivity (MCS) is a condition that affects a growing number of people around the world.

Although the condition was first identified in the mid-20th century, the 2007 medical dictionary contains no reference to MCS or to any of the alternative names by which it is known; these include: Chemical Injury, Chemical Sensitivity, Multiple Chemical Sensitivity Disorder, Environmental Illness and Multiple Allergy. These names are clear indicators of the factors that contribute to the condition, in other words, environmental toxins, especially chemicals; this point is summarised by Nicholas Ashford and Dr Claudia Miller in *Chemical Exposures: Low Levels and High Stakes*,

"Chemical exposures are endemic to our modern industrial society."

The reluctance of the medical establishment to acknowledge the significance of toxic chemicals as causal factors for many conditions of illness, is demonstrated by the paucity of available information about MCS, and by the absence of a WHO fact sheet on the subject. The only information provided by the WHO is a passing reference to MCS in a 2005 Backgrounder article, entitled *Electromagnetic fields and public health*, that refers to EHS (electromagnetic hypersensitivity), which is the topic of the next section in this chapter. Although the article does recognise similarities between EHS and MCS, it does so in a very disparaging manner,

"Both EHS and MCS are characterized by a range of non-specific symptoms that lack apparent toxicological or physiological basis or independent verification."

The article adds that,

"A more general term for sensitivity to environmental factors is Idiopathic Environmental Intolerance..."

The term 'idiopathic' means that the cause is unknown. The use of this term in the context of MCS is disingenuous; the claim that the symptoms lack an 'apparent' toxicological basis does not mean that toxic substances are irrelevant. As previously discussed, the vast majority of chemicals remain untested for all possible adverse effects, and no tests have been conducted to discover the effects from the various combinations of chemicals to which people are exposed on a daily basis.

The condition referred to as 'sensitivity to environmental factors' gained some recognition in the late 1980s, although it had first been mentioned in the 1950s. The physician who brought attention to the problem was Dr Theron Randolph MD, who initiated the discipline called clinical ecology. In *Chemical Exposures*, the authors provide many details about Dr Randolph's work, and report that he referred to chemical sensitivity as the 'petroleum problem', as the result of his observations of a close correlation between the increased use of petroleum-based synthetic chemical compounds and an increased incidence of certain health problems. Correlation is obviously not evidence of causation; but this correlation cannot be easily dismissed. The fact that petrochemicals have been proven to be harmful to health provides corroborative evidence that Dr Theron had made a relevant and undeniable connection.

The failure of the medical establishment to acknowledge the role of toxic chemicals, and other environmental pollutants, in the causation of many forms of ill-health creates a problem for sufferers of conditions like MCS; as explained on the Multiple Chemical Sensitivity website,

"Many features of Multiple Chemical Sensitivity and its effects and the way its effects are described by the sufferer seem altogether unrealistic, impossible or implausible to a conventional and scientifically trained consultant or G.P."

The people who suffer from MCS are poorly served by a medical system that increasingly adheres to an erroneous view, which has become the consensus and been encapsulated into a standardised system of disease recognition and classification. Fortunately, there are some qualified physicians who have expanded their knowledge of health beyond their 'conventional' training, and who therefore possess a better understanding of the role of environmental toxins, as well as MCS and its causes. Dr Carolyn Dean, for example, who explains in *Death by Modern Medicine* that,

"Our toxic environment causes a dramatic new condition in medicine called Multiple Chemical Sensitivity Disorders (MCSD). MCSD patients can be so sensitive to environmental chemicals that they are unable to read a newspaper because they can't tolerate the smell of ink; can't use telephones because they react to plastic; and can't wear synthetic clothing that zaps them of their energy."

The wide variety of symptoms with which a person may suffer, together with the refusal of the medical establishment to recognise MCS as a genuine health problem, means that conventionally-trained physicians are likely to only focus on certain symptoms for which they will prescribe pharmaceutical drugs. Alternatively, some symptoms may indicate the existence of a 'recognised' condition, such as an allergy. Although one of its alternative names is 'Multiple Allergy', MCS is not regarded as a 'true allergy'; allergies are discussed later in this chapter.

Interestingly, the Multiple Chemical Sensitivity website indicates that there are many similarities between the symptoms of MCS and a number of other conditions; it states,

"Also worthy of mention here is the fact that there is no sharp demarcation between the symptoms of MCS and those of ME/CFS/CFIDS/PVFS."

ME is myalgic encephalomyelitis; CFS is chronic fatigue syndrome; CFIDS is chronic fatigue and immune dysfunction syndrome; PVFS is post-viral fatigue syndrome. The absence of a sharp demarcation between the symptoms of these conditions strongly indicates that they are not distinct and separately identifiable disease entities, but should, more correctly, be viewed as different combinations of symptoms with similar, although not necessarily identical causes.

Nevertheless, there is a wide variety of symptoms that can be associated with these conditions. The fact they may include anxiety, confusion, depression and irritability has resulted in a reference to MCS and similar conditions as 'psychogenic'; a term that suggests they are more psychological than physiological. This is an appalling attitude; many people genuinely suffer from this health problem; the fact that it is not 'officially' recognised does not mean that it does not exist. Unfortunately, however, these symptoms and their misunderstood causes can precipitate a referral to a psychiatrist, who may make a diagnosis of 'mental illness' and prescribe one or more of a variety of psychiatric 'medications'. The discussion in chapter one showed that psychiatric drugs are harmful; they clearly cannot correct neurological problems caused by exposures to neurotoxic chemicals.

The multiplicity of symptoms presented by people with MCS is the direct result of exposures to a multiplicity of toxic substances that affect different bodily organs and systems; a point that is substantiated by Dr Sarah Myhill MD, who states, on the web page entitled *Chemical poisoning – general principles of diagnosis and treatment*, that,

"Every bodily system can be adversely affected by toxic chemicals, therefore sufferers present with a multiplicity of symptoms."

Toxicology is the scientific study of poisons and their effects; however, like conventional medicine, conventional toxicology suffers from fundamental flaws, not least of which is the idea that it is only the dose that makes a substance 'toxic'. This particular fallacy has been shown to generate profound consequences for health and especially for MCS, as the authors of *Chemical Exposures* explain,

"One reason MCS has been said to violate accepted principles of toxicology is that it does not appear to follow a conventional dose-response relationship."

It is abundantly clear that significant limitations exist within 'conventional toxicology' as well as 'conventional medicine'; particularly with respect to the failure to acknowledge the toxicological causes of illness, and the role of multiple exposures to chemicals that interact in ways that can increase their toxicity, as the authors of *Killer Clothes* explain,

"The role of chemical synergies in triggering health problems isn't understood by most ordinary consumers, or by many toxicologists and physicians, for that matter."

It is claimed that consumers are provided with information about the ingredients of their products on the labels and that this information is sufficient for consumer protection; but these are unacceptable claims, as explained by Dr Samuel Epstein in *Toxic Beauty*,

"Labels present such an alphabet soup of complex chemical names that most of us need a toxicological dictionary to read them."

Furthermore, as discussed, very few of the chemicals used in most consumer products have been tested for their safety or for the full range of their potential health effects. This fact is referred to in many scientific studies; for example, a 2007 article entitled *Diverse Toxic Chemicals Disrupt Cell Function Through a Common Path* states that,

"Sixty years after the dawn of the petrochemical era, health effects are known for just a fraction of its bounty."

Although the adverse health effects of all petrochemicals remain unknown, because poorly tested, it is widely acknowledged that they are toxic; this acknowledgement corroborates the existence of the connection between petrochemicals and 'environmental illnesses' that was recognised by Dr Theron. It also refutes the medical establishment claim that MCS and other similar conditions are 'idiopathic'.

Although the entire range of chemical combinations to which people are exposed in the real world has not been evaluated, there exists a substantial volume of evidence that demonstrates many of the adverse health effects that result from exposures to multiple toxic chemicals. A July 2011 article entitled *The Search for Reliable Biomarkers of Disease in Multiple Chemical Sensitivity and Other Environmental Intolerances* indicates the lack of understanding by the medical establishment about MCS, but nevertheless refers to the presence of oxidative stress in connection with this condition and states,

"Sustained organic damage occurring from chronic exposure to ambient doses of environmental toxicant presumably involves specific malfunction of detoxification pathways..."

The references to organic damage and to poorly functioning detoxification pathways indicate a serious level of systemic poisoning. The reference to oxidative stress is also extremely significant; as mentioned in the previous section, free radical damage is a contributory factor for most, if not all, diseases. Dr Russell Blaylock explains in *Health and Nutrition Secrets* that,

"...free radicals appear to play a central role in virtually every disease you can name, either directly or secondarily."

Furthermore, the previously cited 2007 article about *Diverse Toxic Chemicals* recognises that,

"...diverse toxicants can make cells more oxidised..."

Cellular damage from high levels of free radicals is a clear mechanism for MCS.

The previous chapter demonstrated that the operations of the chemical industry are extensive and that thousands of chemicals permeate virtually every aspect of life. The consequences of these continual exposures to multiple toxic chemicals have included the increased incidence of 'sensitivities' to chemicals that have presented as conditions such as MCS, ME and CFS, to name just a few.

Most of these conditions result from years of exposures to substances at levels that have been determined to be 'safe'; but no long-term studies of chemicals have ever been conducted to determine that decades of cumulative exposures to multiple chemical combinations are 'safe'. The adherence of the scientific community to the Paracelsus fallacy has caused untold health damage; as poignantly summarised by Rachel Carson in *Silent Spring*,

> "Like the constant dripping of water that in turn wears away the hardest stone, this birth-to-death contact with dangerous chemicals may in the end prove disastrous. Each of these recurrent exposures, no matter how slight, contributes to the progressive build-up of chemicals in our bodies and so to cumulative poisoning."

The solution to any problem must begin with knowledge of its existence and an understanding of its nature, both of which are sadly lacking in the information provided by the medical establishment about MCS. However, chemicals are not the only sources of harmful exposures that cause ill-health, as the following discussion will demonstrate.

Electromagnetic Hypersensitivity

Electromagnetic hypersensitivity (EHS), like MCS, is a condition that affects a growing number of people around the world; it is also a condition for which there is no establishment definition.

The 2005 WHO Backgrounder article entitled *Electromagnetic fields and public health*, referred to in the previous discussion, provides an overview of EHS and states that,

> "EHS is characterized by a variety of non-specific symptoms, which afflicted individuals attribute to exposure to EMF."

The article is a brief summary of the findings from a WHO Workshop held in 2004. Full details of the workshop have been published in a report entitled *Electromagnetic Hypersensitivity*, which recognises that,

> "Whatever its cause, EHS is a real and sometimes disabling problem for the affected persons."

The report, which will be referred to in this discussion as the *Workshop* report, describes some of the allegedly 'non-specific' but very real symptoms that include,

> "...nervous symptoms like headache, fatigue, stress, sleep disturbances, skin symptoms like prickling, burning sensations and rashes, pain and ache in muscles and many other health problems."

The medical establishment clearly recognises the existence of these symptoms but refutes their attribution to EMF exposures. The *Workshop* report refers to the term 'IEI' (Idiopathic Environmental Intolerance) as preferable to 'EHS', because the latter term implies the existence of a causal relationship, whereas, according to the Summary in the *Workshop* report,

"...there is presently no scientific basis to link IEI symptoms to EMF exposure."

Yet again, nothing could be further from the truth.

The discussion in chapter six about non-ionising radiation showed that research had been conducted in the post-WWII period to investigate the effects of exposures to radar and that, at the time, tissue heating was considered to be the only effect. Subsequent research discovered that adverse effects occurred at exposures to radar far below that at which tissues were heated. One notable research study, conducted by Dr John Heller and his colleagues at the New England Institute for Medical Research, is reported by Dr Robert Becker in his 1985 book *The Body Electric: Electromagnetism and the Foundation of Life*, in which he states that the researchers,

"...found major chromosome abnormalities in garlic shoots irradiated with low levels of microwaves. They soon found the same changes in mammalian cells..."

In his 1990 book *Cross Currents: The Perils of Electropollution, The Promise of Electromedicine*, Dr Becker discusses many studies that have reported a number of detrimental health effects resulting from exposures to various forms of EM radiation. Some of those studies relate to effects that will be discussed in later sections of this chapter, particularly those that involve birth defects and cancer.

It is clear therefore, that scientific evidence to the contrary existed long before 2004 when the *Workshop* report made the claim that there was 'no scientific basis' for exposures to EMFs to be causally linked to adverse health effects. Furthermore, the Workshop participants should have been aware that the IARC had classified ELF as a Group 2B carcinogen in 2002.

Nevertheless, the WHO maintains the stance that tissue heating is the main biological effect of exposures to EMFs, despite the classification of RFR as a Group 2B carcinogen in 2011. Although Group 2B relates to 'possible' human carcinogens, it should be noted that cancer is not the only adverse health effect caused by exposures to non-ionising radiation. The web page entitled *Current science on Electromagnetic Sensitivity: an overview* refers to the 2011 IARC decision on RFR and states that,

"Since then, the medical science has advanced significantly, with many hundreds of scientific studies showing adverse health effects, including Electromagnetic Sensitivity, at non-thermal levels."

The exposure levels to EMFs that are considered to be 'safe' are set by ICNIRP (International Commission on Non-Ionizing Radiation Protection), a non-governmental organisation that was chartered in 1992. The 1973 IRPA (International Radiation Protection Association) Congress led to the formation of INIRC (International Non-Ionizing Radiation Committee) in 1977 and to ICNIRP fifteen years later. The structure of ICNIRP includes a central Commission and a 'Scientific Expert Group';

these groups are comprised of scientists from varying disciplines, including medicine and biology. The aim of ICNIRP is stated to be,

"...to protect people and the environment against adverse effects of non-ionizing radiation."

The ICNIRP scientists examine and review existing scientific literature from which they determine appropriate exposure limits. According to the WHO web page entitled *Standards and Guidelines,*

"...EMF exposures below the limits recommended in the ICNIRP international guidelines do not appear to have any known consequence on health."

This claim is unfounded; there is an abundance of evidence that demonstrates the existence of harm to health caused by EMF exposures at levels significantly lower than those determined by ICNIRP to be 'safe'. In addition to the work performed by ICNIRP, is that of the International EMF Project, which was created by the WHO in 1996. This project, according to the WHO *Standards* page,

"...provides a unique opportunity to bring countries together to develop a framework for harmonisation of EMF standards..."

The aim of the EMF Project is,

"...to assess the scientific evidence of possible health effects of EMF in the frequency range from 0 to 300 GHz."

The most recent information on the WHO website about the adverse health effects from exposures to EMFs, is the October 2014 fact sheet entitled *Electromagnetic fields and public health: mobile phones,* which states that,

"To date, no adverse health effects have been established as being caused by mobile phone use."

This claim is refuted by the Group 2B classification of RFR in 2011; this is yet another example of the contradictions contained within the information promulgated by the medical establishment.

The bioelectrical system of the human body and the effects caused by exposures to external EMFs are explained by Dr Neil Cherry PhD in his 2000 paper entitled *Evidence of Health Effects of Electromagnetic Radiation, To the Australian Senate Inquiry into Electromagnetic Radiation,*

"We have natural EMR-based communication systems in our brains, hearts, cells and bodies. External natural and artificial EMR resonantly interacts with these communication systems altering hormone balances and damaging organs and cells."

Dr Cherry specifically discusses the sensitivity of the heart and the brain to external electrical and electromagnetic influences and states that,

"The brain and the heart are especially sensitive because they mediate and regulate primary biological functions that are vital to life..."

The effects on the heart from EMF exposures can manifest as health problems diagnosed as CVDs, as previously discussed. The effects on the brain can manifest as a number of symptoms, including those described as 'nervous symptoms' by the *Workshop* report.

The level of electromagnetic pollution has risen phenomenally in the past few decades. Unfortunately, this level is anticipated to continue to worsen, not only as the result of increased demand for existing applications, such as mobile phones and wireless communications, amongst others, but more specifically, as mentioned in chapter six, for the new 5G systems that are to be introduced globally in the 2020s. There are, however, increasing efforts to introduce 5G ahead of schedule.

A January 2017 IEEE (Institute of Electrical and Electronics Engineers) article, entitled *Everything You Need to Know About 5G*, states that 5G is needed to handle the increasing volume of traffic required for the 'Internet of Things', which mainly refers to 'SMART' technologies. One of the innovations of 5G is the use of millimetre waves that operate in the frequency range between 30 and 300 GHz, which is a major sector of the frequency range under review by the EMF Project. The article states that,

"Until now, only operators of satellites and radar systems used millimetre waves for real-world applications."

As also mentioned in chapter six, the technologies proposed for 5G are virtually untested. On the basis that existing electromagnetic technologies that were claimed to be 'safe' have been proven to be otherwise, the proposed new technologies have raised a considerable level of concern amongst scientists and physicians who are already aware of the existing level of harm caused by EMF exposures. As mentioned in chapter six, Dr Devra Davis PhD founded the EHT (Environmental Health Trust) in 2007; the EHT website contains useful information about the hazards of EMF exposures. With particular reference to 5G, a September 2017 article entitled *Scientists And Doctors Demand Moratorium on 5G* states that,

"Over 180 scientists and doctors from 35 countries sent a declaration to officials of the European Commission today demanding a moratorium on the increase of cell antenna for planned 5G expansion."

The article refers to a study by the US NTP (National Toxicology Program), which has been conducted to determine the effects of mobile phone radiofrequencies on rats and mice, and states that some of the early results show,

"...statistically significant increases in the incidence of brain and heart cancer in animals exposed to cellphone radiation at levels below international guidelines."

There is an increasing level of awareness amongst many scientists and physicians that exposures to both EMFs and toxic chemicals are responsible for many health problems. This awareness has encouraged an increased demand for 'official' recognition of EHS and MCS as genuine health problems; as indicated by a 2015 article entitled *Reliable disease biomarkers characterizing and identifying electrohypersensitivity and multiple chemical sensitivity as two etiopathogenic aspects of a unique pathological disorder* by Professor Dominique Belpomme MD and his colleagues. The article demonstrates that EHS and MCS are not 'idiopathic' but genuine medical conditions.

The study referred to in the article identified certain significant symptoms experienced by many patients who suffer from either EHS or MCS or both; these were inflammation, oxidative stress and reduced melatonin levels.

The coinciding symptoms of oxidative stress and inflammation are a common feature of many ill-health conditions; the latter is discussed in more detail later in this chapter. Melatonin is an extremely important hormone that regulates a number of vital functions, one of which is sleep; low melatonin levels are therefore directly related to sleep disturbances, one of the symptoms recognised by the *Workshop* report. Dr Cherry's 2002 article about reduced melatonin levels caused by EMF/EMR exposures, which was discussed in chapter six, referred to some of the more serious health effects that can result from such exposures.

At a meeting in May 2011, a delegation of scientists and physicians, including Professor Belpomme, presented a petition to the WHO requesting the official recognition of MCS and EHS as genuine environmental illnesses; this petition failed to influence the WHO. Another petition, presented to the medical establishment in 2015, also requested a change to the official position on EHS and MCS. This petition had arisen as a result of the Fifth Congress of the Paris Appeal held in Brussels. Another result of the Congress was the production of the *2015 Brussels International Scientific Declaration on EHS & MCS*, which states that,

> "Following the fifth Paris Appeal Congress, the attending European, American and Canadian scientists unanimously decided to write a Common International Declaration to request an official recognition of these new diseases and of their sanitary consequences worldwide."

The press release that accompanied this Declaration states that,

> "The declaration calls upon national and international bodies and institutions and particularly the WHO, for taking urgently their responsibility for recognizing electrohypersensitivity and multiple chemical sensitivity as real diseases..."

It would seem that this request also failed to influence the WHO; the stance of most of the medical establishment towards EHS and MCS remains unchanged; as indicated by the lack of a WHO fact sheet relating to either of these conditions.

The refusal to acknowledge that these conditions represent genuine health problems means that physicians are not trained to recognise or understand the systemic problem with which their patients suffer; instead physicians are only able to offer 'treatments' for their symptoms. This means that headaches will be treated with painkillers; sleep difficulties with sleeping tablets or benzodiazepines; and depression with antidepressants. However, none of these pharmaceutical drugs is capable of addressing symptoms that have been caused by exposures to EM radiation or to toxic chemicals, or, as is invariably the case, to both.

As stated, the human body functions bioelectrically and biochemically; however, these systems function interdependently, which means that chemicals affect the bioelectrical system and EMFs affect the biochemical system. The effects of exposure to EM radiation on the body's production of melatonin exemplifies this interconnectedness; the close similarities between EHS and MCS should therefore not be surprising.

The discussion about EMFs in chapter six demonstrated the influence of vested interests, especially the military, to suppress information about the adverse health effects from various technologies and the electromagnetic radiation they produce. This influence was recognised by Dr Becker in *The Body Electric*, in which he states that,

"Because industry and the military demand unrestricted use of electromagnetic fields and radiation, their intrinsic hazards are often compounded by secrecy and deceit."

The 'industry' vested interests are mainly those involved in telecommunications and electronic technologies, which, together with the military, seem to exert a powerful influence over ICNIRP and the WHO, both of which deny the existence of proven harm to health; as demonstrated by the Electromagnetic Sensitivity web page about *Current Science* that states,

"A small number of scientists, mainly physicists and those linked with the radio industry and its regulators, such as some members of ICNIRP and WHO EMF Project, still cling to the long invalidated hypothesis of no harm."

The continually increasing level of electropollution in the environment requires awareness of the problem and the understanding that the WHO, despite its claim to be the 'authority' for health matters, fails to acknowledge the huge weight of evidence of harm caused by unnatural EM radiation. The fact that some people are more affected by certain influences than others does not provide an excuse to avoid recognition of the problem or to imply that they may be suffering from a 'psychiatric' condition, as suggested by the *Workshop* report in the statement that,

"There are also some indications that these symptoms may be due to pre-existing psychiatric conditions as well as stress reactions as a result of worrying about believed EMF health effects, rather than the EMF exposure itself."

This attitude is egregious; however, there is an increasing emphasis on 'mental health' problems and diagnoses of a variety of 'mental disorders' that are used to describe a wide range of emotional, but entirely normal, responses to the stresses of life. This important topic has been mentioned in chapter one, but will be further explored in chapter ten.

The adverse health effects from exposures to electromagnetic radiation are real, there are, however, some measures that can be taken to reduce exposures to EMFs and to ameliorate their effects; these are also discussed in chapter ten.

Gulf War Syndrome

The establishment definition of Gulf War Syndrome (GWS) refers to the condition as,

"a variety of symptoms, mainly neurological (including chronic fatigue, dizziness, amnesia, digestive upsets and muscle wasting) that have been attributed to exposure of armed forces personnel to chemicals (e.g. insecticides) used during the Gulf War (1991) or possibly to the effects of vaccines and tablets given to protect personnel against the anticipated threat of chemical and biological warfare during the conflict."

The wording of this definition conveys the impression that these 'chemicals, vaccines and tablets' have not been definitively proven to be relevant causal factors for the symptoms experienced by armed forces personnel; this is however, a mistaken impression. There is demonstrable evidence that these factors have played a direct and highly significant role in the debilitating illness experienced by veterans of the 1990/91 Gulf War.

The military personnel involved in this conflict were not solely American; however, the website of the US VA (Department of Veteran Affairs) provides information about GWS, including a definition of the condition and some of the symptoms suffered; it states, on the page entitled *Gulf War Veterans' Medically Unexplained Illness*, that,

> "A prominent condition affecting Gulf War veterans is a cluster of medically unexplained chronic symptoms that can include fatigue, headaches, joint pain, indigestion, insomnia, dizziness, respiratory disorders and memory problems."

The use of the term 'medically unexplained' to describe the condition demonstrates that the medical establishment attitude towards GWS bears a striking resemblance to their attitude towards MCS and EHS; GWS requires further examination.

On the VA web page entitled *Gulf War Exposures*, is a list of 13 'potential' hazards that troops may have encountered; these hazards include: vaccinations, pyridostigmine bromide, pesticides, chemical and biological weapons, depleted uranium and occupational hazards. For each hazard there are additional web pages that provide more detailed information. Whilst it is unlikely that military personnel would have been exposed to all 13 hazards, there is one hazard to which they were certainly all subjected. All military personnel received a number of vaccinations; these are described on the web page devoted to the topic as,

> "Standard series of inoculations against infectious diseases provided to any US citizen travelling to the Gulf."

Although this 'standard series' is not explicitly detailed, the vaccines administered are stated to have included: yellow fever, typhoid, cholera, hepatitis B, meningitis, whooping cough, polio and tetanus. Some troops received additional vaccines for anthrax and botulinum toxoid, neither of which are part of any 'standard' vaccines for travellers.

On the Institute of Science in Society website is a July 2003 article entitled *Vaccines, Gulf-War Syndrome and Bio-defence* by Dr Mae-Wan Ho PhD and Professor Malcolm Hooper PhD, who report that UK troops received an additional vaccine; an experimental one for 'plague'. The article also states that,

> "Vaccine overload was identified as a significant factor in GWS."

In addition, the article states that the UK MoD (Ministry of Defence) claims that the troops were given 10 vaccines, but that,

> "...records exist to show that some troops received a greater number."

The previous chapters about vaccinations and the 'germ theory' demonstrated that not only were all of the vaccinations unnecessary, but that together they would have introduced a large volume of toxic material into the bloodstream of these people; especially as multiple vaccines were often administered simultaneously or shortly after each other. The neurotoxic ingredients of most vaccines provide an entirely adequate explanation for the onset of neurological problems.

Pesticides are another of the hazards to which troops were exposed; the VA web page lists 4 types: methyl carbamate organochlorine pesticides, DEET, organophosphorus (OP) pesticides and pyrethroid pesticides. Lindane, which is a methyl carbamate organochlorine pesticide, was used to treat uniforms. DEET (diethyltoluamide) is a common insect repellent that is applied directly onto the skin. Pyrethroid pesticides, such as permethrin, were also used to treat military uniforms. As discussed, pesticides are toxic by nature and by intent. Although they have not been fully tested in combination to determine the existence of all possible synergistic interactions, there are some chemical combinations that have been proven to substantially enhance the combined toxicity. The authors of *Killer Clothes* discovered evidence of the existence of synergies as the result of tests conducted on certain substances, including those to which the military personnel were exposed,

"...researchers had discovered that permethrin interacts synergistically with DEET and other chemicals resulting in severe health problems being produced in lab animals."

As discussed in chapter five, animals are not suitable experimental models for humans, but this does not mean that evidence of harm to animals can be ignored. Any substance that causes harm to animals must be regarded as having the potential to be harmful to humans; it is, after all, the purpose of animal experiments to ascertain if a substance has the potential to cause adverse effects. Unfortunately, however, animal testing research studies tend to focus on the determination of 'safe' doses rather than the investigation of the full extent of the adverse health effects that substances may produce.

Another item on the list of hazards is pyridostigmine bromide (PB), which is a pharmaceutical drug that is said to provide a measure of protection against the highly toxic nerve gas 'Soman', when taken prior to exposure and in conjunction with certain antidotes that are taken after exposure. Soman is an organophosphate compound; it is referred to as an acetylcholinesterase (AChE) inhibitor. PB is also an AChE inhibitor, although the effect of the drug is claimed to only be temporary.

The reference to organophosphate pesticides in chapter six explained that cholinesterase is an important enzyme required for the normal functioning of the human nervous system. The inhibition of this enzyme has serious consequences, as explained by Dr Russell Blaylock in *Health and Nutrition Secrets*,

"When cholinesterase is deactivated, acetylcholine over-stimulates muscles, resulting in an inability to control movements."

Gulf War personnel were clearly exposed to a number of compounds that acted as AChE inhibitors; a situation that provides another adequate explanation for some of the neurological symptoms they experienced.

Despite the recognition that military personnel were exposed to various combinations of many different hazardous substances, the medical establishment maintains that no 'medical explanation' exists for the symptoms that veterans continue to experience. The medical establishments of the US and the UK are particularly fervent in retaining a stance that denies the existence of any links between these hazards and GWS.

The attitude of the US establishment is represented by HMD (the Health and Medicine Division of the NAS), formerly known as IOM (Institute of Medicine), in a 2010 report entitled *Health Effects of Serving in the Gulf War*. The conclusion to the report is stated to be that,

> "...current available evidence is not sufficient to establish a causative relationship between chronic multisymptom illnesses and any specific drug, toxin, plume or other agent, either alone or in combination."

The position of the UK government is expressed on the page entitled *Gulf veterans' illnesses*, which refers to an independent review conducted by the MRC (Medical Research Council) in 2003 and states,

> "The MRC report stated that no evidence of a unique syndrome had been found in this country or abroad following research of troops deployed to the Gulf."

These statements highlight the many problems associated with all conditions of this nature; one of which is the idea that a 'unique syndrome' must be identified in order for a variety of symptoms to be 'officially' recognised as a medical condition. Another is the often-repeated claim that there is 'insufficient evidence' of a causal relationship.

By contrast to the medical establishment stance, a November 2008 report entitled *Gulf War Illness and the Health of Gulf War Veterans*, published by the Research Advisory Committee on Gulf War Veterans' Illnesses, discusses different interpretations of the term 'unique syndrome' and states that,

> "However the question of a unique syndrome is interpreted, extensive descriptive and analytic research has clearly demonstrated that an illness, characterized by a complex of multiple systems, resulted from service in the Gulf War."

The report also states under the heading *Findings in Brief* that,

> "Gulf War illness is a serious condition that affects at least one fourth of the 697,000 US veterans who served in the 1990-1991 Gulf War."

It should be clear that it does not require the existence of a 'unique syndrome' to recognise that more than a hundred thousand men and women currently experience serious and debilitating health problems due to certain aspects of their involvement in that conflict.

The failure of the medical establishment to acknowledge the connection between the exposures of military personnel to hazardous substances and their ill-health does not mean that the problem does not exist.

The reasons that the medical establishment continues to maintain this position with respect to GWS are based on factors that include the controlled 'conventional' medical training of physicians and the centralised disease classification system of the ICD. This attitude also owes its existence to the powerful influence of vested interests, especially the military, that seek to prevent public awareness of the real nature of the problem, partly due to their fear of a public outcry and the resulting demand for compensation. This problem is discussed in *Chemical Exposures*,

"In the United States, legal action or liability concerns unfortunately drive much of the acerbic rhetoric and distortions of science that retard the advancement of understanding about chemical sensitivity. The same is also true in parts of Europe, notably Germany and the United Kingdom."

Although this explanation refers to MCS, it can be seen to also apply to GWS.

These fears are, however, only some of the reasons that vested interests within industry and the military seek to prevent a full level of public understanding about the effects of their activities on the health of the public and the environment.

Autoimmune Diseases

An 'autoimmune disease' is defined by the establishment as,

"one of a number of otherwise unrelated disorders caused by inflammation and destruction of tissues by the body's own immune response."

It is claimed that there are in excess of 80 different autoimmune diseases; however, although considered to be 'otherwise unrelated', they are said to share a common feature of an absolutely fundamental nature. They are all claimed to result from the loss of the immune system's ability to distinguish between the body's cells and those of an 'invader'; a situation that causes the immune system to attack and even destroy the body's own cells and tissues 'by mistake'.

It would seem therefore that, according to the medical establishment, the human body is not only a passive receptacle that is attacked by disease, but it also makes mistakes and is capable of self-destruction.

Nothing could be further from the truth.

The medical establishment theories relating to autoimmune diseases are fraught with problems, the main one of which is that these theories are dependent upon erroneous ideas about the immune system, the existence of which is predicated upon the 'germ theory'; a theory that has been shown to be fatally flawed.

The rigid adherence to a flawed theory will inevitably result in a failure to understand and correctly interpret circumstances observed in the real world. This is particularly noticeable in the failure to understand and correctly interpret ill-health conditions diagnosed as autoimmune diseases. The medical establishment does however, admit to a poor level of understanding about these diseases; as acknowledged on the NIAMS (National Institute of Arthritis and Musculoskeletal and Skin Diseases) web page entitled *Autoimmune Diseases* that states,

"No one is sure what causes autoimmune diseases."

Nevertheless, despite this paucity of knowledge, the medical establishment refers to certain 'factors' that are claimed to play influential roles in the onset of autoimmune diseases; the NIAID (National Institute of Allergy and Infectious Diseases) web page entitled *Autoimmune Diseases* states that,

"Although the causes of many autoimmune diseases remain unknown, a person's genes in combination with infections and other environmental exposures are likely to play a significant role in disease development."

The idea that 'genes' or 'infections' are relevant factors to the onset of any disease has been shown to be unfounded; the role of environmental factors is, however, certainly significant, as will be discussed.

The theories underlying 'autoimmunity' were recognised to be problematic more than two decades ago by Dr Peter Duesberg, who states in his 1996 book *Inventing the AIDS Virus* that,

"The autoimmunity hypothesis, however, suffers several fatal flaws."

He proceeds to explain some of those flaws,

"For one thing, autoimmune reactions have been poorly documented in any disease, not to mention AIDS. In fact, they may never occur in an otherwise healthy person. Moreover, the immune system works so well precisely because it has built in (but poorly understood) safeguards that prevent it from attacking its own host body..."

The immune system is comprised of a number of organs, each of which has specific functions; however, according to the medical establishment, the main function of the 'immune system' is to detect, fight and kill invading pathogens. The discussions in chapter three demonstrated that none of the immune system's functions involves the destruction of microbial invaders. As also previously discussed, some organisms can 'invade' the body, but they only do so under certain conditions, which, as Dr Duesberg indicates, do not occur in an otherwise healthy person; parasites are discussed in more detail in chapter eight.

The human body is not inert; it does not make mistakes nor does it try to destroy itself. On the contrary, the human body is a complex, self-regulating organism that constantly seeks to attain and maintain itself in the state of health, and, when harmed, it will make every effort to repair the damage and heal itself.

The establishment definition claims that autoimmune diseases are caused by inflammation; but the establishment defines inflammation as,

"the body's response to injury, which may be acute or chronic."

The definition explains that this response is a 'defensive reaction' that enables healing to take place after injury. The medical establishment therefore appears to attribute two entirely conflicting roles to inflammation; one that is protective and another that is destructive. This is clearly anomalous; but it is an anomaly that has arisen from a fundamental misunderstanding about the processes that induce inflammation. In *Natural Hygiene: Man's Pristine Way of Life*, Herbert Shelton explains that inflammation is protective; it produces an increased blood supply that delivers 'repair materials' to the affected area and enables healing to take place. He further explains that,

"Inflammation, whether in a wound or in a so-called disease, is a remedial, a reparative and, also, a defensive process."

Under normal circumstances the inflammation processes will cease when the repair has been achieved; however, if the damage is extensive and the repair processes are prolonged, inflammation will also be prolonged and may cause damage to the affected tissues. This is explained by Herbert Shelton, who states that,

"Death or mortification of the inflamed part represents the unsuccessful termination of the remedial effort."

It is clear therefore, that the processes that initiate inflammation are not intentionally destructive, and that damage only occurs when the underlying problem has not been resolved. The most common underlying cause of inflammation is the presence of 'poisons', as he further explains,

"Inflammation in any part of the body arises out of the same cause – toxemia."

The claim that toxins cause inflammation and can induce symptoms associated with 'autoimmune diseases' is corroborated by Hal Huggins and Dr Thomas Levy, who explain in *Uninformed Consent* that certain toxic substances are specifically used for autoimmune disease animal research studies. The reason that these toxic substances are used, is because they are known to induce conditions in animals that approximate to those observed in humans diagnosed with certain autoimmune diseases. It should not be surprising to discover that mercury is one of the toxic substances used for the purposes of inducing some of the relevant conditions in animals.

Another toxic substance used in autoimmune disease research is a chemical referred to as TMPD (tetramethylpentadecane), which is described by the chemical industry as 'a hydrocarbon oil adjuvant' and promoted for its ability to act as an 'autoimmune disorder induction reagent'. The use of hydrocarbons for this purpose is discussed in a March 2010 article entitled *Toxicology of Autoimmune Diseases* that states,

"The adjuvant properties of certain hydrocarbons can precipitate inflammatory or autoimmune disease in humans and animals..."

In addition, certain drugs are also known to induce or trigger an 'autoimmune' response, as the article explains,

"The chemicals most often associated with development of autoimmunity in humans are medications."

The article refers to a list of drugs that have been shown to induce certain 'SLE-like' conditions; SLE is systemic lupus erythematosus, which is more commonly referred to as lupus. Most significantly, the article concludes that,

"There is ample evidence that exposure to a variety of drugs and chemicals can lead to autoimmunity."

A December 2002 article, entitled *Environmental chemicals and autoimmune disease: cause and effect*, provides further supportive evidence of the association between certain medications and some autoimmune diseases, including lupus. This association is not merely a 'correlation'; the evidence indicates a direct causative relationship; as the article states,

"These are temporary conditions that resolve when the medication is removed."

The article continues with the comment that,

"There are now over 70 such medications which have been reported related to these autoimmune conditions."

In common with many other types of disease, there are no 'cures' for autoimmune diseases; the medical establishment only offers drug 'treatments' that are claimed to manage these conditions by alleviating symptoms. There are two types of treatment; immunosuppressive drugs and anti-inflammatory drugs.

Immunosuppressive drugs are used on the basis of the idea that the immune system attacks the body's own cells and tissues; but, as discussed, this is an erroneous idea. One of the immunosuppressant drugs prescribed for the treatment of certain autoimmune diseases, particularly lupus and rheumatoid arthritis, is azathioprine. There are some serious 'side effects' associated with this drug, particularly low blood pressure and liver damage; the effects also include vomiting and diarrhoea, all of which are indicative of the drug's toxicity and the body's efforts to expel it. Another immunosuppressive drug used in the treatment of autoimmune disease is methotrexate, which is also used to treat certain cancers. In addition to the 'side effects' of nausea and vomiting, this drug can adversely affect the blood and the liver; these effects are all clear indications of its toxicity.

Immunosuppressive drugs are also used to prevent organ rejection after a transplant operation; however, a better solution needs to be sought for this problem because these drugs are toxic.

The other type of treatment that may be prescribed for autoimmune diseases are anti-inflammatory drugs, which include NSAIDs and corticosteroids, but these are also attended by serious adverse health effects. In *Death by Modern Medicine*, Dr Carolyn Dean reports the result of a survey of French GPs which included the finding that,

"Non-steroidal anti-inflammatory drugs (NSAIDs) rank first among commonly prescribed drugs for serious adverse events."

The fact that a large number of 'medicines' have been shown to induce health problems that can be diagnosed as 'autoimmune conditions' strongly indicates that pharmaceuticals, especially those derived from hydrocarbons, are entirely inappropriate for the treatment of these conditions.

Of further concern is that, despite their poor level of knowledge and understanding about autoimmune diseases and their causes, the medical establishment has created a new category of diseases referred to as 'auto-inflammatory diseases', which are explained on a NIAMS web page entitled *Understanding Autoinflammatory Diseases*. On the web page it is claimed that autoimmune diseases and autoinflammatory diseases are different, but share common characteristics, which are,

"...that both groups of disorders result from the immune system attacking the body's own tissues, and they also result in increased inflammation."

The difference is claimed to be that,

"In autoinflammatory diseases, this innate immune system causes inflammation for unknown reasons."

There is, however, little to differentiate between autoinflammatory diseases and autoimmune diseases, except for the claim that inflammation occurs for 'unknown' reasons in the former. This is yet another unfounded claim, because the medical establishment has a poor understanding of inflammation. The creation of a new category of 'diseases' does not help to better understand these conditions, especially as they are based on a fundamentally flawed theory.

The next few sections examine some of the more common 'autoimmune diseases' to further illustrate the medical misconceptions promulgated by the medical establishment about them.

Diabetes

The establishment defines diabetes as,

> "any disorder of metabolism causing excessive thirst and the production of large volumes of urine."

The term 'diabetes' is, however, predominantly used to refer to the specific form of the condition known as 'diabetes mellitus', which is defined by the establishment as,

> "a disorder of carbohydrate metabolism in which sugars in the body are not oxidised to produce energy due to lack of the pancreatic hormone insulin."

There are two types of diabetes mellitus, known as type 1 and type 2.

Type 1 diabetes is regarded as the more severe condition because the body is said to have lost the ability to produce insulin; this type of diabetes is said to begin in childhood or adolescence.

Type 2 diabetes is regarded as a metabolic disease that generally begins later in life and is regarded as less severe than type 1.

Mortality from diabetes is significant; it is the fourth most serious NCD and claimed to be responsible for the worldwide loss of more than a million lives each year. The incidence of diabetes has grown considerably in the past few decades, as indicated by the October 2018 WHO fact sheet entitled *Diabetes* that states,

> "The number of people with diabetes has risen from 108 million in 1980 to 422 million in 2014."

It is claimed that type 1 diabetes is an autoimmune disease; there is however, a lack of knowledge about certain aspects of this condition, as the fact sheet admits,

> "The cause of type 1 diabetes is not known and it is not preventable with current knowledge"

By comparison, it is claimed that the causes of type 2 diabetes are known and that, according to the fact sheet, this type of diabetes is,

> "...largely the result of excess body weight and physical inactivity."

The reasons for such a distinction between two forms of the same disease are not explained.

One point of particular concern is that type 2 diabetes is increasingly prevalent among children, as the fact sheet indicates,

> "Until recently, this type of diabetes was seen only in adults but it is now also occurring increasingly frequently in children."

Although it is only type 1 diabetes that is categorised as an autoimmune condition, there is a school of thought that suggests type 2 diabetes belongs in the same category. This view is articulated by a June 2015 article entitled *Are obesity-related insulin resistance and type 2 diabetes autoimmune diseases* which refers to type 2 diabetes and CVD as 'chronic metabolic disorders' but makes the familiar statement that,

"Although these disorders affect a significant proportion of the global population, the underlying mechanisms of disease remain poorly understood..."

This poor level of understanding about type 2 diabetes would appear to be inconsistent with the assertion by the WHO that it is 'largely' the result of overweight and inactivity.

In common with virtually all other diseases, the medical establishment can only offer diabetes 'treatments'; as described by the fact sheet,

"Diabetes can be treated and its consequences avoided or delayed with diet, physical activity, medication and regular screening and treatment for complications."

The severity of type 1 diabetes is due to the near or complete failure of the pancreas to produce insulin, an important hormone. It is claimed that the body's insulin deficiency can be rectified by injections that deliver pharmaceutical-based 'insulin' into the body. Until the 1980s, the insulin used to treat diabetes was sourced from animals; it is now 'human insulin', which is described on the web page entitled *Human Insulin* as,

"...the name which describes synthetic insulin which is laboratory grown to mimic the insulin in humans."

This 'human insulin' is claimed to have certain drawbacks; a problem that has been seemingly solved by the creation of 'insulin analogues'. According to the web page entitled *Diabetes Education Online*, these analogues mimic natural insulin,

"However, they have minor structural or amino acid changes that give them special desirable characteristics when injected under the skin."

It should be clear that any changes, however minor, will result in a different substance that is unlikely to act in exactly the same way that 'natural' insulin acts within the body.

Although the WHO fact sheet claims that screening and treatments are effective measures for monitoring diabetes, this claim is contradicted by a January 2017 article entitled *Efficacy and effectiveness of screen and treat policies in prevention of type 2 diabetes: systematic review and meta-analysis of screening tests and interventions*. The article states that the purpose of screening tests is to identify people who are 'at risk'; it refers to two types of screening test currently in use and adds that one was found to be 'specific but not sensitive' and that the other type was found to be 'neither specific nor sensitive'. The article also states that interventions must be efficacious for those who are considered to be 'at risk'; the main interventions for type 2 diabetes involve the use of pharmaceutical drugs. One such drug is metformin, about which an August 2015 article entitled *A Comprehensive Review of Drug-Drug Interactions With Metformin* states,

"Although it is an old drug, its mechanism of action has not yet been clarified and its pharmacokinetic pathway is still not fully understood."

The purpose of the article was, as the title indicates, to review drug-drug interactions; nevertheless, this article contains a significant admission about the lack of knowledge of one of the most commonly used 'treatments' for this serious condition. The article admits to another problem with this drug which is that,

"There is considerable inter-individual variability in the response to metformin."

Although inexplicable to the medical establishment, there are understandable reasons for the variability in the responses to this drug and, in fact to all drugs; these reasons are discussed in more detail in chapter ten.

The reference in the WHO fact sheet to 'overweight' as a major factor in diabetes is misleading. Diabetes does not arise as a direct result of excess weight per se; it occurs as the result of the type of food consumed, amongst other factors. A diet that is mainly comprised of processed food products and drinks that contain substantial amounts of toxic food additives, especially refined sugar, will disrupt many of the normal functions of the body. The WHO does recognise that diet plays a role in diabetes, as indicated by the fact sheet that states,

"Healthy diet, regular physical activity, maintaining a normal body weight and avoiding tobacco use are ways to prevent or delay the onset of type 2 diabetes."

The fact sheet also recommends the avoidance of 'sugar', but fails to differentiate between the different types of sugar, although these different types are discussed in other fact sheets. The role of refined sugar in diabetes is significant, as it affects the body's ability to regulate blood sugar levels, which is the main symptom experienced by people with diabetes, as Dr Carolyn Dean explains in *Death by Modern Medicine*,

"Eating a highly refined diet of white flour and white sugar products...rapidly elevates blood sugar because these non-foods are quickly absorbed as simple sugars into the blood stream."

This aspect of an unhealthy diet is insufficiently emphasised in the diabetes fact sheet; the possible reason for this omission is explained by Dr Dean,

"Both Canadian and American Diabetes Associations receive corporate funding from food and drug companies."

This situation is not exclusive to Canada and America; it applies to any country in which the population consumes a diet that is largely comprised of manufactured 'food products', which contain high levels of refined sugar as well as other food additives. Dr Dean also refers to Dr Betty Martini, whose research included the discovery that aspartame can also precipitate diabetes. It would therefore, be a mistake to believe that the risk of diabetes can be reduced by replacing foods and drinks that contain refined sugars with foods and drinks that contain sugar-free sweeteners, especially aspartame.

Two conditions that are also associated with diabetes are hyperglycaemia, which is an excess of glucose in the bloodstream, and hypoglycaemia, which is a deficiency of glucose in the bloodstream; raised blood sugar is clearly not the only relevant factor for the onset of diabetes. The underlying problems associated with this disease involve disruptions to the body's metabolic processes; as Dr Russell Blaylock explains,

"...the body's metabolism is seriously disrupted leading to significantly increased free-radical generation and lipid peroxidation."

As previously discussed, free radicals are generated as the result of the body's normal metabolic processes. These radicals only become a problem if they are generated at levels that exceed the body's ability to neutralise them with antioxidants. However, free radicals are also produced in the body by many other factors, one of the most significant of which are toxic substances. The relevance of toxicity in diabetes is recognised by Dr Henry Bieler, who explains that,

> "In diabetics there is always a very toxic background and the thyroid gland is usually over-stimulated."

The thyroid gland is one of the organs of the endocrine system, the functions of which include the elimination of toxins from the body.

It is clear that toxins of various types, including 'refined' sugar, play a significant role in the onset of diabetes; the elimination of toxins from the diet would therefore significantly contribute to the amelioration as well as the prevention of this condition.

Multiple Sclerosis

The establishment definition of multiple sclerosis refers to this condition as,

> "a chronic disease of the nervous system affecting young and middle-aged adults. The myelin sheaths surrounding nerves in the brain and spinal cord are damaged, which affects the function of the nerves involved."

This description conveys the impression that MS is a distinct and easily identifiable condition; however, according to the Multiple Sclerosis Society web page entitled *Signs and symptoms*,

> "MS is complex and has many symptoms."

In addition, the National Multiple Sclerosis Society web page entitled *Multiple Sclerosis FAQs* states that,

> "Diagnosing MS can be a challenging process. In early MS, symptoms may be non-specific and suggestive of several disorders of the nervous system."

This diagnostic challenge is not restricted to MS, it applies to all autoimmune diseases, as indicated by a 2012 article entitled *Linkage of Multiple Sclerosis and Guillain-Barre Syndrome: A Population-Based Survey in Isfahan, Iran* that states,

> "Autoimmune diseases are well known for being difficult to diagnose."

Guillain-Barré syndrome is discussed in the next section.

On the MS Society *Signs and symptoms* page is the interesting comment that,

> "There are also other conditions with similar symptoms to MS."

The discussion about MCS referred to similarities between many different conditions; a group to which MS can be added for a number of reasons, not least of which is the lack of knowledge about these diseases and their causes. In common with these conditions, MS is also claimed to be associated with a group of 'risk factors'; as indicated by the MS International Federation (MSIF) web page entitled *Causes* that states,

> "Researchers do not know what triggers the immune system to attack myelin, but it is thought to be a combination of genetic and environmental factors."

The idea that 'genetic factors' are relevant to any autoimmune disease has been discussed and shown to be unfounded. By comparison, 'environmental factors' are relevant; or, to be more precise, certain types of environmental factors are significant to the onset of certain MS symptoms.

In addition, MS researchers claim that there are other factors that may 'trigger' the condition but do not always lead to the onset of disease; however, these 'triggers' cannot be regarded as causal factors. A factor can only be 'causal' if it is present in every single case, with no exceptions.

In common with many of the diseases discussed in this chapter, the Mayo Clinic web page entitled *Multiple Sclerosis* states that,

"The cause of multiple sclerosis is unknown."

Unfortunately, the absence of a known cause does not prevent the medical establishment making certain assertions about the condition, not least of which is the claim that 'infectious agents' are some of the relevant 'environmental factors' involved. But this claim is unfounded; as acknowledged by the MSIF *Causes* page that states,

"Many microbes (particularly Epstein Barr virus) have been proposed as potential triggers for MS, but none have been proven."

Fatigue is one of the most common symptoms associated with MS; however, the MSIF page entitled *Fatigue* states that,

"The cause of fatigue in MS remains unknown."

Despite the many unknown aspects of MS, there are some characteristics of this condition that are known, and are therefore able to assist a better understanding of the actual causes of some of the symptoms associated with it. The most significant feature of MS is that it is usually accompanied by damage to the myelin sheaths that protect nerve fibres. An understanding of this damage requires reference to the body's biochemical pathway called the methylation cycle, which is essential for a number of processes, one of which is the synthesis of myelin basic protein.

Methylation is a process in which a 'methyl group' is added onto another molecule; a methyl group is a carbon atom surrounded by three hydrogen atoms. Dr Amy Yasko PhD explains the importance of methylation on her web page entitled *The Methylation Cycle*,

"Methylation is involved in almost every bodily biochemical reaction and occurs billions of times *every second* in our cells."

It is therefore abundantly clear that anything that disrupts methylation will have serious consequences for the body's biochemical reactions. Dr Yasko further explains that two of the important bodily functions affected by the methylation cycle are detoxification and energy production. The existence of fatigue as a common symptom of MS suggests that the body's energy production system has been disrupted; the link between methylation and MS is, however, even stronger than merely 'suggestive'.

It is claimed that MS is not only lifelong, but also a condition that progressively worsens over time and proceeds almost inevitably to increased disability. A 2012 article entitled *Environmental Risk Factors for Multiple Sclerosis: A Review with a Focus on Molecular Mechanisms* states that there is no effective treatment for this advanced stage of MS, but it also makes the interesting comment that,

"It is hypothesized that loss of axons is the main mechanism underlying progressive disability."

An axon is a nerve fibre that can have a myelin sheath. It has been known for more than two decades that axon damage is one of the main mechanisms involved in MS. Furthermore, aspartame has been implicated in triggering MS in some cases, as mentioned in chapter six. In his 2004 article entitled *The Connection Between MS and Aspartame*, Dr Russell Blaylock writes,

"As far back as 1996 it was shown that the lesions produced in the myelin sheath of axons in cases of multiple sclerosis were related to excitatory receptors on the primary cells involved called oligodendroglia."

One of the constituent molecules of aspartame is methanol, about which Dr Blaylock states,

"Methanol is an axon poison."

Methanol is always metabolised into formaldehyde, which is highly toxic and a known carcinogen.

Dr Woodrow Monte PhD has also conducted research into the dangers of aspartame and written extensively on the subject. He dedicates one chapter of his book entitled *While Science Sleeps* to the topic of MS; in this chapter he states that,

"...the myelin sheath can be damaged at multiple sites in the brain."

He provides a further explanation of the significance of this comment,

"Interestingly, these sites are identical to the sites affected during methanol poisoning."

Unfortunately, but unsurprisingly, the manufacturers of aspartame vehemently deny any connection between aspartame and MS; a denial that has been accepted by the medical establishment and promulgated by the main MS organisations; as demonstrated by the National Multiple Sclerosis Society page entitled *Disproved Theories* that claims,

"No scientific evidence supports the claims that aspartame...causes MS."

This assertion is accompanied by the statement that more information is available from other sources that, ironically, include the website of 'Nutrasweet', the manufacturer of one of the main aspartame-containing sweeteners. Information provided by the manufacturer of a product implicated in the onset of MS cannot be considered independent or impartial.

However, aspartame is not the only source of exposure to methanol; this chemical is a common basic feedstock for materials that are used in the manufacture of many everyday products, as indicated by the Methanol Institute web page entitled *The Chemical* that states,

"Methanol is a key component of hundreds of chemicals that are integral parts of our daily lives."

The page also refers to the fact that methanol is involved in processes that produce formaldehyde for use in the manufacture of many different materials, including plastics, glues and resins, amongst others. On another Methanol Institute page, entitled *What is Methanol*, is the statement that,

"Methanol is used to produce other chemical derivatives, which in turn are used to produce thousands of products that touch our daily lives..."

The products for which methanol is a feedstock include 'health and pharmaceutical products'. Clearly, people can be exposed to methanol from many sources; the increasing incidence of multiple sclerosis should not therefore be entirely surprising.

As discussed in chapter one, cholesterol is essential for a number of functions; an additional point of great significance in the context of MS is that cholesterol is an essential constituent of myelin. Furthermore, cholesterol is soluble in methanol. This fact alone clearly demonstrates that exposure to methanol poses a hazard not only to the cholesterol in the brain but also to the cholesterol in the myelin that protects nerves.

The medical establishment claims that there is no cure for MS, but there are 'treatments', which involve different types of pharmaceutical drugs. One MS drug is teriflunomide, which is referred to as an immunomodulatory drug as it is said to affect the immune system. Its mechanism of action is explained by the MS Society on the web page entitled *Teriflunomide*, which states that it,

"...inhibits the function of specific immune cells that have been implicated in MS."

However, the page also makes the comment that,

"We don't know exactly how teriflunomide works, but it dampens down inflammation."

Inflammation is not the only symptom of MS and teriflunomide is not the only drug used to treat the condition; however, although research is said to be ongoing, it mainly focuses on the creation of new drug treatments rather than understanding and addressing the causes of MS.

Some research involves the investigation of existing drugs used for other conditions to determine if they may be effective in the treatment of MS. One drug that has been the focus of research of this nature is simvastatin, a statin drug commonly used to treat high cholesterol. It is claimed that simvastatin also has 'anti-inflammatory' and 'neuroprotective' effects, which is the reason it is undergoing investigation for its potential use in MS. A March 2014 study article entitled *Effect of high-dose simvastatin on brain atrophy and disability in secondary progressive multiple sclerosis* claims that this drug was able to reduce brain atrophy.

Simvastatin is associated with 'side effects' that include muscle pain, tenderness, weakness and cramps; some of the more serious 'side effects' include severe muscle pain, rashes, and inflammation and pain in the blood vessels and joints. It is a worrying situation that some of these 'side effects' are the symptoms experienced by people diagnosed with multiple sclerosis; which indicates that this drug cannot be a suitable 'treatment'. The action of statin drugs and the hazards they pose were discussed in chapter one.

It is clear that MS is another example of a condition that is largely the result of exposures to toxic 'environmental factors' that disrupt the methylation cycle, which is responsible for regulating the body's detoxification processes. The involvement of 'toxicity' as a key factor in MS means that one of the most effective methods for addressing this condition involves the reduction and elimination of exposures to toxic substances.

Guillain-Barré Syndrome

The establishment definition of Guillain-Barré syndrome (GBS) refers to,

"a disease of the peripheral nerves in which there is numbness and weakness in the limbs."

The October 2016 WHO fact sheet entitled *Guillain-Barré syndrome* states that it is,

"...a rare condition in which a person's immune system attacks the peripheral nerves."

On the basis of this description, it is clear that GBS is considered to be an autoimmune disease. An alternative name for this condition is 'post-infective polyneuropathy', which indicates one of the main factors alleged to precede and 'trigger' the onset of Guillain-Barré syndrome; as indicated by the fact sheet that states,

"Guillain-Barré syndrome is often preceded by an infection. This could be a bacterial or viral infection."

Although may viruses are claimed to precipitate GBS, the fact sheet focuses on the 'Zika' virus, about which it states,

"In the context of Zika virus infection, unexpected increase in cases of Guillain-Barré syndrome has been described in affected countries."

Zika virus is discussed in more detail later in this chapter in the section about birth defects; it should, however, be noted that no viral infection is the cause of GBS.

In common with most of the diseases discussed in this chapter, there are many unknown aspects of GBS, including its cause; as indicated by the NINDS (National Institute of Neurological Disorders and Stroke) *Guillain-Barré Syndrome Fact Sheet* that states,

"The exact cause of GBS is not known. Researchers don't know why it strikes some people and not others. It is not contagious or inherited."

The NINDS fact sheet offers more information about GBS and states that,

"In most cases of GBS, the immune system damages the myelin sheath that surrounds the axons of many peripheral nerves; however, it also may damage the axons themselves."

It is clear that GBS and MS share some common characteristics.

Interestingly, the WHO fact sheet states that,

"Guillain-Barré syndrome may also be triggered by vaccine administration..."

The reason for this comment stems from claims that GBS has been diagnosed after the administration of certain vaccinations, although the medical establishment vehemently denies that this indicates a causal relationship. The CDC web page entitled *Guillain-Barré syndrome and Flu Vaccine* states that the 'background rate' of GBS is 80 to 160 cases per week; which would seem to contradict the notion that it is 'rare'. However, more pertinently, it is stated on the same web page that GBS may occur after a flu vaccination 'on very rare occasions'.

A 2009 article entitled *Vaccines and Guillain-Barré syndrome* refers to the underlying aetiology of GBS as 'not completely understood' but that 'immune stimulation' is involved; the article continues with the comment that,

"Thus, since vaccines have an effect on the immune system it is biologically plausible that immunizations may be associated with subsequent GBS."

Despite the recognition that an association is 'plausible', the article denies the existence of evidence that there is a proven causal relationship between them. However, some cases reported to the VAERS (Vaccine Adverse Event Reporting System) have involved a diagnosis of GBS following certain vaccinations. A 2011 article entitled *Guillain-Barré syndrome after Gardasil vaccination: data from Vaccine Adverse Event Reporting System 2006-2009* refers to the incidence of post-Gardasil GBS as being,

"...higher than that of the general population."

The fact that neurotoxic substances, such as aluminium, formaldehyde and mercury, are ingredients of vaccines offers a more than plausible explanation for damage to nerves following the administration of certain vaccinations.

The fact that GBS and MS both involve damage to the myelin sheath, although at different sites, indicates that they share common characteristics. The article that discussed a 'linkage' between GBS and MS, referred to in the previous section, indicates that the medical establishment regards these conditions as separate disease 'entities' that do not exist concurrently in an individual; however, the article reports that,

"...our findings might be suggestive of a linkage between the two diseases."

Furthermore, the study reported that, although extremely rare, some cases of concurrent GBS and MS were found to exist. One of the main reasons that this is referred to as a rare occurrence is the idea that MS and GBS are distinctly different diseases. Furthermore, once a diagnosis of one condition has been made, it is unlikely that additional symptoms will be considered to indicate the presence of a different disease. The diagnostic difficulties associated with both conditions make it more than likely that additional symptoms will be regarded as a worsening of the original condition.

In common with many conditions discussed in this chapter, there is no 'cure' for GBS, but the medical establishment can offer 'treatments', which unusually are required to be administered within a hospital setting. These treatments are intravenous immunoglobulin and plasma exchange, both of which are firmly based on the theory that claims the disease is due to a faulty immune system that attacks its 'host' body.

It must be emphasised that, as will be discussed in chapter ten, the body is a self-healing organism; the perpetuation of the erroneous belief that it is capable of attacking itself, even by mistake, poses a serious obstacle to a genuine understanding of any of the debilitating conditions referred to as autoimmune diseases.

Allergies

The establishment definition of an allergy refers to,

"a disorder in which the body becomes hypersensitive to particular antigens (called allergens), which provoke characteristic symptoms whenever they are subsequently inhaled, ingested, injected, or otherwise contacted."

The establishment defines an allergen as,

"any antigen that causes allergy in a hypersensitive person..."

The establishment defines an antigen as,

"any substance that may be specifically bound by an antibody molecule..."

The establishment defines an antibody as,

"a special kind of blood protein that is synthesized in lymphoid tissue in response to the presence of a particular antigen..."

Although these definitions explain some of the functions associated with allergies, they provide no information about the underlying mechanisms that precipitate 'allergic' reactions. The reason for this paucity of information is due to the medical establishment's poor level of understanding about allergies, as this discussion will demonstrate.

Allergies are not classified as autoimmune conditions, but they are claimed to involve the stimulation of the immune system in response to 'allergens'; as indicated by the NHS web page entitled *Allergies*, which, under the sub-heading *What causes allergies*, states that,

"Allergies occur when the body's immune system reacts to a substance as though it's harmful."

Nevertheless, the NHS makes the significant admission that,

"It's not clear why this happens..."

The definition of 'allergy' claims that the body becomes 'hypersensitive', but fails to explain the mechanism that induces this 'hypersensitivity'. Also unexplained is the reason that some people suddenly develop allergic reactions to substances to which they had never previously reacted.

Another unexplained phenomenon is that only certain substances are referred to as 'allergens'; as indicated by the AAAAI (American Academy of Allergy, Asthma & Immunology) web page entitled *Allergic Reactions*, which states that,

"It is not yet fully understood why some substances trigger allergies and others do not..."

It is claimed that contact with an 'allergen' stimulates the immune system to produce antibodies known as Immunoglobulin E (IgE); yet people do not all react in the same manner. The reasons that people react differently are largely unknown, as revealed in a 2010 article entitled *Mechanisms of IgE-mediated allergy* that states,

"Knowledge is still lacking about what causes some people to develop allergies while others remain tolerant to environmental allergens."

The reference to 'environmental allergens' is misleading as the term implies that such substances would always trigger allergic reactions, but this is clearly not the case. This does not mean, however, that 'environmental factors' are not relevant to the onset of reactions referred to as 'allergies', because, as this discussion will demonstrate, they are some of the main factors that induce these reactions.

In common with most NCDs, the medical establishment claims that allergies are related to genetic or hereditary factors; as indicated by the previously cited NHS web page, which claims that,

"...most people affected have a family history of allergies..."

This claim is unfounded; if the development of allergies were due to genetic factors, the problem would occur from birth, or soon afterwards. The fact that many people develop 'allergies' much later in life refutes this idea.

A further problem with the medical establishment view of allergies pertains to the role attributed to IgE antibodies; as revealed in a 2012 article entitled *IgE and mast cells in allergic disease* that states,

"Despite many years of intense study, the roles of IgE and mast cells in asthma and other allergic diseases are not fully understood."

It is clear that many aspects of 'allergies' remain unknown or not fully understood; this situation owes its origin to erroneous ideas about the 'immune system' and its alleged functions. These erroneous ideas extend to the notion that the immune system can make 'mistakes' about the nature of substances, with which it comes into contact, and treat harmless substances as if they are harmful.

In common with many of the NCDs discussed in this chapter, allergies are reported to occur in continually increasing numbers; a situation that the NHS *Allergies* web page attempts to explain by the comment that,

"The reasons for this are not understood, but one of the main theories is it's the result of living in a cleaner, germ-free environment, which reduces the number of germs our immune system has to deal with."

This 'theory', which is also referred to as the 'hygiene hypothesis', is highly misleading. Although the environment can correctly be described as 'germ-free', because there are no real 'germs', this is not the meaning intended by the NHS, which, in common with all other mainstream medical organisations, adheres rigidly to the 'germ theory'. Furthermore, as indicated in previous discussions, it is claimed that there are increasing numbers of 'infectious diseases' of increasing severity; this claim clearly and directly contradicts the idea that the environment is 'germ-free'. The suggestion that the environment is 'cleaner' can only be described as egregious; the discussions in chapter six demonstrate that the environment is becoming increasingly polluted; which means it is increasingly less clean.

The idea that the immune system reacts to substances 'as if they are harmful' suggests that these substances are otherwise entirely 'harmless'; however, this too is misleading. The web page provides a list of 'common allergens' and states that,

"Most of these allergens are generally harmless to people who aren't allergic to them."

This statement is highly unsatisfactory; it is essentially a circular argument that merely claims allergens are harmful to people who have allergies. But this clearly fails to explain the reason that 'allergic reactions' occur in the first place, or the reason that the body treats otherwise harmless substances as if they are harmful. The failure of the medical establishment to provide a credible explanation does not, however, mean that a credible explanation does not exist.

It should be noted that the list of 'common allergens' provided by the NHS includes substances such as 'medication' and 'household chemicals'. Part of the problem therefore lies with the use of the term 'allergen' to describe such substances, which, in most, if not all cases, should more correctly be described as 'toxins'.

One of the most common types of 'allergy' is called 'hay fever'; a condition that is also referred to as allergic rhinitis, which is defined by the establishment as,

> "a form of allergy due to the pollen of grasses, trees and other plants, characterised by inflammation of the membrane lining of the nose and sometimes of the conjunctiva."

The main types of treatment offered for allergic rhinitis are antihistamines, which are claimed to block the body's production and release of histamine, a chemical that is said to initiate irritation and inflammation. One of the major 'side effects' of the first generation of antihistamine drugs was drowsiness, although these drugs were also associated with other effects such as impaired thinking and blurred vision. Second and third generation antihistamines are said to be less likely to cause drowsiness, but are still associated with certain 'side effects', such as headaches and nausea. Other treatments for allergic rhinitis include corticosteroids, which are anti-inflammatory drugs.

Allergic rhinitis is claimed to be an 'IgE mediated reaction' that triggers the release of histamine from mast cells, which are located in connective tissue. However, as cited above, the roles of IgE and mast cells remain poorly understood; which therefore raises questions about the veracity of the explanation for this condition and the appropriateness of the treatment.

There is a credible explanation for the occurrence of 'allergic rhinitis' and one that does not involve unknown and unproven reactions by the immune system to substances that are arbitrarily referred to as 'allergens'. This explanation is provided by Dr Henry Bieler who states in *Food is Your Best Medicine* that,

> "Hay fever develops after there is an atrophy of the nasal and sinus mucous membranes."

Damage to the mucous membranes will therefore always precede the irritations and symptoms that may be diagnosed as 'hay fever', as Dr Bieler continues,

> "When there is no catarrhal state, there is no hay fever, no matter what irritant is inhaled."

Although commonly associated with pollen, 'hay fever', like many other 'allergies', is acknowledged to be 'triggered' by various substances, as indicated by the ACAAI (American College of Allergy, Asthma and Immunology) web page entitled *Allergic Rhinitis*, which, under the sub-heading *Symptoms*, states,

> "Symptoms also may be triggered by common irritants..."

Some of these 'common irritants' are: cosmetics; laundry detergents; pool chlorine; and strong odours, such as perfume and hairspray. These 'irritants' are strikingly similar to the substances described by the NHS as 'common allergens'. The body's reaction to such substances should not be surprising; the discussions in chapter six demonstrated that they all contain a variety of chemicals, most of which are toxic. The body does not therefore, make a 'mistake' in identifying these substances as harmful.

Dr Bieler explains that mucus is a protective lubricant barrier for the membranes and that the body increases the production of mucus in certain circumstances. One of these circumstances results from the inhalation of toxic chemicals, especially those of a volatile nature, which include certain chemical ingredients of household products, especially those referred to as 'fragrances'. These chemicals can clearly induce nasal irritation and inflammation, which, if prolonged because the underlying problem has not been resolved, will cause further damage to the tissues. This is explained by Herbert Shelton, who, in *Natural Hygiene: Man's Pristine Way of Life*, refers to catarrhal inflammation and calls it a 'crisis in toxaemia'; he expands on this point and states that,

> "Repeated for months and years, catarrhal inflammations end in chronic catarrh of the nasal passages, ulceration, hay fever and other so-called nasal diseases."

It is only the existence of this 'toxaemic' condition that precipitates the onset of the symptoms diagnosed as 'allergies'; the absence of a toxaemic condition provides a perfectly clear explanation of the reason that some people remain unaffected. However, the increasing use of toxic chemicals as ingredients of most consumer products is one of the main reasons that the incidence of allergies is increasing at an ever-faster rate. The solution to this problem inevitably involves reducing exposures to toxins.

Another allergy that is also increasingly common, especially in children, is 'food allergy', which, according to a 2011 article entitled *Food allergy*, affects approximately 6 per cent of young children; it is therefore a significant problem. The article states,

> "Food allergy is defined as an adverse immunologic response to a dietary protein."

It is suggested that there are two types of food reaction; one is an allergy, the other an 'intolerance'; the main difference between them is that an 'allergy' involves an immune system response and is usually more severe. However, the article fails to explain the reason that the immune system reacts adversely to food proteins, which are an important category of essential nutrients, especially for growing children. Furthermore, the ACAAI page entitled *Food Allergy* refers to the severity of each reaction as 'unpredictable' and adds the interesting comment that,

> "...a food that triggered only mild symptoms on one occasion may cause more severe symptoms at another time."

The idea that the same 'food' may, at different times, produce reactions of differing intensity indicates that the severity of the reaction cannot be an appropriate or reliable indicator of whether a reaction is an 'allergy' rather than an 'intolerance'.

FARE (Food Allergy Research and Education) discusses food allergy on the web page entitled *Food Allergy Research Funding* and refers to it as a 'disease'. The page also makes an increasingly familiar statement that,

> "The numbers are growing and becoming more serious - but there is no clear answer as to why."

The failure of the medical establishment to provide adequate explanations for the increased incidence of reactions to foods does not mean that credible explanations do not exist. The discussion about hay fever referred to the existence of an underlying toxicity; the same applies to food allergy, and indeed to all allergies. They always involve long-term exposure to various 'toxins' that damage tissues, generate inflammation and result in increased 'sensitivity' of the damaged tissues.

Many of the toxins that are likely to contribute to 'food allergy' were discussed in chapter six; the increasing use of synthetic chemicals as food additives in processed food products and drinks provides a more than adequate explanation for this problem, and for its increased incidence especially in children; however, it must be noted that many other factors will also be involved; as discussed in chapter ten.

The problem of 'food allergy' is unlikely to be addressed by the medical establishment whilst it maintains its current stance, and refuses to acknowledge the extensive use of toxic chemicals in all areas of food production. Although the NHS does not recognise the true nature or extent of the problem, the web page makes the statement that,

> "Almost any food can cause an allergic reaction..."

Although reactions are claimed to occur from the consumption of 'almost any food', they will only occur from the consumption of foods that contain toxins of some description. It is therefore interesting to note that most 'food allergies' are claimed to involve reactions to eight types of food, which are eggs, milk, peanuts, tree nuts, fish, shellfish, wheat and soy. One of the most common foods associated with adverse reactions are peanuts, the next topic of discussion.

Peanut Allergy

There is no establishment definition for 'peanut allergy'; however, a basic explanation is provided by the Mayo Clinic web page entitled *Peanut allergy* that states,

> "Peanut allergy occurs when your immune system mistakenly identifies peanut proteins as something harmful."

As with all other allergies, the medical establishment does not know the reason that some people develop a reaction to peanuts whilst other people remain impervious to them. It is, however, a matter of concern that the incidence of this particular 'allergy' has risen dramatically in the past few decades and mainly affects children; as indicated by the FARE web page entitled *Peanut Allergy* that states,

> "According to a FARE-funded study, the number of children in the US with peanut allergy more than tripled between 1997 and 2008."

This situation is not exclusive to the US; the scale of the problem in the US as described by FARE is, however, of particular relevance to this discussion because peanuts have been consumed in America for more than a century;

yet peanut allergy is a relatively recent phenomenon.

People with allergies are generally advised to avoid contact with the substance that precipitates the onset of their symptoms. However, the findings of a new study indicate that this advice is likely to be significantly altered with respect to peanut allergy. The NIAID (National Institute of Allergy and Infectious Diseases) issued a January 2017 news release entitled *NIH-sponsored expert panel issues clinical guidelines to prevent peanut allergy* that states,

> "...recent scientific research has demonstrated that introducing peanut containing foods into the diet during infancy can prevent the development of peanut allergy."

The research referred to is the LEAP (Learning Early About Peanuts) study conducted at King's College London; the web page entitled *LEAP Study results* states that,

> "The LEAP study was based on a hypothesis that regular eating of peanut-containing products, when started during infancy, will effect a protective immune response instead of an allergic immune reaction."

The LEAP web page entitled *Peanut Allergy* claims that, according to many scientists, repeated exposure to peanuts will create 'tolerance' to them. This hypothesis is partly based on the observation that in countries where peanuts are commonly consumed at an early age, there is little, if any, peanut allergy. But this hypothesis directly contradicts the basic definition of a 'food allergy' that refers to an adverse reaction to a food protein; peanuts are a protein-based food. Furthermore, even in countries where peanut allergy is rife, many people consume peanuts without any adverse reactions to them; this also refutes the new hypothesis.

It should be clear from the discussion in the previous section that other factors are required to initiate an adverse reaction to peanuts and that these other factors invariably include a wide variety of 'toxins'. It should also be clear that it is these toxins that are the cause of the body's adverse reactions diagnosed as an 'allergy'.

Peanuts are not true 'nuts'; they are legumes that grow underground and have soft shells, unlike tree nuts that have hard shells.

One of the causes of an allergic reaction to peanuts is claimed to be due to the presence of the *Aspergillus* mould, which is said to release aflatoxins; but this mould will only develop if peanuts are grown or stored in damp conditions. As discussed in chapter six, it is not the mould that is toxic. On the contrary, the presence of mould indicates that the peanuts have begun to decompose; which means they are no longer fit for human consumption; it is therefore, unsurprising that people would become ill after consuming peanuts in this condition.

There is another route by which peanuts can become 'toxic'; this involves the liberal use of toxic pesticides on the peanut plants. Robyn O'Brien, a former food industry analyst, explains in her January 2019 article entitled *Food Allergies: The Hidden Truth About Peanuts* that,

> "Most of the peanuts consumed in the US are now one of the most pesticide-contaminated snacks we eat."

Cotton is frequently grown in rotation with peanuts and pesticides are liberally applied to both crops; but this is not a recent practice; as explained by Rachel Carson who wrote in 1962 that,

> "The most stubborn problems were concerned with peanuts. In the southern states peanuts are usually grown in rotation with cotton, on which BHC is extensively used. Peanuts grown later in this soil pick up considerable amounts of the insecticide."

BHC is benzene hexachloride; a toxic organochlorine that is chemically similar to lindane. The level of pesticide use on cotton plants is an extremely serious problem; the authors of *Killer Clothes* explain the reason and state that,

> "Because cotton isn't a food crop, the herbicides and pesticides and other chemicals used in the production of non-organic varieties aren't regulated by the government."

Clearly, all peanut crops that are grown in rotation with cotton crops will become contaminated with the toxic chemical ingredients of pesticides, which are applied frequently. Robyn O'Brien explains in her article that, according to farmers,

> "It is common to see a conventional peanut crop sprayed with some type of pesticide every 8-10 days during the growing season."

Furthermore, cotton is commonly grown in the US as a GM crop, which may nevertheless be rotated with non-GM peanut crops. This means that the peanut crops will also be exposed to soil residues of pesticides like glyphosate that are applied liberally to GM cotton crops, which are claimed to be 'resistant' to them. Non-GM peanut plants have no such resistance, but they are still exposed to soil residues of this highly toxic chemical that can be absorbed into the plants.

Pesticides are not the only soil pollutant with which peanut and many other plants can be poisoned; the discussions in chapter six identified many sources of soil contaminants that will increasingly affect all food crops. It is therefore unsurprising that there is an increasing incidence of adverse reactions from the consumption of various foods; the scale of the problem is indicated by the FARE web page entitled *Symptoms of an allergic reaction to food*, which states that,

> "Every three minutes, a food allergy reaction sends someone to the emergency room in the US."

It is clear that these reactions occur due to the existence of an underlying body burden of toxins that is exacerbated by the consumption of foods contaminated by toxins. This further intake of toxins is likely to overwhelm the body and reduce its ability to process and effectively expel the toxins; a situation that invariably results in an adverse reaction, which can vary in intensity, from mild to severe. The most serious reaction is known as anaphylaxis, which is potentially fatal.

The most common 'treatment' for allergies is epinephrine, a drug that is delivered by an 'auto-injector', which people with peanut allergy are advised to carry with them at all times for immediate use in the event of a severe reaction. This treatment is a synthetic substance derived from adrenaline (epinephrine), a natural hormone secreted by the adrenal glands. Although this drug is claimed to be life-saving in the event of an emergency, it does not solve the underlying problem. It should be noted that, as previously discussed, synthetic hormones are not the same as natural hormones, however chemically 'similar' they may be.

Robyn O'Brien makes the particularly pertinent comment that,

> "Children with food allergy are two to four times more likely to have other related conditions, such as asthma and other allergies, compared with children without food allergies."

The fact that these conditions are frequently concurrent indicates that they have common features, the main one of which is an underlying systemic toxicity that makes the body 'sensitive' to further exposures to toxic substances.

It should be clear therefore that the body does not mistakenly identify harmless foods as harmful; the reason that the body perceives certain foods to be 'harmful' is because they are actually harmful due to the presence of toxic substances.

Eczema

The establishment definition of eczema refers to,

> "a common itchy skin disease characterized by reddening and vesicle formation, which may lead to weeping and crusting."

The definition refers to eczema as endogenous; which means that,

> "...outside agents do not play a primary role."

In addition, the definition states that the term 'eczema' is often used interchangeably with that of 'dermatitis', which is defined by the establishment as,

> "an inflammatory condition of the skin caused by outside agents."

These definitions suggest that the terms eczema and dermatitis are not synonymous because one is endogenous and the other is not. This is, however, contradicted by the NIOSH web page entitled *Skin Exposures and Effects* that describes eczema in the same terms as those used in the above definition of dermatitis; as indicated by the reference to eczema as,

> "an inflammation of the skin resulting from exposure to a hazardous agent."

Furthermore, the NEA (National Eczema Association) web page entitled *An Overview of the Different Types of Eczema* claims that there are several different types of eczema, four of which are listed as different forms of 'dermatitis'. Nevertheless, the NEA web page makes the familiar claim that,

> "...the exact cause of eczema is unknown..."

The page contains another familiar claim, which is that,

> "...researchers do know that people who develop eczema do so because of a combination of genes and environmental triggers."

The most common form of eczema is referred to as 'atopic eczema', which is not regarded as an allergic condition but is considered to be 'associated with' other allergic conditions, especially asthma, which is discussed in the next section. The term 'atopic' refers to a predisposition to develop an allergy, which suggests that this is a known phenomenon; however, the NHS web page entitled *Atopic Eczema* claims that,

"The exact cause of atopic eczema is unknown…"

This claim is disingenuous; the previously cited *Dermal Exposure* report not only refers to factors that are known to cause 'contact dermatitis', one of the many forms of eczema, it also states quite clearly that,

"Dermal exposure to chemical or physical agents may lead to skin disease."

The term 'physical agents' refers to factors that are said to include ionising radiation and thermal burns.

The report claims that there are two forms of 'contact dermatitis', one of which is 'irritant' and the other 'allergic'. Irritant contact dermatitis is claimed to be the most common occupational 'skin disease', whereas allergic contact dermatitis is claimed to be more common in the general population. But this is misleading, as there is no real distinction between 'irritants' and 'allergens'. This also means, therefore, that there are no distinctly different 'forms' of contact dermatitis or eczema; these conditions are all the result of skin contact with harmful substances.

This assertion is supported by the statement in the *Dermal Exposure* report that the vast majority of cases of occupational 'skin disease' are the result of contact with chemicals or 'wet work'; even though they are described as 'irritants'. Although the report insufficiently emphasises the role of chemicals in precipitating skin diseases, it does make the statement that,

"…an irritant can damage the skin surface, leading to increased percutaneous penetration of the same or other chemicals."

The permeability of the skin was discussed in chapter six.

It is clear therefore, that 'skin diseases', whether referred to as eczema or dermatitis, are the result of contact with harmful substances, especially toxic chemicals, that damage the skin and can also enter the entire bodily system; as indicated by the report that states,

"A systemic effect can be observed in other organs or parts of the body after the chemicals penetrate through the skin and enter the bloodstream."

The source of the problem is indicated by the previously cited *Dermal Absorption* report, which states that,

"…the prevalence of atopic dermatitis in industrialized countries is dramatically increasing."

Many of the factors involved in 'industrialisation' will therefore be contributory factors to 'skin diseases'. This assertion is further supported by the above cited NIOSH web page that refers to exposures to 'hazardous agents' as the cause of skin inflammation.

Occupational exposures to hazardous chemicals, even though protective clothing is worn, are often more intense and more prolonged than domestic exposures. This situation is acknowledged by the NIOSH page entitled *National Occupational Research Agenda*, which, under the sub-heading *Allergic and Irritant Dermatitis*, states that,

"There is virtually no occupation or industry without potential exposure to the many diverse agents that can cause allergic and irritant dermatitis."

Despite the claim that different forms of dermatitis exist, the web page makes an even more pertinent comment, which is that,

> "Irritant contact dermatitis is the most common occupational skin disease, usually resulting from toxic reactions to chemical irritants such as solvents and cutting fluids."

The ingredients of solvents and cutting fluids include some extremely toxic chemicals that cannot be referred to as mere 'irritants'.

The connection between eczema and 'industrialisation' is also recognised by the NEA page entitled *Eczema Causes and Triggers* that lists a number of substances referred to as 'common eczema irritants'; these include soaps and household cleaners, amongst others. The connection between these 'irritants' and certain health problems is demonstrated by the example of triclosan, about which Dr Epstein states in *Toxic Beauty* that,

> "In humans this preservative chemical has been linked to allergies, asthma and eczema."

It is clear that different conditions can be 'triggered' by the same toxic chemical, which indicates that they are not different diseases but, instead, are indicative of systemic 'poisoning' that can involve various symptoms in different parts of the body. It should be noted that a wide variety of chemicals are capable of initiating the symptoms associated with these conditions.

Some of the chemicals that can irritate the skin include those used to create 'fragrances' for cosmetics, personal care products and household cleaning products. This has led to the creation of a new 'disease' referred to as 'perfume allergy', which is said to be associated with both skin problems and respiratory problems. When the symptoms affect the skin, the problem is called 'eczema' and when the respiratory system is affected, it is called 'asthma'. As a consequence of their reactions to these chemicals, people are increasingly advised to avoid products that contain 'perfume' and to source 'fragrance-free' products. Although this supports the assertion that 'perfume' chemicals are harmful to health, they are not the only chemicals capable of initiating reactions.

Eczema is claimed to be associated with a reaction of the immune system, but it is not currently regarded as an autoimmune disease; however, new research indicates that this perspective may be changed. A December 2014 Mount Sinai Press Release entitled *Atopic Dermatitis Found To Be an Immune Driven Disease* states,

> "For the first time, a team led by researchers at the Icahn School of Medicine at Mount Sinai has proven that atopic dermatitis, also known as eczema, is an immune-driven (autoimmune) disease at the molecular level."

The research was conducted using a drug treatment that is claimed to target,

> "...specific immune proteins in atopic dermatitis."

There are a number of problems with the claims made as the result of this research, not least of which is the failure of the medical research community to acknowledge that skin problems are known to be caused by contact with toxic chemicals. The failure of the research community to fully investigate the connection between toxic chemicals and health problems has led to the situation revealed by the *Dermal Exposure* report, which states that,

"For most chemicals, however, the relationship between dermal uptake and health effects observed elsewhere in the body is still poorly understood."

A specific relationship does not need to be 'understood' in order for researchers to recognise and acknowledge that toxic chemicals are hazardous to health. The safety testing procedures that are undertaken to determine a 'safe' level of use for a toxic chemical provides clear evidence that these substances are harmful; otherwise they would not need to be reduced to a 'safe' level. The influence of the Paracelsus fallacy is yet again clearly discernible.

In common with virtually all diseases, it is claimed that there is no 'cure' for eczema, but that there are 'treatments', which mainly involve steroid-based moisturising creams that may help to reduce inflammation and relieve dry skin. Although moisturisers may be able to relieve dry skin, any relief will only be temporary as these creams are unable to address the underlying problem. The most common type of steroids used in these creams are corticosteroids, which are synthetic versions of the hormone cortisol. These steroid-based creams are associated with a number of 'side effects', one of which, according to the NHS, is a burning sensation; this would make it extremely uncomfortable, if not painful, when this cream is applied to skin that is already sore.

Antihistamine drugs may also be prescribed in addition to moisturising creams; these drugs and their effects have been discussed. In addition to creams and drugs, people with eczema are advised to avoid substances that 'trigger' their condition, but this advice needs to be extended to include contact with all products that contain toxic substances.

It is clear that relief from eczema requires an understanding of the underlying causes; Dr Bieler provides the necessary clue in his statement that,

"Skin diseases...are really signs of toxic irritation..."

This underlying 'toxic irritation' is a key feature of many of the health problems referred to as 'allergies', including asthma, as the discussion in the next section will demonstrate.

Asthma

The establishment definition of asthma refers to,

"the condition of subjects with widespread narrowing of the bronchial airways, which changes in severity over short periods of time (either spontaneously or under treatment) and leads to cough, wheezing, and difficulty breathing."

In common with many conditions discussed in this chapter, the August 2017 WHO fact sheet entitled *Asthma* states that,

"The fundamental causes of asthma are not completely understood."

This is a significant admission, because the fact sheet also claims that,

"Asthma is one of the major noncommunicable diseases."

The fact sheet estimates that 235 million people worldwide suffer from asthma, but states that this condition is 'under-diagnosed'. As indicated by the statistics cited at the beginning of this chapter, respiratory diseases, which include asthma, are claimed to be the third group of killer diseases worldwide.

Unlike eczema, asthma is not claimed to manifest in a variety of different forms; although the establishment definition refers to 'bronchial asthma', which, it claims,

"...may be precipitated by exposure to one or more of a wide variety of stimuli..."

This description does not seem to indicate that this is a distinctly different form of asthma. It is interesting to note, however, that the 'stimuli' listed in the definition include drugs, such as aspirin and other NSAIDs, as well as beta blockers. This indicates that respiratory problems are not always due to substances that have been inhaled.

The previous discussion indicated that a close connection exists between eczema and asthma; this is recognised by a May 2009 article entitled *Skin-Derived TSLP Triggers Progression from Epidermal-Barrier Defects to Asthma*, which refers to eczema as AD (atopic dermatitis). TSLP stands for thymic stromal lymphopoietin. The article claims that both conditions are 'allergic' and states that,

"Importantly, a large proportion of people suffering from eczema go on to develop asthma later in life."

Equally important is the failure of the medical establishment to understand the true nature of the connection between these conditions; the article states that,

"...the mechanism underlying the progression from AD to asthma...is unclear."

The idea that eczema 'progresses' to asthma is misleading. They are not separate 'conditions'; but the perception that there is a progression is indicative of an underlying health problem that manifests as a skin condition known as 'eczema', which worsens and develops into a respiratory health problem known as 'asthma'. It should be noted that the skin and lungs act as organs of elimination that assist the kidneys and liver.

Previous discussions have referred to the many consumer products that contain 'fragrance chemicals' that can trigger a variety of respiratory problems. Laundry softeners, for example, contain a number of highly toxic and volatile chemical compounds, as explained by Drs Brian and Anna Clement in *Killer Clothes*,

"These chemicals include toxins like chloroform, benzyl acetate, pentane, and compounds that release formaldehyde."

Fabric softeners also contain 'fragrance ingredients', which, in combination with the softening chemicals, will exacerbate the exposure to irritants. The volatile nature of many of these chemicals means that they 'off-gas', which enables them to be inhaled and drawn into the respiratory system where they cause damage and precipitate inflammation, which can cause the narrowing of the airways associated with asthma.

Another of the key contributory factors for respiratory problems, including asthma, is 'air pollution', which, according to the May 2018 WHO fact sheet entitled *Ambient (outdoor) air quality and health*,

"...is a major environmental risk to health."

The WHO *Asthma* fact sheet acknowledges that,

"Urbanization has been associated with an increase in asthma."

But adds the qualifying statement that,

"...the exact nature of this relationship is unclear."

This is a further indication of the refusal of the medical establishment to recognise the detrimental health effects due to widespread environmental pollution, much of which emanates from industry and from the detrimental living conditions in some urban areas. Although 'outdoor air' is polluted by factors such as vehicle exhaust and industrial emissions, amongst others, 'indoor air' can also be polluted by a variety of factors. The EPA website provides information on various pages under the general heading *Indoor Air Quality*, one of which is entitled *Volatile Organic Compounds' Impact on Indoor Air Quality* and refers to a number of organic chemicals that are widely used in household products. The page states that,

"Paints, varnishes and wax all contain organic solvents, as do many cleaning, disinfecting, cosmetic, degreasing and hobby products."

The toxic nature of solvents has been discussed, but it is pertinent to reiterate that they include some highly toxic chemicals, which include benzene, perchloroethylene and methylene chloride. Many of these substances are also volatile; they can therefore be inhaled and cause damage to the respiratory system. Methanol is another chemical of concern for asthmatics, mainly because it always metabolises into formaldehyde, which, according to the EPA page is,

"...one of the best known VOCs..."

Formaldehyde is categorised as a group 1 carcinogen, but it is also known to produce other adverse health effects, some of which involve the respiratory system, as the authors of *Killer Clothes* explain,

"Even at fairly low concentrations, formaldehyde can produce rapid onset of nose and throat irritation..."

If the exposure is of a short duration, the irritation, which may present symptoms similar to those of 'hay fever' or other 'allergies', may also be of a similarly short duration. Exposures of a longer duration will inevitably induce symptoms of a much more severe nature, as they further explain,

"At higher levels of exposure, it can cause significant inflammation of the lower respiratory tract, which may result in swelling of the throat..."

These symptoms bear a close resemblance to those included in the definition of asthma and they clearly implicate toxic volatile chemicals, such as formaldehyde, as some of the causes of respiratory problems and asthma. It should be noted that swelling of the throat is also a typical symptom associated with anaphylaxis; which therefore implicates exposure to toxic chemicals as the major, if not the sole, cause of this severe reaction.

The group of respiratory diseases claimed to be responsible for the third largest number of deaths includes chronic obstructive pulmonary disease, which is said to be more serious and the cause of more deaths than asthma. Interestingly, the December 2017 WHO fact sheet entitled *Chronic obstructive pulmonary disease (COPD)* claims that,

"Some cases of COPD are due to long-term asthma."

It is clear from this statement that the WHO considers these respiratory problems to be related, especially as COPD is claimed to involve a reduction of airflow. The fact sheet also claims that both indoor and outdoor pollution are major factors for COPD, although it is claimed that smoking is the main contributory factor.

COPD and asthma are both considered to be incurable but 'manageable' with treatment; the fact sheet about asthma claims that,

"...failure to use appropriate medications or to adhere to treatment can lead to death."

A further similarity between asthma and eczema is that 'treatment' involves anti-inflammatory drugs, although people who suffer from asthma are also advised to avoid the offending substances that 'trigger' an asthma attack. One drug used in the treatment of asthma is a synthetic glucocorticoid, which is described as a 'derivative of cortisol', a natural hormone. But, as previously discussed, synthetic hormone derivatives are not the same as the natural hormones produced by the body. Another asthma treatment involves drugs that are administered through an inhaler; as the fact sheet states,

"Medications such as inhaled corticosteroids are needed to control the progression of severe asthma and reduce asthma exacerbation and deaths."

In common with all pharmaceuticals, these drugs are associated with many 'side effects', which can include: tremors, headache, muscle cramps and palpitations. However, the UK NHS website comments on these symptoms and states that,

"These side effects aren't dangerous and should pass within a few minutes."

Whilst the side effects may not be dangerous, they are a clear indication that the substance referred to as 'medicine' is harmful. These 'reactions' also indicate that the body has reacted appropriately to a substance that it has correctly recognised as toxic.

Although the symptoms of asthma mainly occur within the respiratory system, this should not be interpreted to mean that the underlying problem resides solely within that system; as indicated by Herbert Shelton, who states that,

"When there is irritation of the nose, throat, sinuses, and elsewhere, this represents a systemic condition..."

This reference to a systemic condition demonstrates that other health problems will also be present in other organs and systems of the body; this explains the concurrence of eczema, asthma and other 'allergies'. Dr Bieler indicates some of the other organs associated with health problems in the respiratory system in *Food is Your Best Medicine*, in which he refers to asthma as a catarrhal bronchitis. He also discusses the presence of an underlying toxic build-up that initiates an inflammatory response. In most instances, the underlying toxicity affects the endocrine system and the adrenal glands in particular; as he states,

"The adrenal activity in asthma patients is much below normal..."

Furthermore, Dr Bieler counters the establishment claim that asthma is incurable with the statement that,

"...I have found that a rational and often successful treatment depends first upon detoxicating the patient."

The success of his detoxification treatments is a demonstration that asthma is due to an underlying toxicity. Although this undermines the medical establishment claim that asthma is not 'curable', it must be noted that detoxification is only one of the factors that will contribute to improved health; as the discussions in chapter ten will demonstrate.

Arthritis

The general condition known as 'arthritis' is defined by the establishment as,

"inflammation of one or more joints characterized by pain, swelling, warmth, redness of the overlying skin, and diminished range of joint motion."

It is claimed that there are many conditions that affect the joints, spine and limbs; as indicated by the WHO web page entitled *Chronic rheumatic conditions*, which states that,

"Rheumatic or musculoskeletal conditions comprise over 150 diseases and syndromes, which are usually progressive and associated with pain."

There are, however, two forms of arthritis that are claimed to be the most common and to have the greatest impact on morbidity and disability; these conditions are osteoarthritis and rheumatoid arthritis (RA).

The establishment definition of osteoarthritis describes it as,

"a degenerative disease of joints resulting from wear of the articular cartilage..."

The WHO page claims that osteoarthritis is associated with ageing and that it,

"...will most likely affect the joints that have been continually stressed throughout the years..."

Although osteoarthritis is claimed to mainly affect older people, it is not an inevitable consequence of ageing; there are many people of an advanced age who do not suffer from this condition. The reference to long-term 'stress' on joints indicates one of the relevant factors that contribute to the occurrence of this condition in people who are not 'old'. It is reliably reported that many former athletes and dancers are affected by this condition; however, even then it is not inevitable; the role of 'physical activity' and its relationship to health is discussed in further detail in chapter ten.

In common with many NCDs, the incidence of osteoarthritis is reported to have increased to the extent that, according to the WHO,

"Osteoarthritis is already one of the ten most disabling diseases in developed countries."

The other major type of arthritis is called rheumatoid arthritis, which is defined by the establishment as,

"...a disease of the synovial lining of the joints..."

Unlike osteoarthritis, rheumatoid arthritis is considered to be an autoimmune disease, as indicated by the CDC web page entitled *Rheumatoid arthritis* that describes it as,

"...an autoimmune and inflammatory disease, which means that your immune system attacks healthy cells in your body by mistake, causing inflammation (painful swelling) in the affected parts of the body."

The idea that the body makes a 'mistake' and attacks its own healthy cells and tissues has been discussed and shown to be unfounded. However, despite the CDC's assertion that this is the case, the web page also makes the familiar admission that,

"The specific causes of RA are unknown..."

The lack of knowledge about 'specific causes' is not limited to RA; the CDC web pages entitled *Arthritis Basics* include one labelled *FAQs*, which, in response to the question about the causes of arthritis, makes the astounding admission that,

"Experts don't know the cause of many forms of arthritis."

Despite this lack of knowledge, the CDC web pages about rheumatoid arthritis claim that there are many 'risk factors' that trigger this condition. Some of these factors are referred to as 'non-modifiable', a list of which includes 'genetic' factors. The second group of risk factors are referred to as 'modifiable' and this list includes 'infections', about which the CDC web page entitled *Risk Factors* states,

"Many microbial agents, like bacteria and viruses, can infect joints and potentially cause the development of some types of arthritis."

This hypothesis has not, however, been proven, even by the medical establishment; as demonstrated by the NHS web page entitled *Rheumatoid arthritis*, which refers to theories that suggest infections or viruses may precipitate RA but admits that,

"... none of these theories have been proven."

The idea that arthritis mainly affects older adults is further refuted by the fact that it can also affect young people and even children. Although this condition is referred to generically as 'juvenile arthritis', the Arthritis Foundation web page entitled *Juvenile Arthritis* states that,

"Juvenile arthritis (JA) is not a disease in itself."

According to the page,

"JA is an umbrella term used to describe the many autoimmune and inflammatory conditions or pediatric rheumatic diseases that can develop in children under the age of 16."

The most common form of JA is called 'juvenile idiopathic arthritis'; which means that the cause is unknown. The web page also makes the increasingly familiar statement that,

"No known cause has been pinpointed for most forms of juvenile arthritis..."

However, this sentence continues with the claim that,

"...nor is there evidence to suggest that toxins, foods or allergies cause children to develop JA."

This statement is disingenuous; the failure of the scientific community to fully investigate and test the effects of chemicals, including food additives, means that the absence of evidence does not mean that these factors are not relevant to the onset of health problems, including inflammatory conditions diagnosed as arthritis.

It is clear that many features of the conditions referred to under the umbrella term 'arthritis' remain unknown to the medical establishment; nevertheless, despite this paucity of knowledge, it is claimed that they are incurable and therefore lifelong. The consequence is that, as with all other NCDs, the medical establishment only provides 'treatments', most of which invariably involve pharmaceutical drugs. The Arthritis Foundation web page entitled *Drug Types* refers to five main types of drugs, which are: analgesics; biologics; corticosteroids; DMARDs (disease-modifying antirheumatic drugs) and NSAIDs (non-steroidal anti-inflammatory drugs). Analgesics are pain relievers such as paracetamol (acetaminophen); these over-the-counter drugs have been discussed. Other forms of analgesics are 'opioids', which are prescription-only drugs as they are more potent; opioids are not only associated with various 'side effects', they have been shown to be addictive.

Biologics are described on the web page as,

> "...medications genetically engineered from a living organism, such as a virus, gene or protein, to stimulate the body's natural response to infection and disease."

It should be noted that viruses, genes and proteins are not 'living organisms'. The appropriateness of genetic engineering techniques for the production of 'medicines' is highly questionable; especially in view of the lack of certainty and predictability of these techniques, as demonstrated by the discussion about GE foods in chapter six.

DMARDs and NSAIDs are anti-inflammatory drugs; the latter are also pain-relievers. One type of DMARD is methotrexate, which is commonly used to treat adult rheumatoid arthritis and JIA, both of which are considered to be autoimmune conditions. As previously discussed, methotrexate is associated with unpleasant 'side effects'; the web page entitled *DMARDs: Side Effects and Solutions* states that,

> "The most common side effect with DMARDs is stomach upset, especially with methotrexate."

Other 'side effects' referred to on this page include hair loss, fatigue and liver damage; the last of which provides the clearest demonstration of the toxicity of these drugs.

NSAIDs are claimed to suppress inflammation by blocking prostaglandins that in turn inhibit two enzymes known as cyclooxygenase (COX); these are referred to as COX-1 and COX-2. NSAIDs are also associated with adverse 'side effects', including headaches, nausea and dizziness. However, some have also been linked to far more serious effects. One type of COX-2 inhibitor drug, called Vioxx, was discovered to produce an increased risk of heart attacks and strokes, after which it was withdrawn from the market.

The occurrence of pain and inflammation in an 'older person' may lead to a diagnosis of 'arthritis'; however, many people over the age of 60 or even

50 may take a number of 'medicines' as preventives for raised blood pressure or cholesterol, for example. It is highly unlikely that these people will be aware of the possibility that their current 'medications' are the cause of their new symptoms. Dr Carolyn Dean refers to this problem in *Death by Modern Medicine* and states that,

> "Many people who take statins don't know that their new aches and pains and arthritic symptoms are due to statins."

The medical establishment claims that arthritis is not only incurable, but it cannot be prevented; as indicated by the web page entitled *How to Prevent Arthritis* that states,

> "Right now, because scientists don't fully understand the causes or mechanisms behind these diseases, true prevention seems to be impossible."

Although scientists within the mainstream medical research community do not fully understand this condition, there are physicians who have investigated the problem and have established that toxicity is a major factor. One of these knowledgeable physicians is Dr Henry Bieler, who refers to arthritis as the result of toxic overload and calls it a,

> "...vicarious elimination through the middle skin."

The 'middle skin' refers to the middle layer of the skin.

Contrary to the claim made by the Arthritis Foundation, Dr Bieler considers that both toxins and a poor diet are relevant factors for the onset of pain and inflammation that may be diagnosed as one of the many forms of arthritis.

There are many factors that could generate inflammation around the joints; the previous discussions have indicated that damage to the tissues initiates inflammation, which is a 'remedial action', the purpose of which is explained by Herbert Shelton who states,

> "Inflammation is simply a great increase in the amount of blood in a circumscribed area of the body."

He also explains that the increase in the blood supply will produce certain symptoms,

> "The pain, the redness, the swelling, the heat and the impairment of function are all due to the local excess of blood."

These symptoms bear a close resemblance to those referred to in the definition of 'arthritis'. Inflammation is, as discussed, only problematic if the underlying 'toxaemia' is not addressed; but these health problems cannot be solved by pharmaceutical drugs, which contain synthetic chemicals that are toxic to the human body and therefore increase the body burden of 'poisons'.

Endocrine Diseases and Disorders

The establishment definition refers to an endocrine gland as 'ductless' and defines it as,

> "a gland that manufactures one or more hormones and secretes them directly into the bloodstream..."

The page entitled *Overview* on the website of The Endocrine Disruption Exchange (TEDX) describes the endocrine system in more detail,

"The endocrine system is the body's exquisitely balanced system of glands, organs, and hormones that regulates such vital functions as body growth, response to stress, sexual development, production of insulin and utilization of glucose, metabolism, neurodevelopment, intelligence, behaviour, sleep patterns, blood pressure, and the ability to reproduce."

Hormones are 'biochemical messengers', each type of which produces specific 'messages' that are relevant to specific organs, as Dr Hans Selye explains in *The Stress of Life*,

"...each hormone carries instructions in a code which only certain organs can read."

The field of endocrinology is reported to have begun during the 19th century when anatomical investigations first revealed the existence of ductless glands, which were discovered to secrete 'messenger chemicals'. However, it was not until the early 20th century that the first of these chemicals was isolated by Dr E H Starling, who is credited not only with the discovery of secretin, but also with the creation of the term 'hormone' to refer to these chemicals.

Further research in the field of endocrinology revealed that certain health problems were related to an 'incorrect' level of hormones, whether too high or too low. These health problems have been labelled 'endocrine disorders', as indicated by the NIDDK (National Institute of Diabetes and Digestive and Kidney Diseases) web page entitled *Endocrine Diseases* that states,

"If your hormone levels are too high or too low, you may have an endocrine disease or disorder."

There are many different conditions referred to as endocrine diseases or disorders that are said to result from an under- or over-production of a particular hormone. The conditions of this nature listed on the NIDDK page include acromegaly, Cushing's syndrome, Graves' Disease, Cystic Fibrosis and Addison's Disease.

In common with all other health problems, the medical establishment considers that pharmaceuticals are the only method by which 'endocrine diseases' should be addressed. They therefore employ pharmaceutical drugs that are claimed to be able to correct a hormone imbalance by delivering extra hormones if the level is too low, or by inhibiting their production if the level is too high. There are, however, many problems with this approach, not least of which is that pharmaceutical hormones have been shown to differ from hormones naturally produced by the body, despite the assertion that they have the same chemical structure.

Cortisol is a hormone produced by the adrenal glands when the body is under stress; high levels of stress generate high levels of cortisol, but these levels return to normal when the body ceases to be under stress; the topic of stress is discussed in more detail in chapter ten. Cushing's syndrome, which is said to be caused by an excess level of cortisol is, however, reported to mainly result from the long-term use of pharmaceutical corticosteroids, as recognised by the NIDDK page about this condition that states,

"Many people develop Cushing's syndrome because they take glucocorticoids – steroid hormones that are chemically similar to naturally produced cortisol – such as prednisone for asthma, rheumatoid arthritis, lupus and other inflammatory diseases.”

The cortisol in pharmaceutical drugs may be 'chemically similar' but it is not identical to the natural cortisol produced by the adrenal glands.

The level of each hormone naturally fluctuates according to the body's requirements; this is demonstrated by the 'exquisite balance' of the endocrine system that carefully regulates and controls the production and release of hormones.

Pharmaceuticals, by contrast, do not participate in the regulation of all hormones; instead they interfere with and disrupt the endocrine system, which, as the TEDX page states, regulates many of the body's vital functions. In addition, pharmaceutical drugs always contain other ingredients, preservatives for example, none of which are 'natural' components of the human body; which means that they interfere with normal functioning, rather than assist it. As has been discussed, all pharmaceutical-based treatments are acknowledged to be associated with 'side effects'; synthetic hormone treatments are clearly no exception. The 'side effects' of hydrocortisone, a corticosteroid drug, include nausea, headaches and dizziness.

There are many aspects of the endocrine system that are poorly understood by the medical establishment, as indicated by the widespread use of steroid-based treatments for conditions that involve inflammation. One particular characteristic of the endocrine system that is inadequately recognised is that hormones exist in the body in extremely tiny concentrations. Dr Theo Colborn describes this characteristic with reference to the womb environment in her essay entitled *Peace* that states,

> "The endocrine system is so fine-tuned that it depends upon hormones in concentrations as little as a tenth of a trillionth of a gram to control the womb environment, as inconspicuous as one second in 3,169 centuries.”

The existence of hormones in incredibly minute concentrations is not restricted to the womb environment. It is clear, therefore, that any influence that disrupts the 'exquisite balance' of the endocrine system can have serious consequences. Furthermore, hormones do not function in isolation, many of them rely on the production and release of other hormones in the body. Yet, pharmaceutical drugs are intended to only deliver or affect a single hormone, which means that they further disrupt the endocrine system, its balance, and the functions it regulates.

In common with many other chronic health problems, endocrine disorders are increasing in incidence. Unfortunately, the medical establishment possesses a poor level of knowledge about the diseases associated with the endocrine system. The discussion about diabetes demonstrated that, despite the fact that insulin was one of the first hormones to be discovered, this condition remains poorly understood, as indicated by a 2002 article entitled *The endocrine system in diabetes mellitus* that states,

> "The pathophysiology of diabetes mellitus is complex and not fully understood.”

Pathophysiology refers to the functional changes that occur during disease.

Another problematic hormone treatment is HRT (hormone replacement therapy), which is claimed to relieve the symptoms experienced during the 'menopause'; as explained by Dr Carolyn Dean in *Death by Modern Medicine*,

"Labeling menopause a disease due to estrogen deficiency, doctors attempted to 'cure' the condition by introducing estrogen replacement."

Inevitably, as with all pharmaceuticals, HRT is associated with 'side effects', which, according to the NHS web page entitled *Hormone replacement therapy (HRT)*, include nausea, leg cramps, bloating, headaches and indigestion, amongst others. It is clear that the use of HRT merely exchanges one set of symptoms for another. Dr Dean also discusses the Women's Health Initiative study that was intended to demonstrate the efficacy of one type of HRT drug; but, as she explains,

"...the study found an increased incidence of heart attack, stroke and breast cancer in women."

She also reports that the study revealed an increased risk of dementia associated with the use of this particular HRT drug.

Another clear but poignant example of the effects of disruption to the endocrine system is the pharmaceutical drug thalidomide, which was the cause of a variety of birth defects in approximately 8,000 children in 46 different countries. One of the countries in which birth defects did not occur was the US because Dr Frances Kelsey PhD MD, the FDA officer responsible for approving thalidomide, had had reservations about the drug and had decided to withhold FDA approval pending further studies. The reports from other countries about the devastating effects caused by this drug vindicated her decision. Thalidomide was originally prescribed as a general treatment for nausea, but was subsequently extended to treat pregnant women who suffered from morning sickness. In their book *Our Stolen Future*, authors Dr Theo Colborn, Dianne Dumanoski and Dr John P Myers PhD discuss the different abnormalities experienced by babies born to mothers who had taken thalidomide during their pregnancy,

"Some babies were born with hands sprouting directly from their shoulders and no arms at all. Others lacked legs or were no more than a totally limbless trunk."

It is particularly significant that, in addition to the variations in the type of limb deformities that occurred, there were many cases in which different organs had been affected; some babies suffered defects in their heart or other organs. It is also significant that some babies remained unaffected. It is explained in *Our Stolen Future* that these differences bore no relation to the 'dose' of thalidomide that the mothers had taken; the effects were shown to be closely related to the stage of foetal development when the drug was taken. Even a single dose of this drug at a particularly crucial stage in foetal development had been shown to have a major effect on the growth of a limb or organ.

A similar tragedy with less conspicuous, but equally devastating consequences, involved the drug called DES (diethylstilbestrol), which, in this case, had been approved for use in the US. It was believed that DES had an 'oestrogenic' effect, which was claimed to be beneficial for certain problems associated with pregnancy. In *Our Stolen Future* it is explained that DES was prescribed,

> "...to women experiencing problems during pregnancy in the belief that insufficient estrogen levels caused miscarriages and premature births."

Prescriptions for DES were not restricted to pregnant women; as the book also explains,

> "Doctors used it liberally to suppress milk production after birth, to alleviate hot flashes and other menopausal symptoms, and to treat acne, prostate cancer, gonorrhoea in children..."

Like thalidomide, the consequences of DES taken by the mother during pregnancy were visited on both male and female babies; but, unlike thalidomide, the consequences of DES were not discovered at birth. The adverse effects, which often manifested within the reproductive system, were frequently revealed when the affected babies had become adults and wanted to have a family of their own; the effects of DES had sadly made this impossible. It was also discovered that there was an increased incidence of cancer in the children of mothers who had taken DES; although these cancers would also appear later in life. It became clear that, as with thalidomide, it had been the timing rather than the dose of DES that had been the most significant factor.

It should be noted that, despite the adverse health effects with which they are associated, both thalidomide and DES remain in use as treatments for certain cancers; DES, for example, is used as a treatment for prostate cancer.

The examples cited above, although well-known, are not the only pharmaceutical drugs that have been demonstrated to cause serious adverse effects in the endocrine system. Furthermore, pharmaceutical drugs are by no means the only substances that can produce such adverse effects, many chemicals have also been found to affect the endocrine system; these are known as 'endocrine disrupting chemicals', or EDCs.

As has been asserted throughout this book, the vast majority of chemicals have not been tested to determine the full extent of their effects on the human body; however, until relatively recently, none of them had been tested to determine their effects on the endocrine system.

Observations of certain problems within wildlife populations, especially dwindling bird population numbers, were famously brought to the attention of the public by the publication in 1962 of *Silent Spring*. which eventually led to the withdrawal of DDT from use in many, but not all, countries. Although regarded as a 'victory', it was an extremely limited one; DDT was by no means the only toxic chemical in widespread use. Furthermore, the DDT ban was not accompanied by efforts to test the safety of all chemicals in use; nor was it accompanied by the introduction of procedures to test the effects of chemicals on the endocrine system.

Prior to the publication of *Silent Spring*, there was some awareness that chemicals could produce adverse effects on the endocrine system, but this had clearly failed to influence chemical testing procedures. Some progress in expanding the awareness of the problem was made in July 1991, when a meeting of scientists from a variety of fields, including biology, toxicology and endocrinology, was held in a place called Wingspread in the US. One of the participants was Dr Theo Colborn, who subsequently dedicated herself to studying endocrine disrupting chemicals, and exposing the dangers they pose to a wide audience of policy makers and government officials as well as the public. These efforts included the creation in 2003 of the TEDX website, which contains a wealth of information about the adverse effects of EDCs, including scientific research papers on the topic. After Dr Colborn's death in December 2014, the website continued to be updated by TEDX scientists; but these updates ceased in November 2019.

The documents available on the TEDX website include a paper about the Wingspread meeting that declares one of the purposes of this meeting to have been,

> "...to establish a research agenda that would clarify uncertainties remaining in the field."

The paper, which is a statement from one of the work sessions at the Wingspread meeting, is entitled *Chemically-induced alterations in sexual development: The wildlife/human connection*; it expresses the problem under investigation in the following terms,

> "Many compounds introduced into the environment by human activity are capable of disrupting the endocrine system of animals, including fish, wildlife and humans."

The endocrine system has been demonstrated to exhibit similarities across a wide range of animal species, if not all of them. It is for this reason that all endocrine disrupting effects demonstrated by animal research studies are directly relevant to human health. This does not mean that animal experimentation is justifiable; it does, however, demonstrate that EDCs can adversely affect all living organisms in a very similar way.

The participants of the Wingspread session stated in the paper that they had reached a consensus on certain issues, one of which was that the chemicals implicated in the disruption of the endocrine system included,

> "...the persistent, bioaccumulative, organohalogen compounds that include some pesticides (fungicides, herbicides, and insecticides) and industrial chemicals, other synthetic products, and some metals."

The footnote to this paragraph refers to many substances that were known at that time to be endocrine disruptors; those listed in the footnote include: DDT; TCDD and other dioxins; lead; mercury; synthetic pyrethroids; TCDF and other furans.

The fields of toxicology and chemistry both adhere to the notion that it is the dose that makes a substance a poison and that there is therefore a 'safe' dose of all substances, no matter how toxic. It should be clear that the tiny concentrations in which hormones circulate throughout the body means that nowhere is it more imperative that this dangerous myth be destroyed than in the context of the endocrine system, which regulates so many vital functions, including the ability to reproduce.

Dr Colborn and her colleagues expose the 'dose' myth in a 2012 paper entitled *Hormones and Endocrine-Disrupting Chemicals: Low-Dose*

Effects and Nonmonotonic Dose Responses, which states that,

> "For decades, studies of endocrine-disrupting chemicals (EDCs) have challenged traditional concepts in toxicology, in particular the dogma of 'the dose makes the poison', because EDCs can have effects at low doses that are not predicted by effects at higher doses."

The mainstream scientific approach to testing the effects of chemicals has followed the idea that increased doses produced increased effects; this linear association is referred to as the 'monotonic dose-response' relationship. However, many chemicals display a non-linear, 'non-monotonic dose-response' relationship; which means that doses at levels lower than those deemed to be 'safe' under traditional toxicology, can produce far greater effects, especially within the endocrine system, as indicated by the 2012 paper cited above.

One of the greatest consequences from adherence to the 'dose' myth has been the devastating effects of EDCs on the developing baby, the most vulnerable member of the human population. This problem is eloquently expressed by Dr Colborn in her 2000 *Peace* article that states,

> "In our ignorance we assumed that the womb was inviolable while at the same time we produced more and more synthetic chemicals to improve the quality of our lives."

The resources available on the TEDX website include video presentations, one of which is entitled *Endocrine Disrupting Chemicals: Science, Policy, and What You Can Do*. This video is presented by Dr Carol Kwiatkowski PhD, Executive Director of TEDX, who explains that one of the main problems associated with EDCs is that,

> "There are hundreds of thousands of chemicals in existence, most of which have never been tested for endocrine disruption."

The failure to incorporate procedures to test the effects of chemicals on the endocrine system has resulted in their continued production and use in many common household products; the consequences of this are explained on the *Overview* page on the TEDX website, that states,

> "Endocrine disruptors have been found in every person tested, across world populations."

The TEDX team had compiled a list of the EDCs that had been identified by September 2018; this list is available on the web page entitled *TEDX List of Potential Endocrine Disruptors*. Another web page, entitled *About the TEDX List*, states that this list,

> "...identifies chemicals that have shown evidence of endocrine disruption in scientific research."

The first list, compiled in 2011, contained 881 chemicals; by September 2018 the number had increased to 1,484.

This is clearly a very small fraction of the hundreds of thousands of chemicals in existence; however, it would be a mistake to assume that these are the only chemicals capable of causing endocrine disruption. These 1,484 substances are the only chemicals that have so far been tested and proven to disrupt the endocrine system; as Dr Kwiatkowski has stated, most chemicals are untested for their endocrine effects. The chemicals that have been discovered to affect the endocrine system are associated with many adverse health effects, as explained on the TEDX *Overview* page,

> "Endocrine disrupting chemicals have been implicated in numerous adverse health outcomes, including those of the endocrine, reproductive, neurological and metabolic systems."

These adverse health outcomes are clearly related to the many 'endocrine diseases and disorders' described by the NIDDK, NHS and other mainstream health organisations. However, in her TEDX video, Dr Kwiatkowski refers to the increased incidence of other health problems that are not endocrine diseases as such, but are linked to a poorly functioning endocrine system. The health problems referred to include autoimmune disorders, autism, asthma, diabetes, thyroid disorders, ADHD and some forms of cancer. In addition, Dr Kwiatkowski makes the extremely important comment that,

> "Genetic inheritance cannot explain the relatively recent and dramatic increases in many disorders which have been shown to be endocrine related."

The salient point is that the rise in endocrine-related health problems corresponds closely with the 20th century expansion of 'industrialisation', and the accompanying increased production and use of synthetic chemicals, predominantly those based on petrochemicals derived from coal, natural gas and oil; this supports the description by Dr Theron Randolph of modern chronic health conditions as 'the petroleum problem'.

The TEDX page entitled *Oil & Gas Program* refers to oil and gas as 'fossil fuels', a mistaken label for reasons that are discussed in chapter nine. Nevertheless, it is recognised by TEDX that many of the chemicals involved in oil and gas extraction, especially hydraulic fracturing operations, are endocrine disruptors. The discussion in chapter six about fracking indicates the highly toxic nature of many of the chemicals discovered by Dr Colborn and her team to have been used in those operations.

The endocrine system can also be disrupted by harmful influences other than toxic chemicals; these influences include electromagnetic radiation. The discussion about EHS referred to evidence that EMFs can disrupt the production of melatonin, a hormone produced by the pineal gland, which is an organ of the endocrine system. The effects of EMFs on melatonin production are discussed by Dr Robert Becker in *The Body Electric*, in which he refers to a 1980 rat study that,

> "...found that a weak 60-hertz electric field (only 3.9 volts per centimetre) cancelled the normal nightly rise in production of the pineal gland hormone melatonin, the main hormone mediatory of biocycles."

The similarities in the endocrine systems of all animals means that this study result is directly applicable to humans. Dr Becker also refers in his book to the findings of Russian studies conducted in the 1970s which showed that,

> "...radio and microwave frequencies, at power densities well below the American safety guideline of 10,000 microwatts, stimulate the thyroid gland and thus increase the basal metabolic rate."

It was previously demonstrated that an increased metabolic rate is associated with an increased generation of free radicals and oxidative stress, which is associated with an increasing variety of health problems.

It is clear that all disrupting influences, whether chemical or electromagnetic in nature, are able to override the ability of the endocrine system to retain control over all of the body's vital functions it regulates. These disrupting influences inevitably interfere with the body's ability to restore and maintain homeostasis, which is discussed in more detail in chapter ten.

Although some effects of endocrine disruption can be alleviated and even reversed, others cannot be. The examples of DES and thalidomide indicate the extent of the damaging effects that can occur during pregnancy, especially from exposures at a critical stage of development, and can result in permanent 'birth defects', as discussed in the next section.

Birth Defects

The 2007 Oxford Concise Medical Dictionary does not define 'birth defect', but it does define the term 'congenital', which is described as a condition that exists at birth; the definition also refers to 'congenital malformations', about which it states,

> "Congenital malformations include all disorders present at birth whether they are inherited or caused by an environmental factor."

The September 2016 WHO fact sheet entitled *Congenital anomalies*, states that,

> "Congenital anomalies are also known as birth defects, congenital disorders or congenital malformations."

This statement indicates that these terms are used interchangeably, the establishment definition of a 'congenital malformation' therefore applies to all of them.

Birth defects are clearly a distressing topic, but they need to be discussed because there are reasons that they occur, although these reasons are poorly acknowledged by the medical establishment. The fact sheet claims that,

> "Although approximately 50% of all congenital anomalies cannot be linked to a specific cause, there are some known genetic, environmental and other causes or risk factors."

It is claimed that the other causes and risk factors include certain maternal 'infections' such as rubella and syphilis. Infection with the 'Zika' virus has also been implicated in causing a certain type of birth defect called 'microcephaly'; this will be discussed in more detail later in this section. It should be clear however, that no 'infection' can cause a birth defect.

It is disturbing that congenital anomalies are a significant and increasing cause of infant deaths within the first month of life; a stage referred to as 'neonatal'. According to the April 2015 version of the WHO *Congenital anomalies* fact sheet, the estimated worldwide number of neonatal deaths each year due to birth defects was 276,000; the revised fact sheet updated in September 2016, however, states that,

> "An estimated 303,000 newborns die within 4 weeks of birth every year, worldwide, due to congenital anomalies."

Also disturbing is that the CDC web page entitled *Facts about Birth Defects* refers to birth defects as 'common' and usually caused by a mix of factors, but that,

> "...we don't fully understand how these factors might work together to cause birth defects."

The WHO fact sheet refers to the role of genetic factors and indicates that they represent a significant contribution to birth defects in the claim that,

> "Genes play an important role in many congenital anomalies."

This claim is misleading; birth defects have occurred in the absence of a family history of such events; however, the significant increase in the incidence of birth defects in recent years refutes the idea that genetic factors play any role. This refutation is corroborated by Dr Kwiatkowski, whose comment in the TEDX video referred to in the previous discussion deserves repetition,

> "Genetic inheritance cannot explain the relatively recent and dramatic increases in many disorders which have been shown to be endocrine related."

Reproduction, growth and development are all regulated by the endocrine system; birth defects are therefore undeniably 'endocrine-related' conditions.

Despite the misleading claim about the role of genes, the fact sheet also refers to environmental factors as relevant 'risk factors' for congenital anomalies,

> "Maternal exposure to certain pesticides and other chemicals, as well as certain medications, alcohol, tobacco and radiation during pregnancy, may increase the risk of having a fetus or neonate affected by congenital anomalies."

The reference to 'certain' substances would seem to suggest that it is only a relatively small number of pesticides, chemicals and medications that have a recognised association with birth defects. Whilst this may be factually correct, it is a misleading statement, because the full range of adverse effects on the endocrine system of the majority of chemicals remains untested and therefore unknown.

The previous discussion referred to some of the 'medications' that have given rise to birth defects, and to the many different organs and systems in the developing baby that can be affected by toxic pharmaceuticals taken by the mother when pregnant. It was also shown that it is the timing of the maternal exposure to an endocrine-disrupting 'medication' that is the main influence over the extent and nature of the effects produced on the developing baby.

In addition to pharmaceuticals, there are many chemicals that have been identified as having the ability to disrupt the endocrine system; which means that maternal exposure to these EDCs can cause significant harm to the developing baby, as indicated by Dr Colborn in her *Peace* essay,

> "Unfortunately, when development is violated in the womb by man-made chemicals, the newborn is compromised."

These chemicals are, however, truly ubiquitous, as Dr Colborn states,

> "No child born today is free of man-made chemicals."

All substances that are capable of adversely affecting the development of a foetus are called teratogens, the establishment definition of which is,

"any substance, agent, or process that induces the formation of developmental abnormalities in a fetus."

The failure of safety testing procedures to investigate the effects of all chemicals, including pharmaceuticals, on the endocrine system means that only a small percentage of substances have been recognised to be teratogenic. This is particularly significant in respect of drugs used for the treatment of certain conditions, even during pregnancy, as revealed by a 2010 article entitled *Teratogenic mechanisms of medical drugs* which, under the heading *Background*, states,

"Although prescription drug use is common during pregnancy, the human teratogenic risks are undetermined for more than 90% of drug treatments approved in the USA during the past decades."

The reason that the teratogenic effects of most drugs is 'undetermined' is because it is regarded as unethical to conduct drug trials on pregnant women. Yet drugs that have not been tested for human teratogenicity are nevertheless prescribed for use by pregnant women, who are therefore unwitting test subjects. The similarity of the endocrine systems of all animals means that teratogenic effects observed during animal research studies should be recognised as a clear demonstration that the drug, or chemical, will be a definite human teratogen.

Certain conditions, epilepsy for example, are claimed to require the continuation of 'medication', even during pregnancy, in order to manage the symptoms. Other 'diseases' are also claimed to require the continuation of 'medication' in order to prevent the disease being transmitted to the developing baby. Most conditions of this type are 'infectious diseases', such as 'AIDS', which has been discussed. It should be noted, however, that AZT, one of the main drug treatments for 'HIV/AIDS', was originally formulated as a cancer drug, and that virtually all cancer drugs and treatments are teratogenic.

In addition to pharmaceutical drugs, many chemicals have been proven to be teratogenic; the family of phthalates, for example, which are used as coatings on certain drugs as well as in a wide variety of common consumer products. The ubiquitous nature of phthalates has been discussed; their teratogenicity adds another serious concern about their inclusion in a wide variety of products that may be used by pregnant women. Chemicals that have been shown to be teratogenic include pesticides and other agricultural chemicals. A 2009 article entitled *Agrichemicals in surface water and birth defects in the United States* refers to a study that investigated an association between agrichemicals and birth defects. The article reports that a 'significant association' was found by the study and states that this finding is not an isolated occurrence,

"There is a growing body of evidence that agrichemical exposures may contribute to birth defects."

One of the many chemical compounds found to be teratogenic is TCDD, a member of the family of dioxins, which, as discussed, result from the processing of organochlorines. The manufacture of Agent Orange, the organochlorine-based defoliant used in the Vietnam war, caused the final product to be 'contaminated' with TCDD; it was not an intended ingredient. However, the 'contamination' of Agent Orange by TCDD is claimed to have occurred only in 'trace amounts'; the concentration is said to occur in parts per billion, which is not considered to be a significant level. As Dr Colborn has stated, hormones circulate in far tinier concentrations; often in only parts per trillion, which makes the 'trace amounts' of TCDD, or any other teratogen, at parts per billion, a matter of significance and of serious concern.

Organophosphate-based chemicals, such as cholinesterase-inhibiting pesticides, are also teratogenic. The discussion about Gulf War Syndrome indicated that exposures to the combination of organophosphate pesticides and other toxic chemicals had seriously affected military personnel. In addition to the effects suffered by the men and women who served in the military, there has been an increased incidence of birth defects in children conceived after their return from military conflicts in the Gulf and elsewhere. Exposure to organophosphate pesticides has been associated with an increase in a particular type of birth defect, called neural tube defects, which are discussed in the section about spina bifida.

Glyphosate, the pesticide commonly used with GM crops, has also been linked to birth defects. The section about GE foods in chapter six referred to the Argentinian study conducted by Professor Carrasco that was reported by William Engdahl in his October 2010 article entitled *Study Shows Monsanto Roundup Herbicide Link to Birth Defects*. The most significant statement in the article is that,

> "Roundup in far lower concentrations than used in agriculture is linked to birth defects."

This demonstrates, yet again, that endocrine disruption occurs at levels that have been deemed by traditional toxicology to be 'safe'; but these chemicals are clearly unsafe.

Methanol is another teratogenic chemical; this is demonstrated by Dr Woodrow Monte, who explains that, when purchased for laboratory use, methanol carries a warning label that refers to its potential to cause birth defects. As discussed, methanol has many uses; it is present in cigarettes due to the methods used to process tobacco leaves. In *While Science Sleeps* Dr Monte states that,

> "Consequently, methanol is one of the most abundant poisons found in tobacco smoke."

The fact that methanol is an ingredient of aspartame means that this toxic 'sweetener' is also teratogenic; as indicated by Dr Carolyn Dean who quotes Dr Betty Martini's statement that,

> "Aspartame is a teratogen causing birth defects and mental retardation."

The endocrine system also regulates growth and development after birth; which means that any influence that can adversely affect the baby's endocrine system can adversely affect 'normal' development after birth. The use of plastics made with phthalate plasticisers for the manufacture of many baby's toys can be a contributory factor to later 'problems' that may be labelled as ADD, ADHD or autism, for example. In the previous discussion, Dr Kwiatkowski referred to these conditions as being 'endocrine-related'; autism is discussed later in this chapter.

One substance that has been mentioned many times is also appropriate to this discussion, because mercury is also teratogenic. Its deadly nature is explained by Dr Carolyn Dean in *Death by Modern Medicine,*

"Mercury is a neurotoxin, a carcinogen, a teratogen, a nephrotoxin and is life threatening."

Many of the chemicals used as ingredients of cosmetics and personal care products are not only toxic, they are also teratogenic and, again, this often involves members of the family of phthalates. One chemical in this family, called DBP (dibutyl phthalate), is an ingredient of nail polish and implicated in various reproductive problems; as Dr Epstein explains in *Toxic Beauty,*

"The highest levels were recorded in women twenty to forty years of age, the prime childbearing years – a major cause for concern since DBP has been linked to birth defects and reproductive problems."

Other influences that have been proven to be teratogenic include ionising radiation, especially X-rays. In *Secret Fallout,* Dr Ernest Sternglass refers to a study by Dr ML Griem that investigated children whose mothers had been X-rayed whilst pregnant. Dr Griem's data showed that,

"...there was a significant increase in benign tumors and certain types of congenital birth defects..."

Although the expectant mother's exposure to teratogens is a significant contributory factor for birth defects, the father's exposure cannot be ignored, as the example of the male Gulf War veterans has demonstrated. This point is also of significance in the context of exposures to ionising radiation. In *The Plutonium Files,* Eileen Welsome reports details of the nuclear bomb tests that occurred in the late 1940s. Although there were many unknown factors about 'safe levels' of radiation, she explains that, at the time, it was discovered that,

"...as little as 0.5 roentgens per day for three months or less could result in defective children in successive generations."

She also refers to examples of military personnel who had worked in the Manhattan Project, or were present during various nuclear bomb tests, or both. As a result of their duties, many of these men were exposed to radiation and some of their children suffered defects of various kinds.

In *Secret Fallout,* Dr Sternglass also refers to radiation emissions from the everyday operations of nuclear power plants. He reports that, at a particular location near to a nuclear power plant, it was discovered that there was a higher than 'normal' number of infant deaths in the vicinity; in addition to which were some other disturbing discoveries,

"And for each infant dying in the first year of life, it was well known that there were perhaps three to four that would live with serious genetic defects, crippling congenital malformations, and mental retardation..."

Non-ionising radiation, although considered to be less dangerous than ionising radiation, is also capable of causing birth defects. The link between

EMFs and birth defects has been known for decades. In *Cross Currents*, Dr Robert Becker refers to Dr S Nordstrom, who conducted investigations in Sweden in 1983 to discover the effects on men who worked in high-voltage electric switchyards, and who found that,

> "The exposure to the electric-power frequency fields (50 Hz in Europe) produced abnormalities in chromosomes of the sperm of the switchyard workers, which resulted in birth defects in their children."

One of the articles in the BioInitiative Report 2012, referred to in chapter six, is entitled *Electromagnetic Field Exposure Effects (ELF-EMF and RFR) on Fertility and Reproduction*. Although the article is mainly concerned with decreased fertility in men as the result of exposure to EMFs, it also makes the pertinent statement that,

> "Several studies, especially at power frequency 50/60 Hz magnetic field, have found an association of exposure to human health, with emphasis on a range of clinical conditions including childhood leukaemia, brain tumours, genotoxicity and neurodegenerative disease, infertility, birth defects, increased risk of miscarriage, childhood morbidity and de novo mutations."

These effects indicate that EMF exposures have wide-ranging detrimental effects, especially on many of the functions of the endocrine system.

During 2015, reports began to emerge about the outbreak of a new birth defect 'problem'; an unusual cluster of cases of microcephaly had been observed in Brazil. Microcephaly is a 'congenital' condition in which the baby's head or brain, or both, has not fully developed prior to birth. According to the medical establishment, the cause of this outbreak had been discovered to be a previously-known 'virus' called Zika.

Microcephaly is clearly a serious problem, but the symptoms of a Zika 'infection' were, prior to 2015, only associated with mild symptoms that commonly involved a fever, rash, joint pain, muscle pain and headache. However, despite the fact that the causes of most birth defects are unknown to the medical establishment, the idea was promoted that the Zika 'virus' was the cause of these cases of microcephaly. This is demonstrated by the CDC web page entitled *Facts about Microcephaly* that states,

> "CDC scientists announced that enough evidence has accumulated to conclude that Zika virus infection during pregnancy is a cause of microcephaly and other severe fetal brain defects."

It is clear that microcephaly cannot be caused by a virus, but can be caused by toxic chemicals that are teratogenic. It was also reported at the time that certain regions of Brazil had been subjected to intense pesticide spraying programmes, and that these regions included the same areas in which many cases of microcephaly had been discovered. Unfortunately, the medical establishment belief that the Zika virus is spread by mosquitoes has resulted in further pesticide spraying programmes in various countries around the world to 'combat' the Zika problem. Clearly the increased and intensified use of pesticides will only exacerbate the problem, not solve it.

Although the information promulgated by the medical establishment is frequently misleading, it occasionally contains some useful advice; the CDC web entitled *Planning for pregnancy*, for example, includes the recommendation to,

"Avoid toxic substances and other environment contaminants, harmful materials at work or at home, such as synthetic chemicals, metals, fertilizer, bug spray..."

This is good advice, but, as in most instances of the advice offered by the medical establishment, it is woefully inadequate because, it fails to include reference to all of the substances that are teratogenic, including certain pharmaceutical 'medicines'.

Down's Syndrome

Down's syndrome, also called Down syndrome, is defined by the establishment as,

"a condition resulting from a chromosomal abnormality most commonly due to the presence of three copies of chromosome 21 (trisomy 21), which is most likely to occur with advanced maternal age."

The claim that 'advanced maternal age' is a relevant factor for a Down's syndrome baby is misleading, because women of all ages have given birth to babies with this condition; there is however, a reason for the increased likelihood that an older mother may give birth to a baby with Down's syndrome, as this discussion will demonstrate.

The nucleus of most cells contains 46 chromosomes arranged in 23 identical pairs. During the normal course of life, millions of the body's cells die every day and need to be replaced. The replacement process involves a form of cell division called 'mitosis' that entails the generation of two identical daughter cells, each of which contains 46 chromosomes arranged in 23 identical pairs.

The exception to this process occurs in cells referred to as 'germ cells', also called cells in the germ line. In this context, however, the word 'germ' does not refer to a pathogen. Instead, it refers to the primary stage of something. Germ cells are precursors of the reproductive cells of both sperm and ova and are therefore the primary cells from which the human body develops. These germ cells undergo 'meiosis', a form of cell division that entails the generation of four daughter cells, each of which contains 23 unpaired chromosomes. After further processes take place, including fertilisation, these cells become the sex cells and are restored to the full complement of 46 chromosomes, but arranged in 22 identical pairs plus an additional pair that comprise the relevant sex chromosomes. Females have two X chromosomes; males have one X chromosome plus one Y chromosome.

Under certain circumstances, cell division of either type may result in the generation of an 'abnormal' number and arrangement of chromosomes in the daughter cells; a situation that is known as aneuploidy. An extra chromosome that creates a trio instead of a pair is called trisomy; a missing chromosome from a pair is called monosomy.

According to the NDSS (National Down Syndrome Society) web page entitled *Down Syndrome*,

"There is no definitive scientific research that indicates that Down syndrome is caused by environmental factors or the parents' activities before or during pregnancy."

This is erroneous; there is scientific research that has discovered reasons for chromosomal abnormalities to occur.

Dr David Rasnick PhD and Dr Peter Duesberg have studied aneuploidy and its role in health problems, especially cancer, which is discussed later in this chapter. In his article entitled *The aneuploidy theory of cancer and the barriers to its acceptance*, Dr Rasnick refers to the existence of aneuploidy in Down's syndrome and states that,

> "Just one extra copy of the smallest chromosome, with its thousand or so normal genes, is sufficient to cause the syndrome."

The existence of 'normal' genes in the presence of abnormal chromosomes indicates that 'genetic' factors' do not contribute to the occurrence of Down's syndrome.

Although it is not uncommon for babies born with Down's syndrome to grow to full adulthood, many do not survive, as Dr Rasnick indicates in his article,

> "Most Down's foetuses are spontaneously aborted. Nonetheless, the imbalance is small enough (47 chromosomes) to permit occasional live births."

The error in chromosome 21 that results in Down's syndrome occurs in the germ cells, which means that all these cells contain the error. The variation in the 'viability' of a foetus indicates that the factors that influence the occurrence of this chromosomal 'error' are of a varying intensity.

Cell division errors can affect chromosomes other than chromosome 21. These other chromosomal errors produce 'defects' that are also referred to as trisomy, each type of which is identified by the affected chromosome. For example, trisomy 18, which is also called Edwards syndrome, involves an extra copy of chromosome 18.

However, most chromosomal errors other than trisomy 21 generally cause conditions in which there is a much greater level of damage. In the majority of these cases, the foetus is not 'viable' and is spontaneously aborted via a 'miscarriage', which generally occurs in the very early weeks of pregnancy. Occasionally some babies survive to birth, but it is rare that those born with aneuploidy other than trisomy 21 live beyond their first year.

The CDC web page entitled *Facts about Down Syndrome* states,

> "Researchers know that Down Syndrome is caused by an extra chromosome, but no one knows for sure why Down Syndrome occurs or how many different factors play a role."

This claim that 'no one knows' is disingenuous; many researchers do know why it occurs. They also know about some of the substances that have the ability to cause chromosomal damage. The authors of *Uninformed Consent* refer to one substance that is a known teratogen with the ability to interfere with chromosomes,

> "Mercury has been found to produce aberrant chromosome numbers."

The timing of the exposure to mercury, or any other toxic substance, that will affect chromosome numbers will be a crucial factor in determining the extent of the effect. If exposure has occurred and is passed to the foetus in the early weeks of the pregnancy, it can lead to 'aberrant chromosome numbers' that can result in birth defects or to an 'unviable' life that results in a spontaneous abortion or miscarriage.

Another danger posed to the developing baby results from an excess of free radicals, which may be caused by a number of factors, especially of the toxic chemical variety, and by various combinations of these factors. Any substance that generates a high level of free radicals that are not neutralised by an adequate supply of antioxidants in the body can damage cells; as Dr Russell Blaylock explains,

> "...the huge number of free radicals produced by exposure to pesticides and heavy metals, extreme exercise, and prolonged poor nutrition will produce the same cellular damage to the sperm and ova as it does to other cells in the body."

Clearly, damage to the cells of sperm and ova can result in chromosomal damage during meiosis, and lead to aneuploidy and the various birth defects associated with chromosomal errors.

Ionising radiation in the form of X-rays and non-ionising radiation in the form of radar were shown to be associated with Down's syndrome more than half a century ago; as indicated by Dr Becker in *The Body Electric*,

> "In 1964 a group of researchers studying Down's syndrome at the Johns Hopkins School of Medicine, after linking the malady to excess X rays given to pregnant women, found an unexpected further correlation with fathers working near radar."

It has also been known for a few decades that other forms of ionising radiation cause chromosomal damage and certain 'defects'; as Dr Rosalie Bertell states in *No Immediate Danger*, which was published in 1985,

> "If the radiation damage occurs in germs cells, the sperm or ovum, it can cause defective offspring."

Other evidence that non-ionising radiation can cause chromosomal damage is indicated by a 2008 article entitled *Increased levels of numerical chromosome aberrations after in vitro exposure of human peripheral blood lymphocytes to radiofrequency electromagnetic fields for 72 hours*. The title of this article, which is published in the BioInitiative Report 2012, is self-explanatory.

It is clear, therefore, that, contrary to the claim of the NDSS, there are a number of environmental factors that have been proven to cause the chromosomal abnormalities associated with Down's syndrome; these environmental factors are toxins that include chemicals and electromagnetic radiation, both of which generate free radicals. An increased body burden of toxins for either parent produces increased levels of damaging free radicals that can adversely affect the outcome of cell division. A high body burden of toxins that have accumulated over the course of many years is one of the main reasons that 'older' women may be more likely to give birth to babies with Down's syndrome than younger women.

Spina Bifida

The establishment definition of spina bifida refers to,

> "a developmental defect in which the newborn baby has part of the spinal cord and its coverings exposed through a gap in the backbone."

Spina bifida is a condition within the group called 'neural tube defects' (NTDs); these are defined by the establishment as,

"a group of congenital abnormalities caused by failure of the neural tubes to form normally."

The Mayo Clinic web pages about spina bifida include a page entitled *Symptoms and Causes* which, under the heading *Causes*, makes the familiar statement that,

"Doctors aren't certain what causes spina bifida."

This page continues with another familiar statement that,

"As with many other problems, it appears to result from a combination of genetic and environmental risk factors..."

The 'risk factors' referred to include folate deficiency, some medications, diabetes, obesity and a family history of neural tube defects. The claim that genetic factors are relevant is discussed in a 2009 article entitled *Genetics of human neural tube defects* that also reports,

"...rather limited progress in delineating the molecular basis underlying most human NTDs."

It is clear therefore, that the medical establishment possesses a poor level of knowledge about all NTDs, not just spina bifida. According to a number of articles, some NTDs are associated with aneuploidy, as indicated by a 2007 article entitled *Chromosomal abnormalities associated with neural tube defects (1): full aneuploidy*, that states,

"Fetuses with neural tube defects (NTDs) carry a risk of chromosomal abnormalities."

It must be noted that NTDs are not considered to be caused by chromosomal abnormalities, but they have been observed to occur concurrently; which indicates that they may have similar causal factors. In addition, the article refers to an increased incidence of NTDs in spontaneous abortions; which also indicates that the foetus had serious defects and was therefore not 'viable'.

As suggested by the Mayo Clinic, folate deficiency is regarded as one of the 'risk factors' associated with spina bifida. In addition, a 2007 article entitled *Folate and neural tube defects* refers to the protective effects of folate and claims that this effect has been,

"...established by a chain of clinical research studies over the past half century."

Although the benefits of folate are claimed to have been 'established', the article also refers to epidemiological studies of women who followed the recommendation to increase their folic acid intake; but the result of these studies was, according to the article, that,

"...a reduction in NTD births did not follow promulgation of these recommendations..."

Although this does not directly prove that there are no beneficial effects from an increased intake of folic acid, it does demonstrate that the connection between folic acid and spina bifida has not been established beyond doubt. The level of uncertainty of the benefit of folate supplementation is demonstrated by a 2006 article entitled *Neural tube defects and folate: case far from closed*, which states that,

"...the mechanism underlying the beneficial effects of folic acid is far from clear."

This uncertainty is further substantiated by a 2009 article entitled *Not all cases of neural tube defect can be prevented by increasing the intake of folic acid*; the title is self-explanatory.

Folate is an antioxidant; which means that it can neutralise free radicals that may damage a developing baby. There is however, an assumption that folate and folic acid are identical substances; this is a mistaken assumption. Folate, which is one of the B vitamins, occurs naturally in foods; folic acid, by comparison, is a manufactured synthetic substance. Although folic acid supplements are said to be 'based on' folate, they are not the same chemical; this point is clarified by Dr Joel Fuhrman in a March 2017 article entitled *Why You Need Folate and Not Folic Acid* that states,

"Folic acid is chemically different from dietary folate..."

He also makes the point that supplementation is unnecessary because there are plenty of vegetables that contain folate and adds the comment that,

"Pregnancy isn't the only time in life to focus on folate."

It is clear that folate deficiency is not the cause of spina bifida; although nutrient deficiencies may be contributory factors, they are not the main causes of birth defects. It is important to emphasise that attention should be paid to nutrition as a whole, not just to individual nutrients.

The medical establishment considers that, in addition to folate deficiency, certain health conditions that affect the mother increase the risk of her having a baby with spina bifida, as indicated by the NICHD (National Institute of Child Health and Human Development) web page entitled *How many people are affected by or at risk for spina bifida?*

"Women who are obese, have poorly controlled diabetes, or take certain antiseizure medications are at greater risk of having a child with spina bifida."

The causes of diabetes have been discussed and shown by Dr Bieler to be related to a 'toxic background'; obesity may also be related to a diet that mainly comprises processed food products that contain many toxic chemical food additives.

However, the reference to antiseizure medications is of particular significance, as indicated by a 2003 article entitled *Clinical care of pregnant women with epilepsy: neural tube defects and folic acid supplementation*, which acknowledges that there is a higher risk for women with epilepsy to have babies with malformations and especially NTDs. The article states,

"Most antiepileptic drugs (AEDs) have been associated with such risk. Valproate and carbamazepine have been associated specifically with the development of neural tube defects (NTDs), especially spina bifida."

In addition to their use as antiepileptic medications, these drugs, but especially valproate, may also be used to treat bipolar disorder. However, epilepsy and bipolar disorder are both conditions in which drug treatments are recommended to be continued throughout pregnancy. It has previously been shown that most drugs are untested for their human teratogenic effects; furthermore, the NHS web pages about both conditions admits that the causes of epilepsy and bipolar disorder are unknown and the reasons they occur are not fully understood. According to the NHS web page about epilepsy,

"...the electrical signals in the brain become scrambled and there are sometimes sudden bursts of electrical activity."

The discussions about EHS and the dangers of EMFs indicate some of the likely causes of the problems with electrical signals in the brain.

The establishment defines bipolar affective disorder as,

"a severe mental illness causing repeated episodes of depression, mania, or mixed affective state."

Significantly, however, the NHS web page claims that,

"Bipolar disorder is widely believed to be the result of chemical imbalances in the brain."

The discussion in chapter one that referred to the work of Dr Peter Breggin demonstrated that this belief has no basis in science; it is a hypothesis that has never been scientifically established and there are no tests to determine the existence of any such imbalance. It should be clear therefore, that no pharmaceutical drug is able to address epilepsy or bipolar disorder; but more importantly, the drugs used to treat these conditions are proven to be able to cause harm, especially to a developing baby. A 2014 article entitled *Treatment of bipolar disorders during pregnancy: maternal and fetal safety and challenges* expresses the perceived problems, which are that both cessation and continuation of treatments, especially valproate, are associated with harm. The article makes the pertinent comment about the challenges of continuing medication,

"...some of the most effective pharmacotherapies (such as valproate) have been associated with the occurrence of congenital malformations or other adverse neonatal effects in offspring."

Some of the less serious 'side effects' of valproate for the person who takes the drug include nausea and vomiting; more serious side effects include liver dysfunction. All of these effects indicate that this drug is toxic; a fact that is substantiated by evidence that it can cause 'malformations'; which means that it is also teratogenic.

Sudden Infant Death Syndrome

Sudden infant death syndrome (SIDS) is also known as cot death, which is defined by the establishment as,

"the sudden unexpected death of an infant less than two years old (peak occurrence between two and six months) from an unidentifiable cause."

The NHS web page entitled *Sudden infant death syndrome (SIDS)* provides an important additional detail in the reference to SIDS as,

"...the sudden, unexpected and unexplained death of an apparently healthy baby."

It should be noted that the establishment defines a syndrome as,

"a combination of signs and/or symptoms that forms a distinct clinical picture indicative of a particular disorder."

The death of a baby under any circumstances will always be an extremely traumatic experience, a sudden death will be even more so; nevertheless, it is a misnomer to describe the sudden death of an apparently healthy baby as a 'syndrome'.

The medical establishment has, however, recently amended the definition of SIDS, which now only refers to the death of an infant in the first year of life. The sudden and unexpected death of a baby beyond their first birthday is now referred to as SUDC (Sudden Unexplained Death in Childhood). Whatever label may be attached to the sudden and unexpected death of a baby or young child, the medical establishment claims that the causes are largely unknown, but that there are a few 'risk factors'.

The NHS web page explains that most unexpected deaths occur in the first six months of a baby's life and further states that,

"Experts believe SIDS occurs at a particular stage in a baby's development and that it affects babies who are vulnerable to certain environmental stresses."

One of the specific 'environmental stresses' referred to is tobacco smoke; however, although inhaling smoke is certainly detrimental to a baby's health, it cannot be the sole factor, otherwise all babies exposed to tobacco smoke would die. Although rarely, if ever, mentioned by the medical establishment, the many toxic and often volatile chemicals in most household products, including personal care products for babies, can also be contributory factors; especially as people are more fastidious about making sure that everything is 'clean' and 'germ-free' for the new baby.

All health problems are caused by a combination of factors; this includes health problems that affect babies. All of those factors will involve exposures to toxic substances of varying types, but some of the exposures may involve a significant toxin at a particularly important stage of development.

But the 'stresses' to which babies are subjected are not restricted to those in the external environment; virtually all babies are subjected to a particular set of internal stresses, namely vaccinations, many of which are administered within the first few months of their lives; as indicated by the CDC web page entitled *Sudden Infant Death Syndrome (SIDS)* that states,

"Babies receive many vaccines when they are between 2 to 4 months old. This age range is also the peak age for sudden infant death syndrome (SIDS), or infant death that cannot be explained."

It is clear that, as with tobacco smoke, babies do not all die when vaccinated. Nevertheless, vaccines contain many highly toxic ingredients; which means that they cannot be exempted from the category of 'contributory factors'. Unsurprisingly, the concurrence of the peak age for SIDS and the age at which many vaccines are administered is claimed by the medical establishment to be a pure 'coincidence' and that there is absolutely no causal relationship between these two events. This vehement denial of any direct causal relationship is demonstrated by an article entitled *Six common misconceptions about immunization* on the WHO website; one of the 'misconceptions' is stated to be that,

"...vaccines cause many harmful side effects, illnesses and even death."

The idea that this claim is a 'misconception' is egregious for reasons that have been discussed, particularly in chapter two. Nevertheless, the article specifically refers to reported claims about a correlation between the DTP vaccine and SIDS, and states that this is 'a myth that won't go away', but which had arisen,

> "...because a moderate proportion of children who die of SIDS have recently been vaccinated with DTP..."

DTP is not the only vaccine that has been associated with the death of an infant soon after its administration. The ever-increasing number of vaccines that are administered to babies in the routine schedules of most countries has led to many of them being administered simultaneously in ever-larger multiples. For example, the triple DTP has largely been replaced by a hexavalent vaccine that is claimed to immunise against diphtheria, tetanus, acellular pertussis, hepatitis B, inactivated poliovirus and Haemophilus influenzae type B.

The discussion about polio demonstrated the efforts of the medical establishment to deny the existence of an association between vaccines and an adverse event, such as paralysis, which has frequently followed the administration of vaccines, by the creation of a new condition called AFP; the discussions in chapter eight demonstrate that AFP affects an increasing number of babies in countries such as India.

The denial that multivalent vaccines pose an even greater hazard to the baby is demonstrated by a March 2014 article entitled *Sudden infant death following hexavalent vaccination: a neuropathologic study*, which claims that no causal relationship had been proved. Nevertheless, the article added the comment that,

> "However, we hypothesize that vaccine components could have a direct role in sparking off a lethal outcome in vulnerable babies."

The most vulnerable babies are those born prematurely; however, the medical establishment view is that premature babies should still be vaccinated, as indicated by the NHS web page entitled *Vaccinations* that, under the sub-heading *Vaccinations for premature babies*, states,

> "It's especially important that premature babies get their vaccines on time, from 8 weeks after birth, no matter how premature they are."

The NHS states that premature babies need to be vaccinated because they are at a greater risk of developing an 'infection'; yet no exceptions are made for babies that are breastfed, even though they are acknowledged to be better 'protected' against illness, as previously discussed.

It is clear that the 'vaccine components' referred to in the 2014 article above will be a significant contributory factor for the 'lethal outcome' for a baby, especially a premature baby, that dies suddenly and unexpectedly soon after receiving a vaccination.

It is also claimed by the medical establishment that a contributory factor for SIDS is that babies have often had a 'cold' or some other 'infection' prior to their sudden death. The establishment definition of cot death includes the additional information that,

"About half the affected infants will have had a viral upper respiratory tract infection within the 48 hours preceding their death..."

It is likely that babies with an 'infection' will have been treated with medicines such as paracetamol (acetaminophen), the dangers of which have been discussed. However, vaccines can also cause certain symptoms that are similar to those of a 'cold'; as acknowledged by the WHO in the article about 'misconceptions',

"Most vaccine adverse events are minor and temporary, such as a sore arm or mild fever. These can often be controlled by taking paracetamol after vaccination."

But the WHO maintains that there is no connection between vaccines and SIDS,

"As for vaccines causing death, again so few deaths can plausibly be attributed to vaccines that it is hard to assess the risk statistically."

Assessing the risk 'statistically' is wholly inappropriate. The efforts to justify vaccines include the assertion that their 'benefits' outweigh their 'risks'; but for any parent whose baby has died, the 'risk' has been 100 per cent, the 'benefit' zero and the result devastating.

The reference on the above cited NHS web page to SIDS occurring at a particular stage in a baby's development is an important aspect of the link between vaccines and a baby's death. The reason is because, as previously discussed, the endocrine system regulates growth and development and can be adversely affected by EDCs, including the toxic ingredients of vaccines. Dr Viera Scheibner PhD also makes this point in her 2005 article entitled *Vaccination and the Dynamics of Critical Days*, in which she states,

"Scientific evidence shows that babies can have severe adverse reactions to vaccinations at critical intervals following their shots, and that vaccination is the more likely cause of cot death and shaken baby syndrome."

There is an abundance of evidence about infant deaths following vaccinations to implicate them as a major contributory factor to many, if not most, cases of SIDS.

Some research implicates other contributory factors, but indicates that vaccines may play the role of a 'trigger' for SIDS in the presence of these other factors. One of these theories is indicated by the Mayo Clinic web page about SIDS that states,

"Although the cause is unknown, it appears that SIDS might be associated with defects in the portion of an infant's brain that controls breathing and arousal from sleep."

Dr Viera Scheibner and her husband, Leif Karlsson, have studied the significance of breathing difficulties in cases of SIDS. In her 1991 article entitled *Cot Deaths Linked to Vaccinations*, Dr Scheibner refers to 'Stress-Induced Breathing Patterns' that can occur in a baby during illness, teething or other 'insults' to the body, including vaccinations. A baby may also develop breathing difficulties due to exposures to various toxins, including volatile chemicals that are used in many cleaning products for example.

Another factor that has been associated with SIDS is a deficiency of serotonin (5-hydroxytryptamine, 5-HT). A February 2010 article entitled

Brainstem Serotonergic Deficiency in Sudden Infant Death Syndrome describes the problem and reports that,

> "Serotonin levels were 26% lower in SIDS cases..."

The article proposes that SIDS results from an abnormality in the serotonin system that,

> "...causes an inability to restore homeostasis following life-threatening challenges..."

The article reports that the systems involved in homeostasis are still developing during the first year of life; as previously discussed, the endocrine system is part of the system that maintains homeostasis. It should be clear that the toxic ingredients of vaccines would be significant contributors to the 'life-threatening challenges' to which the article refers. Furthermore, the article proposes a 'triple-risk model' for SIDS, which is,

> "...the simultaneous occurrence in the infant of an underlying vulnerability, a critical developmental period, and an exogenous stressor."

Another significant factor for the incidence of SIDS involves serotonin levels that are disrupted by the psychiatric medications known as SSRIs (selective serotonin reuptake inhibitors). A January 2013 report entitled *Adverse Effects on Infants of SSRI/SNRI Use During Pregnancy and Breastfeeding* links the use of SSRI antidepressants by expectant mothers to an increased risk of SIDS. The report discusses the comparison between SIDS deaths and non-SIDS deaths and refers to findings which indicated that SIDS deaths were found to have serotonin abnormalities that were,

> "...in the serotonin pathway in the regions of the brainstem which regulate such basic functions such as body temperature, breathing, blood pressure and heart rate..."

These critical functions are regulated by the endocrine system; this indicates, therefore, that SSRIs are endocrine disruptors. Although the full extent of their endocrine effects has not been studied, SSRIs have been shown to adversely affect certain vital functions associated with the endocrine system. The conclusion to the above cited 2013 report includes the statement that,

> "There is significant evidence that the harm caused to neonates by exposure to and withdrawal from SRIs during pregnancy and after birth can lead to sudden infant death..."

The term SRI includes SNRIs (serotonin and noradrenaline reuptake inhibitors) as well as SSRIs.

The dangers of SSRIs have been discussed in chapter one; it should be obvious that SNRIs will be similarly dangerous. The use of these pharmaceuticals during pregnancy substantially increases the risk of harm to the unborn baby; a situation that could account for an 'underlying vulnerability' that would weaken the ability of a baby's system to resist the effects of the toxins administered by vaccines.

Another point of significance is that serotonin and melatonin are interconnected, as indicated by a 2003 web page entitled *The Pineal Gland and Melatonin* that states,

> "The precursor to melatonin is serotonin, a neurotransmitter that itself is

derived from the amino acid tryptophan."

This clearly indicates the close connection between different hormones as well as other natural body chemicals, such as amino acids. It is for this reason that interference with the production of any single hormone can upset homeostasis and cause many different adverse effects. The problems associated with low levels of melatonin include SIDS, as indicated by a 1990 article entitled *Melatonin concentrations in the sudden infant death syndrome* that states,

> "...CSF melatonin levels were significantly lower among the SIDS infants than those dying of other causes."

CSF is cerebrospinal fluid. The significance of melatonin was discussed in the section about EHS; it is however important to reiterate that newborn babies do not produce and secrete melatonin immediately after birth; they gradually develop this function over the course of time. Nevertheless, babies require melatonin, which is usually provided by the mother through breastfeeding. Melatonin is a powerful antioxidant; which means that it is capable of reducing the adverse effects of the toxic chemical ingredients of vaccines. A low level of melatonin would therefore contribute to a baby's poorly functioning detoxification system.

There are other factors that may contribute to the build-up of toxic matter in a baby's body that cannot be adequately eliminated; these have been discussed, but it must be noted that they will also include many products that are specifically intended for use with babies. For example, some of the toxins that have been implicated in SIDS cases include chemicals used as fire-retardants.

Other hazards to which newborn babies are exposed are the chemicals used in clothing fabrics, as well as those used in dyes and plastics for printed images on clothes; they also include chemicals used in cot mattress materials and bedding. Furthermore, many baby care products contain the same toxic ingredients as adult products; baby shampoos, lotions and powders, for example, contain phthalates.

Chemicals are not the sole source of potential health hazards for babies; exposures to EM radiation are also implicated. The discussion about EHS referred to the work of Dr Neil Cherry who demonstrated that EM radiation reduced melatonin levels; as discussed above, SIDS is often associated with reduced melatonin levels. Dr Cherry also associates EM radiation with increased levels of serotonin; which is certainly indicative of an imbalance in the serotonin/melatonin metabolism.

In view of the variety of hazards to which babies are often subjected it is a testament to the amazing resilience of the human body that the vast majority of them do survive and thrive. Unfortunately, it is becoming increasingly obvious that a significant majority of babies, young children and young adults are far less healthy than they ought to be.

Autism

The establishment defines autism as,

> "a psychiatric disorder of childhood, with an onset before the age of 2½ years. It is marked by severe difficulties in communicating and forming relationships

with other people, in developing language, and in using abstract concepts; repetitive and limited patterns of behaviour; and obsessive resistance to tiny changes in familiar surroundings."

The symptoms associated with autism are diverse; they can manifest in a wide variety of combinations and with varying degrees of severity. Autism is not, however, regarded as a single 'disorder' but as a range of conditions that are categorised under the generic label 'autism spectrum disorder' (ASD). Interestingly, and in common with most of the health problems discussed in this chapter, the medical establishment acknowledges that many aspects of autism, including its causes, are poorly understood or even unknown.

Also interesting is that the CDC web page entitled *What is Autism Spectrum Disorder?* states that,

"Diagnosing ASD can be difficult since there is no medical test, like a blood test, to diagnose the disorders."

A diagnosis of ASD in the US will usually be based on the criteria contained within the DSM-5 (the Diagnostic and Statistical Manual, Fifth Edition, of the American Psychiatric Association). These criteria require doctors to make assessments of various behaviours that a child displays, as the CDC page states,

"Doctors look at the child's behavior and development to make a diagnosis."

A diagnosis of ASD outside of the US may also be based on the criteria within the DSM-5 or it may be based on the criteria within the ICD-10, which is the disease classification system of the WHO; as discussed at the beginning of this chapter.

ASDs are claimed to develop during the early years of life, as indicated by the April 2018 WHO fact sheet entitled *Autism spectrum disorders*, which states that,

"ASDs begin in childhood and tend to persist into adolescence and adulthood."

This means that an adolescent or adult who has been diagnosed with ASD later in life is deemed to have almost certainly had the condition since their childhood, even though it had remained undiagnosed; as the fact sheet indicates,

"In most cases the conditions are apparent during the first 5 years of life."

The fact sheet claims that ASDs affect an estimated 1 in 160 children worldwide and states that,

"Available scientific evidence suggests that there are probably many factors that make a child more likely to have an ASD, including environmental and genetic factors."

The claim that 'genetic factors' may be involved is not, however, corroborated by geneticists; as indicated by Dr Russell Blaylock, who reports in his 2008 article entitled *Vaccines, Neurodevelopment and Autism Spectrum Disorders* that,

"...geneticists were quick to respond that genetic disorders do not suddenly increase in such astronomical proportions."

Dr Blaylock states in his article that the incidence of autism in the US in

1983 was 1 child in 10,000. The CDC web page entitled *Data & Statistics on Autism Spectrum Disorder* contains a table that displays the rates of ASD for 8-year-old children surveyed at 2-year intervals between 2000 and 2014. The table shows that the rate of ASD for 8-year-olds surveyed in the year 2000 was 1 in 150; in 2010 the rate had risen to 1 in 68; by 2014, it had reached 1 in 59. At the time of writing, 2014 is the most recent year for which the ASD rates in the US are available.

The WHO fact sheet refers to the increase in the global prevalence of ASD during the past 50 years and states that,

"There are many possible explanations for this apparent increase, including improved awareness, expansion of diagnostic criteria, better diagnostic tools and improved reporting."

The description of the increase as 'apparent' is disingenuous, as demonstrated by the marked increase in the CDC's acknowledged rate of ASD in the US between the years 2000 and 2014. Furthermore, the factors referred to by the WHO are merely recording tools; they fail to offer a genuine explanation for the existence of autism, its continually increasing incidence or the rapidity with which it continues to increase. This is particularly significant with respect to the US where the incidence of 1 in 59 is far higher than the worldwide incidence of 1 in 160.

The real reasons for the rapid rise in the incidence of autism owe their origin to a variety of 'environmental factors', as this discussion will demonstrate.

Although the establishment definition describes autism as a 'psychiatric disorder', ASD is more commonly referred to as a 'mental disorder'; these terms are, however, regarded as synonymous and often used interchangeably. The CDC website contains many pages about *Children's Mental Health*; the web page entitled *What Are Childhood Mental Disorders?* states that,

"Mental disorders among children are described as serious changes in the way children typically learn, behave, or handle their emotions, which cause distress and problems getting through the day."

One of the mental disorders referred to as 'common' in childhood is ADHD. The page also states that,

"Childhood mental disorders can be treated and managed."

Treatment for these conditions may entail the use of pharmaceutical drugs, although this is not always the case. However, and more disturbingly, the age at which a child can be diagnosed with a 'mental disorder' and treated with drugs has no lower limit, as indicated by a May 2014 CCHR (Citizens Commission on Human Rights) article entitled *Watchdog Says Report of 10,000 Toddlers on ADHD Drugs Tip of the Iceberg*. The article refers to documents obtained by CCHR from IMR Health that report statistics for the US for the year 2013; these statistics state that, in the age range of birth to 1 year there were: 249,669 infants on anti-anxiety drugs; 26,406 on antidepressants; 1,422 on ADHD drugs and 654 on antipsychotics. The number of psychiatric drugs prescribed for 2- to 3-year old toddlers were even higher. In addition, the article reports that the total number of children under the age of 18 who were taking psychiatric drugs were: over 1 million between birth and 5 years of age; over 4 million between the ages of 6 and 12; and over 3 and a half million between 13 and 17.

The reason these drugs are prescribed for children with 'mental disorders' such as ADHD, is because they are claimed to be able to correct a 'chemical imbalance in the brain'; however, as discussed in chapter one, there is no test that is able to determine the existence of any such 'chemical imbalance', and there is no evidence that psychiatric drugs could correct such an imbalance, even if it were to exist. Dr Peter Breggin, who constantly refers to these problems throughout his work, asserts that these drugs are dangerous and eminently capable of producing a variety of adverse effects, including many of the symptoms for which they are commonly prescribed.

Psychiatric drugs may also be prescribed for children diagnosed with ASD. In his February 2014 article entitled *$1.5 Million Award in Child Tardive Dyskinesia Malpractice*, Dr Breggin refers to a case in which he testified as the psychiatric expert and explains that,

> "...the boy was diagnosed with autism as a child and then started on SSRI antidepressants before the age of seven."

Tardive dyskinesia is a condition in which the symptoms include involuntary repetitive movements; it is officially recognised to be associated with the long-term use of certain psychiatric 'medications', which clearly demonstrates that, as Dr Breggin states,

> "...psychiatric drugs do much more harm than good in treating autistic children..."

ASD is also referred to as a 'developmental disability'; the CDC web page entitled *Developmental Disabilities* describes them as,

> "...a group of conditions due to an impairment in physical, learning, language, or behavior areas."

Of particular concern is that, according to the CDC page,

> "About one in six children in the US have one or more development disabilities or other developmental delays."

The page claims that most developmental disabilities, including ASD, exist at birth, but this is not always the case. A substantial proportion of children diagnosed with ASD experience developmental regression, as described by a 2013 article entitled *Evidence of neurodegeneration in autism spectrum disorder*, which states that,

> "Autism spectrum disorder (ASD) is a neurological disorder in which a significant number of children experience a developmental regression characterized by a loss of previously-acquired skills and abilities."

The article explains that a loss of neurological function can be described as neurodegeneration and states that,

> "...the issue of neurodegeneration in ASD is still under debate."

The scale of developmental regression in the US is reported in a 2015 article entitled *Developmental regression in autism spectrum disorder*, which states that,

> "About one-third of young children with ASD lose some skills during the preschool period..."

The importance of developmental regression and neurodegeneration cannot be overstated; together they demonstrate that a loss of previously-acquired skills and abilities is almost certainly the result of disruptions to neurological functioning that occur during the first few years of life when a child's brain and nervous system are at critical stages of development. The most likely causes of disruptions to neurological functions and development will include exposures to neurotoxic substances.

There are various sources of exposure to neurotoxic substances; one of them, however, namely vaccination, is of particular significance with respect to children in their first years of life. Unsurprisingly, the medical establishment vehemently denies that there is any association between autism and vaccines, especially the MMR vaccine; as demonstrated by the WHO fact sheet about ASDs which claims that,

"Available epidemiological data are conclusive that there is no evidence of a causal association between measles, mumps and rubella vaccine, and ASD."

This denial of a causal association is extended to apply to all vaccines, not just the MMR, as the fact sheet also claims,

"There is also no evidence to suggest that any other childhood vaccine may increase the risk of ASD."

These claims are not only disingenuous, they are erroneous. The discussions in chapter two demonstrated that all vaccines pose genuine risks to health due to the toxic nature of many of their ingredients. Whilst it may be virtually impossible to prove beyond doubt that a specific vaccine is the sole cause of a specific adverse health event following its administration, it is beyond doubt that vaccines are eminently capable of 'triggering' the onset of a variety of health problems, including neurological problems, by virtue of the toxic and neurotoxic properties of their ingredients.

Although the exact number may vary according to the country in which a child is born, the majority of vaccines are usually administered before the age of 24 months; an age that closely correlates with the average age at which developmental regression occurs; as indicated by the previously cited 2015 article, which states that,

"...the average reported age of regression was around 20 months of age."

Unfortunately, but unsurprisingly, the medical establishment denies that this correlation is indicative of a causal association; but their denial is disingenuous.

It is indisputable that the number of vaccine doses administered during the first two years of a child's life has increased substantially since the early 1980s. However, the health problems associated with vaccinations are not restricted to ASD or to developmental regression. As the discussions in chapter two demonstrated, vaccines have been causally associated with a variety of adverse health events that include infant mortality. An investigation that compared vaccination schedules and IMR (infant mortality rate) in 34 countries, including the US, is reported in a 2011 article entitled *Infant mortality regressed against number of vaccine doses routinely given: Is there a biochemical or synergistic toxicity?* In the article, Neil Z Miller and Gary S Goldman report their finding that the countries with the lowest IMR were those that administered the fewest vaccines within the first year of a child's life. They discovered that the US, which administers the most vaccines, had the highest IMR.

An additional fact identified by the investigation reported in the article is that the number of premature births in the US had also increased in recent decades. The discussion in this chapter about SIDS indicated that babies born prematurely are particularly vulnerable, but nevertheless receive the standard series of vaccines at the same 'age' after birth as babies born at full term.

The fact that most babies and small children do not experience developmental regression or die soon after receiving a vaccine, does not mean that they have not been harmed by it. In the vast majority of cases, there are no obvious signs of harm; but cells and tissues within the child's body will be damaged by the neurotoxic ingredients of vaccines, although at a subclinical level. The extent of the damage will vary as it depends on a number of factors, as will be discussed in chapter ten; however, in some cases, the damage may contribute to neurological health problems that manifest later in life.

The claim by the medical establishment that there is no causal link between vaccines and autism is said to be 'evidence-based'; but this claim clearly ignores the mounting evidence that there is a very close link between them. In his previously cited 2008 article, Dr Blaylock discusses the issue of 'evidence' and the fact that different standards seem to apply depending on the source of the evidence; he refers to the existence of,

"...an incredible double standard when it comes to our evidence versus theirs."

Nowhere is this double standard more apparent than in its application to evidence relating to vaccines, especially with respect to their safety; as Dr Blaylock states,

"The proponents of vaccination safety can just say that they are safe, without any supporting evidence what-so-ever, and it is to be accepted without question."

The same can be said for statements by the proponents of vaccinations with respect to their efficacy.

The claim that vaccines are based on 'science' was shown in chapter two to be a complete fallacy; a conclusion reached by Dr M Beddow Bayly whose words were quoted in that chapter but bear repetition,

"Of scientific basis or justification for the practice there is none..."

Chapter two referred to a number of vaccine ingredients and, although none of them can be regarded as harmless, three of them are particularly pertinent to autism; these are mercury, aluminium and formaldehyde, all of which are recognised as neurotoxic.

Previous discussions have referred to the acknowledged fact that there is no 'safe' dose of mercury. In *Health and Nutrition Secrets*, Dr Blaylock discusses the processes involved in the development of the human brain, including the production of important enzymes; he continues,

"Mercury, as an enzyme poison, interferes with this meticulous process, causing the brain to be 'miswired'."

445

He expands on the process he refers to as 'miswiring' and explains the consequences,

"The process of miswiring can result in anything from mild behavioral and learning problems to major disorders such as autism and other forms of cerebral malfunction."

The discussion in chapter two also referred to the use of aluminium as a vaccine adjuvant; which means that its purpose is to 'boost' the body's reaction to the vaccine to create 'immunity'. The body does react to vaccines; but not in the way described by the medical establishment. The body's reactions are not the result of the immune system's response to a 'germ'; instead, they are the body's efforts to expel toxins. The consequences of introducing aluminium into the body are explained by Dr Blaylock,

"It is known that aluminum accumulates in the brain and results in neurodegeneration."

Formaldehyde, the third neurotoxic vaccine ingredient, generally receives less attention than mercury or aluminium, but is similarly harmful. The discussions in chapter two indicated that the justification for the use of this carcinogenic neurotoxin in vaccines is based on the claim that the body produces it 'naturally'. However, formaldehyde is recognised to be highly reactive and to display 'strong electrophilic properties'; these properties suggest that its presence in the body does not contribute beneficially to any of the body's normal biochemical reactions. The discussions in chapter six indicated that the presence of formaldehyde in the human body is more likely to be the result of direct exposures to this volatile chemical due to its use as an ingredient of many products; it may also result from the metabolism of other chemicals, such as methanol for example.

There are recognised adverse health effects from exposure to formaldehyde; some of those effects are developmental and therefore relevant to childhood health problems, including ASD. A March 2013 article entitled *Toxic effects of formaldehyde on the urinary system* provides a table of the effects that have been discovered and the systems that have been affected. The article reports that effects on the central nervous system include behavioural disorders and convulsions, both of which are associated with ASD. A November 2015 article entitled *Formaldehyde: A Poison and Carcinogen* published by The Vaccine Reaction highlights the problem,

"One might assume that, since formaldehyde is routinely used in many vaccines given to babies, even tiny and vulnerable premature babies, studies would have looked at whether it is safe to inject this poison into their immature systems."

Unfortunately, however, the article states that,

"No such studies appear to have been done."

In the absence of such studies, there is no basis for the claim that it is safe to inject this toxic substance into the body of any person, but more especially into the vulnerable body of a tiny baby. The vaccines that contain formaldehyde include diphtheria and pertussis, both of which are administered within multivalent vaccines, three doses of which are given to babies prior to the age of six months; the association between the DTP vaccine and SIDS has been discussed.

There is other evidence that formaldehyde is highly likely to be a contributory factor to the onset of autism; this has been demonstrated from the results of animal studies conducted by Dr Woodrow Monte, who noticed that, in addition to birth defects, there were other effects, which he describes in *While Science Sleeps* as,

"…a much more subtle but significant inability to interact normally with the environment, with a general cognitive slowness that might be as close as animal pups can bring us to autism."

It should also be noted that some vaccines, including the MMR, contain MSG, which has been discussed and shown to be neurotoxic.

It is impossible to discuss autism and its association with vaccines without referring to Dr Andrew Wakefield MD, albeit very briefly, as his story serves to demonstrate the atrocious attitude of the medical establishment towards anyone who dares to suggest the possibility that vaccinations may not be as safe and effective as they are claimed to be. Dr Wakefield describes the events in his book entitled *Callous Disregard*, in which he explains that,

"On February 28, 1998, twelve colleagues and I published a case series paper in *The Lancet*, a respected medical journal, as an 'Early Report'. The paper described the clinical findings in 12 children with an autistic spectrum disorder (ASD) occurring in association with a mild-to-moderate inflammation of the large intestine (colitis)."

This now 'infamous' paper has been withdrawn from *The Lancet* and, when reported in the mainstream media, is erroneously referred to as 'discredited' and 'fraudulent'. Although reported as such, the study that was conducted was not an investigation of a possible correlation between the MMR vaccine and autism. Dr Wakefield and his colleagues had investigated the presence of a variety of gastrointestinal symptoms presented by the children diagnosed with 'autism'. It was incidental to the investigation that some of the parents reported that their children's symptoms had begun soon after they had received the MMR vaccine.

Despite the public denial of any link between vaccines and autism, privately the establishment, particularly in the US, has undertaken a very different approach that began seven years before his paper was published; as Dr Wakefield explains,

"…as a matter of fact, the US vaccine court began compensating for cases of vaccine-caused autism starting in 1991, and the US Department of Health and Human Services has been secretly settling cases of vaccine-caused autism without a hearing also since 1991."

Autism is, however, only one of the many vaccine-related 'adverse events' that have been compensated by the Fund, although, as discussed in chapter two, more claims are rejected than accepted for compensation. But the rejection of a claim does not mean that the adverse event was not vaccine-related.

The treatment of Dr Wakefield by the medical establishment, which included his being struck off the medical register in the UK, would seem to indicate that he is being held as an example of what could happen to any other researcher, doctor or scientist who may decide to challenge, or even question, the safety or efficacy of vaccines. The medical establishment has made it abundantly clear that such courage could jeopardise or even terminate a person's career.

It should be clear that 'science' cannot progress amidst a climate of fear; historically it has always progressed through innovative research undertaken by pioneers.

Although courageous in the face of the harsh criticism of his work, Dr Wakefield did not conduct pioneering research; his investigation had discovered the existence of a correlation between children diagnosed with an ASD and inflammation within their digestive systems. The close and causal association between digestive problems and ill-health has been known for centuries; Hippocrates, for example, is credited with stating that 'all disease begins in the gut'.

In her book entitled *Gut and Psychology Syndrome*, Dr Natasha Campbell-Mcbride MD also discusses the problem of inflammation in the gut, and refers to the clinical findings of Dr Wakefield and his colleagues; she mentions that the team,

"...found various stages of chronic inflammation in the gut of these children, erosions of the mucous membranes of the colon and intestines, abscesses filled with pus, ulcers and plenty of faecal impaction."

These are serious digestive system problems, which, as Dr Campbell-Mcbride has also discovered, frequently occur in children with a variety of health problems; she states that,

"I have yet to meet a child with autism, ADHD/ADD, asthma, eczema, allergies, dyspraxia or dyslexia, who has not got digestive abnormalities."

The serious nature of these digestive abnormalities indicates a long-term build-up of toxic material in the body caused by an inability to properly digest and process foods as well as eliminate the waste products of digestion.

The WHO fact sheet also recognises that ASD is frequently accompanied by other health problems and states that,

"Individuals with ASD often present other co-occurring conditions, including epilepsy, depression, anxiety and attention deficit hyperactivity disorder (ADHD)."

The co-occurrence of epilepsy and ASD may seem surprising as they are not perceived to be similar conditions; however, epilepsy clearly involves impairment of neurological functioning that affects the brain, as indicated by the establishment definition that refers to epilepsy as,

"a disorder of brain function characterized by recurrent seizures that have a sudden onset."

The February 2019 WHO fact sheet entitled *Epilepsy* claims that the most common form is 'idiopathic'; which means that it does not have an identifiable cause. However, any disruption to neurological functioning strongly suggests the involvement of neurotoxic substances and influences. Unfortunately, the vast majority of chemicals remain untested with respect to their neurotoxic effects; as discussed in a 2011 article entitled *Environmental neurotoxicants and developing brain*, which states that,

"Only about 200 chemicals out of more than 80,000 registered with the United

States Environmental Protection Agency have undergone extensive neurotoxicity testing, and many chemicals found in consumer goods are not required to undergo any neurodevelopment testing."

The significance of this dearth of neurotoxicity testing cannot be over-emphasised in the context of babies and young children, whose bodily systems and organs are still undergoing development, but can nevertheless be exposed to a variety of neurotoxic chemicals used as ingredients in a wide variety of consumer products. The article refers to the dangers from these exposures and states that,

"The timing and duration of neurotoxicant exposures during development can give rise to a broad spectrum of structural and functional deficits."

The reference in the article to 'deficits' that occur due to the timing of exposures to toxicants is extremely important. As previously discussed, disruptions to the endocrine system can result from exposures to incredibly minute concentrations of chemicals and, when they occur in the body of a pregnant woman, these disruptions may have an adverse impact on the developing baby. In some cases, the effects may not be readily identifiable at birth, but may manifest at a later stage and be triggered by an increased body burden of neurotoxic substances, such as those used in vaccines.

Although the WHO fact sheet correctly indicates that there are many factors involved in generating ASDs, it fails to fully acknowledge the major role of neurotoxic chemicals in the onset of these disorders, due to their ability to disrupt 'normal' development during a child's formative years. There is, however, a growing body of evidence that demonstrates a direct association between exposures to neurotoxins and developmental problems that may be diagnosed as an ASD; as indicated by a 2013 article entitled *The Dynamics of Autism Spectrum Disorders: How Neurotoxic Compounds and Neurotransmitters Interact* that states,

"Accumulating evidence shows that exposure to neurotoxic compounds is related to ASD."

The neurotoxic compounds referred to in the article include phthalates as well as organophosphate and organochlorine pesticides, amongst others. The article states that these neurotoxic compounds are 'hypothesised' to affect certain neurotransmitter systems, including the GABAergic system. The term GABA refers to gamma-Aminobutyric acid. In addition, the previously cited 2013 article that refers to neurodegeneration in ASD states that,

"To date, the etiology of ASD remains under debate. There are, however, many studies that suggest toxicity in children with ASD."

Although the neurotoxic ingredients of vaccines can certainly be included as contributory factors, or even 'triggers', for the onset of ASD, vaccines are not the only sources of childhood exposures to neurotoxic substances and influences. As discussed in chapter six, some of the ingredients of personal care products, including those specifically intended for use on babies and small children, contain toxic substances, including neurotoxic compounds such as phthalates.

The disruptions to normal functions associated with ASD may affect a number of the body's systems, including the endocrine system and the hormones it regulates. As discussed earlier in this chapter, very few chemicals have been tested to determine their effects on the endocrine system; however, disruption to hormone levels has been shown to be associated with ASDs, as indicated by a November 2014 article entitled *The serotonin-N-acetylserotonin-melatonin pathway as a biomarker for autism spectrum disorders*, which states that,

"Elevated whole-blood serotonin and decreased plasma melatonin...have been reported independently in patients with autism spectrum disorders (ASDs)."

The discussion in chapter six about non-ionising radiation explained that melatonin is an extremely important hormone, and that disruption to its production can have significant adverse effects, including sleep disturbance. A 2015 article entitled *Melatonin in Children with Autism Spectrum Disorders: How Does the Evidence Fit Together?* indicates that some of the adverse effects associated with ASD are the result of disturbances to the serotonin-melatonin pathway,

"There is also strong evidence supporting an involvement of the serotonin-N-acetylserotonin-melatonin pathway in the etiology of ASD."

As previously discussed in this section, children of all ages, especially in the US, are increasingly 'medicated' with psychiatric drugs, which include SSRIs (selective serotonin reuptake inhibitors) that are used to treat various 'mental disorders' on the basis of the idea that an increased level of serotonin will help to 'ease' the problem. In common with all pharmaceuticals, SSRIs are associated with a number of 'side effects', including insomnia. However, an excess level of serotonin in the brain can induce symptoms such as agitation; of even greater concern, is that, if the level of serotonin becomes too high, it can lead to extremely serious effects, such as seizures or a loss of consciousness.

It is clear that children may be directly exposed to toxic and neurotoxic substances that may affect their development during the first years of life; however, they may also be exposed to toxic and neurotoxic substances prior to birth if the mother has been prescribed pharmaceutical 'medicines' during pregnancy.

As discussed in chapter one, depression is one of the most common types of 'mental disorder' and, according to the previously cited WHO fact sheet entitled *Mental Disorders*, women are more affected by depression than men. One of the reasons that depression is more frequently experienced by women may be due to maternal depression, which may occur either during or after pregnancy, or both. It is not uncommon, especially in the US, for pregnant women to be prescribed antidepressants, including SSRIs. The justification for the use of antidepressants during pregnancy is explained in a 2008 article entitled *ACOG Guidelines on Psychiatric Medication Use During Pregnancy and Lactation*, which states that,

"Untreated maternal depression is associated with increased rates of adverse outcomes..."

ACOG is the American Congress of Obstetricians and Gynecologists. The article acknowledges that there are also potential risks of adverse outcomes as the result of the treatment of depression with antidepressants, both prenatal and postnatal, and admits that these outcomes may include birth defects,

"There is limited evidence of teratogenic effects from the use of antidepressants in pregnancy and adverse effects from exposure during breastfeeding."

In his 2008 article entitled *Pregnant mothers should not take antidepressants*, Dr Breggin discusses a number of 'effects', including birth defects, that are associated with the use of antidepressants during pregnancy. He also makes the extremely important statement that,

"Newborns also go through withdrawal when their mothers have taken antidepressants during pregnancy."

Dr Breggin strongly recommends that people who wish to stop taking psychiatric drugs should be supervised during the withdrawal process.

Newborn babies whose mothers have taken antidepressants during pregnancy should also be monitored for the effects of withdrawal. These effects are particularly significant with respect to the still developing brain of a newborn baby, as Dr Breggin explains in his article,

"Withdrawal reactions confirm that the brain of the fetus has been bathed in SSRIs and that it has suffered significant functional changes."

The discussion in this chapter about SIDS indicated that the use of SSRIs during pregnancy has been associated with the subsequent death of the baby; but for the babies that survive, the consequences can include potential, if not actual, serious adverse health effects, including autism. In his August 2014 article entitled *Autism, Antidepressants and Pregnancy: The Basics*, Dr Adam Urato MD refers to eight studies that have recently been conducted to investigate a connection between antidepressants taken by the mother during pregnancy and a subsequent diagnosis of autism for the baby. The reason that so few studies have been conducted should be obvious; however, Dr Urato states that the studies that have now been conducted show,

"...that antidepressants use during pregnancy (principally with selective serotonin reuptake inhibitors or SSRIs) is associated with autism in the exposed children."

It should be clear from previous discussions that neurotoxic chemicals, whether in vaccines, psychiatric drugs or everyday household and personal care products, are not the only hazards that can contribute to the onset of autism. There is a great deal of evidence that an association exists between ASD and EM radiation, as discussed by Dr Andrew Goldsworthy PhD in his May 2011 article entitled, *How Electromagnetically-Induced Cell Leakage May Cause Autism*, in which he states that,

"The first effect of non-ionising electromagnetic radiation is to generate small alternating voltages across the cell membranes, which destabilize them and make them leak."

He discusses the role of calcium ions in the cell membranes of the brain and indicates that weak EMR can remove these ions, which can leak into the cell. In his March 2012 article entitled *The Biological Effects of Weak Electromagnetic Fields*, Dr Goldsworthy expands on the problem of electromagnetically-induced membrane leakage and explains that it can result in changes in the way neurons release their transmitters. He states that this can lead to,

"...spurious signals that have no right to be there, which makes the brain hyperactive and less able to concentrate."

Discussions in this chapter have shown that most chronic diseases are associated with the presence of oxidative stress; autism and ASDs are no exceptions. The link between exposure to EMR, oxidative stress and ASD is demonstrated by the BioInitiative Report 2012 article entitled *Findings in Autism (ASD) Consistent with Electromagnetic Fields (EMF) and Radiofrequency Radiation (RFR)*, which states that,

"Autism (ASD) research indicates that oxidative stress may be a common attribute amongst many individuals with autism."

All disease processes involve damage to different organs and systems; but there are many common features, which, in addition to oxidative stress, include disruptions to the body's production and release of important hormones and antioxidants. These features are also common to ASD, as the article indicates,

"At the cellular and molecular level many studies of people with ASD have identified oxidative stress and evidence of free radical damage, evidence of cellular stress proteins, as well as deficiencies of antioxidants such as glutathione."

The role of cellular stress proteins is discussed in chapter ten.

The article also indicates that oxidation of an important enzyme can affect the body's production of the hormones, serotonin and melatonin,

"Of pertinence, tryptophan hydroxylase (TPH$_2$) – the rate limiting enzyme in the synthesis of serotonin, from which melatonin is derived – is extremely vulnerable to oxidation..."

Furthermore, although ASDs are defined in terms of behavioural problems, the article states that they also involve other levels of damage and functional problems and that,

"...under the surface they also involve a range of disturbances of underlying biology that find striking parallels in the physiological impacts of electromagnetic frequency and radiofrequency exposures (EMF/RFR)."

In addition to directly affecting babies and small children, EM radiation exposures can also affect babies before birth as the result of the mother's exposures to EMF/RFR during her pregnancy. Whilst they are not claimed to have been proven to cause autism, these 'disturbances' caused by exposures to EMF/RFR can clearly have a serious adverse effect on the health of babies in their first few years of life.

Another interesting and highly significant comment in the article is that,

"The problem has been that no one such biological feature has turned out to be present in every single person carrying an ASD diagnosis – and they are not specific to ASDs either."

This situation is not exclusive to ASDs; many, if not most, diseases fail to display unique signs and symptoms by which they can be easily identified. The reason for this is because, contrary to the claims of the medical establishment, 'diseases' are not distinct entities. Instead, as will be discussed in chapter ten, diseases are manifestations of different combinations of symptoms that represent the body's efforts to expel toxins, repair damage and restore health. Furthermore, as this chapter has demonstrated, there is increasing evidence that all diseases share a common underlying mechanism, which is the excess generation of free radicals that induce oxidative stress and cause damage at the cellular level.

Although the medical establishment claims that autism is a lifelong condition for which there is no cure, many children diagnosed with ASD have, through certain treatment approaches, achieved a dramatic reduction in their symptoms; some have even achieved a complete recovery. These successes have not, however, been gained through the usual medical establishment treatment methods, as Dr Blaylock explains,

> "Intrepid workers in the shadows, that is outside the medical establishment, have worked many miracles with these children using a multidisciplinary scientific approach completely ignored by the orthodoxy. Some children have even experienced a return to complete physiological normalcy."

It should be clear from the discussion in this section that autism and ASDs are largely, if not entirely, the result of 'environmental factors', the most significant of which are: the toxic and neurotoxic chemicals used in the manufacture of vaccines, pharmaceuticals and many everyday products; and exposure to electromagnetic radiation.

Cancer

The establishment definition refers to cancer as 'any malignant tumour' and states that,

> "It arises from the abnormal, purposeless, and uncontrolled division of cells that then invade and destroy the surrounding tissues."

Although still a dreaded disease, cancer has become almost commonplace; the incidence has increased to the extent that it is currently estimated that 1 in 3 people will be diagnosed with some form of cancer during their lifetime. The September 2018 WHO fact sheet entitled *Cancer* states that it accounts for about 1 in 6 deaths worldwide and that,

> "Cancer is the second leading cause of death globally..."

Statistics obtained from earlier versions of the fact sheet demonstrate that mortality due to cancer has continued to rise; statistics for the year 2008 showed that cancer accounted for 7.6 million deaths, for 2012 it had risen to 8.2 million and by 2015 it had reached 8.8 million. The most recent cancer statistics are reported in the September 2018 IARC Press Release entitled *Latest global cancer data: Cancer burden rises to 18.1 million new cases and 9.6 million cancer deaths in 2018*; the title is self-explanatory.

Although generally referred to as a single disease, the WHO fact sheet describes cancer as,

> "...a generic term for a large group of diseases that can affect any part of the body."

Under the sub-heading *What causes cancer*, the fact sheet states that,

> "Cancer arises from the transformation of normal cells into tumour cells in a

multistage process that generally progresses from a pre-cancerous lesion to a malignant tumour."

This description does not explain the cause of cancer; however, the fact sheet continues with the statement that,

"These changes are the result of the interaction between a person's genetic factors and 3 categories of external agents..."

These three categories of external agents are 'physical carcinogens', 'chemical carcinogens' and 'biological carcinogens', all of which are discussed in more detail later in this section, as are 'genetic factors'.

However, despite the clear reference to carcinogens as relevant to the onset of cancer, the fact sheet claims that cancer also results from the same four 'risk factors' that apply to all NCDs and states that,

"Tobacco use, alcohol use, unhealthy diet and physical inactivity are major cancer risk factors worldwide..."

This claim is highly misleading. There is a proven association between smoking and lung cancer, which, according to the WHO fact sheet, accounts for 1.76 million deaths each year. The main reason that smoking increases the risk of developing cancer is because most tobacco products contain carcinogens, such as benzene, formaldehyde, methanol and arsenic.

Alcohol is also unhealthy; it is closely associated with liver damage that may initially be diagnosed as cirrhosis but may lead to liver cancer. The fact that alcohol affects the liver is indicative of its toxicity.

An unhealthy diet certainly contributes to ill-health, but the association with cancer is rather different from the risk implied by the WHO fact sheet. The foods that contribute to the development of cancer are those that have been produced using substantial quantities of toxic chemicals, such as pesticides and food additives.

The reference to physical inactivity as a risk factor for cancer is, however, totally unfounded; a lack of physical activity in the absence of any other relevant factors does not cause or contribute to cancer.

It is claimed that cancer has an ancient origin because it has been described in the writings of both the ancient Egyptians and Greeks, including Hippocrates. These writings are cited as evidence in efforts to refute the argument that cancer is predominantly a 'modern' disease and the result of industrialisation. These efforts are, however, futile because there is an abundance of evidence that links the carcinogenic products of industrialisation to cancer, as this discussion will demonstrate. Furthermore, the incidence of cancer in ancient times can also be explained by reference to carcinogens, as will also be explained.

Prior to the 20th century, cancer was relatively uncommon; it was not the scourge it has since become. One of the explanations for this phenomenon is based on the theory that cancer is a disease of ageing, as indicated by the fact sheet, which claims that,

"The incidence of cancer rises dramatically with age..."

This is clearly a correlation, but it does not prove a causal relationship, especially as old people do not all develop cancer. The fact sheet does, however, provide a clue to the underlying problems that may explain the increased incidence of cancer in older people, which is that it is,

"...most likely due to a build-up of risks for specific cancers that increase with age."

The reason that cancer is more prevalent in older people is, however, because it results from a build-up of toxins in the body, not a build-up of 'risks'. This fact is acknowledged, albeit to a limited extent, in the WHO fact sheet that states,

"The overall risk accumulation is combined with the tendency for cellular repair mechanisms to be less effective as a person grows older."

The reason that cellular repair mechanisms become less effective is not solely the result of advancing years, but is far more closely related to factors that cause them to become weakened.

The theory that cancer is a disease of ageing is, however, thoroughly refuted by the fact that children and young adults also suffer from the disease. The page entitled *Adolescents and Young Adults with Cancer* on the website of the NCI (National Cancer Institute) indicates that the scale of this problem is significant,

"Cancer is the leading cause of disease-related death in the AYA population. Among AYAs, only accidents, suicide and homicide claimed more lives than cancer in 2011."

The abbreviation 'AYA' refers to the age group between 15 and 39.

The incidence of cancer is also significant in an even younger age range that

includes all children, as indicated by the September 2018 WHO fact sheet entitled *Cancer in Children*, which states that,

"Cancer is a leading cause of death for children and adolescents around the world and approximately 300,000 children aged 0 to 19 years old are diagnosed with cancer each year."

It is clear that 'ageing' is not a relevant factor in the development of cancer.

The incidence of cancer began to increase noticeably in the early 20th century. As this was the period during which the 'germ theory of disease' was in its ascendancy, microbiologists began to investigate the potential role of 'germs' in connection with this disease. However, despite the occasional discovery of a 'virus' in an animal tumour, there was little progress with this field of investigation.

After the creation of the NCI in the US in 1937, a number of different programmes were developed to continue research into the causes of and treatments for cancer. In the 1950s, a programme was established to develop chemotherapy cancer treatments. In 1962, another programme was established to investigate potential carcinogens in the environment. In 1964, investigations returned to the possibility of a connection between viruses and cancer and resulted in the creation of another programme for this field of research.

In *Inventing the AIDS Virus*, Dr Peter Duesberg reports that, for a while, these three programmes ran in parallel, but that the virus programme was preferred by the medical establishment for a number of reasons. The favouritism shown to the virus programme enabled it to receive a larger proportion of the available funding and to eventually over-shadow all the other programmes, which, starved of adequate funding, experienced severe difficulties in pursuing the research studies they had been set up to conduct. The preferential treatment shown to the virus programme proved to be misplaced; the investigations conducted by this programme were unable to discover any virus capable of causing cancer. Eventually this programme was abandoned and some of its researchers transferred to the research programme to investigate HIV/AIDS, as previously discussed.

However, in 1971, while the 'virus-cancer' connection was still under investigation, Richard Nixon famously launched the 'War on Cancer'. The principal objective of this 'war' was to find the elusive cure for cancer; but the use of military-style language encouraged a military-style approach to the problem, and led to the implementation of methods to 'attack', 'fight' and 'kill' the disease. This was not an entirely new approach to tackling disease, especially cancer; the purpose of this 'war' initiative was to intensify the campaign against the most feared human disease.

The continual rise in both morbidity and mortality from cancer demonstrates that this 'war' has been lost. The real reason for its failure is because its approach was based on fundamentally flawed theories about cancer, especially its causes and treatment.

One of the theories about cancer claims that 'genes' play a relevant role in its development; but, despite efforts to link various genes to different forms of cancer, this is a flawed theory. Furthermore, there is ample evidence that demonstrates genes do not account for many of the known aspects of cancer. This extremely important point is explained by Dr David Rasnick in his previously cited 2002 article entitled, *The aneuploidy theory of cancer and the barriers to its acceptance*, in which he states that,

> "There is a growing list of carcinogens that do not mutate genes at all. In addition there are no cancer specific gene mutations. Even tumors of a single organ rarely have uniform genetic alterations. And, in a rebuttal that should be decisive, no genes have yet been isolated from cancers that can transform normal human or animal cells into cancer cells."

As mentioned at the beginning of this section, the WHO claims that cancerous changes involve 'genetic factors' that interact with three types of 'carcinogen'; namely physical, chemical and biological. The role of genetic factors is not adequately explained in the fact sheet, but it is generally claimed by the medical establishment that cancers are caused by mutated genes. However, research conducted by Dr Rasnick and Dr Peter Duesberg provides an indisputable refutation of the claim that there are any cancer specific gene mutations, and of the claim that genes can transform healthy cells into cancerous ones. Their research, which will be discussed later in this section, shows that 'genetic factors' are irrelevant to the development of cancer.

Biological carcinogens are defined in the WHO fact sheet as,

> "...infections from certain viruses, bacteria, or parasites."

The discussions in chapter three provide a clear refutation of the claim that any virus, bacterium or parasite causes any 'infection'; parasites are further discussed in chapter eight. Unfortunately, the rigid but misplaced adherence to the 'germ theory' means that 'microbes' remain a key feature of theories about disease causation, including those that relate to cancer; as demonstrated by a 2014 article entitled *Infection and Cancer: Global Distribution and Burden of Diseases* that states,

"Infection is one of the main contributors to cancer development."

Despite the seemingly authoritative nature of this assertion, nothing could be further from the truth.

Nevertheless, the 'germ theory' has become so firmly entrenched within medical establishment dogma that the IARC Group 1 category of definite human carcinogens includes eleven 'biological agents', seven of which are viruses. Interestingly, six of the 'infectious agents' in this group are claimed to be,

"Indirect carcinogens that act via chronic inflammation."

The theory that biological agents can cause cancer is similarly promoted by the WHO fact sheet that states,

"Approximately 15% of cancers diagnosed in 2012 were attributed to carcinogenic infections, including Helicobacter pylori, Human Papillomavirus (HPV), Hepatitis B virus, Hepatitis C virus and Epstein-Barr virus."

The term 'carcinogenic infection' is meaningless. Firstly, 'germs' do not cause infections; secondly, 'germs' do not transform normal cells into tumour cells that initiate cancer. Thirdly, and more significantly, cancer involves the proliferation of cells, whereas an 'infection' is said to involve the destruction of cells; it is clear that these are entirely different mechanisms of action.

This therefore means that the category of 'biological carcinogens' can be dismissed, as they too are irrelevant to the development of cancer.

The category of 'physical carcinogens' however, cannot be dismissed; the WHO fact sheet acknowledges that this category includes ionising radiation, which is a proven human carcinogen, as discussed in chapter six.

The category of 'chemical carcinogens' also cannot be dismissed. Although the WHO fact sheet only refers to a few examples, such as asbestos and arsenic, this category represents the main group of relevant factors known to cause cancer.

In *The Secret History of the War on Cancer*, Dr Devra Davis refers to the second Cancer Congress in Brussels in 1936. She reports that the discussions that took place revealed a significant level of knowledge about the causes of cancer, including the awareness that certain industrial compounds were carcinogenic. One compound that is specifically mentioned is benzene, the safe level of which was conceded in 1948 by the American Petroleum Institute to be zero. Yet, more than half a century later, benzene remains a widely-used industrial chemical, even though it has been officially classified by the IARC as a Group 1 carcinogen.

Dr Davis also cites a 1949 article written by Groff Conklin and published in the journal *Scientific American*. The article, entitled *Cancer and Environment*, refers to the increase in cancer mortality since 1900; it also refers to investigations that were being conducted in the effort to explain the increased incidence of the disease and states that these were,

> "...being sought in an environment so much more complex than it was in 1900. The investigation is focused on carcinogenic agents..."

The 'environment' has become even more complex and far more polluted in the intervening decades since 1949. However, although most chemicals remain untested, one of the effects most commonly tested for is carcinogenicity, which means that the list of proven carcinogens continues to expand. The list of Group 1 carcinogens includes vinyl chloride, trichloroethylene, PCBs and TCDD, all of which are toxic organochlorines.

Nevertheless, despite their known toxicity and carcinogenicity, these compounds, and many more, continue to be widely used by industry; this means that the workplace is a major source of regular exposure to both toxins and carcinogens. The level of exposure that each person may experience in their workplace will inevitably vary according to the type of industry and the nature of the substances to which they may be exposed; however, certain industries can involve significant risks of exposure; as Dr Epstein explains in *The Politics of Cancer*,

> "Various categories of workers are at high risk of exposure to carcinogens."

Some of the industries he refers to in which workers can be exposed to carcinogens include mining, metal processing and smelting, all of which are industries that have a long history, often over many centuries. However, although the industries of the past utilised very different processes from those of modern industries, they would all entail exposures to a variety of naturally-occurring 'poisons', many of which have been discovered to also be carcinogenic. Gold mining, for example, is known to expose miners to both mercury and arsenic; in addition, the disposal of 'tailing' wastes into the local environment will also expose the residents of mining areas to carcinogenic substances. These exposures have occurred throughout history and therefore provide a credible explanation for the incidence of cancer in the distant past, as well as in the present.

The rapid growth of industrialisation in 'Western' countries has significantly increased the volume and concentration of environmental pollutants, including many that are carcinogenic. However, the increasing complexity of the combinations of toxic and carcinogenic substances that now pervade the environment, makes it impossible to identify any single factor as the main cause of the phenomenal rise in the rate of cancer, especially since the mid-20th century.

There are many difficulties entailed in devising methods to determine whether a particular carcinogen has caused a specific case of cancer; these difficulties arise to a certain extent from the virtual absence of any safety testing procedures conducted prior to the release of a chemical onto the market. The absence of direct evidence that a substance is carcinogenic does not mean it is safe. Proof of harm caused by any substance is frequently obtained from epidemiological studies, which are always conducted in the complex real-world environment after the substance has been released onto the market. Epidemiological studies are often able to indicate the existence of a correlation, but they are rarely able to find direct evidence of a causal relationship.

More importantly, cancer is rarely caused by exposure to a single carcinogen; except in certain circumstances, it will develop as the result of long-term exposures to many different toxic substances. The sources of these exposures can vary widely, as Dr Epstein indicates,

> "The toxic and carcinogenic chemicals to which workers may be exposed at relatively high concentrations in the workplace also are discharged or escape into the air and water of the surrounding community. The worker may be exposed to the same chemical carcinogens through consumer products and the general environment as in his or her workplace."

In the 'real-world' environment, it is the complexity and variety of combinations of toxic substances to which people are regularly exposed, that denies epidemiological investigations the ability to demonstrate the existence of a clear and direct relationship between a specific exposure and the development of cancer in the exposed population. This difficulty was exploited by the tobacco industry for decades in their efforts to refute the claim that there was a direct link between smoking and cancer.

Nevertheless, there has been the occasional incident that has enabled a direct causal association to be proved; one such incident was the disaster that occurred in Bhopal, India. This tragic event involved the exposure of a huge number of people to an extremely high level of a specific and highly toxic gas. As will be further discussed in chapter eight, this event has resulted in a substantially increased incidence of and mortality from a number of different types of cancer in the region.

The difficulties of establishing a direct causal link between cancer and a specific carcinogenic substance allows the relevant industry to claim that there is 'doubt' about such a link, which also means that liability for the harm caused can be avoided. This point is explained by David Michaels in his aptly titled book *Doubt is Their Product*,

> "Except for a few very rare instances in which a disease is unique to an exposure, such as mesothelioma caused by asbestos, epidemiologists cannot state that a specific chemical exposure has definitely caused the cancer of a specific patient."

In addition, people who live in the vicinity of certain industries are also exposed to toxic and carcinogenic wastes discharged into the environment, as Dr Epstein explains,

> "Living near petrochemical and certain other industries in highly urbanized communities increases cancer risks, as evidenced by clustering of excess cancer rates; high levels of toxic and carcinogenic chemicals are deliberately discharged by a wide range of industries into the air of surrounding communities."

The discussions in chapter six showed that the pharmaceutical industry is one of those responsible for polluting the environment with toxic effluent.

Exposure to carcinogens also occurs in the home from the use of everyday consumer products, including those intended for use with babies and small children. Dr Epstein provides one example in *Toxic Beauty*,

> "For instance, many baby soaps, baby shampoos and bubble baths hide a carcinogenic contaminant called 1,4-dioxane in a range of ingredients known as ethoxylates."

Ethoxylates are surfactants that are used in many detergent-type products.

Although 1,4-dioxane is not a member of the family of dioxins, it is listed as a Group B2 carcinogen; which means it is a 'probable human carcinogen' and should not therefore, be an ingredient of any consumer products, especially those intended for babies and small children.

Dr Epstein explains that a number of ingredients commonly used in baby products have been proven to induce cancer in laboratory animals. These are significant findings, because it is widely acknowledged by the scientific research community that any substance shown to induce cancer in animals must be regarded as a potential, if not actual, human carcinogen. Whilst this may tend to argue for the continuation of animal testing, it is a poor argument; mainly because many chemicals remain in use as product ingredients, despite being tested and shown to demonstrate carcinogenicity. The claim that animal testing leads to products that are 'safe' for human use is clearly unfounded.

Talcum powder is another product that is frequently, although not exclusively used on babies; it is also a product that, according to Dr Epstein, has been shown to induce cancer in laboratory animals and is 'strongly linked' to ovarian cancer. But, although the link is only to that particular type of human cancer, the fact that talcum powder is linked to cancer in animals has implications for other forms of cancer of the female reproductive system, such as cervical cancer for example.

There are other personal care products used regularly by girls and women that are of significant concern because of their toxic and potentially carcinogenic ingredients; these products include, but are not restricted to, sanitary towels and tampons plus feminine deodorants and wipes. The ingredients of these products can include bleaching agents, which usually contain chlorine-based chemicals, and 'fragrance chemicals', which commonly contain phthalates, some of which are known to be carcinogenic. These chemicals are far more plausible as factors that contribute to cervical cancer than the non-living particles that have been called 'viruses'.

Any carcinogenic compound that is an ingredient of a product applied to the skin has the ability to promote the development of cancer; as discussed, the skin can absorb chemicals that are able to enter the bloodstream and spread to various organs and systems of the body. It should be clear, therefore, that the problem is not exclusive to women; men and boys who apply products that contain toxic and carcinogenic ingredients to their genital area, can be similarly at 'risk' of developing a form of cancer of the reproductive system; prostate cancer, for example. According to the NHS, the cause of prostate cancer is unknown, although unusually it is not claimed to be linked to any 'infection'.

Interestingly, it was discovered that young chimney sweeps in 18th century England were prone to scrotal cancer, which was shown to be directly linked to their constant exposure to soot from the chimneys; soot contains various hydrocarbons, some of which have since been identified as carcinogenic. It was not solely their exposure to soot; their risk of developing cancer was exacerbated by a combination of factors that included their extremely poor personal hygiene, because they rarely washed, as well as the extremely poor and insanitary conditions in which these boys would invariably have lived. This example further refutes the idea that cancer is a disease of 'ageing'. One of the most common childhood cancers is leukaemia; however, a page entitled *Do We Know What Causes Childhood Leukemia?* on the website of the ACS (American Cancer Society) makes the familiar claim that,

"The exact cause of most childhood leukemias is not known."

Nevertheless, the ACS makes another familiar assertion that the 'risk factors' for leukaemia include a 'genetic factor' as well as environmental risk factors that include 'radiation and certain chemicals'. Leukaemia is a cancer of the blood cells; the most common form of leukaemia is ALL (acute lymphoblastic leukaemia). According to the medical establishment, the causes of ALL are also largely 'unknown'; however, a 2013 article entitled *Acute lymphoblastic leukaemia* published in *The Lancet* states that,

"Ionising radiation is an established causal exposure for ALL..."

Furthermore, the NHS web page about ALL refers to known risk factors that are said to include previous chemotherapy treatments for 'unrelated cancers'; the page also refers to specific chemotherapy 'medicines' that may have been used for those other cancers. The link between chemotherapy 'treatments' and the development of cancer is extremely important and will be discussed later in this section.

After decades of denial, it is now widely accepted by the medical establishment that ionising radiation is extremely dangerous; furthermore, all forms of ionising radiation are classified as Group 1 carcinogens.

Although less dangerous than ionising radiation, non-ionising radiation is also associated with many harmful effects, including cancers, even though this link is still denied by the medical establishment. This denial has been discussed, but it is demonstrated by the CDC web page about childhood leukaemias that contains a section entitled *Uncertain, unproven or controversial risk factors*, which lists one of these factors as 'exposure to electromagnetic fields'. The idea that an association between leukaemia and exposures to EMFs is uncertain, unproven or even controversial is unfounded; there is ample evidence that EM radiation is associated with an increased risk of cancer; as demonstrated by the IARC classification of RFR and EMR as Group 2B carcinogens.

There are, however, known associations between non-ionising radiation and cancers other than leukaemia; as indicated by Dr W Ross Adey MD, who, in his article entitled *Electromagnetic fields, the modulation of brain tissue functions – A possible paradigm shift in biology*, states that,

"Epidemiological studies also suggest a relationship between occupational exposure to environmental EM fields and breast cancer in women and men."

In addition, he makes the salient points that exposures are always multiple and that EM radiation can interact synergistically with chemicals,

"Environmental EM fields may act jointly with exposure to environmental chemicals with known cancer-promoting actions in enhancing brain tumor risks."

The point cannot be over-emphasised that the human body is both biochemical and bioelectrical in nature and that these 'systems' are intimately interconnected; any influence that disrupts one system will inevitably disrupt the other. It is also important to emphasise that disease, especially cancer, is mostly the result of multiple exposures to harmful factors usually over the course of many years, if not decades.

In his previously cited article entitled *Evidence of Health Effects of Electromagnetic Radiation*, Dr Neil Cherry refers to an association between reduced levels of melatonin and cancer. He also discusses the results of studies that he refers to as,

"...sufficient to classify a causal relationship between EMR and breast cancer, with melatonin reduction as the biological mechanism."

The BioInitiative Report 2012 contains many articles that refer to an association between EMF exposures and cancers; for example, a 2003 article refers to aneuploidy that occurred when human lymphocytes had been exposed to EMFs and noted that,

"The effects were non-thermal."

Another BioInitiative Report 2012 article, entitled *Use of Wireless Phones and Evidence for Increased Risk of Brain Tumors*, refers to the vulnerability of children and states that,

"The developing brain is more sensitive to toxins and it is still developing until about 20 years of age."

This is an extremely important point as it highlights the reason that mobile phones pose a far more significant health hazard to children and young people under the age of 20; the article further explains that,

"Children have smaller heads and thinner skull bone than adults. Their brain tissue has also higher conductivity and these circumstances give higher absorption from RF-EMF than for adults."

The *Summary for the Public* section of the BioInitiative Report 2012 contains a reference to the existence of different studies which have shown that,

"...children who start using a mobile phone in early years have more than a 5-fold (more than 500%) risk for developing a glioma by the time they are in the 20-29 year age group."

Gliomas are referred to as 'aggressive malignant tumours'; the establishment definition of a glioma is,

"any tumour of non-nervous cells (glia) in the nervous system."

The definition also states that the term may be used to refer to all tumours in the central nervous system. Although a glioma is different from leukaemia, they are both 'cancers' that have developed in different parts of the body. Leukaemia is defined by the medical establishment as,

"any group of malignant diseases in which the bone marrow and any other blood-forming organs produce increased numbers of certain types of white blood cells."

As previously cited, the ACS states that the exact cause of leukaemia is unknown, but it is claimed to involve 'risk factors' that include 'certain chemicals', which, despite vehement denial by the medical establishment, include the toxic ingredients of vaccines that enter the bloodstream and poison the blood. The link between vaccines and cancer can be demonstrated from two incontrovertible facts. Firstly, at least two vaccine ingredients, namely mercury and formaldehyde, are known carcinogens. Secondly, despite the assertion that vaccines are safe, they are not evaluated for their carcinogenicity; a fact that can be ascertained by reference to vaccine package inserts. The pertinent phrase common to all package inserts is that the relevant vaccine,

"...has not been evaluated for carcinogenic, or mutagenic potential, or potential to impair fertility."

The failure to evaluate the carcinogenic effects of vaccines means that the medical establishment cannot claim there is no association between vaccines and cancer.

Furthermore, the age range during which vaccines are administered is closely followed by the age range in which ALL, the most common form of leukaemia, frequently occurs; as reported on the web page entitled *Acute Lymphoblastic Leukaemia* that states,

"There is a peak in incidence in children aged two to three years; more than half of all children diagnosed with acute lymphoblastic leukaemia are under the age of five years."

An association between mercury and leukaemia was also substantiated by Dr Hal Huggins, as discussed in chapter six in the example of the child whose leukaemia disappeared after the removal of her amalgam fillings.

Although the medical establishment in general has a poor level of knowledge about the processes involved in the development of cancer, some scientists are developing a better understanding of this disease. These scientists include, most notably, Dr David Rasnick and Dr Peter Duesberg who together have investigated the aneuploidy theory of cancer, which states that all cancers develop as the result of chromosomal errors.

This is not a new theory; it was first introduced by David von Hansemann in 1890 and first formally stated by Dr Theodor Boveri in his 1914 book originally published in German and subsequently translated into English in 1929. More information about the development of the theory is available from Dr Rasnick's website.

A clear example of problems caused by chromosomal changes is Down's syndrome; the previous discussion about this condition explained that it is caused by a single error in the smallest chromosome. Chromosomal errors also occur in cancers; however, Dr Rasnick explains the difference between Down's syndrome and cancer in his previously cited article, in which he states that,

"With Down's, the defect occurs in the germ line and so the chromosomal error is present in every cell in the body."

As discussed in the section about Down's syndrome, cells in the germ line are those that develop into the reproductive cells, which are the primary cells from which the human body develops.

In cancer, however, Dr Rasnick explains that the defect,

"...occurs in a particular cell after the body is formed."

This distinction is extremely important.

Drs Rasnick and Duesberg are not the only scientists to have made the connection between aneuploidy and cancer. Although her work mainly focused on exposing the dangers of endocrine disrupting chemicals, Dr Theo Colborn also recognised the existence of aneuploidy. On the Our Stolen Future website is an article entitled *What is aneuploidy and why is it important?* that explains the correlation between aneuploidy and cancer,

"Another type of aneuploidy, 'mitotic' aneuploidy, is associated with virtually all solid tumor cancers."

It is clear therefore, that any disruption to the normal processes of cell division that produce a 'defect' within any of the chromosomes passed to the daughter cells, will result in aneuploidy. Meiotic aneuploidy produces birth defects; mitotic aneuploidy produces cancer. It is also clear that any 'factor' that can cause 'mitotic' aneuploidy must be defined as a carcinogen; as Dr Rasnick states,

"In fact, all carcinogens that have been examined so far do cause aneuploidy."

This does not solely refer to 'chemical carcinogens', it also applies to those referred to as 'physical carcinogens', especially ionising radiation, which has been proven to cause chromosomal damage; in other words, aneuploidy. Ionising radiation is both teratogenic and carcinogenic, which demonstrates the existence of a direct and close relationship between aneuploidy, birth defects and cancer.

Another factor associated with cancer is a high level of 'free radicals', as indicated by the previously cited article entitled *Drug-Induced Oxidative Stress & Toxicity* that states,

"Tumour cells have high levels of ROS, and studies have shown elevated levels of oxidative stress and/or oxidative DNA damage in human malignancies relative to normal cells."

In summary, therefore, the development of cancer involves a combination of interrelated factors, which are toxins, oxidative stress, cell damage and chromosomal errors.

Although the WHO predicts that the incidence of cancer will continue to rise in the foreseeable future, it is not inevitable that this dire prediction will become reality. The WHO is, however, optimistic about achieving a reduced mortality rate in the claim that,

"Cancer mortality can be reduced if cases are detected and treated early."

This claim is misleading; most forms of cancer have poor survival rates after treatment, which means that early detection and treatment does not reduce the risk of mortality or guarantee survival; the main reason for poor survival rates is due to the nature of the 'treatments'. The most common forms of 'treatment' are surgery, chemotherapy and radiation, all of which are based on the erroneous theory that cancer is a disease that must be fought and 'killed'.

Furthermore, two of the 'treatments', namely chemotherapy and radiation, are acknowledged to be carcinogenic, which means they have been proven to cause cancer. The basis for their use as a 'treatment' is that they are believed to 'target' and kill cancer cells; the inability of any treatment to 'target' specific cells, including cancer cells, has been discussed. These treatments are also claimed to be tailored to the patient so that they receive the right 'dose' that will kill the cancer but not them; this is another misguided application of the Paracelsus fallacy. Unfortunately, these treatments do not solve the problem, as demonstrated by the large number of people who have not survived, despite being treated for their cancer. Clearly, some people do survive, but they do so despite the treatment, not because of it.

Chemotherapy is carcinogenic, which means that it can cause cancer, as indicated by the previously cited example in which the NHS claims that many cases of ALL are caused by 'previous chemotherapy'. Cancer that has been caused by carcinogenic substances cannot be 'cured' through the use of carcinogenic substances; these treatments only exacerbate the body burden of toxins, and therefore contribute to a worsening of the problem or to a 'return' of the disease, usually in a more aggressive form.

This highlights another poorly understood aspect of cancer; the 'return' of the disease, or 'metastasis' as it is called; the WHO fact sheet explains that,

> "One defining feature of cancer is the rapid creation of abnormal cells that grow beyond their usual boundaries, and which can then invade adjoining parts of the body and spread to other organs, the latter process is referred to as metastasizing."

Metastasis frequently occurs in a different organ or site from that of the 'primary' cancer; it is for this reason that it is also referred to as a 'secondary' cancer. The medical establishment view of metastasis is that the original cancer was not completely eradicated by the treatment and that the cancer cells have migrated to a new location in the body. However, this cannot be the case; the idea that cancer cells 'spread' to other parts of the body and 'invade' other organs is erroneous as it completely contradicts cell biology. The establishment definition of a cell includes the statement that,

> "Complex organisms are built up of millions of cells that are specially adapted to carry out particular functions. The process of cell differentiation begins early on in the development of the embryo and cells of a particular type (e.g. blood cells, liver cells) always give rise to cells of the same type."

The flawed establishment understanding about metastasis is recognised, albeit to a limited extent, in a January 2017 article entitled *Gene discovery could shed light on how cancer cells spread*, which admits that,

> "...the underlying mechanisms that control how cancer cells spread aren't well understood."

Cell specialisation means that cells of one organ do not 'spread' to another organ.

Interestingly, metastasis does not seem to be a 'natural progression' of cancer in laboratory animals, as explained by Dr Tony Page in *Vivisection Unveiled*,

> "... artificially carcinogen-challenged laboratory animals do not normally develop metastases at all."

This is a significant comment that also highlights one of the major problems with the use of animals in disease research experiments; which is that the disease under investigation is often induced by artificial methods.

This means therefore that researchers are unlikely to be studying the same 'disease'. The creation of artificial diseases means that it is not possible to draw meaningful conclusions for human health from the results of animal experimentation; this is one of the most potent arguments against the use of animals for disease research studies.

One of the most common sites of a 'secondary' cancer is the liver, which, as previously discussed, is the body's major detoxification organ. Liver cancer therefore results from an excess body burden of toxins that the body is losing its ability to process and eliminate; these toxins will include the chemicals used as chemotherapy 'medications'. This means that the 'treatment' invariably contributes to metastasis. Unfortunately, a secondary cancer is frequently 'treated' with further doses of chemotherapy or radiation, or both. This additional toxic onslaught far too frequently results in the death of the patient, who is then reported as having 'lost their battle with cancer'. In reality, the patient has lost their battle against the accumulation of toxins, which include the substances that caused the original cancer, in addition to those used as 'treatments'.

The recognition that these treatments often fail to save the patient encourages the cancer research community to continue the search for the elusive cancer cure. Despite the reference to 'infections' as causal factors of cancer, there are new theories that bizarrely contemplate the use of 'germs' as potential cancer 'treatments'. An October 2015 article entitled *Cancer-fighting viruses win approval* was published as a news item on the website of the journal *Nature*; the article states,

"On 27 October, the Food and Drug Administration (FDA) approved a genetically engineered virus called talimogene laherparepvec (T-Vec) to treat advanced melanoma."

There are many problems with this approach, not least of which is that it involves genetic engineering, a technology that has been shown to be an uncertain, unpredictable and imprecise process that has the potential to be extremely dangerous. The discussion in chapter six indicated that the outcome of genetic engineering experiments cannot be controlled; a problem, which, together with the inability to reach the specified 'target', raises serious concerns about these 'treatments' that are to be introduced into human bodies.

The investigation of 'viral' treatments for cancer arose from observations that tumours would occasionally regress when patients had experienced symptoms of an 'infection', especially a fever. These observations do not prove that viruses are the cause of infections nor do they prove that viral infections can 'cure' cancer. Furthermore, this approach directly contradicts the claim that 'infections' are major contributory factors to the development of cancer.

The symptoms of an 'infection' are indicative of the body's efforts to detoxify and eliminate the toxins as waste. The resulting 'remission' in cancer following an 'infection' demonstrates a number of important points, which are: that cancer is directly related to toxic build up in the body; that detoxification is an important aspect of recovering from cancer; and that the body is capable of self-healing.

Bacteria are similarly implicated as causal factors of cancer; helicobacter pylori for example, is claimed to be a cause of gastric cancer. Yet investigations are also being conducted to determine if bacteria may also have the potential for use as cancer 'treatments'. These investigations also involve genetic engineering methods on the basis that they will be able to express the required property in the bacteria; there are clearly many problems with this area of research.

It is abundantly obvious that the medical establishment has not won the 'war on cancer'. But it was inevitable that they would lose this war, because the approach they employed is based on flawed theories that consider it appropriate to use carcinogenic treatments to 'kill' the disease; an approach that has only succeeded in exacerbating the incidence of and mortality from cancer. Unfortunately, the problem is not exclusive to cancer; the medical establishment possesses a flawed understanding about the mechanisms involved in all chronic diseases; as has been demonstrated by this chapter and as will be further discussed in chapter ten.

It is possible to avoid cancer; but to do so requires a completely different understanding of the disease. As this discussion has demonstrated, cancer develops mainly as the result of long-term exposures to a variety of toxic, as well as carcinogenic, substances and influences, most of which are the products, wastes and emissions of a wide variety of industries; as Dr Epstein explains in *Toxic Beauty*,

> "...a strong body of scientific evidence demonstrates that, apart from carcinogenic ingredients in consumer products, the predominant cause of the modern cancer epidemic is directly related to petrochemical and nuclear industry technologies and their environmental pollutants."

It should be noted that non-ionising radiation must also be included as a contributory factor to the 'modern cancer epidemic'.

It is imperative that the flawed medical establishment approach to cancer is replaced by an approach based on a genuine understanding of the disease, in order to prevent the anticipated continual rise in the incidence of and mortality from this disease.

Furthermore, it must be recognised that cancer is not a 'disease entity' that attacks the body; but, instead, is a manifestation of damage within the body.

In *Natural Hygiene: Man's Pristine Way of Life*, Herbert Shelton provides an exquisitely simple explanation of cancer in the statement that,

> "Cancer does not attack. Cancer evolves."

He expands on this by adding,

> "Cancer does not develop in a normal body. This is to say, a genuinely healthy body will not evolve cancer."

The meaning of the phrase 'genuinely healthy body' has implications for all 'diseases'; as the discussions in chapter ten will reveal.

Chapter Eight

Global Issues: The Wider Perspective

*"Economic development can proceed without a concomitant
decrease in environmental quality if it is based on an
appropriate, ecologically benign production technology."*

Barry Commoner

The United Nations (UN) was founded in 1945 at the end of WWII; its
Charter was signed by the representatives of 51 countries that became the
first group of Member States. UN Membership has grown in the post-war
years to the extent that it now includes virtually every country recognised
to be a sovereign state. At the time of writing, there are 193 UN Member
States and 2 Non-Member States with observer status. The original central
mission of the UN is stated on the web page entitled *What We Do* to have
been,

"...the maintenance of international peace and security."

Although there has not been a world war since 1945, there have been many
conflicts throughout various regions of the world that have involved
military personnel from many countries. It cannot, therefore, be claimed
that the UN has been entirely successful in maintaining international peace.

It is beyond the intended scope of this chapter to discuss war, except to
emphasise that its consequences are always detrimental for the
overwhelming majority of people. In addition to the physical damage it
causes, war also causes serious damage to the people who survive; it
adversely affects both the physical and mental health of civilian populations
as well as participating troops.

The UN mission, like its membership, has also grown; the web page
entitled *Overview* in the series of pages entitled *About the UN*, explains its
wide-ranging functions,

"Due to the powers vested in its Charter and its unique international character,
the United Nations can take action on the issues confronting humanity in the
21st century, such as peace and security, climate change, sustainable
development, human rights, disarmament, terrorism, humanitarian and health

emergencies, gender equality, governance, food production, and more."

In addition to the core UN body, the UN system includes many organisations and agencies that are listed on the web page entitled *Funds, Programmes, Specialized Agencies and Others*. The group listed under the sub-heading *Programmes and Funds* includes UNDP (United Nations Development Programme), UNICEF (United Nations Children's Fund), WFP (World Food Programme), UNFPA (United Nations Population Fund), UNCTAD (United Nations Conference on Trade and Development) and UNEP (United Nations Environment Programme). The group listed under the sub-heading *UN Specialized Agencies*, which are described as 'autonomous organizations that work within the UN', includes the World Bank, IMF (International Monetary Fund), WHO and FAO (Food and Agriculture Organization). The most significant organisation under the sub-heading *Other Entities* is UNAIDS (Joint United Nations Programme on HIV/AIDS). The group entitled *Related Organizations* includes IAEA (International Atomic Energy Agency), WTO (World Trade Organization), CTBTO (Preparatory Commission for the Comprehensive Nuclear-Test-Ban Treaty Organisation) and OPCW (Organization for the Prohibition of Chemical Weapons).

The all-encompassing nature of the UN's mission statement, together with its almost total global membership, means that UN policies issued for the purposes of implementing the 'actions' deemed necessary to address the various issues claimed to confront humanity, will affect virtually all aspects of life for the entire population of the world.

The idea that these issues are 'global' is used to justify the implementation of 'global' solutions that follow a coordinated strategy based on a 'consensus' about each of these problems. However, problems can only be resolved when their nature is fully understood and their root causes have been correctly identified; it is for this reason that the UN policies that are intended to resolve the issues that confront humanity, should involve strategies that will address and rectify their root causes. But, as the discussions in this chapter will demonstrate, a number of these issues are not fully understood and their root causes have not been correctly identified. Solutions based on a flawed understanding of a problem and its causes will not only fail to resolve it, they will almost inevitably exacerbate the problem.

One of the key aspects of many current UN strategies is 'development', which is perceived to be synonymous with 'civilisation' and an improved quality of life; the main UN organisations concerned with the issue of 'development' are UNDP and UNCTAD. UNDP was established in 1965 from the merger of the United Nations Expanded Programme of Technical Assistance and the United Nations Special Fund. According to the UN web page that describes the various programmes and funds, UNDP works,

> "...to eradicate poverty, reduce inequalities and build resilience so countries can sustain progress."

The page explains the role of UNDP in development policies and strategies,

"As the UN's development agency, UNDP plays a critical role in helping countries achieve the Sustainable Development Goals."

UNCTAD was created in 1964 and is described on the UN page as,

"...the United Nations body responsible for dealing with development issues, particularly international trade – the main driver of development."

The *About UNCTAD* page on the UNCTAD website states that,

"We support developing countries to access the benefits of a globalized economy more fairly and effectively."

The problems with the view that 'globalisation' is the driving force behind development and is beneficial to 'developing' countries are discussed in a number of sections within this chapter.

The addition of the adjective 'sustainable' to the term 'development' is claimed to have originated from the 1972 Club of Rome publication entitled *Limits to Growth*. Although regarded as only one of the major issues facing humanity in the 21st century, 'sustainable development' is central to many UN programmes, as it is claimed to be interconnected to virtually all of the other issues that need to be resolved.

Countries have all been categorised according to their stage of development and are all referred to as either 'developed' or 'developing'; the latter term was originally created to describe countries that had not achieved 'industrialisation'. In addition, the term 'least developed country' (LDC) was created in the 1960s as a means of identifying countries that were regarded as 'in most need'. The term LDC remains in use; in 2017, according to the UN website, 47 countries were listed as LDCs. Countries are also categorised according to their 'income', which refers specifically to GNI (Gross National Income) per capita. This classification system, produced each year by the World Bank, contains four categories; low, lower-middle, upper-middle and high.

The failure of a country to achieve an adequate level of 'development' is generally perceived to be the result of its 'primitive' nature; but this is a mistaken perception, as Barry Commoner explains in *Making Peace With the Planet*,

"Their characteristic condition – large and rapidly growing populations; grinding poverty; desperate efforts for economic development, now hampered by huge debts – is not the outcome of a 'primitive' past."

A key characteristic of countries referred to as 'developing' or 'least developed' is that many of them are former colonies of European countries; as Dr Commoner also explains,

"...a fact about developing countries that is often forgotten: they once were, and in the economic sense often still remain, colonies of more developed countries."

One of the main activities of colonising countries involved the appropriation of the resources of the colonised country; these resources were then utilised or traded, or both, for the benefit of the colonisers. In many instances, these resources, or the profits from trading them, were transferred out of their country of origin, which not only depleted the resources of the colonised countries, it also impoverished the indigenous population. A number of 'developed' countries have achieved their advanced level of development, in part at least, as the result of the resources of their former colonies.

One of the many examples of such an exploitation of resources is the conquest of 'America' by Europeans, especially the Spanish, Portuguese and British, as discussed in chapter four. The plunder of valuable materials, especially gold and silver, and their removal to European countries, as well as the brutal treatment of the native population, substantially depleted the resources and peoples of these regions, many of which remain 'economic colonies' of developed countries, as described by Dr Commoner.

Another example is the plunder of India's resources by the British; initially by the East India Company (EIC) and later by the British establishment when India became part of the British Empire. It is widely recognised that, prior to the arrival of the EIC, India had a variety of thriving industries, all of which were substantially diminished, if not totally destroyed during the colonial period. The wealth of the EIC and the British establishment was gained at the expense of the Indian people.

The colonisation of a number of African countries during the 'Scramble' of the 19th century, mainly by Britain, France, Germany and Belgium, provides further examples of the exploitation of resources for the benefit of colonising countries at the expense of the native populations. The plunder of many African countries had, however, begun a few centuries prior to the 19th century when African people had been enslaved. Although colonisation cannot be held solely responsible for the current difficulties of most African countries, it is certainly a significant contributory factor; the majority of countries categorised by the World Bank as 'low-income' are within Africa and many of them are former colonies of European countries.

These are by no means the only examples of plunder and exploitation of a country's resources for the economic benefit of another country, but they are sufficient to illustrate that a lack of development in former colony countries cannot be attributed to their 'primitive' past or people. The 'failure' to develop owes its origin, to a certain extent at least, to the rapacious and acquisitive nature of small groups of people who perceive it to be perfectly acceptable to seize power, in order to gain control over the resources of another country and to also make immense personal fortunes in the process.

It is important to emphasise that this exploitation of resources by small groups of people has not ceased; it remains an ongoing process although in a different guise, as the discussions in this chapter as well as chapter nine will demonstrate.

Regardless of their stage of 'development', all UN Member States have agreed to the implementation of the UN 'sustainable development' agenda. This agenda began in 1992 with Agenda 21, was followed in 2000 by the Millennium Development Goals (MDGs) and in 2015 by the Sustainable Development Goals (SDGs), all of which are briefly outlined below.

Agenda 21

The United Nations Conference on Environment and Development (UNCED) was held in June 1992 in Rio de Janeiro, Brazil. The main outcome of this conference, also known as the Earth Summit, was 'Agenda 21', which, according to the UN web page entitled *Agenda 21*,

> "...is a comprehensive plan of action to be taken globally, nationally and locally by organizations of the United Nations system, Governments and Major Groups in every area in which human impacts on the environment."

The *Preamble* to the Agenda 21 document, available from the UN website, begins with the profound statement that,

> "Humanity stands at a defining moment in history. We are confronted with a perpetuation of disparities between and within nations, a worsening of poverty, hunger, ill health and illiteracy, and the continuing deterioration of the ecosystems on which we depend for our well-being."

This is immediately followed by an overview of the measures claimed to be necessary to address this dire situation in the statement that,

> "However, integration of environment and development concerns and greater attention to them will lead to the fulfilment of basic needs, improved living standards for all, better protected and managed ecosystems and a safer, more prosperous future. No nation can achieve this on its own; but together we can - in a global partnership for sustainable development."

The desire to improve the living standards for everyone is indeed a noble and worthwhile goal; but whatever measures have been implemented under Agenda 21 since 1992, they have largely failed. Living standards have improved for a few, but not for the overwhelming majority of people who still suffer from poverty, hunger and ill health. The disparities within nations between the 'rich' and the 'poor' have not been addressed by Agenda 21; instead, there is an ever-widening wealth gap in virtually every country. The number of extremely wealthy people has grown to the extent that, according to reports, there are more than 2 million millionaires and in excess of 2,000 billionaires in the world. But, in contrast to this wealth, is the more than 1 billion people who are reported to live not just in poverty, but in extreme poverty.

The 351 pages of Agenda 21 detail the many diverse areas that are perceived to require attention in order to achieve the UN's 'developmental and environmental' objectives. Of particular importance to health is chapter 6, which is entitled *Protecting and Promoting Human Health* and begins with the statement that,

> "Health and development are intimately interconnected."

The chapter discusses a number of activities that relate to health matters and refers to the WHO as the appropriate international organisation to coordinate all health-related aspects of the agenda. Two of the programme areas listed as requiring attention are 'control of communicable diseases' and 'reducing health risks from environmental pollution and hazards'. The section entitled *Control of communicable diseases* makes the familiar but erroneous claim that,

> "Advances in the development of vaccines and chemotherapeutic agents have brought many communicable diseases under control."

The rigid adherence to the 'germ theory' is one of the medical establishment's major flaws. The retention of the belief in 'pathogenic microorganisms' has not only prevented an understanding of the true nature of disease, it has also prevented the identification of the real causes of disease. The failure to understand diseases and their root causes has inevitably led to the use of totally inappropriate measures to address them.

Interestingly, the section entitled *Reducing health risks from environmental pollution and hazards* recognises that environmental pollution and health are related to development in the statement that,

"The overall objective is to minimize hazards and maintain the environment to a degree that human health and safety is not impaired or endangered and yet encourage development to proceed."

This dilemma is common to a wide variety of issues, including the use of toxic substances to kill 'pathogens' as well as the many vectors claimed to carry 'pathogens'; vector-borne diseases are discussed later in this chapter.

Human health hazards and environmental degradation are not inevitable consequences of 'development', as indicated by Barry Commoner's quote that opens this chapter. These hazards only exist as the result of 'development' that has entailed the use of toxic substances and hazardous technologies and been accompanied by a blatant disregard for the environmental and health consequences of their use and disposal.

Although other plans have been introduced since 1992, they are not entirely new ones as they all effectively expand upon and extend the 'comprehensive plan of action' of Agenda 21.

Millennium Development Goals (MDGs)

The next phase of the 'development agenda' was introduced in September 2000 when the Millennium Declaration was signed and the Millennium Development Goals (MDGs) were adopted. The eight goals and their related targets were intended to specifically address some of the key issues of the 21st century and to be achieved over the course of a 15-year period.

The UN web page about the Millennium Development Goals refers to these goals as,

"...a blueprint agreed to by all the world's countries and all the world's leading development institutions."

However, although agreed to by all UN Member States, this 'blueprint' was intended for implementation only in 'developing' countries. Under the heading *Values and Principles*, the Millennium Declaration claims that,

"We recognize that developing countries and countries with economies in transition face special difficulties in responding to this central challenge."

The 'central challenge' referred to was,

"...to ensure that globalization becomes a positive force for all the world's people."

It would seem that the UN clearly does not acknowledge that many 'developing' countries may not have faced such a daunting challenge had a significant volume of their resources not been appropriated by colonising countries.

The failure of Agenda 21 to resolve the problem of poverty, especially in 'developing' countries, is demonstrated by the first of the MDGs, which aimed to 'eradicate extreme poverty and hunger'. Of the eight MDGs, three relate to health matters; these are: MDG 4 that aimed to 'reduce child mortality'; MDG 5 to 'improve maternal health'; and MDG 6 to 'combat HIV/AIDS, malaria and other diseases'. It is clear however, that these goals were not achieved; these problems are claimed to persist in many countries and efforts to address them continue to feature in the agenda.

Despite this lack of success, the *Millennium Development Goals 2015 Report* nevertheless claims that, at the expiration of the MDGs, there are reasons to celebrate because,

"Thanks to concerted global, regional, national and local efforts, the MDGs have saved the lives of millions and improved conditions for many more."

This claim cannot be substantiated; one of the key problems highlighted in the report, and acknowledged to require attention, is the continuing lack of adequate data, which clearly raises serious questions about the veracity of the statistics quoted in the report as 'evidence' of the successes and achievements of the MDGs.

Sustainable Development Goals (SDGs)

In September 2015, UN Member States agreed to the next phase of the development agenda; they announced a new Declaration and produced a document entitled *Transforming our World: The 2030 Agenda for Sustainable Development*. This document describes the 17 SDGs and 169 targets of this plan, which will be referred to as the 2030 Agenda. As the title indicates, these goals are to be achieved by the year 2030; however, unlike the MDGs, the SDGs are to be implemented by all UN Member States, not just 'developing' countries. It is for this reason that everyone needs to be aware of the measures that are to be introduced for the attainment of the 2030 Agenda goals. The *Preamble* to the *Transforming our World* document states that the SDGs,

"...seek to build on the Millennium Development Goals and complete what these did not achieve."

The allocation of a mere 15 years for the achievement of 17 goals is certainly ambitious, considering the little that was achieved under the previous plan that only contained 8 goals. Nevertheless, the effort to accomplish these goals is to be intensified, as indicated by the *Introduction* to the document that states,

"We commit ourselves to working tirelessly for the full implementation of this Agenda by 2030."

Under the sub-heading *Our Vision* is the statement that,

"In these Goals and targets, we are setting out a supremely ambitious and transformational vision. We envisage a world free of poverty, hunger, disease and want, where all life can thrive."

This noble-sounding 'vision' certainly recognises some of the fundamental issues that the overwhelming majority of people around the world face on a daily basis. But the key to the success, or otherwise, of this vision is totally dependent on the measures introduced to address those issues; these goals and targets can only be achieved if the proposed measures are able to address the real root causes of the problems to be solved.

Unfortunately, it is unlikely that the world will be freed from 'poverty, hunger, disease and want' by the UN, WHO and other global institutions, because they do not understand the nature and causes of the problems they purport to solve. The reasons for this situation are complex, but are mostly due to the influence exerted by a relatively small group of vested interests, as will be demonstrated in this and the next chapter.

The problems that confront humanity can be resolved, but to do so requires a completely different approach; one that does not rely on global organisations.

It is beyond the intended scope of this chapter to discuss the entire 2030 Agenda. It is, however, necessary to examine a number of goals that have an indirect impact on health as well as those that directly relate to health, in order to demonstrate why these goals cannot be achieved. It should be noted that some of the discussions refer to subjects that have previously been discussed, but are re-examined in this chapter with reference to the wider perspective of the 'global agenda'.

Good Health and Well-Being

The core aim of Goal 3 of the 2030 Agenda is to,

"Ensure healthy lives and promote wellbeing for all at all ages."

This Goal contains 13 targets, each of which pertains to a specific issue deemed necessary to be addressed for the attainment of the overall objective of 'health for all'.

The UN web page that refers to specialised agencies, describes the WHO as,

"...the directing and coordinating authority on international health within the United Nations system."

The *About WHO* page on the WHO website states that,

"We are building a better, healthier future for people all over the world."

As previously cited, the WHO defines health as,

"...a state of complete physical, mental and social well-being and not merely the absence of disease or infirmity."

It may be assumed from all of the above statements, that the WHO has the concomitant knowledge and competence to ensure that the proposed measures will be able to achieve all of the targets of Goal 3 of the 2030 Agenda. This would however, be a mistaken assumption.

As previous discussions have shown, the medical establishment, of which the WHO is the leading 'authority', has, and even admits to having, a poor understanding about chronic diseases, including their causes. Previous discussions have also shown that the medical establishment is mistaken in their belief in 'germs' as the causes of many other diseases. Furthermore, the measures employed are unable to improve health; they cannot 'ensure healthy lives'; nor can they facilitate a 'healthier future' for people.

One of the main reasons these measures cannot succeed is because they rely on an approach that almost exclusively employs pharmaceutical medicines and vaccines to treat and prevent disease; but these products are unable to deliver 'health'. The lack of efficacy of this approach is demonstrated by the increasing incidence of and mortality from disease. More disturbingly, the WHO anticipates that disease morbidity and mortality will continue to rise into the foreseeable future.

It may also be assumed that the goal of 'health for all' is intended to be for the benefit of all; but this too is a mistaken assumption. The underlying purpose of this goal is based on the idea that health and development are interconnected; that the population of a country needs to be healthy to enable 'development' to proceed. The people are therefore viewed purely in terms of their economic usefulness to the country, as indicated by the WHO web page entitled *Health and development* that states,

"...healthy populations live longer, are more productive, and save more."

This statement suggests that, by extension, unhealthy people are less productive, or even unproductive if they are unable to work at all; and that this means they are not only less able to contribute to the country's economy but a financial burden to the country when they require healthcare services. The existence of a significant number of unhealthy people within the population is therefore considered to be an impediment to a country's development and economic growth. This notion is, however, based on a number of assumptions, most notably the assumption that the main purpose of life is solely to contribute to the economy of the country in which a person lives; this is however, a seriously flawed assumption.

Another similarly flawed assumption is that 'health' can only be delivered by 'healthcare systems' that include the provision of pharmaceutical medicines and vaccines, which are promoted as essential as well as safe and effective; as indicated by target 8 of SDG 3 that states the aim to,

"Achieve universal health coverage, including financial risk protection, access to quality essential health-care services and access to safe, effective, quality and affordable essential medicines and vaccines for all."

It is claimed that the provision of 'healthcare services' imposes a financial burden on the economy of a country and that the high cost of healthcare imposes a financial burden on individuals. These financial burdens are claimed to be addressed by universal health coverage; as indicated by the January 2019 WHO fact sheet entitled *Universal health coverage* that states,

"UHC means that all individuals and communities receive the health services they need without suffering financial hardship."

The reason for the inclusion of financial risk protection as a core feature of UHC is that it will enable people to afford the cost of healthcare services when they need them, without precipitating them into poverty or extreme poverty. However, most forms of financial risk protection, through insurance or taxation for example, entail ongoing costs that may still be beyond the means of a significant proportion of the world population; especially the billion or more people who live in extreme poverty. The fact sheet claims the reason for universal health coverage is because,

"At least half of the world's population still do not have full coverage of essential health services."

It is claimed that people in 'poor' countries lack the resources and facilities that are available to people in 'rich' countries, and this encourages the notion that the former should be assisted financially by the latter through 'aid'; as indicated by the WHO web page entitled *Aid for health* that states,

"A key goal of many development agencies, including WHO, is to increase the amount of aid provided by rich countries to poor countries."

The purpose of 'aid' is to provide financial assistance, not only for the creation of facilities, such as hospitals and clinics, but also for the purchase of 'essential medicines and vaccines'. The idea that these 'healthcare services' will have a direct and beneficial impact on the health of the people in poor countries is fatally flawed; better access to 'healthcare services' does not correlate with better health.

The point to be emphasised is that the health of an individual person bears no relationship whatsoever to the state of the economy of the country in which they live. An illustrative example is America, which is classified as a 'rich' country yet millions of Americans suffer poor health despite the huge sums of money spent on healthcare services. Health is not a direct and inevitable consequence of wealth, nor is ill-health an inevitable consequence of poverty. Although poverty and ill-health are related, it is a complex relationship, as will be discussed later in this chapter.

In addition to physical structures such as hospitals, 'health care' also requires sufficient numbers of people who are suitably qualified and capable of providing and administering all of the appropriate services; this requirement is highlighted by SDG 3.7 that aims to,

"Substantially increase health financing and the recruitment, development, training and retention of the health workforce in developing countries."

Most people who join the 'health workforce' do so because they want to help others. However, no matter how well-meaning they are, these health workers will invariably have been educated within the medical establishment system. They will therefore believe in and perpetuate flawed theories, especially with respect to the use of medicines and vaccines in the treatment and prevention of disease. Unfortunately, the 2030 Agenda proposes to commit even greater levels of funding to the development of new pharmaceutical products, as demonstrated by SDG 3b that states the aim to,

"Support the research and development of vaccines and medicines for the communicable and non-communicable diseases that primarily affect developing countries..."

This target clearly intends to ensure that 'medicines and vaccines' remain key components of the 'healthcare services' deemed essential for everyone, everywhere, but especially for people in 'developing' countries.

Medicines for all

The medical establishment claims that 'medicines' are a key component of 'healthcare'; that they are not only appropriate in the treatment of disease, but that they are the only means by which diseases can and should be treated. This claim is, however unfounded. Although the problems with 'medicine' have been discussed in chapter one, they require further examination in the context of the 2030 Agenda.

The chemicals required by the human body to support the biochemical processes that sustain life, need to be the 'right' chemicals and in the 'right' form to be utilised by those processes; chemicals that are not the right ones or are not in the right form cannot be utilised by the body's processes and therefore cannot promote health or sustain life.

Pharmaceutical 'medicines' are not employed for the purpose of providing support to the body's biochemical processes. Instead, they are synthetic compounds produced within the laboratories of the chemical industry for the sole purpose of interfering with certain bodily functions that are believed to be involved in disease processes. But, as previously discussed, any substance that interferes with the body's normal functioning is, by definition, a poison.

It is indisputable that pharmaceutical 'medicines' produce effects, it is their intended purpose to produce an 'effect' on the processes of disease. They are also recognised to produce unintended or unexpected effects, which are referred to as merely 'side effects'; but, as has been discussed, this label is a misnomer. The effects produced by medicines are always detrimental, as can be demonstrated by a perusal of the list of possible 'side effects' with which they may be associated. Although medicines are claimed to produce beneficial effects, this is illusory; as will be discussed in chapter ten.

The failure to fully investigate and understand the functions of the human body means that the medical establishment also fails to appreciate the detrimental effects that result from the use of pharmaceuticals. The onset of new symptoms, in addition to those for which a 'medicine' has been prescribed, is generally regarded as a new condition or disease that requires 'treatment' with yet another 'medicine'. The discussion in chapter one referred to reports about the incidence of iatrogenesis in the US where healthcare is the most expensive in the world, yet many thousands of people are harmed and die every year due to 'medicines' administered correctly; in other words, medicines have been shown not to be safe or effective in one of the richest countries in the world.

Although most studies have investigated the extent of the problem in the US, iatrogenesis is not exclusive to that country; it also occurs in Europe, as indicated by Professor Donald W Light PhD, who states in his 2014 article entitled *The Epidemic of Sickness and Death from Prescription Drugs* that,

> "About 330,000 patients die each year from prescription drugs in the United States and Europe."

Although death is clearly the most extreme outcome, it is not the only one; there are many adverse effects of differing intensity that can be attributed to 'medicines' and they affect a huge number of people'; as indicated by the article that refers to,

> "...about 80 million medically minor problems such as pains, discomforts and dysfunctions..."

These 'minor' problems will be regarded merely as 'side effects' that are likely to be regarded as symptoms that can be treated with other medicines. The use of more than one 'medicine', whether prescription or over-the-counter, is referred to as polypharmacy, which is another increasingly common phenomenon, as previously discussed. Although 'medicines' are claimed to have been subjected to rigorous safety testing, many have been withdrawn from the market when they have been found to produce serious adverse effects that were not discovered prior to their release onto the market. This clearly raises questions about the claims that they had been proven to be safe.

Certain drug combinations have been tested to determine their effects, however, very few have been tested in all of the possible combinations that may be used by patients, especially as increasing numbers of people suffer multimorbidity. The drug interactions that are known may be included on the package insert or the information may be provided by the prescribing physician. There are however, many thousands of pharmaceuticals on the market, including those available over-the-counter, which means that there are innumerable combinations, the overwhelming majority of which are entirely untested.

The pharmaceutical industry claims that the development of a new 'medicine' takes many years. However, the study on which FDA approval of a new drug is based may be conducted over a relatively short period of time and may only involve a relatively small population size; as indicated by a May 2017 article entitled *Postmarket Safety Events Among Novel Therapeutics Approved by the US Food and Drug Administration Between 2001 and 2010* that states,

"The majority of pivotal trials that form the basis for FDA approval enrol fewer than 1000 patients with follow-up of 6 months or less, which may make it challenging to identify uncommon or long-term serious safety risks."

The use of the word 'may' to describe the challenge of identifying the risks is disingenuous; a short-term study by definition cannot identify adverse effects that will occur from long-term use of any pharmaceutical product. Furthermore, most adverse effects caused by pharmaceuticals are identified in the post-marketing period from epidemiological studies or adverse event reports; in other words, the full range of 'iatrogenic' effects are only identified after the 'medicines' have been introduced into the market and taken by large numbers of people.

The failure of the medical establishment to acknowledge that pharmaceutical drugs always produce effects that are not merely 'side effects', means that physicians are not taught to recognise that a patient's new symptoms are almost certain to be the result of their 'medicine'. Although adverse health effects are often notified to an appropriate regulatory agency, notification systems are mostly voluntary and far from comprehensive. However, even when an adverse health event is recognised to have been caused by a pharmaceutical 'medicine', this does not automatically result in its removal from the market. The May 2017 article referred to above discusses the problem and states that,

"Among 222 novel therapeutics approved by the FDA from 2001 through 2010,

71 (32.0%) were affected by a post-market safety event."

But these 'safety events' resulted in only 3 product withdrawals. Interestingly, the pharmaceuticals most affected by a 'post-market safety event' are reported to have included biologics and psychiatric therapeutics. As discussed in chapter seven, biologics are described as medications genetically engineered from a living organism. This is not the only study to have discovered the existence of adverse health effects; a December 2015 article entitled *FDA Safety Reviews on Drugs, Biologics and Vaccines: 2007-2013* found that,

"There were 6930 serious adverse event reports in 181 reviews."

The process of monitoring these 'events' is stated to facilitate,

"...detection of safety concerns that may not be identified in prelicensure clinical trials."

It is abundantly clear therefore, that 'medicines' are not fully tested for all potential adverse health effects during the clinical trials conducted prior to their release onto the market; yet all pharmaceuticals that have been approved by the FDA are claimed to be both safe and effective.

In the drive to provide 'medicines for all', the pharmaceutical industry continues to develop an ever-increasing number of products that are claimed to treat a variety of diseases. The PhRMA web page entitled *Medicines in Development* claims that,

"Since 2000, more than 500 new medicines have been approved by the FDA, helping patients live longer, healthier lives."

This claim fails to recognise that many 'medicines' have been removed from the market due to their harmful effects; it also fails to recognise the existence of 'iatrogenesis'.

The page also contains links to various reports about 'medicines' that are being studied or developed by various American biopharmaceutical research companies. The web page entitled *Medicines in Development for Biologics 2013 Report* claims that 907 medicines and vaccines are in development for biologics that 'target' more than 100 diseases. The PhRMA fact sheet about biologics refers to them as 'large molecule medicines' that are,

"Made by or from living cells and structurally complex..."

The processes by which biologics are derived from living organisms are claimed to involve the production of a 'recombinant protein in living cells', which indicates that they create novel protein structures that do not exist in nature. This means that biologics are not compatible with the body and will not therefore support the biochemical processes that support health and sustain life, even though they are made from 'normal' components of the body. The fact sheet states that,

"Their active ingredients are mainly proteins, such as hormones, antibodies, cytokines, and insulin."

Proteins are essential to sustain life; they are involved in virtually every function within the human body, but they too are incompletely understood by the medical establishment. The fact sheet also makes the important comment that biologics,

"...can never be exactly reproduced or copied like generics."

The significance of this point is discussed later in this section.

The PhRMA page entitled *Medicines in Development for Rare Diseases 2016 Report* reports that,

"...30 million Americans, or 10 percent of the population, have one of the 7,000 known rare diseases..."

In this context, 'rare' means that fewer than 200,000 Americans suffer from the disease in question. As has been discussed, polypharmacy is common in the US, which, if 'medicines' truly worked, ought to mean that Americans would be some of the healthiest people; yet, as the above indicates, many Americans are far from healthy.

As new diseases continue to be discovered, the pharmaceutical industry continues to not only develop new medicines, but to also develop new types of medicine, such as biologics. The creation of new medicines often involves a method called 'high-throughput screening', which utilises highly sophisticated and expensive technology and equipment, including robotics. This method enables a huge number of tests to be conducted at a very rapid rate, which is claimed to facilitate a much quicker identification of an active compound that has a positive effect on a particular 'biomolecular pathway'.

The pharmaceutical industry claims that most investigations do not lead to the development of a new medicine and that this low 'success rate', together with the high costs of the technology and the long development period of each new medicine, justify the high cost of the medicines that do reach the market. The industry also claims that high prices of successful medicines are necessary to ensure the ongoing innovation and drug development essential to the viability of the industry. It should be noted however, that the pharmaceutical industry is an extremely profitable one. In addition to the development and sale of products, the largest pharmaceutical companies maintain their profitability through patents and intellectual property rights, which are discussed in chapter nine; but it should be noted that they both impose restrictions on other pharmaceutical manufacturers, especially those in 'developing' countries that mostly manufacture generic drugs.

There are various debates about the best way to solve the problem of inadequate access to affordable medicines for people who live in 'developing' countries. One solution to the dual problem of inadequate access and high prices has been for 'developing' countries to establish their own pharmaceutical industry. This is perceived to be beneficial for a number of reasons that include: the creation of employment opportunities; economic growth and development; and increased access to affordable medicines claimed to be essential for diseases that primarily affect 'developing' countries.

The creation of a pharmaceutical manufacturing facility requires a huge initial outlay to cover the costs of the manufacturing plant, laboratory equipment and appropriately qualified staff, amongst others; these costs are said to be prohibitive for most 'developing' countries. These difficulties are, however, not insurmountable; many countries categorised as 'developing' have an established pharmaceutical industry. One prominent example is India, which had developed a pharmaceutical manufacturing industry in the early 20th century long before the World Bank classified the country as 'developing'. The pharmaceutical industry in India manufactures mostly generic drugs that are not subject to patents and are therefore more reasonably priced, which makes them more affordable, although not for those who live in extreme poverty, a condition endured by many millions of Indian people.

Another Asian country that has pharmaceutical manufacturing facilities is Bangladesh, which is currently categorised as a 'least developed country', but is reported to be undergoing rapid economic growth that may precipitate a change of status out of this category in the near future. The Bangladeshi pharmaceutical industry will not, however, help to improve the health of the Bangladeshi people, even if they were able to afford the medicines produced by them.

A number of companies in African countries have also been able to overcome the difficulties and establish pharmaceutical manufacturing facilities; as demonstrated by an October 2014 article entitled *Boosting drugs manufacture in developing countries will improve health outcomes, UN investment forum told* that states,

"According to UNCTAD data, South Africa has about 79 pharmaceutical factories, Nigeria 75, Ghana 23, Kenya 17 and Uganda 10 factories."

Despite the fact that industrialisation is regarded as a key component of 'development' and that pharmaceutical manufacturing is a profitable industry, these countries all continue to retain the status of 'developing' countries.

The increased development of biologics, which the PhRMA fact sheet claims cannot be exactly reproduced like generics, will have a significant impact on pharmaceutical manufacturing in 'developing' countries as they will not be able to produce these new types of medicine. This, in turn, will reduce access to 'essential medicines' for the poor people in those countries; which is clearly inconsistent with the goal of the 2030 Agenda to increase access to affordable medicines for people in 'developing' countries.

This does not mean that 'developing' countries should continue to produce affordable medicines, because pharmaceuticals are not only ineffective, they are also harmful. They do not facilitate good health; instead they contribute to ill-health.

A problem of significant concern for 'developing' countries is that pharmaceutical manufacturing utilises toxic raw materials and produces toxic effluent. The NRDC report entitled *Dosed Without Prescription*, cited in chapter six, explains that, despite the existence of stringent environmental regulations in 'developed' countries, pharmaceutical production facilities nevertheless discharge their toxic effluent into local bodies of water, such as rivers. The discussion in chapter six revealed that the high level of consumption of pharmaceuticals in 'developed' countries generates high concentrations of pharmaceutical metabolites and by-products in sewage wastes. The NRDC report in particular, revealed that no available technologies are capable of detoxifying water supplies from the toxic wastes of the pharmaceutical industry.

The problem of water pollution due to pharmaceutical industry effluent will be intensified in countries that lack the ability to prevent the contamination of local bodies of fresh water and lack adequate sanitation facilities. The increased use of medicines will increase the contamination of water, especially bodies of water used by the local population for drinking, which will inevitably exacerbate health problems, not solve them.

It is argued by many people that the 'poor people' of the world ought to be allowed to have easy access to affordable 'medicines'; they also argue that high prices are the major obstacle and that the 'greedy' pharmaceutical companies are mainly to blame for this situation. Although these arguments may seem reasonable, they do not focus on the real issues. All arguments that focus solely on the cost and accessibility of 'medicines' fail to acknowledge that there is a fundamental problem with 'medicines'; that they do not resolve health problems because they are neither safe nor effective; a problem that applies equally to vaccines, the other component of SDG 3.8.

Vaccines for all

The WHO page entitled *10 Facts on Immunization* claims that,

"Immunization prevents between 2-3 million deaths every year."

The July 2018 WHO fact sheet entitled *Immunization coverage* claims that,

"An additional 1.5 million deaths could be avoided, however, if global vaccination coverage improves."

Although bold, these claims cannot be substantiated; they do however, support the aim of the 2030 Agenda to expand vaccination coverage and achieve the ultimate goal of 'vaccines for all'. The main efforts are focused on increasing vaccination coverage in 'developing' countries where 'infectious diseases' are claimed to be more prevalent and the people, especially children, are urgently in need of 'life-saving vaccines'.

It is claimed that an association exists between a country's stage of development and the type of diseases experienced by its population; as indicated by the 2009 WHO *Global Health Risks* report that states,

"As a country develops, the types of diseases that affect a population shift from primarily infectious, such as diarrhoea and pneumonia, to primarily non-communicable, such as cardiovascular disease and cancer."

The logical conclusion from this statement is that highly 'developed' countries ought to experience an extremely low level of 'infectious diseases', if at all; but this clearly is not the case, as revealed by a UK Government paper entitled *UK Trends in Infectious Diseases* that states,

"Infectious diseases are a significant health and economic burden in the UK..."

The UK is categorised as a highly developed country, which means that it should not experience infectious diseases as a significant health problem.

Although there is no explanation for the existence of a relationship between 'infectious diseases' and a low stage of development in a country, the *Global Health Risks* report claims that the 'shift' away from infectious diseases is the result of three factors, one of which refers to 'public health interventions' that include vaccination programmes. One of the reasons these interventions are claimed to be related to 'development' is because their costs require a country to have a sufficient level of 'income' to afford them, but 'developing' countries are said to be unable to meet these costs. This is, however, unfounded; as can be demonstrated by the example of India, where vaccination programmes, have existed since the beginning of the 19th century; yet India was, and still is, categorised as a 'developing' country and currently has a 'lower-middle' income status.

One of the many organisations that promote the 2030 Agenda goal to increase access to affordable vaccines in order to save lives, especially for people in 'developing' countries, is GAVI (Global Alliance for Vaccines and Immunizations), now referred to as the Gavi Alliance, which is described on the web page entitled *About GAVI* as,

> "...a global Vaccine Alliance, bringing together public and private sectors with the shared goal of creating equal access to new and underused vaccines for children living in the world's poorest countries."

The Gavi Alliance includes the WHO, UNICEF and the World Bank.

African countries, especially those in the sub-Saharan region of the continent, are particular targets for increased vaccine coverage; as demonstrated by a 2015 article entitled *WHO strives to provide universal access to immunization in the African Region by 2020*, which states the aim to,

> "...ensure that every child in the African Region has access to life-saving vaccines."

The article also claims that,

> "It is estimated that over three million children under five years of age die each year in the Region and a significant number of these deaths could be prevented by vaccines."

As previously discussed, vaccines do not prevent death; they have however, been proven to be dangerous for babies and small children whose health has been compromised by the unhealthy conditions in which they live. This has been demonstrated by physicians who have worked in parts of the world where people live in such conditions. In a 1995 interview, Dr Archie Kalokerinos MD, who worked with the Aboriginal people and children of Australia, stated that,

> "You cannot immunise sick children, malnourished children, and expect to get away with it."

It would seem that the medical establishment does expect to 'get away with it'; as demonstrated by the drive to increase vaccination coverage in 'developing' countries where millions of sick and malnourished children live. The health problems that are often considered to be indicative of 'infectious diseases', but are in fact associated with and often the direct result of poor living conditions, are not exclusive to 'developing' countries; they are increasingly common within the urban slums of 'developed' countries.

Surprisingly, the medical establishment promulgates conflicting advice about whether children who are unwell should be vaccinated. The UK NHS web page entitled *Myths about children's vaccines* states as a 'fact' that,

> "...you should postpone your child's jab if they are ill and have a fever (high temperature)."

By contrast, the US CDC web page entitled *Vaccines when your child is sick* refers to the recommendation that,

> "...children with mild illness can usually receive their vaccinations on schedule."

'Mild illness' is described as including a 'low grade fever'.

In addition to the claim that 'infectious diseases' are associated with a low stage of development, is the idea that they are associated with poverty; as indicated by a 2012 report entitled *Global Report for Research on Infectious Diseases of Poverty*, which was prepared by the TDR (Special Programme for Research and Training in Tropical Diseases) in association with the WHO. This report, which will be referred to as the *Infectious Diseases of Poverty* report, makes the interesting and significant claim that,

> "Infectious diseases of poverty are not restricted to low and middle-income countries, but manifest in poor populations globally."

The report states that almost 9 million people, including many children under the age of five, are killed by these diseases each year. In addition, the report states that more research is needed on the basis of the claim that,

> "Stepping up research into their causes and how to effectively treat them and prevent them from spreading could have an enormous impact on efforts to lift people out of poverty and to build a better world for future generations."

Although the report recognises that certain diseases are associated with 'poor living conditions', it makes the erroneous claim that this association occurs because 'germs' thrive in such conditions and that the proliferation of these 'germs' enables them to spread throughout the population. The efforts to prevent these diseases will inevitably include vaccination programmes.

It should be noted that the 'germs' alleged to be the causes of the diseases prevalent in 'developing' countries include various bacteria, many of which have been found within the bodies of healthy people. For example, respiratory infections, especially pneumonia, are claimed to be a significant health problem for children in 'developing' countries. One of the main 'pathogens' claimed to be responsible for pneumonia is *Streptococcus pneumoniae*, a bacterium that is admitted to be found in healthy children and therefore cannot be the cause of pneumonia. Nevertheless, a March 2015 joint press release by the WHO, GAVI, UNICEF and GPEI (Global Polio Eradication Initiative) entitled *Children in Bangladesh to benefit from dual vaccine introduction* states that,

> "Pneumonia is one of the leading causes of child mortality in Bangladesh..."

This claim cannot be substantiated because autopsies are not a common practice in Bangladesh; furthermore, according to a 2001 article entitled *Causes of childhood deaths in Bangladesh: an update,*

"...very few deaths are attended by a qualified physician."

The article states that the causes of death in Bangladesh are ascertained from 'verbal autopsy reviews' that provide information about the symptoms suffered by the child prior to death. But these 'reviews' cannot substantiate the claim that the disease had been caused by the relevant bacterium nor can they prove that the death can be definitively attributed to 'pneumonia'. Nevertheless, the belief that 'pneumonia' is a major health problem for children in Bangladesh resulted in the introduction, during 2015, of the PCV (pneumococcal conjugate vaccine) that is claimed to prevent pneumonia caused by *Streptococcus pneumoniae*.

Despite the claim that vaccines prevent disease and save lives, there is a large and growing body of evidence that demonstrates vaccines are significant contributory factors to illness and death. Most cases of illness and death after the administration of vaccines involve babies and small children under the age of five, who are subjected to ever-increasing numbers of vaccines that are claimed to protect them from disease.

The medical establishment vehemently denies that vaccines cause damage, except in very 'rare' cases, and justifies this with reference to the millions of vaccines that are administered each year without any adverse effects. This denial is disingenuous; it fails to recognise that the reactions referred to as 'normal', such as fever and pain at the injection site, are evidence of harm caused by the vaccine; these effects are not a sign that the vaccine is 'working' but a sign that the body has reacted to a substance that it regards as toxic. Furthermore, a single exception to a rule invalidates the rule. The death of a single child from a procedure claimed to be protective is a profound tragedy.

In addition to this most extreme outcome, are the many other 'effects', which can vary from subtle and barely perceptible to severe and serious, such as those that may be labelled as 'autism', ADD or ADHD. Some effects may become noticeable soon after the administration of the vaccine; others may not become apparent until weeks, months or even years have elapsed. The most important point to emphasise is that the introduction of toxic and neurotoxic materials into the body can only be detrimental to health.

The purpose of 'immunisation' is to eradicate 'infectious diseases'; yet, despite the practice having existed for more than two centuries, the only human 'infectious disease' that is claimed to have been successfully eradicated is smallpox. But this is hardly a cause for celebration, as the number of 'infectious diseases' claimed to exist has risen dramatically over the same period of time.

Nevertheless, as the discussions in chapter two indicated, the medical establishment claims that polio is very close to eradication. According to the March 2019 WHO fact sheet entitled *Poliomyelitis*, there were 33 reported cases in 2018; interestingly however, earlier versions of the fact sheet indicate that this does not represent a continuing decline in numbers; the April 2017 fact sheet reported the number of cases at 37; whereas the number of cases reported in the March 2018 fact sheet was 22. It is nevertheless claimed that there has been an overall decrease of 99 per cent in the number of cases since 1988 when the intensive polio vaccination campaign was launched. The 2019 fact sheet also makes the bold claim that,

"Polio vaccine, given multiple times, can protect a child for life."

The 'success' of the polio vaccine is said to be illustrated by the example of Pakistan, which had been regarded as the most polio-endemic country. According to the web page entitled *Polio in Pakistan*, this country has experienced a vast reduction in cases of paralysis due to 'wild poliovirus'; the numbers have fallen from 306 in 2014, to 20 in 2016 and only 3 in 2017.

Unfortunately, the WHO fact sheet, as well as other sources that report the 'success' of the polio eradication campaign, fail to refer to the phenomenal increase in the incidence of AFP and, more recently, NFAFP (non-polio acute flaccid paralysis) in many countries. This problem is highlighted by a 2012 article entitled *Polio programme: let us declare victory and move on*, written by two Indian medical doctors and published in the Indian Journal of Medical Ethics; the article states that,

"...while India has been polio-free for a year, there has been a huge increase in non-polio acute flaccid paralysis (NPAFP)."

The doctors refer to NFAFP in their article as being,

"Clinically indistinguishable from polio paralysis but twice as deadly..."

The information reported in the article was compiled from the National Polio Surveillance Project, which is claimed to show,

"...that the non-polio AFP rate increases in proportion to the number of polio vaccine doses received in each area."

The OPV contains 'live' but attenuated viruses; this is claimed to mean that the vaccine can shed viruses, which may spread to other people and cause further cases of polio and paralysis. But viruses are not living organisms; they cannot 'infect' people; they cannot cause disease; they cannot cause paralysis.

Although viruses are not the cause, it must not be assumed that oral vaccines cannot cause paralysis; the discussion in chapter two showed that many vaccine ingredients are neurotoxic and therefore eminently capable of producing neural damage and paralysis. The fact that the OPV is not injected does not mean it is incapable of causing neurological damage and paralysis. The risk of paralysis following the oral polio vaccine is acknowledged by a May 2014 WHO information sheet entitled *Observed Rate of Vaccine Reactions. Polio Vaccines* that states,

"Despite its many advantages, OPV carries the risk of vaccine-associated paralytic poliomyelitis (VAPP) particularly among infants..."

The situation has been exacerbated by the creation of yet another 'condition', called acute flaccid myelitis (AFM), which is regarded as a different form of AFP. The CDC web page entitled *Acute Flaccid Myelitis* states that it affects the nervous system and has,

"...a variety of causes such as viruses..."

The CDC makes the claim that this condition can be prevented by certain actions,

"...such as staying up-to-date on vaccines..."

Although some cases of paralysis have occurred after the administration of the polio vaccine, other cases have occurred after the administration of other 'medicines'. A February 1997 article entitled *Paralytic poliomyelitis in a rural area of north India* reported in the *National Medical Journal of India* refers to the identification of 37 cases of paralysis during a study conducted between 1990 and 1991 and states that,

"Of these...60% had a history of intramuscular injections preceding paralysis."

These injections were administered for the control of fevers. Although 37 is a relatively small number of cases of paralysis, the fact that 60 per cent had received a prior injection is not insignificant. Furthermore, the article also states that,

"The prevalence of paralytic poliomyelitis in the villages surveyed was high despite a stepping up of the national immunization programme."

There are other substances, in addition to vaccines, antibiotics and drugs, that contain neurotoxic substances and are capable of inducing paralysis that may be labelled 'polio', AFP, NPAFP or AFM; these include pesticides and toxic chemicals, such as formaldehyde. It should be noted that DDT was not banned in India and that formaldehyde is one of the products of the Indian chemical industry. Lead is another neurotoxic substance capable of inducing paralysis; it is also ubiquitous in India. A July 2013 article entitled *Lead poisoning affects 20% Kolkata kids* reported the results of a study conducted in Kolkata, which had discovered that,

"...at least 20% of the city's children are affected by lead poisoning, which is turning out to be a bigger threat than anyone imagines."

One of the main culprits, according to the article, is the leaded paint used on children's toys, although, as previously discussed, there are many sources of exposure to lead. Dr Herbert Needleman states in his 2004 article entitled *Lead Poisoning* that,

"Patients with high blood levels may present with severe intractable colic, motor clumsiness, clouded consciousness, weakness and paralysis."

Unsurprisingly, polio has been described as one of the most feared diseases in industrialised countries, which indicates that it has an association with 'industrialisation'; a connection that is assiduously avoided by the medical establishment. However, increased 'industrialisation' within 'developing' countries will inevitably lead to increased exposures to many toxic and neurotoxic substances.

The promotion of the goal to achieve 'vaccines for all' clearly presents vaccine manufacturers with lucrative opportunities, not only to increase profits from increased sales of vaccines for known diseases, but to develop new vaccines for lesser-known diseases. A January 2017 article entitled *Vaccines for three deadly viruses fast-tracked* refers to the thoughts of scientists on this issue and states that,

"Scientists have named three relatively little-known diseases they think could cause the next global health emergency."

These diseases have been chosen from a list of ten that, according to the article,

"...the World Health Organization (WHO) has identified as potentially causing the next major outbreak."

On the basis of fear-mongering claims of this nature, the pharmaceutical industry continues to develop vaccines to prevent and even, in some cases, to 'treat' a variety of different 'diseases'; as indicated by the PhRMA web page entitled *Medicines in Development for Vaccines 2017 Update* that states,

"Today, there are 264 vaccines in development by America's biopharmaceutical companies to both prevent and treat diseases."

Although vaccines are claimed to be able to prevent 'infectious diseases', only 137 of the 264 new vaccines are for this type of disease; surprisingly, 101 of them are being developed for different cancers.

There is an increasing level of awareness that vaccines are not as safe or as effective as they are claimed to be, but the overwhelming majority of people nevertheless retain the belief that vaccines are necessary to prevent 'infectious diseases', if only they could be made 'safer'. This false belief is based on the equally erroneous theory about 'herd immunity', which claims that 'infectious diseases' can be prevented on the proviso that a sufficiently large percentage of the population has been immunised.

The rigid adherence to the 'germ theory' and to the fallacy that vaccines are 'safe and effective' renders the medical establishment incapable of addressing the real causes of the health problems mistakenly identified as 'communicable diseases', especially in 'developing' countries' where they are claimed to be most prevalent, as the next series of discussions will demonstrate.

Communicable Diseases

Target 3 of SDG 3 aims to,

"By 2030, end the epidemic of AIDS, tuberculosis, malaria and neglected tropical diseases and combat hepatitis, water-borne diseases and other communicable diseases."

It is claimed that the 'communicable diseases' specifically referred to in SDG 3.3 are particularly prevalent in 'developing' countries; a claim that is entirely consistent with the idea expressed in the *Global Health Risks* report which, as cited in the previous section, refers to a correlation between a country's stage of development and the type of diseases that affect its population. By contrast, however, and as also cited in the previous section, the *Infectious Diseases of Poverty* report states that diseases of this nature affect 'poor populations globally'; this means therefore, that they are not exclusive to the poor in 'developing' countries. The term 'infectious diseases of poverty' is stated in the report to refer to,

"...a number of diseases which are known to be more prevalent among poorer populations rather than a definitive group of diseases."

This description is somewhat vague and decidedly unhelpful in identifying the diseases to which it is intended to refer; nevertheless, the report indicates that 'poor people' are more vulnerable to certain diseases due to their 'social and economic deprivation', which is claimed to mean that these people,

"...have a greater exposure to the risk factors for disease..."

On the web page entitled *Risk factors* the WHO describes a 'risk factor' as,

"...any attribute, characteristic or exposure of an individual that increases the likelihood of developing a disease or injury."

The 'risk factors' referred to on the web page are: underweight; unsafe sex; high blood pressure; tobacco and alcohol consumption; and unsafe water, sanitation and hygiene. It should be obvious that these 'factors' are not exclusive to 'developing' countries, nor are they exclusive to poor people. The reference to 'risk factors' as necessary for the development of a communicable disease is not consistent with the 'germ theory', which claims 'germs' are the causes of disease and can infect anyone, anywhere; it does not state that 'risk factors' must also be present. Furthermore, the purpose of vaccination is to stimulate the body to produce antibodies against the 'germs' claimed to be the causes of disease; vaccines are not claimed to have any effect on the 'risk factors' that contribute to the development of communicable diseases.

There are clearly many anomalies, inconsistencies and contradictions within the 'information' promulgated by the medical establishment about communicable diseases; but the problem is even more fundamental than this. In all fields of scientific enquiry, empirical evidence should always take priority; theories are supposed to explain phenomena in the 'real world'. The 'germ theory' and the prevailing narratives about 'infectious diseases' do not correlate with or provide explanations for the evidence garnered from the real world, and especially from 'developing' countries.

A 2014 article entitled *The contribution of vaccination to global health: past, present and future* states that the majority of deaths from infectious diseases during the 1960s occurred in the 'developing world' where vaccine coverage was low; it also states that the vaccines that were administered were,

"...restricted largely to children of the small, wealthy section of the community, the group at least risk of a serious outcome from an infection such as measles."

Although the article fails to explain why children in the wealthy section have a much lower risk of 'a serious outcome from an infection', it does acknowledge, albeit in a limited manner, that the decline in child mortality in 'industrialised' countries is not attributable to vaccines, but that it is,

"...associated with improvements in housing, nutrition and sanitation."

The contribution to improved health from these and other measures introduced into 'developed' countries was discussed in chapter two. It would therefore seem that these measures, in addition to others discussed in this chapter, are the 'factors' that ought to be promoted by health organisations such as the WHO for urgent implementation in 'developing' countries. Measures that are known to be associated with improved health should certainly be given a far higher priority than vaccines, which are proven to be hazardous to health, not supportive of it.

Unfortunately, the medical establishment continues to produce large numbers of voluminous reports that refer to an unacceptably high level of morbidity and mortality from various diseases, especially 'communicable diseases', for the purpose of promoting 'medicines and vaccines for all'. The *Infectious Diseases of Poverty* report is a pertinent example, as it claims that almost 9 million people died in 2008 from 'infectious diseases'; however, and most significantly, the report adds the revealing comment that,

> "Given the sketchy data, misdiagnosis and under-detection that are typical of health systems in impoverished areas, these numbers are almost certainly underestimated."

The existence of 'sketchy data' is further supported by the statement in the report that,

> "...in November 2011, Dr Margaret Chan, Director-General of the World Health Organization stated that "At present, some 85 countries, representing 65% of the world's population, do not have reliable cause-of-death statistics.""

The paucity of data about mortality and the causes of death remains a problem that is further substantiated by the *WHO World Health Statistics 2017* report that states,

> "...only 38% of all global deaths are currently reported to the WHO Mortality Database..."

These statements raise fundamental questions about the veracity of mortality statistics quoted by health organisations, especially the WHO; they also raise questions about the reliability of statistics about the incidence of specific disease conditions, many of which are acknowledged to be difficult to diagnose accurately. Although statistics are admitted by the medical establishment to often be estimates, the most significant point is that people in 'developing' countries who suffer ill-health cannot be restored to health by pharmaceutical products; the provision of 'medicines and vaccines for all' will lead to an increased incidence of iatrogenic illness and death, it will not lead to improved health.

Although a number of 'infectious diseases' were discussed in chapter four, those specifically referred to in SDG 3.3 as 'epidemic' require further examination, especially with respect to their prevalence in 'developing' countries. These discussions will also examine some of the genuine health problems suffered by people who live in these countries, in order to ascertain their real causes and thereby provide suggestions for some of the measures by which ill-health can be properly addressed.

As with earlier chapters, the definition of each disease referred to as the 'establishment definition' are from the 2007 edition of the Oxford Concise Medical Dictionary, unless otherwise stated.

Hepatitis

The establishment definition of hepatitis refers to,

> "inflammation of the liver caused by viruses, toxic substances, or immunological abnormalities."

The definition also refers to 'infectious hepatitis', which is regarded as the most common form of the disease and usually caused by one of five 5 different types of 'hepatitis virus' identified by the letters A to E. Each type

491

of hepatitis infection, which is determined by blood tests that detect 'antibodies' specific to each type of virus, is associated with different symptoms and outcomes. The most significant infections are those claimed to be caused by hepatitis B and hepatitis C viruses; as indicated by the WHO web page entitled *Hepatitis* that states,

"...viral hepatitis B and C infections are key causes of primary liver cancer – the second most common cancer in the world."

The July 2018 WHO fact sheet entitled *Hepatitis C* states that,

"Hepatitis C virus (HCV) causes both acute and chronic infection."

The fact sheet indicates that 'acute' HCV infection is not a serious health problem,

"Acute HCV infection is usually asymptomatic, and is only very rarely (if ever) associated with life-threatening disease."

An 'asymptomatic infection' is a contradiction in terms; the medical establishment defines an infection as an invasion by a pathogen, which, by definition, causes a disease, which, by definition, involves recognisable signs and symptoms.

Unlike acute infection, 'chronic' HCV infection is claimed to be serious; but even this does not always lead to a life-threatening disease, as the fact sheet also states,

"Of those with chronic HCV infection, the risk of cirrhosis of the liver is between 15-30% within 20 years."

There is no explanation for the claim that a 'chronic infection' can take up to two decades to develop into a serious health problem; liver problems can, however, be explained by other causal factors, most notably 'toxic substances', as indicated by the establishment definition.

The fact sheet refers to the three remaining 'viruses' and claims that hepatitis A does not cause chronic liver disease; that hepatitis E is mainly self-limiting; and that hepatitis D only occurs in the presence of hepatitis B. It would seem therefore that the hepatitis B virus is the cause of the most serious form of liver 'infection'; a view that is confirmed by the July 2018 WHO fact sheet entitled *Hepatitis B* that refers to it as a 'major global health problem' and states that,

"Hepatitis B is a potentially life-threatening liver infection caused by the hepatitis B virus (HBV)"

Vaccines have, so far, only been developed for hepatitis A and B; but only the latter is included in most routine infant vaccination schedules, as the fact sheet states,

"The hepatitis B vaccine is the mainstay of hepatitis prevention. WHO recommends that all infants receive the hepatitis B vaccine as soon as possible after birth, preferably within 24 hours."

The reason for the urgency to administer this vaccine is based on the idea that the virus is often transmitted from the mother to the baby at birth.

The web page entitled *Hepatitis B Vaccine* indicates that the HBV vaccines used in the UK contain 'a small amount of aluminium' and may also contain 'tiny traces' of formaldehyde. Previous discussions have referred to the hazardous nature of both of these substances. The page also reveals that the

HBV vaccine contains a viral protein produced using recombinant DNA technology; in other words, genetic engineering. The discussion about GMOs in chapter six demonstrated that genetic engineering is imprecise and unpredictable and has been associated with serious health effects. The long-term health consequences of injecting material produced using genetic engineering techniques into the bodies of newborn babies have yet to be revealed; the use of such technology for vaccines is a relatively recent phenomenon.

It is reported that hepatitis B infection is potentially 'life-threatening'; yet the fact sheet makes the surprising statement that,

"Most people do not experience any symptoms during the acute infection phase."

It is claimed that 'acute' infection can, however, cause extremely unpleasant symptoms for some people and these may include: yellowing of the skin and eyes (jaundice), extreme fatigue, nausea and vomiting. These symptoms are certainly indicative of liver problems, but they are not caused by any 'virus'. Surprisingly, the fact sheet states that there is no specific treatment for the acute stage of hepatitis B infection, but the recommendation by the WHO is to provide 'adequate nutritional balance' and to replace lost fluids. It should be noted that chronic HBV infection is not diagnosed by the presence of the virus, but by the persistent presence of the hepatitis B 'antigen'; and that, according to the fact sheet, chronic HBV infection only develops into cirrhosis or cancer in 'some' cases.

Unlike acute infection, the chronic form is said to be treatable with 'medicines', including oral antivirals such as tenofovir and entecavir, both of which are recommended by the WHO. Tenofovir is a drug that is more commonly prescribed for the treatment of 'HIV infection', although it is claimed to be equally 'effective' for HBV. However, according to the AIDSinfo pages on the NIH website, this drug,

"...can cause serious life-threatening side effects."

One of the serious 'side effects' of tenofovir involves 'severe liver problems'; the fact that this drug is known to cause liver damage would indicate that tenofovir is entirely unsuitable for use as a 'treatment' for liver disease. The common side effects associated with entecavir are no better; they include nausea and vomiting, which are two symptoms commonly associated with hepatitis B; this drug is also reported to cause 'severe liver symptoms'. Yet again, this is a drug that can cause the very symptoms it is intended to 'treat'. These drugs are both clearly dangerous, but they do not even have the ability to 'cure' the disease; as the fact sheet states,

"In most people, however, the treatment does not cure hepatitis infection, but only suppresses the replication of the virus. Therefore, most people who start hepatitis B treatment must continue it for life."

The parts of the world considered to be most affected by infection with the hepatitis B 'virus' are the WHO Western Pacific Region and the WHO African Region; it is claimed that approximately 6 per cent of the populations in each of these regions are 'infected' with hepatitis. The Western Pacific Region, which includes countries such as Australia, Cambodia, China, Japan, Malaysia, Singapore and New Zealand, is said to bear the highest burden of hepatitis B. According to the WPRO web page, the Western Pacific region is home to approximately 25 per cent of the world's population, but,

"...it accounts for more than 50% of the hepatitis-related deaths worldwide."

Statistics of this nature are used to justify the introduction of hepatitis B vaccination programmes that are claimed to have been 'successful'; as indicated by the WPRO web page entitled *7 Million Deaths Averted through Hepatitis B Vaccination*. This 'success' is stated to be a step towards the achievement of the 2030 Agenda goal to eliminate hepatitis. Another WPRO article entitled *Delivering additional interventions to eliminate mother-to-child transmission of hepatitis B in the Western Pacific* states that the elimination of hepatitis B infection will occur with the attainment of the target of,

"...0.1% hepatitis B surface antigen (HBsAg) prevalence among children..."

The article also claims that the three doses of the vaccine induce,

"...protective antibody levels in more than 95% of infants. However, perinatal infection still occurs, especially among infants born to mothers with high hepatitis B viral load."

The main concern about 'infection' with hepatitis B is that it is claimed to lead to liver cancer; however, previous discussions have demonstrated that the mechanism of action of cancer is completely different from that attributed to an 'infection'.

The liver is the body's main detoxification organ; a 'problem' within this organ therefore indicates that its ability to function normally has been impaired, most likely as the result of an excess body burden of toxins. The liver problems caused by an excess of toxins can be illustrated by the known association between a high consumption of alcohol over a prolonged period of time and cirrhosis, which can progress to liver cancer. However, alcohol is by no means the only toxic substance that adversely affects the liver; others can cause more serious damage far more quickly than alcohol.

Although the medical establishment claims that the infectious form of hepatitis is far more common, it is clear that 'toxins' contribute significantly to liver damage and that exposures to 'carcinogens' are able to precipitate primary liver cancer, without the need to invoke the existence of a 'virus'. The liver is recognised to have many different and extremely important functions, including detoxification; interestingly, a June 2012 article entitled *Toxic hepatitis in occupational exposure to solvents* identifies this role as applying equally to 'drugs',

"The liver is the main organ responsible for the metabolism of drugs and toxic chemicals..."

The article also states that occupational exposures to hepatotoxins are numerous and that these substances include organic solvents, some of which have previously been discussed and shown to be the source of health hazards from occupations such as dry cleaning. The article refers to a few more occupations in which exposures to solvents can occur; they include chemists, health care workers and nurses. The idea that these occupations are hazardous to health may be surprising, considering that the nature of the work is to assist people to a better state of health. The hazards associated with these occupations arise predominantly from the hazardous nature of the chemicals, including solvents, with which 'medicines' are manufactured. In addition, the article refers to a number of industrial processes that involve the use of, and therefore exposures to, organic solvents. The article adds that,

"...a number of industrial chemicals are known to be hepatotoxins..."

Some of the chemicals identified as hepatotoxic are trichloroethylene (TCE), xylene, toluene and chloroform, amongst others.

Interestingly, the article also refers to inflammation as a common feature of toxicity and to oxidative stress as the mechanism by which pathological changes occur.

There are also a number of 'medicines' that have been shown to be hepatotoxic. Although referring to 'hepatitis', the Mayo Clinic web page entitled *toxic hepatitis* lists many 'drugs' that are hepatotoxic, they include: over-the-counter pain relievers, such as paracetamol/acetaminophen, aspirin and ibuprofen, as well as prescription medications such as statins, azathioprine and certain antivirals, such as tenofovir, which is used in the treatment of hepatitis B infection.

The fact that many of the chemicals and solvents recognised to be hepatotoxic are commonly used in industrial processes means that increased 'industrialisation' within 'developing' countries is likely to be accompanied by increased levels of genuine liver problems.

Influenza

Influenza is not one of the diseases specifically referred to in SDG 3.3, but it is claimed to be a global phenomenon, as indicated by the November 2018 WHO fact sheet entitled *Influenza (Seasonal)* which states that,

"Seasonal influenza is an acute respiratory infection caused by influenza viruses which circulate in all parts of the world."

The fact sheet also states that,

"Worldwide, these annual epidemics are estimated to result in about 3 to 5 million cases of severe illness and about 290,000 to 650,000 respiratory deaths."

As discussed in chapter four, it is claimed that the epidemic referred to as the '1918 Flu' was a 'global health problem'; that an estimated 500 million people worldwide were 'infected'; and that the number of people who died is estimated to range between 20 and 50 million. These estimated numbers of infections and deaths are therefore far in excess of those usually associated with influenza; the 1918 'pandemic' was clearly not one of 'seasonal' influenza. However, the revelation that the medical establishment does not have reliable mortality and cause-of-death statistics in the early 21st century raises serious questions about the veracity of the statistics quoted for the influenza 'pandemic' of the early 20th century.

Nevertheless, whatever the accuracy, or otherwise, of the statistics pertaining to the numbers of infections and deaths, the refutation of the 'germ theory' means that the illness referred to as 'influenza', whether of the 'seasonal' or '1918' variety, cannot be caused by a virus. Although some of the factors that contributed to illness and death during 1918 have been discussed, they were mainly those that affected people in Europe and America; the global nature of the 'pandemic' therefore requires further examination to ascertain the factors that would have affected people in other parts of the world.

One of the most significant aspects of the 'pandemic' is that it occurred in the fourth year of the very first 'world' war; a circumstance that cannot be dismissed as irrelevant; this point is highlighted in the *Infectious Diseases of Poverty* report, which makes the extremely important and revealing comment that,

> "Infectious diseases are prevalent among populations living in conflict and war zones."

The 'germ theory' offers no credible explanation for a correlation between 'infectious diseases' and 'conflict and war zones'; the idea that 'germs' flourish amidst death and destruction cannot be substantiated. Although bacteria are saprotrophic, and therefore assist the decomposition of dead matter, they do not cause disease.

One of the factors that can induce morbidity and mortality during war is 'stress', or, more accurately, distress, as will be discussed in chapter ten. Although rarely included in most discussions about the '1918 Flu', the stresses of combat experienced during WWI are discussed in a 1918 article entitled *War Neuroses, Shell Shock and Nervousness in Soldiers* that states,

> "The longer the war goes on, the more it becomes evident how widespread are the effects of functional nervous disease both in combatant troops and in patients hospitalised for any cause."

It is clear therefore that soldiers were not the only people affected by the traumatic experiences of war, nor was the suffering restricted to the war zones. Furthermore, some of the methods used to treat people suffering from shell shock and other nervous conditions were hardly conducive to the restoration of 'health', as indicated by a March 2012 article entitled *Anaesthetic and other treatments of shell shock: World War 1 and beyond* that states,

> "Some British doctors tried general anaesthesia as a treatment (ether and chloroform), while others preferred application of electricity."

Chloroform was abandoned as an appropriate form of anaesthesia when it was discovered to be toxic; it has since been found to be both neurotoxic and hepatotoxic.

One of the main 'treatments' for 'influenza' during that period was aspirin, also known as acetylsalicylic acid. An extract from a November 2009 article entitled *Salicylates and Pandemic Influenza Mortality, 1918-1919 Pharmacology, Pathology and Historic Evidence* was cited in chapter four, but deserves repetition,

> "Pharmacokinetic data, which were unavailable in 1918, indicate that the aspirin regimens recommended for the 'Spanish influenza' predispose to severe pulmonary toxicity."

Severe pulmonary problems were some of the main symptoms experienced by many people who are said to have suffered from 'influenza'; aspirin use therefore contributed to the worsening of people's health. Unfortunately, the article does not specify the use of aspirin beyond America and Europe; it does, however state that,

> "The loss of Bayer's patent on aspirin in February 1917 allowed many manufacturers into the lucrative aspirin market."

The discussion in chapter four also referred to another 'epidemic' that coincided with that of 'influenza', namely lethargic encephalitis (LE), which, according to Dr Peter Breggin, affected more than a million people and caused hundreds of thousands of deaths. The significance of the LE epidemic is that it is referred to as a neurological disease, which indicates exposures to neurotoxic substances that would have included the materials used in munitions, as well as the ingredients of nerve gases and vaccines. Shell-shock, lethargic encephalitis, vaccine damage and exposures to neurotoxins are clearly not 'influenza', but it would seem that all conditions of illness during that period, from whatever causes, have been conflated and labelled under the single heading of '1918 Flu'; a disease that is said to have claimed more lives than the war itself.

The war of 1914-1918 was truly a world war; it involved troops that had been recruited from many different countries, most of which were colonies of the major European combatants; especially, Britain and France. The main war zone involved hundreds of miles of trenches across France and Belgium, but many other conflicts also took place, for example, in the Middle East and North Africa, as well as in some of the countries in Eastern and Southern Africa that had been colonised by Germany.

Although many countries are said to have been affected by the '1918 Flu', it is claimed that India was the most affected; as indicated by a 2014 article entitled *The evolution of pandemic influenza: evidence from India 1918-19* that states,

> "The focal point of the epidemic in terms of mortality was India, with an estimated death toll range of 10-20 million..."

In 1918, India was part of the British Empire and also had an established pharmaceutical industry, both of which are likely to have influenced the enthusiasm for the implementation of vaccination programmes in India; as indicated by a 2014 article entitled *A brief history of vaccines and vaccination in India* that states,

> "The early twentieth century witnessed the challenges in expansion of smallpox vaccination, typhoid vaccine trial in Indian personnel, and setting up of vaccine institutes in almost each of the then Indian states."

Cholera and plague vaccines were also used in India, although the extent of their coverage is unknown. However, the claim that vaccine institutes were set up in most of the Indian states indicates that vaccination programmes are likely to have been contributory factors for some of the cases of illness and death attributed to 'flu' in India. The article also refers to one of the common explanations for the alleged 'spread' of the flu throughout the population in the comment that,

"The pandemic is believed to have originated from influenza-infected World War
I troops returning home."

The use of the word 'believed' indicates that there is little, if any, evidence
to support this claim; but there is a major flaw in the idea that returning
troops were responsible for the spread of the '1918 Flu'. This disease is
claimed to have been so deadly that it could kill within days, or even hours.
It is clear therefore that Indian soldiers afflicted by this deadly form of
'influenza' would not have survived the long journey from a European war
zone back to India. Another major flaw in this argument is the lack of data
about the number of Indian people who are claimed to have been 'infected';
as the article reveals,

"Data on influenza cases, while desirable, are unavailable..."

Although data about the incidence of 'influenza' are unavailable, the article
refers to mortality statistics and states that,

"These data show a steep spike in fever mortality in late 1918..."

A 'spike' in fever mortality does not provide conclusive evidence of the
existence of an epidemic of 'flu'. There are many reasons for a fever to occur;
it is one of the body's natural processes to eliminate toxins of some
description.

Indian soldiers were deployed to various parts of the world to assist the
British in the conflict, including Europe where they were also employed in
building and defending trenches. The appalling conditions endured in the
trenches were discussed in chapter four and require no repetition; however,
these conditions must be included as contributing to the illness and death
of men from many different countries, not just Europe; these countries
include India, Africa, the West Indies and China.

Another significant factor is that India experienced what has been
described as a 'crippling drought' during 1918-19; a situation that is said to
have been the result of the El Niño Southern Climatic Oscillations (ENSO),
as reported in a December 2014 article entitled *Malaria's contribution to
World War One – the unexpected adversary* that states,

"The ENSO for 1918-1919 was one of the strongest in the twentieth century."

Malaria is discussed in greater depth later in this chapter, however, a few
details about this disease are relevant to the current discussion. According
to the article, malaria was a significant disease that also existed in 'epidemic'
proportions during the war years; although generally,

"...malaria has received little emphasis..."

The article also proposes that the trenches provided ideal conditions in
which mosquitoes would breed and that this encouraged their proliferation
and therefore the spread of the disease, particularly in Europe where
malaria was not considered to be endemic. The eruption of this disease in
such areas resulted in the introduction of various 'treatments', including,
but not limited to, quinine, which was also used prophylactically. In
common with all pharmaceutical products, quinine produces 'side effects'
that include fever, chills, weakness and breathing difficulties, all of which
are symptoms that have also been associated with the form of 'influenza'

referred to as the '1918 Flu'.

India is not, however, the only country to be affected by the ENSO whenever it occurs, nor was it the only country to have been affected by the strong ENSO of 1918-19; many regions in the southern hemisphere were also affected. Parts of Australia, for example, are reported to have experienced severe droughts between 1918 and 1920. Other regions known to have been affected by the ENSO of 1918-19 include Brazil, Central America, Indonesia and the Philippines, as well as parts of Africa. Adverse health problems in these countries are attributed to influenza; as indicated by a July 2013 article entitled *Mortality from the influenza pandemic of 1918-19 in Indonesia*, which states that,

"For Indonesia, the world's fourth most populous country, the most widely used estimate of mortality from that pandemic is 1.5 million."

Indonesia is an archipelago comprised of many thousands of islands; yet the article offers no explanation why the people of those islands would have been affected by the 'virus'; it merely calculates population losses and indicates that the death toll may have been even greater than the original estimate. The article makes no reference to the ENSO of 1918-19, even though it is widely reported in scientific articles that the ENSO is known to have an effect on the rainfall in Indonesia.

Men from African countries that were colonies of the European countries involved in the war were also drawn into the conflict; as discussed in an article entitled *War Losses (Africa)* that refers to the,

"...vast mobilization of African soldiers and laborers for service in Europe between 1914 and 1918..."

The article states that it was mainly the French who recruited men from their African colonies; however, soldiers and labourers were not the only casualties; the article also claims that,

"...very large, but unknown numbers of African civilians perished during the war."

Some of the reasons that African civilians died include,

"...famine prompted by a lack of manpower to till the fields, and diseases exacerbated by malnourishment..."

The problems created by the recruitment of the strongest and healthiest men from African villages into the war were not solved when hostilities ceased in 1918; they persisted long afterwards, especially in the villages to which the men never returned. Although a paucity of data from Africa means that the actual numbers of casualties and deaths due to the war remain unknown, they are estimated to be approximately one million; a figure that is comprised of more than 250,000 soldiers and labourers plus approximately 750,000 civilians.

The conditions that related to India and Africa during the early 20th century have been discussed in order to serve as examples of the different circumstances that would have given rise to illness and death that is usually, but erroneously, attributed to 'influenza'. These conditions would also have been experienced to varying degrees in other parts of the world affected by the war and the factors referred to in this discussion. It should be clear from the above together with the discussion in chapter four that there are many credible explanations for the morbidity and mortality that have been incorrectly attributed to a viral infection.

The perpetual reference to the huge numbers of deaths due to this 'deadly pandemic' does however serve a purpose; the previously cited claim that all subsequent influenza outbreaks have been caused by descendants of the virus claimed to have caused the 1918 influenza pandemic, enables the propagation of fear and the continued promotion of influenza vaccines in order to prevent a reoccurrence of this 'mother of all pandemics'. The propagation of fear certainly benefits vaccine manufacturers.

It is important to emphasise that the circumstances that existed during the war years were complex and varied; they were however, unique.

HIV/AIDS

The previous discussion about HIV/AIDS revealed that the underlying theory, which claims that a virus called 'HIV' is the cause of a disease called 'AIDS', is fundamentally flawed. Nevertheless, the medical establishment maintains the stance that HIV/AIDS remains 'a major global public health issue'; as indicated by the inclusion of 'AIDS' in SDG 3.3 as one of the epidemics to be 'ended' by 2030.

Although the first 'outbreak' occurred in the US, it is claimed that Africa, and especially sub-Saharan Africa, is the main region in which 'HIV infection' occurs, as the July 2018 WHO fact sheet entitled *HIV/AIDS* states,

> "The WHO African Region is the most affected region, with 25.7 million people living with HIV in 2017. The African region also accounts for over two thirds of the global total of new HIV infections."

One of the most important aspects of 'HIV/AIDS' in Africa is that, in the 1980s and for many years afterwards, a diagnosis of 'AIDS' was based on different criteria from those used in most other countries. Prior to the 'discovery' of AIDS, African people who experienced a significant loss of weight were considered to be suffering from a condition known as 'slim'; but after the 1980s a significant weight loss was perceived to be indicative of 'AIDS'. Although HIV tests were introduced into many countries from the mid-1980s onwards, they remained absent from Africa until relatively recently. The reason for this delay is claimed to be that African countries not only lacked the infrastructure and facilities to conduct widespread testing, they also lacked the finances needed to fund the expensive equipment to process the tests.

The criteria on which a diagnosis of 'AIDS' in Africa was to be made, were, however, determined soon after the initial reports arose about this new 'epidemic'; these criteria were established at a workshop held in Bangui, Central Africa in October 1985. The 'Bangui definition' developed at the workshop claimed that a diagnosis of AIDS relied on the existence of three out of four major clinical signs, one of which was a loss of body weight that exceeded 10 per cent; the others were chronic asthenia, chronic fever and chronic diarrhoea. Asthenia means weakness. In addition to these major signs were six minor symptoms, one of which was a chronic cough. These were not, however, particularly unusual symptoms for African people; as indicated by Professor Charles Geshekter PhD, who states in his 1997 article entitled *Reappraising AIDS in Africa* that,

"Millions of Africans have long suffered from severe weight loss, chronic diarrhea, fever and persistent coughs."

The claim that a combination of these symptoms represented 'AIDS' in an African person, despite the absence of a confirmatory 'HIV test', contrasts vividly with a diagnosis of 'AIDS in virtually every other country, where a positive HIV test result was required before a diagnosis of AIDS could be confirmed. This point is corroborated by Dr Eleni Papadopulos-Eleopulos and Dr Valendar Turner of the Perth Group, who state in their 1995 article entitled *AIDS in Africa?* that,

"Unlike the West, AIDS in Africa is diagnosed without any laboratory tests."

The article refers to a WHO report, which claimed that in the mid-1990s, 2.5 million sub-Saharan Africans had AIDS, but the article adds that,

"However, there is no convincing evidence that millions of Africans are infected with HIV..."

Another 1995 article, entitled *AIDS in Africa: distinguishing fact and fiction*, which was co-authored by Dr Papadopulos-Eleopulos and three colleagues, explains that,

"The evidence for the existence of HIV in Africa is based on the random testing of Africans for the presence of HIV antibodies."

As discussed in chapter four, HIV tests do not detect the presence of a 'virus', they only detect the presence of 'antibodies', which are proteins. That discussion also explained that the main proteins claimed to be associated with HIV, namely p24 and p41, are not specific to HIV, nor are they specific to illness. This means therefore, that the detection of these proteins is meaningless with respect to a person's state of health.

The majority of tests conducted in Africa prior to 2001 were performed in antenatal clinics, as indicated by a 2013 report entitled *Demographic Patterns of HIV Testing Uptake in Sub-Saharan Africa* that states,

"Before 2001, HIV prevalence was estimated from sentinel surveillance systems that monitored HIV rates in pregnant women attending antenatal care."

According to the WHO website, the meaning of 'sentinel surveillance' is that it,

"...deliberately involves only a limited network of carefully selected reporting sites."

The previous discussion explained that pregnancy is one of the 'conditions' known to produce a 'false positive' HIV test result. The selection of antenatal clinics as suitable 'reporting sites', from which to gather information about the prevalence of 'HIV infection' in the general population, can only be described as egregious. The use of data that contain an unknown proportion of 'false positive' HIV test results, has distorted the statistics that form the basis of the claims that Africa is still in the midst of a serious 'HIV infection' crisis. The many conditions that can produce 'false positive' HIV test results include tuberculosis and malaria, both of which are regarded as prevalent in sub-Saharan Africa, but neither of which is caused by the 'infectious agent' with which it is normally associated, as the discussions in the next two sections will demonstrate.

The above cited 2013 report about HIV testing uptake also states that,

> "By 2001, international organizations were examining ways to rapidly increase HIV testing on a global scale and to link HIV-positive individuals to treatment and care."

The expansion of HIV testing has been facilitated by the development of rapid diagnostic test (RDT) kits, which are simpler and do not require expensive technical equipment; they are therefore more easily available to 'resource-poor' areas, such as African countries. However, a 'positive' result on a rapid test is not deemed to be definitive; it is claimed to indicate that further confirmatory tests should be conducted.

In the early 21st century, AIDS is still viewed as a potentially devastating disease in Africa, as indicated by a 2006 article entitled *Understanding the Scourge of HIV/AIDS in sub-Saharan Africa* that states,

> "Sub-Saharan Africa is the epicentre of the HIV/AIDS pandemic and faces an unprecedented devastation."

The prediction of imminent devastation faced by the population of Africa, and especially sub-Saharan Africa, has been a constant theme of the 'information' promulgated since the mid-1980s. The population census reports from many of the African countries claimed to be most affected by 'AIDS' demonstrate otherwise; the evidence from census reports shows that population numbers in these countries have grown, they have not declined as the result of the deadly 'scourge' of AIDS. This evidence is reported by Dr Claus Köhnlein and Torsten Engelbrecht in their 2007 book entitled *Virus Mania*, in which they refer to,

> "...the extreme discrepancy evident between perpetual predictions of horror ('Africa will be depopulated by AIDS') and actual population increases."

The failure of AIDS to decimate the populations of African countries is claimed by the medical establishment to be attributable to the availability of simpler rapid tests, which have enabled increased numbers of people to be tested, and to better and faster access to 'treatment' for those people whose test result is said to be 'positive'.

In September 2015, the WHO issued guidelines that made two recommendations, one of which was that ART (antiretroviral therapy) should be given to everyone 'living with HIV' whatever their CD4 cell count. The second recommendation was for the use of ART as a preventive, by means of PrEP (pre-exposure prophylaxis). This strategy is referred to as 'scaling-up' ART, part of the reason for which is to create a 'standardised approach'; as described in an October 2014 article entitled *Simplification of antiretroviral therapy: a necessary step in the public health response to HIV/AIDS in resource-limited settings*, which states that,

> "...simplified prescribing practices support task shifting of care to nursing and other non-physician clinicians..."

The result of increased testing and treatment is discussed in a 2016 article entitled *HIV Infection and AIDS in sub-Saharan Africa: Current Status,*

Challenges and Opportunities that refers to,

"...major advances in treating HIV, as the availability and rapid scale up of antiretroviral therapy (ART) has transformed what was inevitably a fatal disease to a chronic manageable condition..."

The 'success' of increased access to ART is also reported by the WHO in the fact sheet that states,

"Between 2000 and 2017, new HIV infections fell by 36%, and HIV-related deaths fell by 38% with 11.4 million lives saved due to ART in the same period."

The discussion in chapter four revealed that ART is highly toxic; this 'treatment' cannot save lives.

Nevertheless, the WHO claims that continuing to expand access to ART is at the heart of the efforts to achieve the SDG aim to end the AIDS epidemic by 2030. The idea expressed in the 2016 article cited above that ART has transformed a 'fatal disease' into a 'manageable condition', encourages the notion that people no longer suffer from 'AIDS', but instead are 'living with HIV', the scale of which is still claimed to be considerable; as indicated by the WHO fact sheet that states,

"There were approximately 36.9 million people living with HIV at the end of 2017..."

Although perceived as authoritative, these statistics are not based on actual data. The UNAIDS website contains a July 2017 page entitled *Accurate and credible UNAIDS data on the HIV epidemic: the cornerstone of the AIDS response*, which admits that,

"We don't count people. We can't – many people who are living with HIV don't know that they are, so can't be counted."

The claim that there are people who are 'living with HIV' but unaware of it, is used to instil fear, so that people will be more likely to undergo an 'HIV test' in order to 'know their status'. The discovery of a 'positive' status will then lead to the commencement of 'treatment' with antiretroviral drugs, the purpose of which is claimed to be the suppression of viral replication, which needs to be continued and 'treatment' therefore becomes lifelong. The drugs recommended by the WHO fact sheet for use as ART include dolutegravir, efavirenz, raltegravir, darunavir and ritonavir. The AIDS Info website provides information about these drugs and refers to them all as being able to cause 'serious life-threatening side effects' that may include liver problems; in other words, they are all inherently toxic. Yet these highly dangerous drugs are claimed to be 'life-saving' and able to protect people from an 'infection' with a 'virus', that has never been scientifically proven to cause any disease.

One of the significant effects associated with the use of ART is referred to as IRIS (immune reconstitution inflammatory syndrome), which is described in a 2011 article, appropriate titled, *The Immune Reconstitution Inflammatory Syndrome*, which refers to it as,

"A paradoxical clinical worsening of a known condition or the appearance of a new condition after initiating antiretroviral therapy in HIV-infected patients..."

The article claims that the incidence of IRIS is 'largely unknown' and states,

"Despite numerous descriptions of the manifestations of IRIS, its pathogenesis remains largely speculative."

There is, however, a very clear explanation for the 'paradoxical' phenomenon referred to as IRIS; which is that it occurs as the direct result of the ingestion of toxic drugs; it is therefore not a 'paradox', nor should it be referred to as a 'syndrome'.

Unfortunately, the fact that pregnancy can give rise to a 'false positive' HIV test result, means that many pregnant women are inappropriately diagnosed as 'living with HIV' and 'treated' with highly toxic drugs, as the WHO fact sheet states,

"Global ART coverage for pregnant and breastfeeding women living with HIV is high at 80%."

Against this seeming 'success' must be contrasted the evidence that ART does not save lives, but instead these drugs cost lives; as indicated by a 2008 article entitled *Early mortality among adults accessing antiretroviral treatment programmes in sub-Saharan Africa* that refers to,

"...early mortality rates in sub-Saharan Africa are very high; between 8% and 26% of patients die in the first year of ART, with most deaths occurring in the first few months."

Although these deaths are attributed to a variety of causes, including other diseases, this is obfuscation, as it diverts attention from the logical conclusion that these deaths are the direct result of ART. Whilst toxic drugs may not be the sole cause, they cannot be dismissed as irrelevant to an 'early mortality' that occurs soon after the initiation of 'treatment' with drugs that are known to be toxic.

There are many reasons that people in Africa and other 'developing' countries experience a variety of illnesses; poverty, malnutrition, lack of clean water and lack of basic sanitation are some of the contributory factors, as are toxic medications, but these are not the only relevant ones. One particularly significant factor that is generally omitted from discussions about the prevalence of 'disease' in 'developing' countries, is exposure to a wide variety of toxic chemicals produced and used by various industries. A May 2001 article entitled *The ticking time bomb: toxic pesticide waste dumps* states that,

"Huge stocks of toxic pesticide waste are a serious problem in almost all developing countries..."

The stocks referred to are not merely excess pesticide stock intended for use against the pests of these countries, they also refer to pesticides that have been dumped in 'developing' countries, because they have been banned in 'developed' countries or because they have passed their expiry date. These banned, old or obsolete pesticides are often delivered to 'developing' countries under the guise of 'aid', but this is also used as a ploy by donor corporations to avoid the proper, but expensive disposal of these highly toxic chemicals. The article also states that,

"The waste sites contain some of the most dangerous insecticides in existence. They include aldrin, chlordane, DDT, dieldrin, endrin and heptachlor, which have been banned in most countries, along with organophosphates."

The article refers to pesticide waste sites that are frequently situated near farms, wells, dwellings, food stores and markets. Unsurprisingly, the article reports that people living in the vicinity of these sites have experienced a variety of health problems. Pesticides are, of course, only one group of toxic substances to which people in 'developing' countries are exposed; but they are particularly relevant to the measures used to control 'vector-borne' diseases, such as malaria, that are claimed to be prevalent in Africa and particularly in sub-Saharan Africa; a number of these types of disease are discussed later in this chapter.

The existence of ill-health in Africa and all other 'developing' countries is more than adequately explained by a wide variety of contributory factors, including many of those discussed in chapter six that also affect people in 'developed' countries; however, none of the factors that cause illness is a 'virus' known as HIV.

The plight of people who are genuinely ill, but have been assigned a misleading label of 'living with HIV' as the result of a meaningless test, is a tragedy of immense proportions; it is, however, an even greater tragedy that healthy people, including pregnant women, are also assigned this label for which they too are poisoned with toxic drugs that have the potential to cause ill-health and even an early death.

Tuberculosis

Tuberculosis is another of the diseases specifically referred to in SDG 3.3 as an epidemic to be 'ended' by 2030. The magnitude of this 'epidemic' is indicated by the September 2018 WHO fact sheet entitled *Tuberculosis*, which claims that approximately 1.6 million people died from the disease in 2017. This mortality figure means that tuberculosis is now considered to be the greatest 'killer' disease caused by a single 'infectious agent'.

The theory that TB is caused by a bacterium has been shown to be fatally flawed; the reason for a further discussion about this disease is because, like HIV/AIDS, it is said to primarily affect 'developing' countries, as the fact sheet states,

"Over 95% of cases and deaths are in developing countries."

Although HIV/AIDS has previously been promoted as the disease that posed the greatest threat to humanity, this is clearly no longer the case. The fact sheet claims, however, that there is an association between TB and 'HIV' and states that,

"People living with HIV are 20 to 30 times more likely to develop active TB disease than people without HIV."

It should be noted that the original theory about HIV/AIDS claimed that a positive HIV test result would override a prior diagnosis of another condition. In other words, a diagnosis of TB with a negative HIV test result would remain a case of tuberculosis; whereas a diagnosis of TB in the presence of a positive HIV test result would become a case of 'AIDS', which has since been replaced by the category 'living with HIV'.

The claim that TB and HIV commonly co-exist is highly anomalous for a few reasons. One reason is that the HIV/AIDS fact sheet claims that globally

36.9 million people were 'living with HIV' at the end of 2017 and of that total 25.7 million, or almost 70 per cent, were in the African Region, whereas the TB fact sheet claims that 62 per cent of the new cases of TB in 2017 occurred in the South East Asia and Western Pacific Region.

Another reason is that TB is referred to as a bacterial disease whereas HIV/AIDS is 'viral'. It is claimed that the relationship between them is that an 'HIV infection' causes the immune system to become weak and therefore vulnerable to an opportunistic infection, the most common of which is TB; this is, however, a misleading claim. A more plausible reason for a relationship between them is because, as previously discussed, TB is one of the conditions that can produce a 'false positive' HIV test result.

Although tuberculosis mainly affects 'developing' countries, it is not entirely absent from 'developed' countries, some of which have experienced a resurgence of TB in recent years; as reported in a 2003 article entitled *The world-wide increase in tuberculosis: how demographic changes, HIV infection and increasing numbers in poverty are increasing tuberculosis*. Interestingly, the article reports that the increased incidence of TB in some 'developed' countries began in the mid-1980s, a date that coincides with the early years of the so-called 'AIDs epidemic'. It would seem therefore that the 1980s was a period during which there was an overall increasing incidence of ill-health. The article predicts that the incidence of TB will continue to rise and bases this prediction on the three influences referred to in its title. The third factor that is claimed to influence the rise of TB cases globally is of particular significance; the article states that,

> "...as more and more people are forced to live in poverty, where poor nutrition and crowded conditions lead to the spread of tuberculosis, the disease risk will be compounded."

These conditions are commonly associated with TB; other sources, however, posit a different view, one that claims these conditions are not relevant to the onset of TB. This latter view, which is based on the erroneous belief that TB is caused solely by a bacterium, is expressed in a 2011 article entitled *Tuberculosis: current situation, challenges and overview of its control programs in India* that states,

> "Surprisingly, in India, people are still under the impression that TB is a disease of poor people, mostly of those living in slums."

The article claims that rich people are also 'at risk' from the disease because, for example, their 'staff', who may appear to be healthy, may be 'asymptomatic carriers', about which the article states,

> "Since the immune system in healthy people walls off the causative bacteria, TB infection in healthy people is often asymptomatic."

As discussed in chapter four, 'asymptomatic carriers' are said to be able to transmit disease, whereas people with 'latent TB infection' cannot. This is clearly anomalous, and poses a direct challenge to the basic assumption that infection with TB bacteria is the cause of tuberculosis, which is a communicable disease. The medical establishment fails to explain the absence of symptoms or the idea that 'TB infection' can give rise to two mutually exclusive outcomes; nevertheless, the WHO fact sheet claims that,

"About one-quarter of the world's population has latent TB..."

The lifetime 'risk' that people with 'latent TB infection' (LTBI) will develop active TB disease is claimed to be between 5 to 15 per cent, although this risk is said to be dependent upon other factors, as the fact sheet also claims,

"...persons with compromised immune systems, such as people living with HIV, malnutrition or diabetes, or people who use tobacco, have a much higher risk of falling ill."

The WHO *Global Tuberculosis Report 2017*, which will be referred to as the *TB Report*, discusses the phenomenon of latent TB infection and defines it as,

"...a state of persistent immune response to *M. tuberculosis* without clinically manifested evidence of active TB disease."

Interestingly, a diagnosis of LTBI is made using the same 'tests' as those used to diagnose tuberculosis, except that LTBI is not accompanied by the symptoms of 'active disease'. It is important to note that these tests do not detect the presence of TB 'germs'; as the fact sheet states, they only indicate,

"...the presence of an immunological response to TB bacteria."

The *TB Report* admits that the tests for LTBI have limitations, one of which is that they cannot determine whether a person is likely to progress to active TB disease or not. Despite the limitations of the tests, the WHO recommends that certain individuals who have tested positive for LTBI should receive treatment in order to avoid the risk that they will develop active TB disease. The people considered to be 'most at risk' include those who are said to be 'living with HIV'; people with this spurious label are not only in danger of being poisoned with toxic antiretroviral drugs, they are also at risk of being poisoned with toxic antibiotic drugs. Yet neither of these so-called 'treatments' is able to address underlying health problems.

Isoniazid, one of the most common antibiotic drugs used to treat 'TB disease', is also used to treat LTBI; as previously discussed, isoniazid is associated with many adverse health effects. A 2014 article entitled *Adverse effects of isoniazid preventative therapy for latent tuberculosis infection: a prospective cohort study* refers to hepatotoxicity as a recognised 'side effect' of IPT (isoniazid preventative therapy) and adds that,

"However, a wide variety of less well-documented adverse effects have been observed in association with IPT, including acneiform and other rashes, gastrointestinal adverse effects, peripheral neuropathy, drowsiness and alopecia..."

The article reports that the most common adverse effects of isoniazid are gastrointestinal, which is a clear indication of its innate toxicity. However, the treatment for LTBI is usually a regimen that involves a combination of drugs, mainly isoniazid, rifapentine and rifampicin, that are claimed to reduce the risk of developing active TB disease by about 60 per cent. The reason that they are used in combinations is based on the idea that TB bacteria have developed 'resistance' to certain drugs when used individually. However, the *TB Report* makes the important statement that,

"...safety concerns exist, mainly related to the development of hepatotoxicity."

The recognition that antibiotics cause liver damage is a matter of serious concern, especially for an infection that is said to lead to active disease in only 5 to 15 per cent of cases. Furthermore, damage to the liver means that the body's ability to process and eliminate toxins has been severely impaired; this can only lead to worsening health problems. The efforts to address the problem of 'latent TB' are based on the notion that 'reactivation TB', which is the development of active disease, accounts for the greatest number of new cases in regions with low prevalence. In regions where there is a high prevalence of tuberculosis, the medical establishment concentrates its efforts on interventions that involve the treatment of the disease, on the basis that, according to the TB Report,

"Most deaths from TB could be prevented with early diagnosis and appropriate treatment."

The TB Report also claims that approximately 53 million deaths were averted between 2000 and 2016 due to 'successful' treatment, but adds that,

"...there are still large gaps in detection and treatment."

The efforts to fill these 'gaps' will produce yet another massive boost to the profits of the pharmaceutical industry, but they will not enable people to be restored to health.

The claims of the successful treatment of TB and of the millions of lives that have been saved, must be contrasted with the increasing incidence of 'drug resistance' and the condition referred to as MDR-TB, which is described in the WHO fact sheet that states,

"Multidrug-resistant TB (MDR-TB) remains a public health crisis and a health security threat."

The fact sheet claims that MDR-TB is caused by,

"...bacteria that do not respond to isoniazid and rifampicin..."

Rifampicin is another common antibiotic used to treat TB. Although the fact sheet refers to MDR-TB as 'treatable', the success rate of treatment is admitted to be only about 54 per cent, which is unsurprising considering that these treatments involve drugs of even greater toxicity that are used over an extended period, often up to two years. The unsuccessful treatment of MDR-TB is also claimed to be due to 'drug resistance' and assigned the label XDR-TB (extensively drug-resistant TB). The success rate of the treatment for XDR-TB is, however, even lower at only 30 per cent; but this should not be surprising either, considering that it involves treatment with extremely toxic drugs.

It should be clear that the failure to 'cure' tuberculosis is not because bacteria have developed 'resistance' to the drugs. The reason for the failure of these treatments is because they are based on a fatally flawed theory that TB is caused by a bacterium that needs to be killed with toxic drugs. Tuberculosis, in common with all other diseases, is poorly understood; this has been admitted in the previously cited 2011 article entitled *Tuberculosis: Current Situation, Challenges and Overview of its Control Programmes in India* that states,

"Even though tubercle bacilli were identified nearly 130 years ago, a definitive understanding of pathogenesis of this disease is still defective."

There are clearly many factors that can contribute to the pulmonary condition diagnosed as tuberculosis; some of these were discussed in chapter four. One of these factors relates to the statement in the fact sheet that people with LTBI are more likely to develop 'active disease' if they also have diabetes. The previously cited 2009 article entitled *Tuberculosis and diabetes mellitus: convergence of two epidemics*, referred to in the discussion in chapter six about sugar, states that,

"The link between diabetes mellitus and tuberculosis has been recognised for centuries."

Although the article refers to 'industrialisation' and 'urbanisation' as factors that lead to increased rates of obesity and diabetes, it also states that,

"Several studies show that coaffliction with tuberculosis and diabetes mellitus is common both in low-income and high-income countries."

The idea that the onset of a disease is related to the income level of the country in which a person lives is highly misleading; a person's state of health is directly related to a number of factors that include their personal circumstances, their diet and the external influences to which they are exposed. The importance of diet is discussed further in chapter ten, but the consumption of processed foods containing large quantities of refined sugar is directly related to diabetes, as has been discussed. Previous discussions have also indicated that toxic substances contribute to the development of tuberculosis and that refined sugar is a toxic substance that has been described as 'the sweetest poison of all'. This means that it should not be surprising to find the coexistence of TB and diabetes mellitus (DM); a situation that has been found to occur in India, as discussed in an October 2012 article entitled *High Diabetes Prevalence among Tuberculosis Cases in Kerala, India* that states,

"India, the nation with the highest number of TB cases in the world, is also undergoing epidemic growth in DM rates."

Although India is said to have the largest number of TB cases, it should be noted that India has the second largest population, which, in early 2018, is reported at approximately 1.354 billion people; a population size that is only exceeded by China, which has approximately 1.415 billion inhabitants and is reported to have the second largest number of new TB cases.

There is a long history of sugar consumption in India, which provides a partial explanation for the long history of tuberculosis in that country. According to a 2014 article entitled *Sugar Intake, Obesity and Diabetes in India*, India is not only the second largest producer, it is also the largest consumer of sugar. However, sugar is not the only factor that is involved in the development of both TB and diabetes.

The increased influence of the food industry through vast advertising and marketing campaigns in the widespread promotion of manufactured food products and drinks, referred to as 'fast foods', have changed the eating habits of large numbers of people in many 'developing' countries. Some people have abandoned their traditional foods and replaced them with processed foods and drinks, which, although cheaper, have been shown to contain a variety of toxic food additives, in addition to sugar.

Tuberculosis, as has been discussed, is largely a condition that results from an accumulation of toxins that need to be expelled from the body. When toxins cannot be easily eliminated through the normal processes that involve the liver and kidneys, the lungs provide assistance as an additional channel, as Dr Bieler has explained.

Malaria

The establishment definition of malaria refers to,

> "an infectious disease due to the presence of parasitic protozoa of the genus *Plasmodium* within the red blood cells. The disease is transmitted by the *Anopheles* mosquito and is confined mainly to tropical and sub-tropical areas."

Malaria is another of the 'epidemic' diseases specifically referred to in SDG 3.3 that are to be 'ended' by 2030. Although the definition refers to malaria as 'infectious', it is not transmissible between people; it is, however, considered to be a major health problem, as indicated by the March 2019 WHO fact sheet entitled *Malaria* that states,

> "In 2017, there were an estimated 219 million cases of malaria in 87 countries."

The fact sheet also reports that,

> "The estimated number of malaria deaths stood at 435,000 in 2017."

It is interesting to note that both of these statistics refer to 'estimated' numbers.

Although malaria is reported to kill fewer people than TB or 'HIV', it is nevertheless said to pose an extremely serious threat to billions of people, as the fact sheet claims,

> "In 2017, nearly half of the world's population was at risk of malaria."

The people considered to be most 'at risk' are those who live in 'developing' countries, especially African countries, as the fact sheet indicates,

> "The WHO African Region carries a disproportionately high share of the global malaria burden. In 2017, the region was home to 92% of malaria cases and 93% of malaria deaths."

The acknowledged paucity of available data with respect to disease morbidity and mortality in 'developing' countries raises serious questions about the veracity of the WHO statistics relating to malaria, even though they are admitted to be estimated. Furthermore, a close examination of the 'information' about malaria promulgated by the medical establishment, and widely accepted as 'fact', reveals the existence of many anomalous claims. Together, these anomalies pose a powerful challenge to the veracity of these 'facts' and provide a compelling argument that the 'malaria theory' is seriously, if not fatally, flawed; as the following discussion will demonstrate.

According to the fact sheet,

> "Malaria is caused by *Plasmodium* parasites. The parasites are spread to people through the bites of infected female *Anopheles* mosquitoes, called 'malaria vectors'."

This claim highlights two major anomalies. The first is that *Anopheles* mosquitoes inhabit every continent with the sole exception of Antarctica; the second is that the *Plasmodium* parasites claimed to be transmitted by these mosquitoes are also ubiquitous on every continent, except for

Antarctica. Yet malaria is said to be largely 'confined' to tropical and sub-tropical regions.

One attempt to explain this anomaly is the idea that malaria is not transmitted by all species of *Anopheles* mosquito; as indicated by a 2015 article entitled *Highly evolvable malaria vectors: the genomes of 16 anopheles mosquitoes*, which states that *Plasmodium* parasites,

> "...are transmitted by approximately 60 of the 450 known species of anopheline mosquitoes."

More significantly, however, the article states that although *Anopheles* is the only genus of mosquito that transmits malaria,

> "...not...even all members of each vector species are efficient malaria vectors."

This does not, however, explain the anomalies referred to above. The admission that they are not all 'efficient' malaria vectors' casts serious doubt on the claim that disease transmission only requires a female mosquito to have been 'infected' with the parasite for her to be able to transmit the disease. Further doubts are cast on the basic theory by a January 2017 article entitled *Probability of Transmission of Malaria from Mosquito to Human is Regulated by Mosquito Density in Naïve and Vaccinated Hosts*. The article states that the prevailing assumption is that 'infected' mosquitoes are equally 'infectious', but adds that,

> "...this has never been rigorously tested."

The article refers to scientific findings that claim the greater the number of parasites, the more likely the 'infected' mosquito will transmit disease; but this does not correspond to the underlying theory, as expressed in the definition, which states that 'disease' is caused by the presence of parasites in the blood; it does not state that disease is caused by a specific concentration of parasites in the blood.

Malaria is a disease that is said to have existed for many thousands of years; historical records that are claimed to describe malaria refer to two main symptoms; fever and an enlarged spleen. Malaria has also been known by other names, most notably marsh fever and ague, all of which have been recorded to have occurred in various parts of the world, including many regions that are neither tropical nor sub-tropical.

One particularly notable example is an area in the east of England, still referred to as the Fens, which, in the past, was extensively covered by marshes. A 2014 article entitled *Malaria in the UK* states that,

> "From the 15th century, malaria was endemic along the coasts and marshlands of South-East England, Fenlands and Northern England."

England is neither tropical nor sub-tropical; however, of even greater significance is that malaria was endemic in England during the era referred to as the 'Little Ice Age'; a period in which the winter temperatures in England were substantially colder than they are in the early 21st century. Surprisingly, this is admitted on a CDC web page entitled *From Shakespeare to Defoe: Malaria in England in the Little Ice Age* that states,

> "From 1564 to the 1730s – the coldest period of the Little Ice Age – malaria was an important cause of illness and death in several parts of England."

However, the CDC web page entitled *Where Malaria Occurs* states that,

"Temperature is particularly critical."

The reason for this is, according to the CDC, because the parasite cannot be transmitted at temperatures below 20 degrees C (68 degrees F). Yet the temperatures during the Little Ice Age were substantially colder, especially during the winters when the River Thames was covered by a sufficiently thick layer of ice that it enabled 'frost fairs' to take place. However, despite the recognition that malaria occurred in England during this extremely cold period, the CDC page claims that,

"Malaria is transmitted in tropical and subtropical areas..."

The English climate in the 21st century is far warmer than that of the 'Little Ice Age', yet malaria is claimed to no longer occur in England; as the UK NHS website clearly states,

"Malaria is not found in the UK."

Nevertheless, despite the extensive drainage programmes conducted during the 17th century, some marshes still cover parts of eastern England and *Anopheles* mosquitoes are still resident in England. Yet a 2014 article entitled *Study: UK cities becoming mosquito-friendly habitats* makes the bold claim that,

"UK mosquitoes are human disease-free..."

It may be assumed from this claim that the *Anopheles* mosquitoes that currently reside in England belong to the many species that do not transmit malaria, but this assumption ignores the claim that malaria was endemic in England, which means therefore that 'malarial mosquitoes' must have been present at that time. Although the marshes were partially drained, it is unrealistic to assume that every single 'malaria-carrying' mosquito and all of their parasites would have been destroyed during these drainage programmes. This means that 'UK mosquitoes', or at least some of them, must be descendants of 'malarial mosquitoes'; which raises the question of why malaria is claimed to not be found in the UK.

Of greater concern is that the article refers to one of the study authors who is cited to state that,

"...the *Anopheles* mosquito we found is a human-biting species and it can transmit malaria."

Although UK mosquitoes are said to be 'disease-free', the study authors are reported to state that an outbreak of malaria in the UK is 'possible' if the disease is brought into the country. But no explanation is offered for how the UK's human-biting mosquitoes lost their disease-causing parasites or their ability to transmit malaria.

America is another country where malaria has occurred in the past but has been eradicated, despite the continuing presence of *Anopheles* mosquitoes. The CDC web page entitled *Elimination of Malaria in the United States (1947-1951)* claims that this was achieved through a programme that,

"...consisted primarily of DDT applications to the interior surfaces of rural homes..."

The CDC reports that more than 4 million homes in the US had been sprayed during the 4-year period and adds that the programme also included,

"...drainage, removal of mosquito breeding sites and spraying (occasionally from aircraft) of insecticides."

Malaria is also reported to have occurred in Europe but to have been similarly 'eradicated' during the 20th century; as indicated by a June 2016 article entitled *Malaria in Europe: emerging threat or minor nuisance?* that states,

"Malaria was eradicated from Europe in the 1970s..."

The article claims that the measures responsible for this 'success' involved,

"...a combination of insecticide spraying, drug therapy and environmental engineering."

These are virtually the same measures as those employed by the English and American programmes; however, the article makes a revealing comment, which is that,

"Several *Anopheles* species capable of transmitting malaria occur widely all over Europe."

Yet again, although malaria is referred to as having been 'eradicated', the mosquitoes capable of transmitting the disease have not been completely annihilated. The likelihood that every single *Plasmodium* parasite was destroyed during eradication campaigns that failed to destroy every single mosquito is zero. The fact that mosquito species capable of transmitting malaria still inhabit England, America and Europe means that some must still be 'infected' with the parasite. The claim that the disease has been eradicated from these parts of the world is therefore highly anomalous. The article attempts to explain the anomaly and states that,

"In time, anopheline numbers recovered, giving rise to a phenomenon known as 'anophelism without malaria', which essentially means that anopheline mosquitoes are present in formerly malarious areas of Europe where malaria no longer occurs."

The phenomenon of 'anophelism without malaria' bears a close resemblance to that of 'latent TB infection'; but these phenomena are not merely anomalous, they represent serious contradictions to the underlying theories about these diseases. Previous discussions have exposed the erroneous nature of theories relating to TB, which strongly suggests that there is a similarly serious and fundamental problem with the theory about malaria, which claims that it is caused by *Plasmodium* parasites that are transmitted to humans by *Anopheles* mosquitoes.

The previously cited 2014 article entitled *Malaria's contribution to World War One – the unexpected adversary* states that Europe experienced a resurgence in cases of malaria during the war years and that this was due to,

"Deployment of large numbers of troops from tropical Africa and India..."

The article claims that malaria was 'spread' to civilians by these troops, but this is misleading as malaria is not directly transmissible between people; it requires the intervention of a 'vector'.

Malarial parasites are said to be transmitted to humans by 'infected' female mosquitoes and that transmission occurs during a blood 'meal', but the use of the word 'meal' is misleading. Male and female mosquitoes both 'feed' on plant nectar; the reason that female mosquitoes draw blood, whether from humans or animals, is to incubate her eggs. It is claimed that female mosquitoes are born 'parasite-free' but they become 'infected' through the ingestion of a parasite in their first 'blood meal' drawn from an infected person. Once 'infected', female mosquitoes transmit the parasites to humans, or other animals, through their salivary glands whenever they subsequently draw blood. The seemingly simple nature of this explanation conceals the extremely complicated nature of the processes claimed to be involved.

Malarial parasites belong to the genus *Plasmodium*, of which there are more than 100 species, although the WHO fact sheet states that only 5 of these species cause malaria in humans. It is, however, the complex nature of the life cycle of these parasites that poses one of the major challenges to the underlying theory about the development of malaria. A web page entitled *Life Cycle* states that,

> "The malaria parasite has a complex, multistage life cycle occurring within two living beings, the vector mosquito and the vertebrate host."

The life cycles of the different *Plasmodium* species claimed to infect humans are not identical; two species are said to produce 'hypnozoites' that may lie dormant and harmless in the liver, whereas a third species does not produce hypnozoites. The idea that allegedly 'pathogenic' parasites can lie dormant and harmless in the liver is anomalous; but it is not the most significant anomaly. The main anomalies arise from the explanations about the processes involved in the transmission of 'infection' between the mosquito vector and the human host and about the different stages of the parasite's life cycle in both mosquitoes and humans.

Malaria is said to result from a bite from a female *Anopheles* mosquito infected with a *Plasmodium* parasite; however, because female mosquitoes are born without parasites they therefore need to 'acquire' them, which is said to occur when she takes her first 'blood meal'. This is, however, an overly simplistic explanation. Firstly, it ignores the fact that each mosquito can only draw a few drops of blood, yet this tiny quantity is said to contain an 'infective' parasite. Secondly, the parasite must be at exactly the 'right' stage of its highly complex life-cycle and be delivered by the body's moving bloodstream to the exact part of the body that the mosquito intends to bite. Furthermore, once the mosquito has drawn blood and been 'infected' with the parasite, it plays 'host' to the next stage of the parasite's complex life-cycle. When this stage has been completed, the mosquito obligingly assists the parasite again by transferring it into a human host when taking her next blood 'meal'.

The stages of the parasite life-cycle that are said to occur within the human host are even more complex; a diagram of the entire parasite life-cycle is available on the CDC web page entitled *Biology* in the series of pages entitled *About Malaria*. One particularly interesting comment on the page is that,

"Differently from the human host, the mosquito vector does not suffer from the presence of the parasites."

The idea that a minute parasite can cause serious harm and even death to the larger of the two organisms, whilst the smaller organism is entirely unaffected, remains unexplained. Also problematic is the idea a parasite initiates processes that can damage or even kill its host, because the purpose of inhabiting the human body is said to be to progress its life-cycle.

The CDC claim that mosquitoes are not affected by parasites is, however, contradicted by a September 2010 article entitled *How Mosquitoes Fight Malaria*, which refers to a study conducted at the NIAID that discovered some mosquitoes do succumb to the parasites, but that others can 'fight' the infection; yet the article also states that,

"...researchers don't know exactly how insects do this."

The development of disease is said to result from the presence of parasites in the blood, as indicated by the CDC *Biology* page that states,

"Blood stage parasites are responsible for the clinical manifestations of the disease."

Although this may seem to explain why the 'liver stage' does not produce symptoms, it would be a mistake to make this assumption; the liver is the most important organ of elimination that assists detoxification, as has been discussed.

The 'disease' stage of malaria is said to result from the release of thousands of parasites into the bloodstream. However, although this may seem to be a serious level of 'infection', it must be noted that the human body is estimated to contain approximately 20 trillion red blood cells. An analogy that puts these huge numbers into their true perspective is that a few thousand parasites within 20 trillion red blood cells is as insignificant as one day in approximately 600,000 years.

The fact that thousands of 'infected' cells are insignificant compared to the total number of red blood cells, raises the extremely important question of how so few 'infected' cells can produce such a serious disease. Another equally important question it raises is the likelihood that a female *Anopheles* mosquito will ingest at least one 'infected' cell in the few drops of blood she draws. The probability is extremely low.

An interesting revelation is made in a 2010 article entitled *History of the discovery of the malaria parasites and their vectors*, which states that,

"...apart from the initial discovery of parasites in the blood, every subsequent discovery has been based on studies on non-human malaria parasites and related organisms."

The article explains that the discovery of malaria was originally the result of observations made by Alphonse Laveran, a French army officer. Early theories about malaria included suggestions that it was caused by a bacterium that had been shown to produce fevers and enlarged spleens when injected into rabbits. However, the bacterial cause of malaria was abandoned when Alphonse Laveran discovered granules of black pigment in the spleens of people diagnosed with malaria; he regarded these pigments as specific to malaria. The article states that Alphonse Laveran had observed,

> "...several different forms of erythrocytic organism, including crescents, spherical motionless bodies with pigment, spherical moving bodies with pigment..."

His observations led to the discovery that these 'organisms' were protozoa, not bacteria; but, due to the belief, both then and now, that the blood is a sterile environment and therefore free from any type of 'contaminant', it was assumed that the presence of these 'bodies' meant that the blood had been invaded. The belief that blood is a 'sterile' environment is however, erroneous. The discussion about protozoa in chapter three referred to a July 2011 article which includes a statement that bears repetition,

> "...many people infected with known parasites...are asymptomatic."

The WHO *World Malaria Report 2018*, which will be referred to as the *Malaria Report*, states that,

> "Patients with suspected malaria should have prompt parasitological confirmation of diagnosis, with either microscopy or RDT before antimalarial treatment is started."

RDTs are rapid diagnostic tests. It is claimed that microscopy is the 'gold standard' test but the cost of the necessary equipment to process the tests is prohibitive for many 'developing' countries, especially in 'poor' sub-Saharan African countries where malaria is said to be most prevalent. As with the RDTs used for 'HIV', those for malaria do not detect the actual parasite; they are claimed to detect antigens said to be specific to the parasite that the body has produced in response to a prior infection. However, as previously discussed, the presence of antibodies is interpreted in two different ways. One is that they indicate immunity; the other is that they indicate disease. Although mutually exclusive, these interpretations are both incorrect.

Although tests are recommended by the WHO as a method of determining whether a person has been 'infected', a 2002 article entitled *Rapid Diagnostic Tests for Malaria Parasites* makes a significant observation that,

> "Malaria presents a diagnostic challenge to laboratories in most countries."

This applies to all types of test; even so-called 'gold standard' microscopy tests are not without their difficulties. On the English translation pages of the website based on an Italian book entitled *Atlas of Human Malaria* is a page entitled *Artifacts that may be confused with malaria or other blood parasites*, which begins with the interesting comment that,

> "Inexperienced microscopists may have difficulty in examining thin and especially thick film because of contaminating elements that can be accidentally present in stained samples."

The types of 'contaminants' to which the book refers include: bacteria, skin dirt, vegetable spores, yeasts or moulds in the air. The reference to bacteria as 'contaminants' reveals the authors' belief in the 'germ theory'; however, they make another revealing comment, which is that,

> "The presence of malaria parasites in a blood sample is an indication of infection, but not necessarily of disease."

The presence of 'infection' by parasites in the absence of disease is also acknowledged on the CDC web page entitled *Malaria Diagnosis (United States)* that states,

"In some malaria-endemic areas, malaria transmission is so intense that a large proportion of the population is infected but not made ill by the parasites."

The idea that a person can be 'infected' with parasites without experiencing any ill-effects contradicts the definition of malaria which states that it is caused by the presence of parasites in the blood. One of the 'explanations' offered for this phenomenon is that some people have developed 'immunity', or at least 'partial immunity'; this point is addressed by the statement in the *Atlas of Human Malaria* book that,

"Individuals who live in malaria endemic areas and are subject to repeat plasmodium infection develop a special type of immunity..."

This comment is supported by the WHO *Malaria* fact sheet that states,

"Human immunity is another important factor, especially among adults in areas of moderate or intense transmission conditions."

The fact sheet also states that,

"Partial immunity is developed over years of exposure..."

This is all highly anomalous; the mechanism by which people develop 'immunity', whether partial or otherwise, is inadequately explained, but there are clear similarities with the anomalous claims about immunity to 'infectious diseases'. The failure of the medical establishment to provide plausible explanations for these anomalies is due to their poor level of understanding about the mechanisms involved; as indicated by a 2009 article entitled *Acquired Immunity to Malaria* that refers to the protection offered by 'naturally acquired immunity' but adds that,

"There is no clear concept about how this protection works."

The previously cited 2010 article about the history of the discovery of the malaria parasite provides a description of the symptoms associated with the illness regarded as the early form of malaria,

"The early Greeks...were well aware of the characteristic poor health, malarial fevers and enlarged spleens seen in people living in marshy places."

This view is supported by the writings of the Greek physician Hippocrates, particularly in his work entitled *On Airs, Waters and Places*, in which he refers to the waters in marshes and states that,

"...those who drink them have large and obstructed spleens, their bellies are hard, emaciated and hot..."

Fever and an enlarged spleen remain two of the symptoms associated with malaria; fever is regarded as a symptom of the acute form of malaria, whereas an enlarged spleen is a symptom of the chronic form of the disease.

It is claimed that one of the functions attributed to the spleen is to defend the body against 'pathogens', which indicates that it would also be involved in defending the body against parasites. The main functions of the spleen include cleaning the blood and removing 'abnormal' red blood cells, which indicates that the spleen would be involved in the processes that remove red blood cells that have been 'infected' by parasites. It should be noted that red blood cells are not long-lived; their lifespan is approximately 120 days, which means that the death and removal of RBCs from the body is a normal and ongoing process. The malaria fact sheet describes the symptoms of acute malaria,

"The first symptoms – fever, headache, and chills – may be mild and difficult to recognize as malaria."

In a 'Western' country, these symptoms are more likely to be regarded as a cold or the 'flu'. In other countries, especially those referred to as 'developing', these symptoms are likely to be regarded as 'malaria' that would need to be confirmed by a test, the accuracy of which is questionable.

Malaria has been particularly associated with Africa since Europeans began to explore the continent in the 19th century; one of the most famous explorers was David Livingstone, a medical doctor. A 2013 article entitled *What is David Livingstone's legacy, 200 years after his birth?* contains an extract from his writings, in which Dr Livingstone is claimed to have stated,

"I have drunk water swarming with insects, thick with mud and putrid with rhinoceros urine and buffaloes' dung, and no stinted drafts of either."

These contaminants are more than capable of producing severe illness and symptoms such as fevers and an enlarged spleen. However, Dr Livingstone was a conventional medical doctor and a keen proponent of the use of 'medicines' for the treatment of diseases, including malaria with which he is claimed to have suffered. One of the earliest 'medicines' used as a preventive for 'malaria' was quinine, the 'medicine' with which Doctor Livingstone treated his own illness. Quinine was first isolated by chemists in the early 19th century; it is an active substance of the cinchona bark, a plant native to South America. It remained one of the main 'medicines' for the treatment of malaria for more than a century; as indicated by the previously cited article about malaria during WWI that states,

"Clinical treatment primarily depended on quinine, although efficacy was poor..."

This poor level of efficacy is claimed to be because different malarial parasites are said to require different treatments; but this idea ignores the more important fact, which is that quinine is toxic. In *Natural Hygiene: Man's Pristine Way of Life*, Herbert Shelton refers to quinine as a 'protoplasmic poison' and states that,

"Untold thousands of nervous systems have been wrecked by quinine; deafness and blindness have been caused by it and no case of malaria was ever cured by it..."

He adds that quinine substitutes are equally unsuccessful in their ability to either prevent or cure malaria.

The medical establishment does not dispute that quinine is toxic; it is acknowledged to be associated with hepatotoxicity; a clear indication of its inherently toxic nature. The article about malaria during WWI states that quinine was not the only 'medicine' used in the treatment of malaria during that period and refers to other 'medicines' that contained either arsenic or strychnine. The 'effects' of arsenic have been discussed; it is however important to note that they include vomiting, diarrhoea and abdominal pain as well as anaemia. Strychnine is also highly toxic; it can produce adverse effects in the central nervous system, painful muscle spasms and death from respiratory arrest.

Interestingly, another effect of arsenic poisoning is referred to as 'black water urine'. This effect is also associated with a condition known as 'Blackwater Fever', which is claimed to be a 'complication' of malaria. The establishment definition of blackwater fever states that,

"The condition is probably brought on by inadequate treatment with quinine..."

It is however, far more likely that 'blackwater fever' occurs due to the treatment of malaria with quinine, rather than 'inadequate' treatment with this toxic substance; quinine-based drugs are associated with severe adverse effects, as the CDC admits,

"Overdose of anti-malarial drugs, particularly chloroquine, can be fatal."

Chloroquine is a derivative of quinine.

The medical establishment claims that 'treatment' is nevertheless essential, as indicated by the *Malaria Report* that states,

"Prompt diagnosis and treatment is the most effective way to prevent a mild case of malaria from developing into severe disease and death."

The report also recognises the reduced efficacy of chloroquine (CQ) and advises that,

"Where there is a high treatment failure rate with CQ (>10%), countries are encouraged to change their first-line treatment to an ACT."

ACT refers to artemisinin-based combination therapy.

Chloroquine had been the main treatment for malaria until relatively recently, but, according to a 2012 article entitled *Diagnosis of Malaria Infection with or without Disease*, it has become,

"...increasingly ineffective against Plasmodium falciparum due to the spread of selected resistant strains."

Artemisinin is a synthetic chemical derived from sweet wormwood; the 'natural' and synthetic substances are both associated with nausea and vomiting, which indicates that the body regards them both as toxic. Nevertheless, artemisinin is considered to be highly effective against malaria; it is claimed to reduce the concentration of the 'blood-stage' parasites that cause disease. The reason that artemisinin is used in combination with other drugs is because it has a short half-life of about one hour in the human body; the longer-lasting drugs, with which it is combined include: amodiaquine, mefloquine and sulphadoxine-pyrimethamine, all of which are associated with adverse 'side effects'. Amodiaquine has been linked to hepatotoxicity; mefloquine has been found to cause brain damage. The 'side effects' associated with Sulphadoxine-pyrimethamine (SP) include nausea, vomiting and diarrhoea.

The *Malaria* fact sheet claims that certain groups are at a 'considerably higher risk' of developing malaria than others and states that,

"These include infants, children under 5 years of age, pregnant women and patients with HIV/AIDS, as well as non-immune migrants, mobile populations and travellers."

It is considered that infants, children under the age of five and pregnant women are those at greatest risk, although their increased risk of contracting malaria is not explained. Nevertheless, this 'risk' is given as the justification for the use of toxic drugs as interventions claimed to be necessary for the achievement of the goal to end the 'epidemic' of malaria.

In areas where malaria transmission is said to be moderate or high, the WHO recommends that IPTp (intermittent preventive treatment of pregnant women) with SP is introduced and administered during scheduled antenatal clinic appointments. However, SP is not administered during the first trimester as it has been associated with teratogenic effects when taken during this stage of pregnancy. The WHO also recommends that, in these areas, infants and children between the ages of 3 and 59 months should receive SP for IPTi (intermittent preventive treatment for infants). It is said that these treatments can be administered during scheduled visits to immunisation clinics. The simultaneous administration of toxic 'medicines' and toxic vaccines will invariably produce a variety of adverse effects, even if some of them are not immediately noticeable.

In areas where seasonal transmission of malaria is claimed to be high, which is said to occur in areas of the Sahel sub-region of Africa, the WHO recommends SMC (seasonal malaria chemoprevention) as an 'additional prevention strategy'. The fact sheet describes this strategy and states that it involves,

> "...the administration of monthly courses of amodiaquine plus sulphadoxine-pyrimethamine to all children under 5 years of age during the high transmission season."

These drugs are not administered during visits to immunisation clinics; according to the *Malaria Report*,

> "Implementation of SMC was scaled up from 2015, and delivery is primarily door-to-door in most countries..."

It is reported that *Plasmodium falciparum* has also begun to develop resistance to artemisinin-based 'medicines'. 'Resistance' in this context is said to mean that there is a noticeable reduction in the rate that parasites are cleared from the blood, on the basis that their presence in the blood is indicative of disease; but this has been shown to not always be the case.

Although malaria is not an 'infectious disease', it is claimed that a person can develop 'immunity' to the disease; this has clearly been one of the reasons that the pharmaceutical industry has been encouraged to develop a vaccine that would induce an 'immune response' to the malaria parasites. To date, only one vaccine has made progress through various stages of testing; the *Malaria* fact sheet states that,

> "RTS,S/AS01 (RTS,S) is the first and, to date, the only vaccine to show partial protection against malaria in young children."

The WHO page entitled *Q&A on the malaria vaccine implementation programme (MVIP)* claims that this vaccine has been shown in trials to be 'well tolerated', even though it is associated with the 'usual' adverse reactions that include pain and swelling at the site, as well as fever. However, RTS,S is also associated with some more serious adverse effects, as admitted on the *Q&A* page that states,

> "During the Phase 3 trial, an increased risk of febrile seizures was seen within 7 days of the administration of any of the RTS,S vaccine doses."

Nevertheless, the fact sheet states that this vaccine is to be introduced into three countries in 2019; these are Ghana, Kenya and Malawi. In common with all other vaccines, the RTS,S will contain toxic ingredients, such as adjuvants and preservatives. Furthermore, on the basis that no vaccine has been proven to be either safe or effective, the malaria vaccine will be no exception; like all other vaccines, it will induce serious adverse health effects, in addition to febrile seizures, for the young children in the three African countries in which it is to be introduced.

The strategies recommended for the eradication of malaria also involve methods to destroy the mosquito; these methods are referred to as 'vector control' and entail the use of pesticides for two applications; insecticide-treated mosquito nets (ITNs) and indoor residual spraying (IRS) with insecticides. The class of insecticides most commonly used for ITNs are pyrethroids, which have been discussed and shown to be highly toxic; as indicated by the Beyond Pesticides fact sheet that states,

> "While pyrethroids are a synthetic version of an extract from the chrysanthemum, they were chemically designed to be more toxic with longer breakdown times, and are often formulated with synergists, increasing potency and compromising the human body's ability to detoxify the pesticide."

There is a clear potential for serious health problems to occur as the result of exposures to toxic pyrethroids for adults and children who sleep under the treated nets. The main concern of the WHO would seem to be that the insects and parasites are developing 'resistance' to these chemicals, as indicated by the *Malaria Report* that states,

> "Resistance to pyrethroids – the only insecticide class currently used in ITNs – is widespread..."

Three other classes of insecticides are also used in malaria vector control, although they are mainly used for indoor residual spraying (IRS); these insecticides are carbamates, organophosphates and organochlorines. Carbamates have a similar mechanism of action to organophosphates and therefore produce similar adverse health effects; the toxicity of organochlorines and organophosphates have been discussed. It should be noted that one of the organochlorines used for IRS is DDT.

The toxic 'medicines' used to kill parasites in the human body and the toxic insecticides used to kill the mosquitoes that transmit parasites have clearly failed to 'control' the disease; the use of even stronger chemicals, whether as 'medicines', insecticides or vaccines, will similarly fail to solve the problem.

It is clear that the 'malaria theory' contains many anomalies, not least of which is that the presence of the parasites, the purported causal agent of the disease, is not necessarily accompanied by disease. These anomalies are strikingly similar to those of all other 'infectious diseases' and show that the 'malaria theory' is similarly erroneous; this, in turn, raises serious questions about a number of other diseases claimed to be caused by parasites.

Neglected Tropical Diseases

SDG 3 of the 2030 Agenda includes the aim to end the epidemic of neglected tropical diseases (NTDs), which are described on the WHO web page entitled *Neglected Tropical Diseases* as,

"...a diverse group of communicable diseases that prevail in tropical or subtropical conditions in 149 countries..."

Although referred to as 'neglected', these diseases do not have an insignificant impact; the page states that they,

"...affect more than one billion people and cost developing economies billions of dollars every year."

In common with many of the 'communicable' diseases that are claimed to be prevalent in tropical or subtropical regions, NTDs are said to mainly affect certain sectors of the population; as the page also states,

"Populations living in poverty, without adequate sanitation and in close contact with infectious vectors and domestic animals and livestock are those worst affected."

It is claimed that one of the reasons that 'infectious agents' invade the human body is to facilitate microbial replication; this does not however, explain the reason that microbes prefer to invade the bodies of poor people who live in unhygienic conditions.

The microorganisms claimed to be the main causes of neglected tropical diseases are bacteria, fungi and protozoa.

However, bacteria, fungi and protozoa are also the microorganisms that comprise the body's normal microbial inhabitants. The 4th edition of a leading cell biology textbook, entitled *Molecular Biology of the Cell*, contains a chapter entitled *Pathogens, Infection and Innate Immunity*, which refers to the human body as a complex ecosystem that,

"...contains about 10^{13} human cells and also about 10^{14} bacterial, fungal, and protozoan cells, which represent thousands of microbial species."

The book describes these microbial species as the body's 'normal flora' and states that,

"Pathogens are usually distinct from the normal flora."

One of the main differences between the body's normal flora and pathogens is that the latter are claimed to be invading microbes that cause disease. Although the body's normal microbial inhabitants are claimed to be harmless and even beneficial, the book indicates that, under certain conditions, they may become harmful,

"Our normal microbial inhabitants only cause trouble if our immune systems are weakened..."

The reason that the body's normal flora would alter their normal functioning to become harmful is not explained.

The book claims that a weakened immune system is not necessary for 'pathogens' to be able to cause disease; as indicated by the statement that,

"...dedicated pathogens do not require that the host be immunocompromised or injured."

This statement is not, however, consistent with the information provided

522

by the 2011 article about microbial eukaryotes, previously cited in chapter three, which states that,

"Opportunistic parasites are a significant source of morbidity in immune compromised patients, although these same taxa may be present in healthy people without apparent consequence."

The presence of these 'parasites' in the absence of symptoms is not consistent with the claim that they are a source of morbidity.

These inconsistencies further demonstrate the problems inherent within the 'germ theory' that remain unexplained by the medical establishment. The rigid adherence to the belief that microorganisms are 'germs' that invade the body and cause disease remains a serious obstacle to efforts to address human health problems.

One of the main consequences of the perpetuation of this erroneous belief is the implementation of strategies to destroy microorganisms and, where appropriate, the vectors claimed to transmit them. The inappropriate nature of these strategies and their inability to address the genuine health problems of people claimed to be affected by neglected tropical diseases are discussed in the following sections.

Leprosy

Leprosy is one of the 'bacterial' diseases included on the WHO list of NTDs; the discussion in chapter four demonstrated that historically leprosy was not confined to tropical regions of the world. The March 2019 WHO fact sheet entitled *Leprosy* claims that the disease was eliminated as a 'public health problem' in the year 2000, although it is said to still affect many people,

"There were 211,009 new leprosy cases registered globally in 2017..."

The reason for a further discussion of this disease is due to the claim that leprosy is prevalent in three 'developing' countries: namely Brazil, India and Indonesia. According to the *Global Leprosy Strategy 2016-2020* report,

"Together, these three countries account for 81% of the newly diagnosed and reported patients globally."

As previously discussed, the information promulgated by the medical establishment about leprosy contains many anomalies, one of which is that *Mycobacterium leprae*, the bacterium purported to be the cause of leprosy, is said to be 'slow multiplying'; *M. leprae* is also said to have a highly variable incubation period, as reported by the WHO fact sheet that states,

"Symptoms may occur within 1 year, but can also take as long as 20 years or even more to occur."

This anomaly is not explained.

Despite the assertion that leprosy is caused by *M. leprae*, this bacterium does not always cause disease and is not always accompanied by serious symptoms. The previously cited November 2011 article about a leprosy vaccine includes a statement that deserves repetition,

"M. leprae infection does not always cause disease, and it is estimated that anywhere between 30-75% of infections are spontaneously cleared without causing significant symptoms."

This statement is another contradiction of the basic assumption of the 'germ theory' and is a violation of Koch's first Postulate. Furthermore, the medical establishment admits to a poor level of understanding about leprosy; as indicated by the CDC page entitled *Transmission* that states,

"It is not known exactly how Hansen's disease spreads between people."

Yet another anomaly is that, according to the CDC page,

"...more than 95% of all people have natural immunity to the disease."

It is, however, said to be curable, as the WHO fact sheet states,

"Leprosy is curable with multidrug therapy (MDT)."

MDT involves three antibiotic drugs; namely, dapsone, rifampicin and clofazimine. There are said to be two forms of leprosy, referred to as paucibacillary and multibacillary, each of which requires a slightly different form of treatment. The WHO recommends that all leprosy patients receive treatment with dapsone and rifampicin, but that patients with the multibacillary form of the disease should also receive clofazimine in their treatment regimen. The reason that multiple drugs are used is because, as with all antibiotics, it is claimed that the bacteria have developed 'resistance' to them and that they are therefore less effective when used individually.

Dapsone was first introduced as a 'breakthrough' treatment for leprosy during the 1940s. Rifampicin is also used for the treatment of TB on the basis that *M. Leprae* closely resembles *M. tuberculosis*, even though these bacteria are said to be responsible for two entirely different diseases with very different symptoms. In common with all other pharmaceutical drugs, these three antibiotics produce 'side effects', or, more accurately, 'effects'. Dapsone is associated with nausea, loss of appetite and liver inflammation; rifampicin is associated with hepatoxicity; and clofazimine with some skin effects, but also with nausea, vomiting and diarrhoea. These drugs are all toxic.

The reference to leprosy as a 'neglected' disease would seem to be misleading; it certainly has not been neglected as far as the provision of treatment is concerned; as the WHO fact sheet explains,

"Since 1995 WHO has provided MDT free of cost."

Leprosy is said to affect a number of different parts of the body; as the fact sheet states,

"The disease mainly affects the skin, the peripheral nerves, mucosa of the upper respiratory tract, and the eyes."

One of the most devastating effects associated with leprosy is nerve damage that can lead to numbness and even a total loss of feeling, which, when it occurs in the hands and feet is referred to as 'peripheral neuropathy'. A 2017 article entitled *Epidemiology of Peripheral Neuropathy: An Indian Perspective* states that almost 60 per cent of the worldwide incidence of leprosy occurs in India and that leprosy is the cause of most cases of neuropathy. More importantly, the article refers to a variety of factors that can also cause peripheral neuropathy; these include exposures to neurotoxic substances such as arsenic, lead and mercury. In addition to these 'natural' neurotoxins are many 'unnatural' toxins; the article refers to,

> "...different chemotherapeutic agents with a propensity to affect peripheral nerves."

In other words, certain 'medicines' are neurotoxic and eminently capable of causing peripheral neuropathy.

Leprosy is also said to affect the skin; one of these effects involves a loss of skin pigmentation, also known as vitiligo, or leucoderma as it more formally called. A November 2000 article entitled *High prevalence of vitiligo in lepromatous leprosy* makes the interesting comment that,

> "Vitiligo frequently occurs in lepromatous patients, an observation rarely reported in the literature."

Although the cause of vitiligo is referred to as 'unknown', there are some known causes; as indicated by a 2010 article entitled *Chemical leucoderma: Indian scenario, prognosis and treatment* that states,

> "Chemical leucoderma is an industrial disorder in developed countries and the common causative chemicals are phenols and catechols."

Phenols and catechols are both petrochemical derivatives.

It is inappropriate to refer to 'chemical leucoderma' as a problem restricted to 'developed' countries; the continuing expansion of many industries, especially those that involve the use or manufacture of petrochemicals, into 'developing' countries will be accompanied by the same occupational health problems experienced in 'developed' countries. Hazardous chemicals and industrialisation are discussed in the context of their relevance to 'developing' countries later in this chapter. However, the use of the adjective 'chemical' to suggest that there is a separate form of leucoderma that can be caused by chemicals is inappropriate.

The frequent, but rarely reported, co-occurrence of leucoderma and leprosy indicates that they are both associated with exposures to 'chemicals'. This association is further supported by the comment in the article that a wide variety of chemicals are known to be toxic to melanocytes, the cells that produce the skin pigment melanin; these chemicals include mercury and arsenic, both of which are also associated with neuropathy, another symptom of 'leprosy'. It is widely reported that the groundwater in many regions within the Indian subcontinent is contaminated with arsenic.

The article also refers to traditions within Indian culture that involve the application of colourful substances to the body and face, but reports that the traditional mineral- and vegetable-based dyes have been increasingly replaced by synthetic chemical-based dyes, especially azo dyes, which, as previously discussed, are known to be neurotoxic. Azo dyes are another class of chemicals associated with leucoderma. It is clear, therefore, that there are many toxic substances that can produce the symptoms associated with leprosy; some are 'naturally-occurring' such as lead, arsenic and mercury and others are entirely synthetic, such as phenols, catechols and azo dyes.

In the attempt to eliminate leprosy, the medical establishment has also administered the BCG vaccine as a preventive, on the basis that *M. leprae* is similar to *M. tuberculosis*. However, there are efforts to develop a vaccine specifically for leprosy, as the BCG is claimed to only confer 'partial protection'; previous discussions have shown that it confers no protection. The dedicated leprosy vaccine, which was developed by IDRI (Infectious Disease Research Institute) is currently undergoing trials. An October 2017 press release by IDRI is entitled *Promising New Leprosy Vaccine Moves into Human Trials*; the title is self-explanatory. At the time of writing, there are no further reports on the progress of this vaccine.

It is clear from the discussions in chapter two that no vaccine has ever been proven to be either safe or effective; the leprosy vaccine will be no exception, for the simple reason that no disease is caused by a bacterium. The above discussion indicates that exposures to toxic substances provide far more credible explanations for the symptoms attributed to the disease known as leprosy.

Parasitic Diseases

The discussion about 'other germs' in chapter three included reference to parasites, which are defined by the establishment as,

"any living thing that lives in or on another living organism."

The medical establishment claims that, with few exceptions, parasites are pathogenic; however, the previously cited 2011 article about 'microbial eukaryotes' states that the functions of these organisms within the human body are rarely studied and therefore largely unknown. The idea that they are 'pathogenic' is due to the rigid adherence to the 'germ theory' and the consequent failure of the medical establishment to study diseases without reference to 'germs'. The general view, as demonstrated by the CDC web page entitled *Parasites*, is that these organisms can cause a number of diseases commonly regarded as 'tropical', in other words, NTDs. Nevertheless, the page includes the interesting comment that,

"The burden of these diseases often rests on communities in the tropics and subtropics, but parasitic infections also affect people in developed countries."

Although the establishment definition refers to bacteria and viruses as examples of 'parasites', the CDC does not. The CDC web page entitled *About Parasites* claims that there are only three types of 'pathogenic parasite'; protozoa, helminths and ectoparasites. The page states that protozoa are found in the intestines or in the blood and tissues; those found in the intestines are claimed to be transmitted through the faecal-oral route; those found in the blood and tissues are said to be transmitted by vectors. The CDC describes helminths as,

"...large multicellular organisms that are generally visible to the naked eye in their adult stages."

There are three types of helminth: flatworms, thorny-headed worms and roundworms. Flatworms include trematodes, also known as flukes. Roundworms, also known as nematodes, are microscopic, but one of their main functions is to act as 'decomposers'. Most references to this role discuss it in the context of the decomposition of dead organic matter within the soil; however, whether nematodes are part of the 'normal flora' or whether they are 'invaders', their presence in the human body cannot be attributed to a function other than their 'normal' function of the decomposition of dead matter.

The establishment definition of an ectoparasite refers to it as,

"a parasite that lives on the outer surface of its host."

This class of parasite includes ticks, fleas, lice and mites, some of which are claimed to directly cause disease and others are claimed to be the vectors for various pathogenic organisms. One 'ectoparasite' is the tick claimed to be the carrier of the bacterium *Borrelia burgdorferi*, which is said to be the cause of Lyme disease; previous discussions have indicated the erroneous nature of the idea that this disease is caused by bacteria.

A healthy human body employs self-protective mechanisms that prevent the entry of invaders; the presence of parasites is a clear indication that a person's health has been compromised, which means that the body's functions, including the elimination of parasites, have been impaired; as explained by Herbert Shelton who states in his article entitled *Intestinal Parasites* that,

"When you start homesteading parasites, you may know that your tissues and secretions have become so impaired that the parasites find residence in them possible."

This also applies to ectoparasites, the presence of which is most commonly associated with poor hygiene, especially infrequent washing of the body and clothes. Parasites of this type, such as lice for example, are easily eradicated by regular bathing.

The solution, according to the medical establishment, is to utilise methods and treatments that will kill the parasites, including external parasites, it is for this purpose that DDT was originally used. But this strategy will not resolve the problem, mainly because it will increase exposures to toxic substances that will further compromise health and impair the body's ability to initiate its normal defence mechanisms against parasites.

Trypanosomiasis

The establishment definition refers to trypanosomiasis as,

"any disease caused by the presence of parasitic protozoans of the genus *Trypanosome*."

The definition also states that,

"The two most important diseases are Chagas disease (South American trypanosomiasis) and sleeping sickness (African trypanosomiasis)."

These forms of trypanosomiasis are considered to be distinctly different diseases; the WHO has produced a fact sheet for each of them.

The April 2019 WHO fact sheet entitled *Chagas disease (American trypanosomiasis)* claims that most of the 6 to 7 million cases of Chagas disease occur in Latin America. The disease is said to be caused by a parasite called *Trypanosoma cruzi* that is transmitted by a 'triatomine bug', which is also known as a 'kissing bug' as it is said to mainly bite people around the mouth. The fact sheet states that there are two phases of the disease and that during the first or 'acute' phase,

"...a high number of parasites circulate in the blood but in most cases symptoms are absent or mild and unspecific."

The absence of symptoms in the presence of a high number of parasites is not consistent with the definition of the disease; it is also a violation of Koch's first Postulate.

The symptoms that may manifest during the first phase include breathing difficulties and chest pain, neither of which can be referred to as 'mild'. It is during the second or chronic phase that the symptoms become serious because the parasites are said to 'hide' in the heart muscles and cause a potentially fatal cardiac condition.

The fact sheet claims, however, that,

"Trypanosoma cruzi infection is curable if treatment is initiated soon after infection."

Chagas disease is treated with two drugs, namely benznidazole and nifurtimox, the 'side effects' of both of which include polyneuropathy, nausea, vomiting, dizziness and headache. These effects demonstrate that both drugs are toxic and neurotoxic.

It should be clear that Chagas disease is not caused by the *T. cruzi* parasite, and that the real causes of the symptoms attributed to this disease will involve exposures to a variety of toxic substances, most of which are produced by various industries that operate in South America. Some of the significant industries in the region include mining and smelting, both of which have been discussed and shown to cause serious health hazards in addition to environmental pollution.

Other industries common throughout the region include the manufacture of pesticides and petrochemicals. Previous discussions have indicated that these industries and their products are associated with many hazards to human health and with the environmental pollution that exacerbates the hazards. The high level of agriculture in many regions of South America has inevitably entailed the increased use of pesticides, which contaminate the food as well as the environment.

The April 2019 WHO fact sheet entitled *Trypanosomiasis, human African (sleeping sickness)* states that this disease is endemic in 36 countries within sub-Saharan Africa. There are said to be two forms of the disease depending on the type of parasite involved, although the parasite called *Trypanosoma brucei gambiense* is said to be responsible for 98 per cent of all cases. The vector claimed to be responsible for the transmission of the parasite is the tsetse fly, although it is only 'infected' females that are said to transmit the disease when they take a blood 'meal'. In common with female *Anopheles* mosquitoes, the female tsetse flies are not all infected, but, according to the fact sheet, they,

"...have acquired their infection from human beings or from animals harbouring human pathogenic parasites."

This claim is clearly anomalous; the human disease is claimed to be caused by 'infection' with the parasite transmitted through the bite of an infected tsetse fly, yet the fly must first be infected as the result of biting a human. Another anomalous feature common to virtually all 'parasitic diseases' is that the vector remains unaffected by the parasites that they carry within their tiny bodies, whereas the far larger human 'host' can be seriously harmed and even die due to their presence in the body.

There are two stages of human African trypanosomiasis; the first stage, which is said to involve the invasion of the tissues and blood, produces 'mild' symptoms such as fever, headaches and joint pains. The second stage is more serious; as the fact sheet states,

"In the second stage the parasites cross the blood-brain barrier to infect the central nervous system."

The symptoms produced in the second stage are the reason this disease is also known as sleeping sickness, as they include confusion, sensory disturbances, poor coordination and disturbance of the sleep cycle. Human African trypanosomiasis is also claimed to be treatable, but the fact sheet states that,

"Diagnosis and treatment of the disease is complex and requires specifically skilled staff."

The 'treatment' involves five drugs, which the WHO distributes free of charge to all countries in which the disease is considered to be endemic. Two of these drugs are used during the first stage; these are pentamidine and suramin. The three drugs used during the second stage are melarsoprol, eflornithine and nifurtimox. All of these drugs are inherently toxic; the purpose for which they are used is to kill parasites. It is therefore unsurprising that they are all associated with adverse 'side effects', which include chest pain and breathing difficulties, vomiting and diarrhoea, gastrointestinal problems and polyneuritis, amongst others. Melarsoprol is derived from arsenic, which has a long history of use in the treatment of this disease. A 2013 article entitled *Arsenic – the 'Poison of Kings' and the 'Saviour of Syphilis'* refers to the use of arsenic-based drugs for the treatment of trypanosomiasis in the early 19th century and states that,

"...its effectiveness was outweighed by its neurotoxicity..."

This raises the serious question of why the treatment for a disease that is said to affect the CNS involves a substance that has long been known to be neurotoxic.

As discussed in chapter four, an epidemic of lethargic encephalitis (LE) coincided with that of '1918 Flu'. The discussion indicated that LE is also known as 'sleepy sickness' in order to distinguish it from 'sleeping sickness' or human African trypanosomiasis. This distinction would seem to be irrelevant because both conditions are neurological; therefore, a far more plausible explanation for both of them would include exposures to toxic and neurotoxic substances.

The operations of many industries located in Africa are capable of producing adverse neurological health effects; these include mining and especially large-scale gold mining that invariably entails exposures to mercury, a known neurotoxin. Exposure to mercury also results from small-scale gold mining, also known as artisanal small-scale gold mining (ASGM) that has expanded in many 'developing' countries, particularly within Africa. The report entitled *The World's Worst Pollution Problems 2016* ranks ASGM as 5th in the list of *Top 10 Polluting Industries*. The most significant pollutant associated with ASGM is mercury, which is used during the extraction process and is a recognised cause of serious health problems; as indicated by a 2017 article entitled *Global Burden of Disease of Mercury Used in Artisanal Small-Scale Gold Mining*, which states that,

"Gold miners are highly exposed to metallic mercury and suffer occupational mercury intoxication."

Although miners are the most affected, they are not the only people to be exposed to mercury; people who live in the vicinity of gold mines will also be adversely affected by mercury and all other pollutants released into the environment. Exposure to mercury is only one factor amongst many that can cause damage to the nervous system; exposures to varying combinations of different toxic and neurotoxic substances provide a far more compelling explanation for neurological health problems than a 'parasite'.

Leishmaniasis

The establishment definition refers to leishmaniasis as,

"a disease, common in the tropics and subtropics, caused by parasitic protozoans of the genus *Leishmania*, which are transmitted by the bite of sandflies."

There are said to be many hundreds of sandfly species, but only some of them are claimed to be vectors of the *Leishmania* parasite, as the March 2019 WHO fact sheet entitled *Leishmaniasis* states,

"Over 90 sandfly species are known to transmit *Leishmania* parasites."

There are also many species of parasite, as the fact sheet states,

"Leishmaniasis is caused by a protozoa parasite from over 20 *Leishmania* species."

In common with other 'parasitic' diseases, leishmaniasis is said to be caused by the transmission of a parasite through the bite of an 'infected' female when she takes a blood 'meal'. However, the discussion about leishmaniasis in chapter three referred to the claim by the WHO that, in most cases, 'infection' with the parasite does not result in disease; this is corroborated by the CDC FAQ web page about the disease that states,

"Some people have a silent infection, without any symptoms or signs."

It is claimed that there are three distinct forms of the disease; they are referred to as visceral, cutaneous and mucocutaneous.

Visceral leishmaniasis (VL), which is also known as kala-azar, is the most serious and is said to be fatal in the vast majority of cases, unless treated. The symptoms of VL, which is said to be 'highly endemic' in India and East Africa, include anaemia and enlargement of the spleen and the liver. Cutaneous leishmaniasis (CL) is said to be the most common form; the main symptoms are skin lesions, usually in the form of ulcers. Mucocutaneous leishmaniasis (ML) is said to involve the destruction of the mucous membranes of the nose, mouth and throat.

There is, however, no explanation for the manifestation of three distinctly different groups of symptoms that are claimed to be caused by members of the same species of parasite. The CDC web pages about leishmaniasis include one entitled *Biology* that presents a diagram of the life-cycle of the parasite. Interestingly, the page states that,

> "Parasite, host, and other factors affect whether the infection becomes symptomatic and whether cutaneous or visceral leishmaniasis results."

The web page provides no further details about the 'other factors' said to be involved; nor does it provide an explanation for the role of the 'host' in the development of disease. The WHO fact sheet, however, does provide some clues about these 'other factors' in the statement that,

> "The disease affects some of the poorest people on earth, and is associated with malnutrition, population displacement, poor housing, a weak immune system and lack of financial resources."

The reason that sandflies would choose to only 'bite' and 'infect' poor people who are malnourished remains unexplained. However, as previously cited, the *Molecular Biology of the Cell* textbook states that 'dedicated pathogens' do not require the host to have a weakened immune system.

The fact sheet refers to leishmaniasis as treatable and curable, but that the treatment,

> "...requires an immunocompetent system because medicines will not get rid of the parasite from the body..."

This indicates that the people most affected by the disease cannot be treated.

Although the fact sheet does not provide details of the 'medicines' recommended by the WHO, this information is available in a 2017 article entitled *Diagnosis and Treatment of Leishmaniasis* that provides clinical practice guidelines and states that,

> "The only Food and Drug Administration (FDA) approved medications for the treatment of leishmaniasis are intravenous liposomal amphotericin B (L-AmB) for VL and oral miltefosine for CL, ML and VL caused by particular species."

In common with all drugs, those recommended for leishmaniasis are toxic and produce many adverse effects. Liposomal amphotericin is associated with nephrotoxic effects and liver damage. Miltefosine is associated with nausea, vomiting and diarrhoea; it can also cause liver and kidney problems. It should be noted that previous treatments for leishmaniasis have included, and in some cases still include, antimony-based drugs; antimony is a known toxin.

The claims about leishmaniasis, like all other 'parasitic' diseases, are highly anomalous; none of them provides an adequate explanation for the mechanism by which microscopic organisms can cause serious and potentially fatal health problems for humans but produce no ill effects in the tiny insect vector. There is also no explanation for the claim that 'infection' is not always accompanied by symptoms. There is however, a plausible explanation for the symptoms associated with this disease; like all other diseases, this includes exposure to a variety of toxic substances.

Schistosomiasis

The establishment definition of schistosomiasis, also known as bilharzia, refers to, "a tropical disease caused by blood flukes of the genus *Schistosoma*."

Schistosoma blood flukes, also known as trematodes, are a type of worm; the vector claimed to be responsible for their transmission is a freshwater snail, as the April 2019 WHO fact sheet entitled *Schistosomiasis* states,

"People become infected when larval forms of the parasite – released by freshwater snails – penetrate the skin during contact with infested water."

The infestation of water is claimed to occur when people 'infected' with the disease contaminate the water with their faeces, which contain the eggs of the *Schistosoma* parasites that require fresh water in order to hatch. The CDC web pages entitled *Schistosomiasis* include one entitled *Biology* that claims there are three main species of parasite that 'infect' humans; it also provides a diagram of the parasite's life-cycle.

There are said to be two forms of the disease, one of which is intestinal and produces symptoms that include abdominal pain, diarrhoea and blood in the stool. The symptoms of the advanced form of the disease include enlargement of the liver; however, according to the WHO fact sheet,

"Symptoms of schistosomiasis are caused by the body's reaction to the worm's eggs."

It is clear that the symptoms described above can result from the body's reactions to exposures to toxic substances; the fact sheet also claims that,

"In children, schistosomiasis can cause anaemia, stunting and a reduced ability to learn..."

There is no explanation for the mechanisms by which a parasite is able to produce such a wide variety of symptoms that include impaired growth and development, which, as previously discussed, are functions regulated by the endocrine system.

Unsurprisingly, and like the other 'parasitic' diseases discussed in this chapter, schistosomiasis mainly affects certain sectors of the population, as the fact sheet states,

"Schistosomiasis is prevalent in tropical and subtropical areas, especially in poor communities without access to safe drinking water and adequate sanitation."

Also, like the other parasitic diseases, the fact sheet claims that schistosomiasis can be controlled through 'medicines',

"The WHO strategy for schistosomiasis control focuses on reducing disease through periodic targeted treatment with praziquantel..."

The populations targeted for this 'preventive' treatment are those people who live in the 'highly endemic' areas, which are predominantly within Africa. Praziquantel is also used in the treatment of a number of other parasitic infections. However, like all treatments of this type, the purpose of praziquantel is to kill parasites; this drug is therefore inherently toxic; it is, unsurprisingly associated with adverse health effects such as abdominal pain, vomiting and headache. More serious effects include dizziness, fatigue and vertigo.

Another similarity with the other 'parasitic' diseases is that the *Schistosoma* parasites do not appear to affect the vector, in this case, the water snail; although the process is unexplained, it is claimed that the snails are 'equipped' to defend themselves. This would suggest that, yet again, the small vector remains unaffected by a parasite that can cause serious harm to the much larger human hosts, who are believed to be incapable of defending themselves.

But, contrary to this belief, humans are not defenceless; the human body has a number of self-protective mechanisms. The existence of these mechanisms is corroborated by a 2017 article entitled *Nitric oxide blocks the development of the human parasite Schistosoma japonicum*; the title is self-explanatory. However, the body's protective mechanisms may be impaired when health has been compromised as the result of poor living conditions and malnutrition, for example.

The likely causes of the symptoms associated with schistosomiasis, which is claimed to be transmitted through 'infested' water, will include pesticides, such as larvicides to control mosquito larvae, that are applied directly into or near bodies of fresh water. In addition to these toxins, are many other water contaminants, such as toxic industrial wastes discharged into these bodies of water.

Noncommunicable Diseases

Target 4 of SDG 3 aims to,

> "By 2030, reduce by one third premature mortality from non-communicable diseases through prevention and treatment and promote mental health and well-being."

Although noncommunicable diseases were discussed in detail in chapter seven, they require a further, albeit brief, discussion in the context of their prevalence in 'developing' countries, because, as the WHO June 2018 fact sheet entitled *Noncommunicable diseases* states,

> "NCDs disproportionately affect people in low- and middle-income countries..."

This statement is not consistent with the claim that communicable diseases are more prevalent in 'developing' countries. It is also inconsistent with the statement in the *Global Health Risks* report that the types of diseases change from communicable to noncommunicable as countries 'develop'. The populations of 'low- and middle-income' countries would seem to be 'disproportionately affected' by disease of all types.

The idea that any disease disproportionately affects people in 'developing' countries needs to be placed into the correct context with reference to two circumstances, the first of which is that the overwhelming majority of the world population lives in countries categorised as 'developing'. The second is that, as the medical establishment has admitted, most 'developing' countries do not have adequate, if any, systems for recording and reporting disease morbidity and mortality. The statistics provided by the medical establishment and reported in fact sheets do not reflect exact numbers, but instead, are predominantly estimates generated by computer models.

Nevertheless, the WHO fact sheet claims that certain sectors of the population are more likely to become ill,

> "Vulnerable and socially disadvantaged people get sicker and die sooner than people of higher social positions..."

The reasons are claimed to be because 'low-income' countries in particular lack the resources to provide adequate 'healthcare services', and because most people in those countries lack the income to be able to afford the few services and 'treatments' that are available. Therefore, according to the fact sheet,

"Poverty is closely linked with NCDs."

It should be clear that 'poverty' is not unique to the populations of 'developing' countries. More importantly, however, an individual person's state of health is not related to the stage of development or the income of the country in which they live; their individual personal circumstances exert a far greater influence over their health. These circumstances involve a wide variety of factors that are unique to each person, as will be discussed in more detail in chapter ten.

The previously cited *Global Action Plan* report, states that,

"Four main shared risk factors—tobacco use, unhealthy diet, physical inactivity and harmful use of alcohol—are the most important in the sphere of noncommunicable diseases."

The reference to these risk factors as 'behavioural' and 'modifiable', as well as the 'most important' in respect of the onset of NCDs, is intended to suggest that people who engage in these 'behaviours' are mostly responsible for their own illness when they have been diagnosed with an NCD. Although three of these factors do contribute to ill-health, they are by no means the only factors relevant to NCDs, as the discussions in chapter seven demonstrated.

People are, to a large extent, responsible for their own health and ill-health, as will be further discussed in chapter ten; however, it is disingenuous of the medical establishment to repudiate any share of the responsibility for the escalation of ill-health around the world. The phenomenon of iatrogenesis demonstrates that 'modern medicine' is a major contributory factor to illness; pharmaceutical drugs are not conducive to improved health.

The four major NCDs said to cause the highest mortality are: cardiovascular diseases, cancer, chronic respiratory diseases and diabetes, all of which are claimed to significantly affect the populations of low- and middle-income countries; as indicated by the May 2017 WHO fact sheet entitled *Cardiovascular diseases (CVDs)*, which states that,

"At least three quarters of the world's deaths from CVDs occur in low- and middle-income countries."

CVDs are said to be caused by the same four behavioural risk factors that apply to all NCDs. These factors are referred to as modifiable, which is intended to indicate that CVDs are therefore preventable through the modification or avoidance of the relevant behaviours. It is claimed that these behaviours cause CVDs because they precipitate the development of 'intermediate risk factors', such as raised blood pressure, which, according to the medical establishment, should be treated. However, as the discussion about CVDs in chapter seven indicated, blood pressure-lowering drugs cause additional health problems and often fail to prevent a heart attack or stroke.

The burden of cancer in 'low- and middle-income countries' is claimed to be substantial; as indicated by the September 2018 WHO fact sheet entitled *Cancer* that states,

"Approximately 70% of deaths from cancer occur in low- and middle-income countries."

In addition to the four main 'risk factors', the fact sheet claims that certain 'infections' are particularly relevant to the onset of cancer in 'developing' countries,

"Cancer causing infections, such as hepatitis and human papilloma virus (HPV), are responsible for up to 25% of cancer cases in low- and middle-income countries."

As previously discussed, cancer and 'infections' involve completely different mechanisms of action. Unfortunately, the belief that viruses are pathogens that can also cause cancer, has encouraged the development of various vaccines claimed to be able to provide protection against 'cancer-causing infections'; according to the fact sheet,

"Vaccination against these HPV and hepatitis B viruses could prevent 1 million cancer cases each year."

As previous discussions have shown, this claim is unfounded; the overwhelming body of evidence demonstrates that vaccines cannot prevent any disease, including cancer.

The WHO web page entitled *Chronic respiratory diseases (CRDs)* claims that the most common CRD is asthma; the WHO August 2017 fact sheet entitled *Asthma* states that 235 million people suffer from asthma and that,

"Most asthma-related deaths occur in low- and middle-income countries."

The previous discussion about asthma indicated that one of the major causes of the condition involves inhalation of toxic irritants, whether air pollution, VOCs or other airborne contaminants. It is interesting, therefore, that one of the less common CRDs is referred to as 'occupational lung disease', which is clearly the result of workplace exposures to substances that irritate and damage the respiratory system; but it is inappropriate to describe such damage as a 'disease'. The expansion of industrialisation in, as well as the increasing relocation of polluting industries to, 'developing' countries contribute to an ever-greater incidence of many health problems, including those that affect the respiratory system.

Diabetes is the fourth major NCD; it is another disease that is anticipated to continue to increase in incidence. Furthermore, according to the WHO October 2018 fact sheet entitled *Diabetes*,

"Diabetes prevalence has been rising more rapidly in middle- and low-income countries."

The fact sheet claims that excess body weight is a major risk factor for type 2 diabetes and that a healthy diet is one method by which this condition can be prevented. However, although the WHO recommends an increased intake of fruit and vegetables, the fact sheet fails to acknowledge the full extent to which an unhealthy diet that mainly consists of processed foods and drinks made with high levels of refined sugars, contributes to the disease. The previous discussion about diabetes included the reference by

535

Dr Henry Bieler to the existence of a 'toxic background' in people with this condition; the discussion also referred to the role of refined sugar, which is described as the 'sweetest poison of all'. The increased consumption of highly-processed food products and drinks by people in 'developing' countries will exacerbate their health problems.

The measures deemed necessary to address the burden of disease caused by all types of NCDs are briefly referred to in the *Global Action Plan* report, the *Foreword* of which declares that,

> "WHO and other UN Organizations will support national efforts with upstream policy advice and sophisticated technical assistance, ranging from helping governments to set national targets to implement even relatively simple steps which can make a huge difference, such as raising tobacco taxes, reducing the amount of salt in foods and improving access to inexpensive drugs to prevent heart attacks and strokes."

It has been shown historically that raising taxes on tobacco or alcohol, or both, is virtually ineffective as a deterrent. Price increases rarely discourage the vast majority of consumers from continuing to purchase tobacco products or alcohol; they will however, succeed in causing greater hardship and deepening poverty. A more appropriate and responsible measure would be for the medical establishment to properly inform the public about the serious health hazards from the factors discussed in chapter six; the reasons this is unlikely to happen are discussed in chapter nine.

In common with all aspects of medical establishment practices, the recommended measures to address the health problems due to NCDs are claimed to be scientifically established and based on the latest evidence, as the *Global Action Plan* report states,

> "Scientific knowledge demonstrates that the noncommunicable disease burden can be greatly reduced if cost-effective preventive and curative actions, along with interventions for prevention and control of noncommunicable diseases already available, are implemented in an effective and balanced manner."

However, as the report states, the recommended measures are also to include actions to improve access to drugs claimed to prevent heart attacks and strokes. One of these suggested drugs is acetylsalicylic acid, better known as aspirin, for the prevention of acute myocardial infarction. The report also recommends hepatitis B vaccinations for the prevention of liver cancer. Previous discussions have demonstrated that neither of these measures are preventive or curative and that they are both associated with adverse health effects.

The burden of NCDs is considered to be of such a magnitude, especially for 'developing' countries, that, according to the WHO fact sheet,

> "NCDs threaten progress towards the 2030 Agenda for Sustainable Development..."

The high level of mortality due to NCDs is said to pose a serious threat to the 'economy' of countries as well as to their 'sustainable development'. The premature deaths of millions of people in their 'productive' years is said to impose a significant economic burden on all countries, but especially on those countries categorised as 'developing'. This burden is compounded by the cost of healthcare services and the interventions required to treat people who have been diagnosed with an NCD. Although these people remain alive, their illness incapacitates them, which means they are unable to work and therefore unable to contribute to the economy.

It is for this reason that interventions are required to be 'cost-effective'; in other words, it is claimed that the actions to be taken should not cost more than a person is able to contribute to the economy; this view is expressed by the *Global Action Plan* report in the statement that,

> "There are interventions for prevention and control of noncommunicable diseases that are affordable for all countries and give a good return on investment generating one year of healthy life for a cost that falls below the gross domestic product (GDP) per person..."

The interventions proposed by the medical establishment, however 'cost-effective' they may be, will not generate a 'healthy life' for any person, nor will they reduce the incidence of NCDs.

Many 'interventions' claimed to prevent and control NCDs have been successfully introduced into the health services of 'developed' countries; a strategy that is to be expanded, so that similar interventions can be introduced into the health services of all 'developing' countries. These interventions include a variety of 'medicines' and vaccines, the increased production of which will inevitably generate a massive boost to the income and profits of pharmaceutical manufacturing companies. Unfortunately, but equally inevitable, is that, if successfully implemented, interventions of this nature will generate a substantially increased incidence of iatrogenic illness and death in 'developing' countries.

Mental Health

In addition to the reduction of NCDs, the aim of SDG 3.4 is to promote mental health and well-being, which is recognised to be as important as physical health and well-being. Mental health has been discussed in chapter one and will be discussed again in chapter ten, but requires a brief discussion in this chapter in the context of how mental health and well-being for everyone, everywhere is to be achieved.

Good mental health, like good physical health, is perceived to be important so that people can be 'productive units'; as indicated by the *Mental Health Action Plan 2013-2020* report, which states that,

> "Good mental health enables people to realize their potential, cope with the normal stresses of life, work productively, and contribute to their communities."

The medical establishment considers that poor mental health is indicative of a 'mental health problem', or 'mental disorder', as they are more commonly labelled. As previously cited in chapter one, the April 2018 WHO fact sheet entitled *Mental disorders* claims that,

> "There are many different mental disorders, with different presentations."

Although the reason remains unexplained, the medical establishment claims that the incidence of 'mental disorders' is rising and that these conditions affect people in all countries, whether 'developed' or 'developing'; as the fact sheet states,

> "The burden of mental disorders continues to grow with significant impacts on

health and major social, human rights and economic consequences in all countries of the world."

One of the major consequences of the continually growing incidence of 'mental disorders' is, according to the fact sheet, that,

"Health systems have not yet adequately responded to the burden of mental disorders."

The failure of 'health systems' to adequately respond means that they have insufficient numbers of staff, especially suitably qualified psychiatrists, to provide the necessary services for people who have 'mental disorders'. These poor staffing levels are claimed to have a more profound effect in 'developing' countries; as indicated by the *Mental Health Action Plan* report that states,

"The number of specialized and general health workers dealing with mental health in low-income and middle-income countries is grossly insufficient."

Another of the major concerns expressed in the report is that,

"People with mental disorders experience disproportionately higher rates of disability and mortality."

This claim requires further examination. Like a 'physical illness', a 'mental illness' is said to be diagnosed by the manifestation of certain symptoms; however, unlike a physical illness, the symptoms associated with a mental illness are rather nebulous. Although previously cited, the WHO fact sheet states that 'mental disorders' are,

"...generally characterized by a combination of abnormal thoughts, perceptions, emotions, behaviour and relationships with others."

There is, however, no clear definition of what constitutes 'normal' with respect to a person's thoughts, perceptions, emotions, behaviours and relationships. Furthermore, as discussed in chapter one, there are no scientifically established criteria or tests to determine the existence of an 'abnormal' mental state; the interpretation of 'abnormal' is highly subjective.

The most important aspect of the claim that the burden of 'mental disorders' is increasing is that these conditions are generally considered to require 'treatment'; but these treatments are not readily available to everyone perceived to be in need of them. The fact sheet reports that one of the consequences of the inadequate response by health systems has been that,

"...the gap between the need for treatment and its provision is wide all over the world."

The fact sheet claims that in 'high-income' countries, this 'gap' may affect between 35 and 50 per cent of people with mental disorders; but in 'low- and middle-income' countries, this gap is far worse and may affect between 76 and 85 per cent of people with mental disorders.

Specific treatments are not mentioned in the report or the fact sheet, although both refer to non-pharmacological approaches as well as to 'medicines'. The claim that there are gaps between treatment and its provision would seem to justify the concerns about the inadequate levels of staff in the field of 'mental health'; however, psychiatry is increasingly biased towards the use of pharmacological approaches in preference to non-pharmacological ones. The discussion in chapter one about psychiatric medications indicated that, not only are they entirely inappropriate as 'treatment' for conditions labelled as 'mental disorders', but they are also eminently capable of causing a great deal of harm, including a worsening of the symptoms they are claimed to manage.

In addition to pharmaceutical products, the treatment of 'mental disorders' may include therapies such as 'electric shock' treatments, which are reported to be undergoing a revival, although under the label ECT (electroconvulsive therapy), and mainly used in the treatment of depression. Previous discussions have referred to the bioelectrical nature of the body, and to the evidence that exposures to certain electromagnetic fields produce detrimental effects on many of the body's functions. The direct application of an unnatural electric current to the brain, one of the two major organs that function bioelectrically, has the ability to cause serious harm. The increased use of 'treatments', both chemical and electrical, will clearly exacerbate the incidence of iatrogenic morbidity and mortality; they do not contribute to good mental or physical health and well-being.

As previously cited, the fact sheet states that,

> "Stress, genetics, nutrition, perinatal infections and exposure to environmental hazards are also contributing factors to mental disorders."

Stress is a significant factor; the many circumstances that can induce stress include wars and conflicts; the effects of the stresses of war on soldiers have been recognised and assigned labels such as 'shell shock' and PTSD (post-traumatic stress disorder); but it is not solely those involved in the fighting that are affected by war. The nature of war has changed dramatically since WWI as have the types of weapons used. However, although the world has not been at war since 1945, many smaller wars and conflicts have taken place in many different regions of the world, including those within 'developing' countries. Some of these conflicts have been of a long duration and have created many humanitarian crises involving large numbers of refugees who have had to flee their homes in order to survive. These refugees clearly exist in a perpetual state of severe stress, but they cannot be regarded as suffering from a 'mental disorder'.

There are many reasons that people may exhibit the symptoms associated with a 'mental disorder', including, as the fact sheet acknowledges, 'exposure to environmental hazards'. These hazards include unnatural electromagnetic radiation and a wide variety of neurotoxic substances, all of which are known to affect the functions of the brain. Common neurotoxins include aluminium, mercury, lead, aspartame, methanol and fluoride, to name just a few; these neurotoxic substances can be found in various everyday household products as well as pesticides, 'medicines' and vaccines.

It is clear therefore, that the increased rates of disability and mortality claimed to be associated with 'mental disorders' are the direct result of the same factors that cause virtually all conditions of illness.

Reproductive Health

There are two aspects relating to 'reproductive health'; the first refers to maternal mortality, which is the subject of target 1 of SDG 3 that aims to,

"By 2030, reduce the global maternal mortality ratio to less than 70 per 100,000 live births."

The scale of this problem is indicated by the February 2018 WHO fact sheet entitled *Maternal mortality*, which states that,

"Every day, approximately 830 women die from preventable causes related to pregnancy and childbirth."

The fact sheet also states that,

"99% of all maternal deaths occur in developing countries."

Significantly, the fact sheet claims that more than half of these maternal deaths occur in sub-Saharan Africa and that they mainly affect the poor in rural areas. The veracity of these statistics is questionable on the basis of the admission that most 'developing' countries lack adequate mortality data collecting systems.

The main cause of maternal mortality is attributed to 'complications' that are largely preventable, but occur because women in 'developing' countries, unlike their counterparts in 'developed' countries, lack access to 'healthcare services', especially those provided by antenatal clinics. The inequity of this situation is used to justify demands that pregnant women in 'developing' countries receive the same level of antenatal and postnatal care as women in 'developed' countries; as indicated by the fact sheet that states,

"All women need access to antenatal care in pregnancy, skilled care during childbirth and care and support in the weeks after childbirth."

It would seem that, according to this attitude, the medical establishment perceives pregnancy and childbirth to be 'medical conditions' rather than part of the natural processes of human life. Whilst it certainly is important for women to receive an appropriate level of care during pregnancy and childbirth, women have successfully carried, given birth to and cared for babies for tens, if not hundreds of thousands of years with the assistance of other women acting as midwives. Although, in the past, many women have died during childbirth, reductions in maternal mortality are mainly due to the same factors that have contributed to overall health, such as nutrition and improved living conditions, for example.

It is acknowledged that complications may occur and that they will require the application of certain skills to protect both mother and baby, but these complications do not occur in sufficient numbers to necessitate intervention in all cases. The purpose of most interventions is to prevent a potential problem rather than address an existing problem; the discussions throughout this book indicate that most medical 'interventions' are unnecessary and many are decidedly harmful.

Three of the 'complications' specifically referred to are: severe bleeding, 'infections' and high blood pressure, all of which are claimed to require interventions as preventive measures; for example, the fact sheet claims that,

"Injecting oxytocin immediately after childbirth effectively reduces the risk of bleeding."

Oxytocin is a hormone; the injected form is a synthetic derivative, which, like all pharmaceutical hormones is known to produce 'side effects'. The effects associated with injected oxytocin include nausea and vomiting, which are indicative of its toxic nature. It should be noted that oxytocin is also used to induce labour and to induce an abortion.

Antenatal clinics provide a variety of services, including blood tests, to detect the existence of underlying conditions that may pose a problem during the pregnancy or childbirth. Unfortunately, one of those tests is to determine a pregnant woman's 'HIV status', which is of particular concern in 'developing' countries, but especially in African countries where 'HIV' is claimed to be most prevalent. However, as previously discussed, pregnancy is one of the 'conditions' that can give rise to a 'false positive' HIV test result. Nevertheless, a positive test result is very likely to lead to 'treatment' with toxic ARV 'medicines' for the mother, both during and after her pregnancy, and for the baby after birth; the toxicity of these drugs has been discussed.

Postnatal care also involves various services, some of which may involve certain interventions for the baby as well as the mother; the main interventions offered to newborn babies are 'immunisations', the problems and hazards with which have been discussed at length.

The second aspect of 'reproductive health' refers to a wider range of issues that are incorporated into target 7 of SDG 3, the aim of which is to,

"By 2030, ensure universal access to sexual and reproductive health-care services, including for family planning, information and education and the integration of reproductive health into national strategies and programmes."

The justification for interventions in respect of 'reproductive health' is indicated by the February 2018 WHO fact sheet entitled *Family planning/contraception*, which, under the sub-heading *Slowing population growth*, states that,

"Family planning is key to slowing unsustainable population growth and the resulting negative impacts on the economy, environment, and national and regional development efforts."

The idea that population growth is 'unsustainable' is based on the theory attributed to Thomas Malthus, which claims that, if unchecked, the rate of growth of the population will always exceed the rate of growth of food production. This theory has been interpreted to mean that population growth rates should therefore be 'controlled'; the topic of 'population control' is discussed in chapter nine. However, the mistaken belief that this idea represents a bona fide theory has had profound consequences, not least of which has been the promotion of fear-based claims that the world is in imminent danger of becoming 'overpopulated' and unable to provide sufficient food for the burgeoning population. According to the Population Reference Bureau (PRB) web page entitled *2017 World Population Data Sheet*, the world population is projected to reach 9.8 billion by 2050. Furthermore, the page claims that,

"...Africa's population will more than double to 2.6 billion by 2050..."

The purpose of this statement is to instil fear into people; it is intended to convey the impression that such a population increase would create a huge 'problem', but this claim fails to recognise that Africa, a resource-rich region of the world, is the second largest continent with a land area of approximately 30.3 million km². It also fails to recognise that, even if this population growth were to occur, the continent would not be overcrowded, nor would Africans be unable to feed themselves; the topic of food production in Africa is discussed in more detail later in this chapter. The main UN organisation responsible for matters relating to 'population' is UNFPA, which is described on the *About us* web page as,

"...the United Nations reproductive health and rights agency. Our mission is to deliver a world where every pregnancy is wanted, every childbirth is safe and every young person's potential is fulfilled."

The mission of UNFPA is related to 'sexual health' as well as 'reproductive health', and the importance of both to 'development, as the web page entitled *Sexual and reproductive health* states,

"UNFPA works to ensure sexual and reproductive health and rights remain at the very centre of development."

The concern about 'sexual health' is almost entirely related to 'infections' that are claimed to be sexually transmitted and to cause serious health problems, even death; as the UNFPA indicates on the same page that states,

"More than a million people acquire an STI every single day. Without diagnosis and treatment, some STIs, such as HIV or syphilis, can be fatal."

In addition, UNFPA claims that these 'infections' can affect pregnancy and childbirth, as indicated by the statement that,

"STIs can also cause pregnancy-related complications, including stillbirth, congenital infections, sepsis and neonatal death."

The claims in both of the above statements are unfounded; they are also erroneous. Previous discussions have demonstrated that no disease is caused by 'pathogenic organisms'; that no disease is sexually transmitted; and that the treatments used for these diseases are harmful. Previous discussions have also indicated that many factors are able to cause the wide variety of health problems erroneously attributed to 'infections'; these factors include, but are not restricted to, exposures to chemicals and electromagnetic radiation that can disrupt the mother's endocrine system and adversely affect her developing baby.

It should be clear that health problems caused by toxic chemicals or EM radiation cannot be prevented by better access to 'healthcare services' that include the administration of medicines and vaccines. Furthermore, some of the proposed 'solutions' are likely to be contributory factors; for example, the WHO family planning fact sheet claims that,

"Some family planning methods, such as condoms, help prevent the transmission of HIV and other sexually transmitted infections."

This claim fails to acknowledge the existence of health risks associated with the use of certain types of contraceptives. The materials used to make condoms include latex, which has been associated with 'allergic' reactions; a clear indication that this material is an irritant. In addition, condoms are generally used in conjunction with a lubricant and a spermicide; one of the chemicals used as an ingredient of condom lubricants is benzene; a known carcinogen. A common ingredient of spermicides is a substance called nonoxynol-9, which is also reported to be an irritant. As previously discussed, the definition of a 'poison' includes reference to a substance that causes irritation to the body's tissues; the materials and chemical ingredients used in condoms can therefore be described as 'toxic', although spermicides are toxic by intention. The application of toxic substances to the genital area or inside the body is therefore, eminently capable of causing irritations and other unpleasant symptoms that may be mistakenly interpreted to indicate the presence of an 'infection'.

The causes of reproductive health problems cannot be separated from the causes of all health problems; but none of them can be addressed by most of the recommended interventions provided through 'health services', especially those that treat pregnancy and childbirth as if they were 'medical conditions' rather than natural processes.

Hazardous Chemicals

The harmful effects of exposures to 'hazardous chemicals' are recognised in target 9 of SDG 3 that aims to,

"By 2030, substantially reduce the number of deaths and illnesses from hazardous chemicals and air, water and soil pollution and contamination."

The measures by which the goals of the 2030 Agenda are to be achieved, are generally incorporated into a variety of programmes to be administered by organisations within or associated with the UN system; in the case of health matters, this will invariably involve the WHO. One such programme is the IPCS (International Programme on Chemical Safety), which is administered by the WHO. The WHO web page about the IPCS describes its function and states that, through IPCS,

"...WHO works to establish the scientific basis for the sound management of chemicals, and to strengthen national capabilities and capacities for chemical safety."

The web page also provides links to related topics, one of which is a page entitled *Ten chemicals of major public health concern*. These ten chemicals, or groups of chemicals, are: air pollution; arsenic; asbestos; benzene; cadmium; dioxin and dioxin-like substances; inadequate or excess fluoride; lead; mercury; and highly hazardous pesticides. With the sole exception of 'inadequate fluoride', these substances have all been proven to be extremely hazardous to health.

Air pollution is produced by a number of substances; some of the major air pollutants are discussed in a 2010 WHO report entitled *WHO Guidelines for indoor air quality: selected pollutants*. The pollutants referred to include: benzene, formaldehyde, radon, polycyclic aromatic hydrocarbons and trichloroethylene, amongst others; the report states that all of the listed pollutants,

"...have indoor sources, are known in respect of their hazardousness to health and are often found indoors in concentrations of health concern."

The report also states that only the effects of individual chemicals are considered, but recognises that exposures are always to combinations of pollutants; nevertheless, the report admits that,

"Data dealing with the effects of co-exposure to air pollutants are very limited..."

The existence of limited information about the hazards from exposures to combinations of multiple substances is common to all 'hazardous chemicals', not just air pollutants.

The WHO web page about the IPCS also provides a link to a page entitled *Public health impact of chemicals: knowns and unknowns*, which refers to a 2016 report with the same title. The web page provides some information about the contents of the report including an *Overview* that refers to the loss in 2012 of more than one million lives,

"...due to exposures to selected chemicals."

It has been acknowledged by the scientific and medical research communities that there is a dearth of information about the hazards caused by most chemicals; this paucity of data is also recognised by the WHO on the *Overview* page that states,

"...data are only available for a small number of chemical exposures and people are exposed to many more chemicals every day."

The report claims that 'unintentional poisonings' are responsible for an estimated 193,000 deaths annually, most of which are said to be preventable, which suggests that they mainly result from accidental exposures to 'poisons'; the report states that,

"Chemicals such as heavy metals, pesticides, solvents, paints, detergents, kerosene, carbon monoxide and drugs lead to **unintentional poisonings** at home and in the workplace."

One of the recommended solutions for the problem of unintentional poisonings in the home is to store medicines and cleaning products 'out of reach', although this presumably refers to the reach of small children. The number of deaths from accidental poisoning represents only a small fraction of the total number of people who are harmed or killed by regular, long-term exposures to the plethora of toxic ingredients of a wide variety of products used regularly in the home and workplace, a number of which were discussed in chapter six.

Despite the acknowledged paucity of data about the full extent of the adverse health effects that can be caused by exposures to hazardous chemicals, the prevailing view is that the impact on human health and the environment can be minimised through the implementation of 'sound management' practices; as demonstrated by target 4 of SDG 12 that aims to,

"By 2020, achieve the environmentally sound management of chemicals and all wastes throughout their life cycle, in accordance with agreed international frameworks, and significantly reduce their release to air, water and soil in order to minimize their adverse impacts on human health and the environment."

It is interesting to note that this target is anticipated to be achieved by 2020 and therefore a full decade earlier than most other 2030 Agenda goals; this is extremely ambitious considering the magnitude of the problem. However, merely 'managing' toxic chemicals is not an appropriate solution, as it permits industry to continue manufacturing them; which will continue to pollute the environment and contribute to human health problems.

The main 'global authority' within the UN system for matters relating to the environment is UNEP, or UN Environment as it is now referred to; according to the web page entitled *About UN Environment*,

"The United Nations Environment Programme (UN Environment) is the leading global environmental authority that sets the global environmental agenda, promotes the coherent implementation of the environmental dimension of sustainable development within the United Nations system, and serves as an authoritative advocate for the global environment."

The UNEP-led 'international framework' that governs policies in respect of the management of chemicals includes ICCM (International Conference of Chemicals Management), which is referred to as the 'governing body' of UNEP's SAICM, which is described on the web page entitled *SAICM Overview*,

"The Strategic Approach to International Chemicals Management (SAICM) is a policy framework to promote chemical safety around the world."

In 2015, UNEP produced a brochure entitled *Strategic Approach to International Chemicals Management: Good Chemistry, Together*, which refers to chemicals as,

"...the building blocks of many things we use, eat and wear."

The brochure also states that,

"From food and clothing to transport and technology and virtually everything in between, chemicals are part of daily life."

This claim is intended to convey the impression that chemicals are normal components of virtually everything and that it therefore makes no difference whether chemicals are 'natural', derived from natural substances or synthetically produced; the discussions throughout this book indicate otherwise.

The *Healthy Environments* report recognises that the condition of the environment influences the health of the people who inhabit that environment and claims that approximately 23 per cent of all deaths are,

"...due to modifiable environmental factors."

These 'environmental factors' are admitted to include chemicals; however, as previously discussed, the vast majority of chemicals remain entirely untested for the full range of their potential adverse health effects. This means that the scientific community has an extremely limited knowledge about the full extent of the harm that individual 'hazardous chemicals' can cause. The limited extent of this knowledge is compounded by the virtual absence of tests conducted to determine the adverse health effects from exposures to multiple combinations of 'hazardous chemicals'. This situation is further exacerbated by the existence of 'trade secrets' that permit the chemical composition of compounds and products to be categorised as 'proprietary information', and therefore inaccessible to independent assessment of their safety or potential adverse health effects.

Although different sources report different numbers of chemicals on the market, the SAICM brochure states that,

"Around 100,000 chemical substances are found in products or are on the market."

The brochure also acknowledges that,

"...chemical safety is an urgent issue that increasingly affects us all."

Yet again, it is claimed that certain populations are more affected by 'environmental factors' than others; fact number six on the WHO web page entitled *10 facts on preventing disease through healthy environments* states that,

"Low- and middle-income countries bear the greatest share of environmental disease."

The reason for this increased burden of 'environmental disease' is claimed to be that it results from the production and use of chemicals in 'developing' countries; however, according to the SAICM brochure,

"It is estimated that by 2020, developing countries will produce 31 per cent of global chemicals and use 33 per cent of global chemicals."

Although expanded chemical production in 'developing' countries is regarded as an important aspect of 'development', and therefore to be encouraged, the SAICM brochure sounds a note of caution in the statement that,

"If improperly managed, chemicals and the pollution linked with their manufacture, use and disposal come at a cost to the economy, human health and the environment."

The 'costs' to human health and the environment are not merely the result of chemicals that have been 'improperly managed'; instead, they are the direct result of the ubiquitous manufacture, use and disposal of toxic chemicals. Furthermore, pollution of the environment due to 'hazardous chemicals' is not exclusive to 'developing' countries.

The SAICM brochure refers to an initiative, called the Quick Start Programme, that is intended to assist 'developing' countries to better manage chemicals. This would seem to imply that the 'improper management' of chemicals is a far more extensive problem in those regions of the world, and that UNEP 'experts' know how chemicals should be managed because 'sound management' is practiced in 'developed' countries; but this clearly is not the case, environmental pollution due to 'hazardous chemicals' is ubiquitous.

In addition, the problem of 'hazardous chemicals' in 'developing' countries does not exist solely as a consequence of their low stage of 'development'; it is almost entirely due to the continuing production, use and disposal of toxic chemicals with little or no consideration for their detrimental consequences. This is, however, a global problem and largely the result of the increasingly global nature of the chemical industry; as indicated by the SAICM *Overview* page that states,

"The consumption of chemicals by all industries and modern society's reliance on chemicals for virtually all manufacturing processes make chemicals production one of the major and most globalized sectors of the world economy."

It has become increasingly common for large multinational corporations, including those within the chemical industry, to relocate some or all of their manufacturing facilities to 'developing' countries, primarily to take advantage of less restrictive regulations and lower costs, including cheaper labour, and to therefore increase their profitability. It should be clear that all industries that produce and utilise 'hazardous chemicals' should implement procedures that ensure their 'sound management', regardless of the location of the facilities or the existence of safety regulations. It should be equally clear that the responsibility for all matters that relate to 'health and safety' lies with the management of the corporations.

The disingenuous suggestion that 'improper management' is solely due to the 'developing' nature of the country in which 'hazardous chemicals' are produced, can be demonstrated by the example of the tragedy that occurred in 1984 in Bhopal, India; an event that is regarded as one of the worst industrial disasters of the 20th century. Union Carbide Corporation (UCC), a US company, was founded in 1917; Union Carbide India Limited (UCIL) was established in 1934, when UCC 'invested' in India and built a factory in Bhopal to manufacture carbamate pesticides in the belief that India would be a suitable market for their product.

The web page entitled *Union Carbide's Disaster* explains that the pesticide failed to sell in sufficient quantities to make the business viable and UCIL ceased active production in the early 1980s. However, for reasons that are not explained, large volumes of hazardous chemicals remained on the factory site. The page also states that, although some employees remained on the premises, maintenance had fallen into disrepair. On the night of 2nd December 1984, a leakage is reported to have occurred, but the safety systems that were supposed to have prevented such a leak failed to operate. This failure led to the release of a huge volume of methyl isocyanate (MIC), a highly toxic gas, into the atmosphere. The result of this leak has been that,

"Half a million people were exposed to the gas and 25,000 have died to date as a result of their exposure."

The release of this highly toxic gas remains an ongoing problem for the population of Bhopal because, according to the web page,

"The site has never been properly cleaned up and it continues to poison the residents of Bhopal."

In 2001, Dow Chemical purchased Union Carbide thereby inheriting this situation; however, the web page states that Dow Chemical,

"...has steadfastly refused to clean up the site..."

Although categorised as 'developing', India has a thriving chemical industry, which is described by the FICCI (Federation of Indian Chambers of Commerce and Industry) as,

"...a critical part of the Indian economy."

Furthermore, India takes the issue of the safe management of chemicals seriously because, according to the page entitled *Responsible Care* on the website of the Indian Chemical Council,

"The Govt. of India is a signatory to SAICM..."

Although the vast majority of the approximately 100,000 chemical substances in use remain untested, many chemicals that have been tested have been found to be extremely hazardous and to cause many serious adverse health effects. A number of these hazardous chemicals belong to the group known as POPs, the dangers of which are acknowledged in the UNDP report entitled *Chemicals and Waste Management for Sustainable Development*, which states that,

> "Exposure to POPs can lead to serious health effects, including certain types of cancer, birth defects, developmental problems, dysfunctional immune and reproductive systems, and greater susceptibility to disease."

Although recognising the serious health hazards associated with exposures to POPs, the report nevertheless makes the claim that,

> "Chemical products such as medicines, insecticides, repellents and larvicides help prevent millions of deaths each year."

This claim is unfounded; these products contain highly toxic chemical ingredients; which means that they contribute to illness and death. The hazards associated with 'medicines' are demonstrated by the phenomenon of iatrogenesis, as previously discussed; the hazards associated with exposures to all types of pesticide are well-documented and have also been discussed at length.

The report also claims that UNDP, the UN development agency, has helped to eliminate thousands of tonnes of POPs, including DDT. However, as previously discussed, DDT is permitted for use for 'indoor residual spraying' in malaria-endemic countries to control mosquitoes claimed to transmit the malaria parasite. It should be noted that this use of DDT is the only application permitted by the 2004 Stockholm Convention on POPs, on the basis of the claim that the benefits outweigh the risks. But this claim is unfounded for two reasons, the first of which is that DDT is not only toxic it is extremely persistent, which means that it continues to cause harm for years after it has been sprayed inside homes. The second reason is that the theory that malaria is caused by parasites transmitted by mosquitoes has been shown to be seriously flawed. It is therefore, highly questionable whether the use of DDT, even if it does kill mosquitoes, can be associated with the prevention of malaria and the reduction of deaths caused by this 'disease'. This means that the risks far outweigh the benefits, if there are indeed any benefits.

It is clear therefore, that there are many flaws in the claim that the number of deaths and illnesses from exposures to 'hazardous chemicals' can be reduced by the implementation of an approach that relies on 'sound management' practices. One of the problems with this approach is the reliance on the belief that there can be a 'safe' dose of, or exposure to, any hazardous chemical.

The scientific experiments conducted to ascertain the 'safe' dose of a chemical do not include experiments to tests its effects when combined with other chemicals to which people are exposed in the real-world environment. Importantly, as has been discussed, some chemicals are known to interact synergistically; the lack of testing of the majority of the 100,000 or more chemical substances in current use, leaves an immense gap in the knowledge possessed by the scientific research community about the real nature of the 'hazardous chemicals' they claim can be made 'safe' through the implementation of 'sound management' practices.

The fundamental problem is that 'sound management' practices do not prevent 'hazardous chemicals' from being manufactured, used and discharged into the environment; they do not therefore reduce the environmental pollution these substances generate. These chemicals continue to be included as ingredients of a plethora of products used on a regular, if not daily basis by billions of people worldwide.

Furthermore, 'sound management' practices fail to incorporate the precautionary principle, which states that a chemical substance or product should be proven to be safe prior to its introduction onto the market. In this context, the word safe means absolutely safe, not relatively safe as is currently the case.

The incorporation of the precautionary principle into the chemical management practices of all industries would provide one part of the solution to the problem. Another part of the solution is for manufacturers to create products that contain non-toxic ingredients; as discussed in chapter ten.

Industry & Development

Industrialisation is claimed to be an important aspect of 'development'; the more 'industrialised' a country, the more 'developed' it is said to be. It is also claimed that many benefits accrue from industrial development; the populations of 'developed' countries are said to enjoy greater prosperity, a better standard of living and better health than those of 'developing' countries; this is, however, a misleading claim.

The idea that 'industrial development' leads to greater prosperity is demonstrated by a UNIDO (United Nations Industrial Development Organization) document entitled *Introduction to UNIDO* that claims,

"Industrialization helped lift hundreds of millions of people around the globe out of poverty over the last 200 years."

This claim cannot be substantiated; although industrialisation may have provided employment for millions of people, it has not necessarily lifted them out of poverty; as indicated by EF Schumacher, who, in his book entitled *Small is Beautiful*, states that,

"The result of 'development' is that a fortunate minority have their fortunes greatly increased, while those who really need help are left more helpless than ever."

The idea that 'development' leads to better health is also problematic. As previously discussed, the WHO claims that as a country 'develops', the nature of the diseases suffered by the population changes from 'communicable' to 'noncommunicable'. It should be clear that a change from acute to chronic health problems is not indicative of improved health, as NCDs are some of the major 'killer diseases'.

Nevertheless, the idea that 'development' is the key to 'progress' is a fundamental aspect of the plans to address the issues that are said to confront humanity in the 21st century. The *Preamble* to the previously cited

Transforming Our World document that introduces the 2030 Agenda demonstrates this view in the statement that,

"This Agenda is a plan of action for people, planet and prosperity."

As indicated by its title, the 2030 Agenda emphasises 'sustainable' development; it also encourages sustainable 'industrialisation', as indicated by SDG 9 that aims to,

"Build resilient infrastructure, promote inclusive and sustainable industrialization and faster innovation."

The countries that were first to embrace the Industrial Revolution and become 'industrialised' comprise the majority of those categorised as 'developed'; the remainder of the world's countries being categorised as 'developing'. However, the idea that each of the world's countries can be clearly identified as belonging solely to one of these two categories according to their level of 'industrialisation', represents an oversimplification of the nature of corporate operations in the early 21st century. The trend over the past few decades has involved a rapid acceleration of 'globalisation'; which means that large corporations have increasingly expanded their operations across the globe and many have become huge multinational conglomerates.

The complex nature of these multinational organisations precludes an easy identification of the country to which the 'industrialised development' can be said to belong. This complexity can be demonstrated by the example of the Tata Group, which is described on the web page entitled *Tata group Business Profile* as,

"...a global enterprise, headquartered in India, comprising 30 companies across 10 verticals."

Although headquartered in India, the page states that the Tata Group operates in more than 100 countries across six continents. The 'verticals' include: IT; steel; automotive; telecom and media; and tourism and travel. The page reports that the revenue of Tata companies for 2017-18 totalled $110.7 billion. It should be noted that the Tata Group is only one example of the thriving industrialisation currently taking place in India; yet, India continues to retain the status of a 'developing' country.

Furthermore, industrialisation is not a process that has only recently been introduced into India. Indian politician and author, Shashi Tharoor reports in his book entitled *Inglorious Empire*, that, at the beginning of the 18th century,

"...India's share of the world economy was 23 per cent, as large as all of Europe put together."

The Indian economy of this period comprised various manufacturing industries, including, but not restricted to, textiles, pottery, engineering and shipbuilding. However, the invasion of India by the EIC and the later incorporation of the country into the British Empire, had a seriously detrimental impact on the country; not only was the size of the Indian economy substantially reduced, but Indian manufacturing became the source of the Industrial Revolution in Britain; as Shashi Tharoor explains,

"Britain's Industrial Revolution was built on the destruction of India's thriving manufacturing industries."

He also explains that the first industry to suffer destruction by the British was the Indian textile industry, the raw materials of which were used to expand the British textile industry,

> "Ironically, the British used Indian raw materials and exported the finished products back to India and the rest of the world..."

Also ironic is the stark contrast in the early 21st century between the thriving industrial development taking place within India and the rapidly declining industrial activity within Britain. Although there remain many differences between the two countries, the criteria used to categorise India as 'developing' and Britain as 'developed' are increasingly difficult to discern.

In contrast to the claim that many benefits are gained when a country achieves 'industrial development', is the reality that a variety of adverse consequences accompany this 'progress'. One of the most notable consequences is that the condition of the environment suffers a decline in quality. As discussed, the WHO recognises that environmental degradation is a contributory factor to human morbidity and mortality, but claims that increased 'development' only causes a change in the type of illnesses suffered. The erroneous nature of this idea can be illustrated by the example of tuberculosis, which is claimed to be a communicable disease that predominantly affects 'developing' countries. However, according to a March 2018 article entitled *Tuberculosis rates in England fall by third in six years*,

> "The most recent data on infection rates show parts of London still have higher rates of TB than some developing countries, such as Iraq, Libya and even Yemen."

This astounding admission demonstrates not only that tuberculosis should not be described as a disease that predominantly affects 'developing' countries, but also that 'communicable' diseases continue to have a major impact in 'developed' countries. The data that show tuberculosis as only occurring in 'parts of London' is a further demonstration of the fact that TB is not caused by bacteria that are transmitted through the air when 'infected' people sneeze and expel their 'germs'. In addition, it should be noted that Iraq, Libya and Yemen have all been severely affected by war during the early 21st century. These conflicts have inevitably had a seriously detrimental impact on the health of the populations of those countries; Yemen, for example, is reported to have suffered an outbreak of cholera that began in October 2016; cholera is discussed in more detail later in this chapter.

One of the many industrial causes of environmental pollution involves the operations of the extraction industry, which has a very long history in many parts of the world. These operations, which include mining, smelting and quarrying, are responsible for the release of a wide variety of pollutants into all parts of the environment; the air, ground and water are all affected. Mining operations, as discussed, can involve the release of vast quantities of naturally-occurring, but highly toxic heavy metals such as lead, mercury and cadmium. It is therefore unsurprising that mining is recognised to be responsible for a variety of occupational health problems; the nature of the miners' illnesses will vary according to the nature of the toxic substances to which they have been exposed. Occupational Knowledge International, (OK International) recognises some of these problems and describes, on the *About Us* web page, that their work involves efforts to,

"...build capacity in developing countries to identify, monitor, and mitigate environmental and occupational exposures to hazardous materials in order to protect public health and the environment."

The website identifies mining as one of the major polluting industries and, on the page entitled *Environmental Impacts of Mining and Smelting*, states that,

"The mining sector is responsible for some of the largest releases of heavy metals into the environment of any industry."

One of the reasons that 'developing' countries are increasingly affected by pollution caused by mining, can be attributed to the increasingly common practice that involves the relocation of certain aspects of mining operations from 'developed' countries to 'developing' countries; as described on the web page, which states that,

"In recent decades, the US has gradually shifted the most polluting aspects of the mining industry to developing countries."

In addition to being the repositories of some of the polluting activities of industries based in 'developed' countries, many 'developing' countries are also the source of a variety of valuable natural resources, such as gold, for example. This means therefore, that resource-rich 'developing' countries will continue to be affected by extraction industries, whether owned by native industrialists or those from other countries, until the resources have been depleted or are no longer commercially viable.

It is inevitable therefore, that 'developing' countries will continue to suffer environmental degradation, especially by extraction industries, and that their populations will continue to suffer the resulting adverse health effects. Unfortunately, health problems due to environmental degradation by the operations of virtually all industries will, almost certainly, be erroneously identified by the medical establishment as 'communicable diseases' that are claimed to disproportionately affect 'developing' countries, and to be treatable or preventable with medicines and vaccines.

Also unfortunate is that health problems due to industrial activities in 'developing' countries are often attributed to inadequate safety procedures, particularly a lack of regulatory controls, which, if implemented, are claimed to be able to 'mitigate' problems by the reduction of exposures to hazardous materials. However, this idea suffers from the same flaw as the idea that 'hazardous chemicals' can be made 'safe' if they are 'soundly managed'.

The problem with measures aimed at merely 'controlling' pollution is that they permit the continued production and release of pollutants. It is, however, the continuing release of pollutants and toxic substances into the environment that is the major issue. Despite the recognition of the importance of a healthy planet, establishment organisations do not propose to introduce measures that would curtail polluting industrial activities, such as fracking, for example, that cause serious harm to both the environment and human health.

Quarrying operations, which involve the extraction of non-metallic substances, also have a long history, and are also associated with occupational health problems; as indicated by a 2012 article entitled *Effects of Quarry Activities on Some Selected Communities in the Lower Manya Krobo District of the Eastern Region of Ghana* that states,

> "A very high degree of respiratory morbidity is associated with this industry. Fine rock and mineral dust of many kinds have been shown to be carcinogenic when inhaled."

It is likely that the respiratory health problems experienced by quarry workers will be identified as one of the less common CRDs (chronic respiratory diseases), referred to as 'occupational lung disease'. However, these respiratory problems are the direct result of the long-term inhalation of rock and mineral dust. As discussed, a 'poison' is defined as a substance that interferes with normal functioning; which means that, because they interfere with the normal functions of the respiratory system, all types of rock 'dust' must be described as 'toxic'. The fact that some types of rock and mineral dusts have been identified as carcinogenic, indicates that they are certainly detrimental to health.

There are many industries that are responsible for the transfer of their polluting activities to 'developing' countries; including the textile and clothing industry. The two Greenpeace reports referred to in the discussion about clothes in chapter six, were mainly concerned with environmental pollution caused by textile manufacturing facilities in China. But, as mentioned in that discussion, the problem lies with the toxic nature of the materials used by the industry, which means that the same environmental pollution will be produced by all textile manufacturing facilities that utilise the same manufacturing processes and the same toxic substances; the location of the manufacturing facilities is not a key factor.

It is clear, however, that poorly applied safety regulations will certainly exacerbate the problem, but, as discussed, the failure to adhere to practices that protect workers and prevent the discharge of pollutants into the surrounding environment is not exclusive to 'developing' countries. Despite their existence in 'developed' countries, safety regulations and pollution controls are not a guarantee of safe working conditions or a pollution-free environment, because they are not always fully implemented or rigidly observed. The comparatively weak regulatory systems that exist in 'developing' countries are, however, easier to circumvent; a situation that provides one of the incentives for industries of 'developed' countries to relocate their polluting activities to other parts of the world.

Although said to mainly occur in China, the release of toxic textile manufacturing wastes into the environment also occurs in other 'developing' countries; as demonstrated by a July 2015 article entitled *Food chain fouled by industrial waste*, which refers to environmental problems in some parts of Bangladesh caused by certain industries, especially dyeing factories, and states that,

> "For instance, dyeing factories have been set up in many corners of the country though they usually discharge massive amounts of liquid waste into nearby canals and rivers without treating them, thus contaminating the water and the soil."

The nature and causes of environmental pollution are recognised, to a certain extent at least, by some environmental organisations. For example, in 2016 Pure Earth and Green Cross Switzerland prepared a report entitled *World's Worst Pollution Problems: The Toxics Beneath Our Feet*. This report, which will be referred to as the *Pollution* report, is the 11th in the annual series that exposes the most polluting industries in the world. According to the *Pollution* report, the top ten polluting industries in 2016 were: ULAB (used lead acid battery) recycling; mining and ore processing; lead smelting; tanneries; ASGM (artisanal small-scale gold mining); industrial dumpsites; industrial estates; chemical manufacturing; product manufacturing; and the dye industry. In common with many of the problems discussed in this chapter, the countries said to be most affected by pollution are those categorised as 'developing'.

The ten industries deemed to be the most polluting are ranked according to the 'burden of disease' with which they are reported to be associated. Although the *Pollution* report claims that the pollutants produced by these industries are only associated with certain diseases, this is misleading. These pollutants are toxic and therefore inherently harmful; they are some of the main contributory factors to a variety of serious ill-health problems and even death. This is in stark contrast to the WHO claim that tobacco, alcohol, unhealthy diet and a lack of exercise are the main 'risk factors' for noncommunicable diseases. Significantly, but unsurprisingly, the *Pollution* report recognises that,

> "Chemical manufacturing is a large source of pollution worldwide..."

This means therefore, that chemicals are recognised to also be a source of pollution in 'developed' countries, which undermines the UNEP claim that 'sound management' practices operate in respect of chemical manufacturing in 'developed' countries. The *Pollution* report attributes the causes of environmental pollution to the failure to comply with 'environmental standards' and states that,

> "Due to globalization and efforts to incentivize manufacturing, some countries have been slow to apply regulations and/or have not been vigorous in ensuring that companies comply with environmental standards."

The problem of pollution cannot be solved by the introduction of regulations, no matter how strictly they may be enforced; the problem with 'regulations' and their failure to ensure the implementation of appropriate protections for people and the environment are further discussed in chapter nine. It must be emphasised, however, that most regulations rely on the erroneous idea that it is possible to establish a 'safe' level of exposure to a toxic substance.

The increasingly common practice of relocating polluting industrial operations to 'developing' countries owes its origin largely to the escalation of 'globalisation', under which it is claimed that industrial development will generate 'benefits' for 'developing' countries and their populations. However, in reality, the populations of these countries rarely benefit from any of the purported advantages, but invariably suffer from the many detrimental consequences, not least of which are the adverse health effects that accompany environmental pollution.

However, the governments of some 'developing' countries have welcomed industrial relocations, in the belief that the influx of capital investment will generate benefits for the local population by providing them with employment, which will improve their standard of living to a level similar to that believed to be enjoyed by the populations of 'developed' countries. In his book entitled *Green Backlash* Andrew Rowell explains that,

> "Third World governments, lured by the illusion of trickle-down capital and tempted by the dreams of technology transfer, have actually encouraged this corporate and capital flight into the deregulated zone, by setting them up in their own countries."

The nature of such 'deregulated zones' means that they certainly generate benefits, but these are enjoyed almost exclusively by the corporations, with the country, its people and environment suffering the consequences; as he also explains,

> "…numerous countries have established free trade zones (FTZs) or export processing zones (EPZs) which offer lax or non-existent environmental legislation, lenient or non-existent tax regimes and ridiculously low wage costs from underpaid non-unionised workers."

In addition, he quotes the words of environmentalist Paul Hawken who anticipates that the effects of the continuing globalisation of industrial development will be,

> "…that the world becomes a large, non-unionised hiring hall, with poorer countries lining up for plum investments, willing to donate land, resources and environmental quality and cheap labour as their cost of achieving economic 'development'."

One of the main 'costs' of the welcome afforded to industrialisation by 'developing' countries will be deteriorating health, which, in 'developing' countries, especially in sub-Saharan Africa, will be erroneously attributed to 'communicable' diseases, such as HIV/AIDS, tuberculosis and malaria, the three major 'epidemics' to be ended by 2030. The real nature of these diseases has been discussed, and shown to be attributable to a wide variety of toxins that include pharmaceutical medicines and vaccines used in the prevention and treatment of disease. Environmental pollution from industrial activities also needs to be recognised for its detrimental impact on health.

In addition to the pollution that results from industrial operations, is the pollution that results from the disposal of wastes, including the disposal of products at the end of their useful lives. One of the main methods of dealing with waste involves its disposal into huge landfill sites that are extremely hazardous as well as unsightly. Target 5 of SDG 12 recognises the problems caused by waste and aims to,

"By 2030, substantially reduce waste generation through prevention, reduction, recycling and reuse."

There are many forms of 'waste'; these range from plastic containers and food wrapping to liquid and food wastes to large household machines and equipment, to name just a few. Although waste recycling is clearly preferable to disposal into landfill sites, the reference to 'prevention' is even more significant, as prevention avoids the problem occurring in the first place. Furthermore, emphasis on prevention would place greater responsibility onto manufacturers to create products that are not hazardous and do not pollute the environment, either during or at the end of their useful lives. Unfortunately, most manufacturing industries have yet to understand the importance of 'prevention'.

The disposal of the products of some of the fastest growing industries, most notably the electronics and telecommunications industries, is a major source of environmental pollution, because they invariably contain hazardous materials, especially heavy metals and rare earths, as previously discussed. Although hazardous, these materials are valuable, which has encouraged the establishment of operations to recycle 'electronic waste', also referred to as e-waste. Unfortunately, these recycling operations are almost invariably located in 'developing' countries; which further exacerbates environmental degradation and worsening health problems in these regions. The volume of e-waste is immense, as is its value; as indicated by a May 2015 article entitled *Illegally Traded and Dumped E-Waste Worth up to $19 Billion Annually Poses Risks to Health, Deprives Countries of Resources, Says UNEP Report*, which states that,

"Each year, the electronic industry – one of the world's largest and fastest growing – generates up to 41 million tonnes of e-waste from goods such as computers and smart phones."

As the electronics and telecommunications industries continue to grow, the problem of e-waste will inevitably worsen for 'developing' countries; as the article states,

"Africa and Asia are key destinations for large-scale shipments of hazardous wastes for dumping, and sometimes for recycling."

The impact on human health resulting from the processing of e-waste that contains hazardous materials is discussed in a 2017 article entitled *Toward a More Sustainable Trajectory for E-Waste Policy: A Review of a Decade of E-Waste Research in Accra, Ghana*. Although the article refers to the situation in only one region of Ghana, it summarises the types of problems that are common to all e-waste recycling operations,

"Weak e-waste regulations and limited use of safety measures for e-waste workers in Accra, Ghana, foster an exploitative environment within the industry, and pose health risks for those working and living near e-waste processing sites."

The article also refers to the phenomenon of 'built-in obsolescence', which is an increasingly common attribute of electronic equipment and is clearly beneficial for the manufacturer. In addition, the manufacturers of electronic products, especially mobile phones, continually introduce new versions of their devices, the sole purpose of which is to generate a major boost to sales and profits. But the manufacturers benefit at the expense of the environment, especially as they are not held responsible for the safe disposal of the products they produce; as the article states,

"Electronics producers lack accountability in solving the e-waste predicament."

The lack of accountability, or responsibility, of the manufacturers of goods and products that contain toxic materials, is a fundamental aspect of environmental pollution and the associated adverse health effects for all living organisms, as well as humans. It must be noted that the expansion of the electronics industry has also increased the levels of electromagnetic radiation in the environment, which, if 5G technology is implemented globally, will substantially increase the hazards to human health.

It is natural for people in 'developing' countries to want their countries to 'develop'; but if these countries introduce the same type of 'industrial development' that exists in 'developed' countries, they will experience the same levels of environmental pollution and suffer the same adverse health consequences. Although the health problems that prevail in 'developed' countries are called NCDs, they are predominantly caused by exposures to toxic pollutants, whether chemical or electromagnetic in origin.

It is possible for countries to develop without the accompanying adverse effects on the environment or human health. The quote by Barry Commoner that opens this chapter is pertinent in this context and bears repetition,

"Economic development can proceed without a concomitant decrease in environmental quality if it is based on an appropriate, ecologically benign production technology."

The challenge for the innovators of the 21st century is to develop methods by which products can be created utilising non-toxic materials and benign technologies; there are signs that this challenge has been accepted and non-toxic products are being developed. The most significant contribution that the general public can make is to change their purchasing habits and to create a demand for non-toxic products.

Poverty

Poverty is one of the major issues that confront humanity in the 21st century; it is an issue of such significance that the previously cited *Transforming Our World* document contains the following bold statement,

"We are committed to ending poverty in all its forms and dimensions, including by eradicating extreme poverty by 2030."

The term 'extreme poverty' is defined as living below the 'international poverty line', which, when the 2030 Agenda was prepared, was an income of $1.25 per day; as indicated by target 1 of SDG 1 that states the aim to,

"By 2030, eradicate extreme poverty for all people everywhere, currently measured as people living on less than $1.25 a day."

In October 2015, however, the World Bank amended the 'international poverty line' to $1.90 per day; an amendment that inevitably increased the number of people categorised as living in 'extreme poverty'.

The World Bank, which was established as the result of the 1944 Bretton Woods conference, is a 'specialised agency' of the UN. The World Bank mission, according to the web page entitled *Who We Are*, is comprised of two goals, the first of which is,

> "To end extreme poverty: by reducing the share of the global population that lives in extreme poverty to 3 percent by 2030."

Although a reduction in the number of people living in 'extreme poverty' to only 3 per cent of the world population would be an achievement, this cannot be regarded as synonymous with the 'end' of extreme poverty. The section of the World Bank website that relates to Data Topics provides information about each of the 17 SDGs. The web page that refers to SDG 1, entitled *No poverty*, claims that, in 1990, 1.8 billion people lived in 'extreme poverty', but indicates this number has been reduced because,

> "An estimated 766 million people, or 10.7 percent of the world's population, lived in extreme poverty in 2013."

The region claimed to be most affected by 'extreme poverty' is sub-Saharan Africa.

In common with most statistics, those that relate to the number of people living in poverty are compiled from data that are collected through a sample of surveys, and then extrapolated using computer modelling techniques to apply to the entire population. Although surveys are common sources of data for statistics, the information they provide may not accurately reflect the real conditions of life experienced by the population. The problems associated with the poverty statistics of the World Bank are highlighted by Professor Michel Chossudovsky PhD in his book entitled *Globalization of Poverty and the New World Order*, in which he states that,

> "Poverty assessments by the World Bank and the United Nations are largely office- based exercises conducted in Washington and New York, with insufficient awareness of local realities."

This situation certainly raises questions about the poverty statistics quoted by UN organisations. Furthermore, an October 2015 World Bank press release entitled *World Bank's New End-Poverty Tool: Surveys in Poorest Countries* makes a revealing admission about the paucity of actual data collected in the statement that,

> "Poverty-fighting efforts have long been constrained by a lack of data in many countries."

The extent of the problem is reported in the press release to be that, during the period between 2002 and 2011, there were no poverty data for 29 countries and that, during the same period, only one poverty survey had been conducted in each of a further 28 countries. The almost total lack of poverty data available from these 57 countries, which together represent almost 30 per cent of the total of 195 countries, is so significant that it directly challenges the veracity of the poverty statistics claimed to accurately reflect the conditions for people who live in the poorest countries.

In addition to being categorised according to the stage of development they have achieved, countries are also categorised according to their level of 'income'; a criterion that is based on World Bank calculations of GNI (gross national income) per capita. As previous discussions have indicated, there are four 'income' groups; namely low, lower-middle, upper-middle and high. Although GNI may be a reasonable representation of a country's total income, the 'per capita' amount merely represents an averaging calculation; but one that does not realistically represent the actual incomes earned by the population of the country. Interestingly, even the World Bank recognises that the measure of 'GNI per capita' has limitations, one of which is that it does not reflect income inequalities within a country; 'GNI per capita' also fails to indicate the actual incomes earned at each extremity.

The extent of income inequalities can be demonstrated by two examples. The first example involves the US, which is categorised as a 'high income' country and is the home of a large number of millionaires and an increasing number of billionaires. Yet America is a country of contradictions; as indicated by a December 2017 report issued by the US Department of Housing and Urban Development that claimed the existence of more than half a million homeless American people, which represented an increase over the number for the previous year.

The second example involves India, which is categorised as a 'lower-middle income' country and is the home of many millions of people who live in a state of extreme poverty. Yet India is also a country of contradictions; there are more than two hundred thousand Indians who are rupee millionaires, as reported in a July 2015 article entitled *61,000 millionaires left India in the last 14 years*. Although rupee millionaires are not dollar millionaires, the article also reports the existence of a growing number of rupee billionaires, whose wealth does equate to millions of dollars.

The *Transforming Our World* document recognises the problem of inequalities in the statement that,

"We resolve, between now and 2030, to end poverty and hunger everywhere; to combat inequalities within and among countries..."

The examples discussed above that relate to the US and India demonstrate, however, that income inequalities within countries are not being addressed. In reality, the 'wealth gap' that exists within these and virtually all other countries around the world is not narrowing; instead it is continuing to widen and at an increasingly rapid pace. This situation is one that poses yet another serious challenge to the claim that the number of people living in 'extreme poverty' has been substantially reduced.

It is often argued that poverty is 'relative' and varies with respect to certain factors, not least of which is the country in which it is said to exist; this argument is incorporated into target 2 of SDG 1 that states the aim to,

"By 2030, reduce at least by half the proportion of men, women and children of all ages living in poverty in all its dimensions according to national definitions."

The relevance of 'national definitions' is illustrated by Professor Chossudovsky, who cites in his book that the 'poverty threshold' in the US in 1996 was $16,036 for a family of 2 adults and 2 children, which equates to almost $11 per person per day. This amount greatly exceeds the 2015 'international poverty line'; but it was considered to be an amount that represented 'poverty' for an American family in the 1990s.

It is clear that poverty, although mainly referred to with respect to a sum of money or a level of income expressed as a daily amount, in reality, has a much wider meaning. In this wider context, 'poverty' more accurately represents an inability to access 'basic needs', the most important of which are food and water, without which life cannot be sustained.

However, there are other requirements considered to be 'basic needs' that also vary according to 'national definitions', as described in SDG 1.2. This point is also explained by the World Bank *No poverty* web page that states,

> "National poverty lines typically reflect a threshold below which a person's minimum nutrition, clothing, and shelter needs cannot be met, consistent with the country's economic and social circumstances."

It is these 'circumstances' that are said to justify the different 'poverty lines' that apply to different regions and even different countries around the world.

The expansion of 'globalisation', however, has meant that there are far fewer differences in the economic circumstances that prevail in different regions of the world. One of the most significant effects of globalisation has been on prices, and especially the price of food, one of life's most important 'basic needs'. The problem is explained by Professor Chossudovsky who states that,

> "Increasingly, the domestic prices of food staples are brought up to their world market levels."

The consequence of increased food prices without a corresponding increase in income is an inevitable deepening of poverty; as explained by Ellen Brown in her February 2011 article entitled *The Egyptian Tinderbox: How Banks and Investors are Starving the Third World*, in which she states that,

> "In poorer countries, as much as 60 to 80 percent of people's incomes go for food compared to just 10 to 20 percent in industrialised countries."

Although food is one of the most important, it is not the only 'basic need', nor is it the only commodity that has continued to increase in price. Clearly, increased prices on their own are not necessarily problematic; it is only when price increases occur in the absence of increased income that there are serious consequences; a situation that has become increasingly common with the imposition of policies that demand a freeze on wages. Yet the prices of basic necessities have been permitted to increase; as indicated by Professor Chossudovsky in his June 2008 article entitled *The Global Crisis: Food, Water and Fuel. Three Fundamental Necessities of Life in Jeopardy*, in which he states that,

> "In recent years, the prices of these three variables have increased dramatically at the global level, with devastating economic and social consequences."

Poverty can also produce devastating consequences for health; the WHO web page entitled *Poverty and health* states that,

> "Poverty creates ill-health because it forces people to live in environments that make them sick, without decent shelter, clean water or adequate sanitation."

This statement is, however, rather misleading. Although it correctly identifies the existence of a link between unhealthy environments and illness, it fails to correctly identify the main factors that contribute to those unhealthy environments, as it fails to acknowledge the role of environmental pollutants and contaminants produced by industrial activities.

The World Bank also refers to an association between a lack of money and a lack of health on a page with the same title, *Poverty and health*, which states that,

> "Poverty is a major cause of ill health and a barrier to accessing health care when needed. This relationship is financial; the poor cannot afford to purchase those things that are needed for good health, including sufficient quantities of quality food and health care."

This statement is also rather misleading. Although it correctly identifies 'quality food', the World Bank uses this term mainly with reference to the 'energy' content of food, rather than its nutritional content. Furthermore, the World Bank use of the term 'health care' refers to the services provided by the medical establishment system that employs medicines and vaccines, which, as demonstrated throughout this book, are not requirements for 'good health'.

The WHO expands on the idea that an association exists between poverty and illness in the claim that poverty in 'developing' countries is a major contributory factor to 'infectious diseases'; as indicated by the previously cited *Global Report for Research on Infectious Diseases of Poverty* that defines the term 'infectious diseases of poverty' as referring to,

> "...a number of diseases which are known to be more prevalent among poorer populations..."

The reason these diseases predominantly affect 'poor' people is erroneously claimed in the report to be that,

> "Poverty creates conditions that favour the spread of infectious diseases and prevents affected populations from obtaining adequate access to prevention and care."

The failure of the medical establishment to investigate the true nature and causes of 'disease', combined with the rigid adherence to the fatally flawed 'germ theory', means that they are unable to provide effective methods of prevention or treatment for the illnesses that are said to predominantly affect poor people; this failure is demonstrated by the statement in the report that,

> "Research has revealed that the control of infectious diseases of poverty is more complex than previously thought."

The consequences of the erroneous medical establishment theories relating to the causes of the illnesses that affect poor people are explained in the report to be that,

> "Social, economic and biological factors interact to drive a vicious cycle of poverty and disease from which, for many people, there is 'no escape'."

Until the medical establishment relinquishes the belief in 'biological factors' and the 'germ theory', they will continue to fail to resolve this vicious cycle.

It has been demonstrated that one of the factors that exert a major influence over human health is the condition of the environment in which people live; this has been recognised by the previously cited *Healthy Environments* report. However, contrary to the claims of the WHO, unhealthy environments, as well as poverty and disease, also exist in most, if not all 'developed' countries; these conditions are not exclusive to 'developing' countries. There are, however, reasons that these conditions are more prevalent in 'developing' countries; in most instances the reasons owe their origins to the fact that these countries are former colonies; as indicated by Dr Barry Commoner, whose words were quoted at the beginning of this chapter, but deserve repetition,

"...a fact about developing countries that is often forgotten: they once were, and in the economic sense often still remain, colonies of more developed countries."

As previously discussed, colonialism invariably involved widespread exploitation of the natural resources and indigenous populations of colonies. The nature of the exploitation varied, but often entailed the expulsion of the indigenous people from their land, and the subsequent transformation of that land from traditional agriculture into plantations of single crops, such as coffee and sugar for example, grown specifically for the export market. This foreign 'ownership' of the land and the resources it contained, including valuable metals, such as gold in South Africa for example, not only restricted the volume of food produced for domestic consumption, it also hampered the countries' efforts to 'industrialise' and therefore to 'develop'. The result of these exploitative actions has been the continued impoverishment of the indigenous populations; as succinctly described by Eduardo Galeano in *Open Veins of Latin America*, in which he states that,

"...we Latin Americans are poor because the ground we tread is rich..."

One of the reasons that poverty continues to persist throughout the world is due to the nature of the 'international monetary system' and the bankers and industrialists who virtually control that system. The 'world money system' is discussed in chapter nine, but requires some discussion in this section in the context of its effect on poverty, which, in contrast to the World Bank claim, is worsening, not improving.

At the end of WWII, most European countries were in debt as the result of the military expenditures they incurred during the war. One of the countries that emerged from that period virtually unscathed financially was the United States of America, which had been one of the main providers of loans to many of the European combatants in WWII. The US was therefore in a very strong financial position; a situation that was to be exploited by the wealthiest and most influential bankers and industrialists, who desired the goal of making the US the dominant 'world power'.

One of the earliest mechanisms by which they sought to achieve their goal involved the creation of the Marshall Plan that was to provide 'aid' to countries in western Europe in order to enable 'reconstruction'. However, this 'aid' was always subject to certain conditions, one of which was the requirement for the recipient country to 'open' its markets to US products; a situation that provided a significant boost to American industries. The details of the Marshall Plan are explained by F. William Engdahl in his book entitled *Gods of Money: Wall Street and the Death of the American Century*, in which he states that,

> "The Marshall Plan also opened the way for large US corporations to invest in the industries of Western Europe at bargain prices as European currencies were heavily depreciated in dollar terms after 1945 under the parities set under initial IMF rules in relation to the dollar."

The IMF is another specialised agency of the UN, which, like the World Bank, was established as the result of the 1944 Bretton Woods conference; the IMF website claims that its primary purpose is,

> "...to ensure the stability of the international monetary system..."

This purpose is further explained on the web page entitled *How the IMF Promotes Global Economic Stability* that states,

> "Promoting economic stability is partly a matter of avoiding economic and financial crises..."

Since the formation of the IMF, there have been many economic and financial crises that have increased in intensity, which indicates that the IMF has failed to implement the appropriate measures to achieve 'economic stability' and avoid crises. The IMF claims that its other functions are to,

> "...facilitate international trade, promote high employment and sustainable growth, and reduce poverty around the world."

It is interesting to note that the facilitation of international trade is listed before the reduction of poverty.

During the post-WWII period, many colony countries sought to gain their independence, especially from Britain, France and Germany, all three of which had emerged from the war with a significant level of debt and were no longer able to afford the costs of administering their colonies. In addition, there were many other countries, both 'developing' and 'developed', that had also accumulated large debts, for which they required assistance from the newly-created IMF and World Bank.

Under the guise of assisting these countries to achieve 'economic stability', the loans provided by the IMF and World Bank required the recipients to accept the imposition of certain conditions, including the implementation of structural adjustment programmes (SAPs). But, according to Professor Chossudovsky, these SAPs have not generated improved economic stability; instead they have,

> "...contributed largely to destabilizing national currencies and ruining the economies of developing countries."

In addition, he states that these programmes have,

> "...led to the impoverishment of hundreds of millions of people."

The SAPs have clearly failed to achieve their intended purpose but instead, have achieved the complete opposite. Professor Chossudovsky states that,

> "...since the early 1990s...the IMF-World Bank policy prescriptions (now imposed in the name of 'poverty alleviation') have become increasingly harsh and unyielding."

One of the harsh and unyielding policies that have become increasingly common in most countries around the world, especially after the financial crisis of 2007-2008, has involved the imposition of austerity measures. These measures have been imposed on 'developed' as well as 'developing' countries and have led to the impoverishment of unknown millions of people around the world; a situation that clearly raises fundamental questions about the World Bank claim that more than a billion people were lifted out of the condition of 'extreme poverty' between 1990 and 2013.

It is generally claimed that employment is one of the key processes by which people can lift themselves out of poverty or extreme poverty; however, even the UN acknowledges that this is not necessarily the case. The page about SDG 1 on the UN website provides a section entitled *Progress of Goal 1 in 2017* that states,

> "In 2016, just under 10 per cent of the world's workers were living with their families on less than $1.90 per person per day..."

Although the UN claims this represents a reduction from 28 per cent in 2000, it is an outrage that people who have employment income nevertheless live in 'extreme poverty'. One of the main causes of this appalling situation are the low wages paid by some of the multinational corporations that relocate to 'developing' countries with the specific intention of taking advantage of lower costs, lax regulations and the virtual absence of labour unions, or any other organisations that would protect the rights of workers to earn a decent living wage.

As discussed above, one of the conditions of the SAPs imposed by the IMF and World Bank prior to providing financial 'aid', is that the country implements a policy that ensures wages are kept at a low level. The argument used by these institutions to justify this policy is that wage increases are inflationary and cause harm to the country's economy. However, the prices of 'basic needs' such as food, are permitted and even encouraged to increase to market levels, despite the 'low wage' policy; a situation that inevitably exacerbates poverty and is, therefore, in direct contradiction to the stated aims of the UN organisations to reduce poverty and eradicate extreme poverty.

A further consequence of the relocation of the manufacturing facilities of multinational corporations to 'developing' countries, are the difficulties experienced by small local businesses; as they are unable to compete and are often forced to close; as Professor Chossudovsky explains,

> "In developing countries entire branches of industry producing for the internal market are driven into bankruptcy..."

These business failures significantly add to the problem of poverty as the owners of failed businesses and their employees become unemployed and are forced to accept poorly-paid employment, which is often insufficient to meet their 'basic needs'. These people therefore bolster the numbers living in poverty and even in 'extreme poverty'. Yet this situation is entirely avoidable; it has only been brought about by globalisation policies that favour 'international trade' conducted by huge multinational conglomerates.

The ongoing and deepening economic crises that affect virtually all countries around the world in the early 21st century pose serious challenges to the UN efforts to fulfil the goal of ending poverty before 2030. It should be clear that, in order to achieve this goal, the existing policies of UN institutions, especially the IMF and World Bank, must be abandoned and replaced with those that genuinely address the problem of poverty.

The policies imposed by the IMF and World Bank in the name of 'economic stability' also have a profound effect on human health. Many of the small businesses that have been driven into bankruptcy, have included local food producers and suppliers that have been replaced by multinational food manufacturers, supermarkets and 'fast-food' chains that predominantly supply processed 'food products', which contain few, if any, real nutrients. Although these 'food products' are cheap in terms of their money cost, they are expensive in terms of their adverse impact on health.

Hunger & Malnutrition

Hunger, like poverty, is one of the major issues said to confront humanity in the early 21st century; as indicated by the *Transforming Our World* document that states,

"We resolve, between now and 2030, to end poverty and hunger everywhere…"

Hunger and its associated problems are the topics of SDG 2, the aim of which is to,

"End hunger, achieve food security and improved nutrition and promote sustainable agriculture."

Agriculture and food security are discussed in the next section.

The terms 'hunger' and 'malnutrition' are closely related but not synonymous. Although the word 'hunger' is commonly used to express a desire to eat, its meaning in the context of this discussion refers to an insufficient intake of food over a long period of time. The aim of SDG 2.1 is to,

"By 2030, end hunger and ensure access by all people, in particular the poor and people in vulnerable situations, including infants, to safe, nutritious and sufficient food all year round."

Hunger almost invariably coexists with poverty, especially in the presence of rising food prices that are not matched by increased incomes. This combination is increasingly prevalent in 'developed', as well as 'developing', countries as the global economic conditions in the early 21st century continue to worsen. Although financial assistance is provided by the IMF and the World Bank, it is always accompanied by conditions that require the imposition of harsh austerity measures that fail to address the real problems, and therefore fail to achieve a reduction in either poverty or hunger. Nevertheless, on a web page entitled *Progress of Goal 2 in 2017*, the UN claims that,

"Efforts to combat hunger and malnutrition have advanced significantly since 2000."

This is, however, contradicted by the previously cited September 2017 WFP Press Release entitled *World Hunger Again On The Rise, Driven By Conflict And Climate Change, New UN Report Says* that states,

"After steadily declining for over a decade, global hunger is on the rise again…"

The UN report referred to in the press release is entitled *The state of food security and nutrition in the world*; it was produced jointly by FAO, IFAD (International Fund for Agricultural Development), WHO, WFP and UNICEF, all of which are organisations within the UN system. The report, which will be referred to as the *Food Security* report, claims that conflicts are one of the key drivers of worsening hunger. In addition, although incorrectly attributed to 'climate change', extreme weather conditions, such as droughts and floods, are recognised to adversely influence food production; they are also acknowledged to be influenced by the regular occurrence of the climate phenomenon known as El Niño. The report indicates that the current economic situation, which is referred to as an 'economic slowdown', has adversely impacted food availability and caused food prices to increase. These factors are all claimed to affect 'food security', which in turn has an impact on hunger and malnutrition; the *Food Security* report recognises the connections between these factors and states that,

"...we will not end hunger and all forms of malnutrition by 2030 unless we address all the factors that undermine food security and nutrition."

These problems, like all others, cannot be solved unless their underlying causes have been correctly identified; unfortunately, UN organisations have failed to understand the underlying nature of the problems and correctly identify their causes. This means they are unlikely to be able to eliminate or even substantially reduce hunger and malnutrition.

The correct definition of the word malnutrition is 'bad nutrition', which, as previously discussed, can occur in people who eat a sufficient quantity of food; it is for this reason that malnutrition is not synonymous with 'hunger'. Malnutrition is the topic of SDG 2.2 that states the aim to,

"By 2030, end all forms of malnutrition, including achieving, by 2025, the internationally agreed targets on stunting and wasting in children under 5 years of age, and address the nutritional needs of adolescent girls, pregnant and lactating women and older persons."

Stunting and wasting are the result of malnutrition; they are conditions that primarily affect children in 'developing' countries who are severely malnourished during the most important stages of their growth, or even prior to their birth. These children fail to thrive because they do not consume foods with all the nutrients necessary for the proper functioning and development of their bodies. However, 'malnutrition' is not restricted to children or even adults who live in 'developing' countries; it affects anyone whose diet is comprised of nutrient-poor foods, even if the quantity of food is sufficient to prevent 'hunger'. The February 2018 WHO fact sheet entitled *Malnutrition* claims that,

"Malnutrition refers to deficiencies, excesses, or imbalances in a person's intake of energy and/or nutrients."

As previously discussed, this claim is misleading; the 'energy' value of a food is not related to its nutritional value. Some of the consequences of malnutrition are described in the fact sheet that states,

"Malnutrition, in all its forms, includes undernutrition (wasting, stunting, underweight), inadequate vitamins or minerals, overweight, obesity, and resulting diet-related noncommunicable diseases."

The fact sheet identifies overweight and obesity as conditions that can result from 'malnutrition' but claims that,

"Overweight and obesity result from an imbalance between energy consumed (too much) and energy expended (too little)."

This explanation places too great an emphasis on a food's 'energy' value, as measured in calories, that must be balanced by an adequate level of physical activity to prevent overweight and obesity; although commonly assumed to be correct, this view is mistaken; nutrition is discussed in more detail in chapter ten.

One of the main reasons that the incidence of overweight and obesity continues to rise is because dietary habits have changed; large numbers of people no longer consume nutrient-rich foods, they have replaced their traditional foods with nutrient-poor processed 'food products' that are not conducive to good health. This is not a situation that exists solely in 'developed' countries; it is increasingly a global phenomenon, as the fact sheet states,

"Globally, people are consuming foods and drinks that are more energy-dense (high in sugars and fats) ..."

The changing nature of diets is also recognised by the *Food Security* report, which makes the revealing comment that,

"As large companies increasingly dominate markets, highly processed foods become more readily available, and traditional foods and eating habits are displaced."

It is important to note that, although the WHO contributed to this report, which is critical of 'processed food products', it is a core member of JECFA, the organisation that approves chemical food additives as suitable for use in 'food products' that are becoming 'more readily available' in countries where hunger and malnutrition are common. This situation is also recognised in the February 2018 WHO fact sheet entitled *Obesity and overweight*, which states that underweight is a more significant problem than overweight for children in 'developing' countries but that,

"At the same time, these children are exposed to high-fat, high-sugar, high-salt, energy-dense, and micronutrient-poor foods, which tend to be lower in cost, but also lower in nutrient quality."

The reference to these foods as 'energy-dense' means that they provide sufficient calories, but their almost total lack of nutrients contributes to 'malnutrition', whether the child suffers from underweight or overweight. However, as the WHO recognises, these 'food products' are invariably lower in cost than nutrient-rich foods, which is one of the reasons that they appeal to people who live in poverty. It also explains why malnutrition and poverty often co-exist, as the *Malnutrition* fact sheet states,

"Poverty amplifies the risk of, and risks from, malnutrition."

It should be abundantly obvious that a diet comprised of low-cost 'food products' that are energy-dense, but low in nutrients will not solve the problem of malnutrition. Instead, a diet of this nature will exacerbate existing health problems and lead to overweight in the presence of malnutrition, as indicated by the *Overweight and obesity* fact sheet that states,

"It is not uncommon to find undernutrition and obesity co-existing within the same country, the same community and the same household."

The WHO refers to different nutrients, such as vitamins and minerals, and also to 'micronutrients', which are defined on the web page entitled *Micronutrients* as substances that are essential, but required in only miniscule amounts; the page also states that,

"As tiny as the amounts are, however, the consequences of their absence are severe."

However, the WHO makes the further claim that,

"Iodine, vitamin A and iron are most important in global public health terms; their lack represents a major threat to the health and development of populations the world over..."

Although important, these are neither the only nor the most important nutrients, the lack of which pose a major threat to health; many other nutrients are equally, if not more important. More significantly, nutrients should not be considered in isolation. Yet the WHO, the agency responsible for human health, fails to provide adequate information about a major factor that influences health. The reason that the medical establishment has a poor level of knowledge about this extremely important topic is due to the almost total lack of medical school training on the subject of nutrition.

Ill-health is not uncommon in people, especially children, who are underweight, although the health problems they suffer are often erroneously categorised as 'infections', as the previously cited *Global Health Risks* report indicates,

"Around one third of diarrhoea, measles, malaria and lower respiratory infections in childhood are attributable to underweight."

This statement is highly misleading. The 'germ theory' attributes infections to pathogenic microorganisms, not to underweight. There is, however, no explanation offered for the claim that only one third of these 'infectious diseases' are attributable to underweight; if underweight were a causal factor, it would apply in all cases.

Malnutrition that manifests as underweight is not only a problem for children, it can also be problematic for pregnant women and their developing babies, as indicated by the WHO web page entitled, *10 facts on nutrition*, 'fact' number 5 of which states,

"Maternal undernutrition, common in many developing countries, leads to poor fetal development and higher risk of pregnancy complications..."

Malnutrition that manifests as overweight, in both 'developed' and 'developing' countries, can be similarly problematic for pregnant women and their developing babies.

Maternal malnutrition, whether it manifests as underweight or overweight, can also affect the health of the baby after birth. Nursing mothers need to be adequately nourished otherwise the quality of the milk can be reduced, which will inevitably affect the health of the baby. The WHO recommends that babies should be exclusively breastfed for at least the first six months of life, after which it is recommended that they should be introduced to 'complementary' or family foods, in addition to the continuation of breastfeeding. Despite this recommendation, the February 2018 WHO fact sheet entitled *Infant and young child feeding* admits that,

"Few children receive nutritionally adequate and safe complementary foods..."

According to the fact sheet, the main reason for this is due to a lack of 'dietary diversity' and a lack of 'feeding frequency', for which the WHO recommends that children are fed more frequently with a variety of complementary foods that are nutritionally adequate. Whilst this is clearly good advice, families that live in extreme poverty are unlikely to be able to follow it. It is widely recognised that 'undernourishment', especially in 'developing' countries, is a serious problem that requires attention. The main UN organisation tasked with providing food assistance is WFP (World Food Programme), which also, inevitably, promotes the 2030 Agenda goal to 'end hunger'.

The WFP recognises that nutrition is important and that malnutrition can manifest as underweight or overweight; however, like the WHO, the WFP does not have a full understanding of 'nutrition' and places too great an emphasis on the 'energy' value of foods. The nature of the WFP's work includes humanitarian assistance and the provision of food aid during disasters, such as famines and droughts; however, these emergency situations are not the sole focus of their activities. The WFP also provides assistance through a number of programmes that involve the distribution of a variety of products, as indicated by the web page entitled *Specialized nutritious foods* that states,

"The World Food Programme (WFP) uses a wide range of specialized foods to improve the nutritional intake of the people we assist around the world."

These products include: Fortified Blended Foods (FBFs); Ready-to-Use Foods (RUFs); High Energy Biscuits (HEBs); Micronutrient Powder or 'Sprinkles'; and Compressed Food Bars. A few examples will suffice to indicate the real nature of these 'products' that WFP refers to as 'foods'. The first products, called Fortified Blended Foods, are described on the web page as,

"...blends of partially precooked and milled cereals, soya, beans, pulses, fortified with micronutrients (vitamins and minerals)."

The main type of FBF used in WFP programmes is called CSB (Corn Soya Blend), although WSB (Wheat Soya Blend) is also sometimes used. The next products, referred to as Ready-to-Use Foods, are described as likely to contain,

"...vegetable fat, dry skimmed milk, malt dextrin, sugar and whey..."

One variety of RUF, called 'Plumpy', contains peanut paste. The third products, called High Energy Biscuits, are listed as having the following ingredients,

"Wheat flour, Hydrogenate Vegetable Shortening, Sugar, Soyflour, Invert Syrup, High fructose Corn Syrup, Skimmed Milk powder, Sodium and Ammonium, Bicarbonates, Salt..."

It should be clear from the descriptions and ingredient listings that these are all highly processed 'food products' that contain unhealthy ingredients, including sugar and salt. Although claimed to be 'fortified' with vitamins and minerals, these products clearly do not contain the full range of nutrients required by the body to function optimally; it is therefore inappropriate to describe these products as 'nutritious foods'.

The use of these food products in an emergency situation, such as a famine, would certainly help to provide immediate relief from starvation, but only on a temporary basis until real foods become available. However, the WFP also claims that these 'food products' assist in providing education about nutrition and nutritious foods, but this is disingenuous; a more accurate description of these products would include reference to them as 'energy-dense' but 'nutritionally-poor', which means that they are precisely the types of 'foods' that contribute to malnutrition. This highlights the misleading nature of information provided by the WFP, which like the WHO, is a contributor to a report critical of 'processed food products', yet simultaneously promotes processed food products as 'nutritious foods'.

One of the reasons that hunger is said to persist, especially in 'developing' countries, is claimed to be due to food scarcity that is caused by the inability of food production to keep pace with the increasing size of the world population; but this is a false claim. The world does not suffer from a scarcity of food; this point is succinctly explained by authors Frances Moore Lappé and Joseph Collins, who state in their 1977 book entitled *Food First: Beyond the Myth of Scarcity* that,

"While hunger is real, scarcity is an illusion."

Two years prior to the publication of their book, the authors founded the Institute for Food and Development Policy, which is also known as Food First. The current information provided on the Food First website shows that little has changed in the intervening decades. The web page entitled *The Myth: Scarcity. The Reality: There IS enough food* states that,

"Abundance, not scarcity, best describes the supply of food in the world today."

The reasons that hunger persists in a world of abundant food production are discussed in the next section.

Agriculture & Food Security

The UN anticipates that the world population will continue to grow into the foreseeable future, as indicated by a June 2017 web page entitled *World population projected to reach 9.8 billion in 2050, and 11.2 billion in 2100*; the title is self-explanatory.

One of the concerns that arise from projections of this nature relates to 'food security', which essentially refers to the ability to ensure that an adequate supply of food is available for everyone all year round. Concerns about food security had been raised by Agenda 21, specifically in Chapter 14, in which it was claimed that the capacity of existing resources to provide sufficient food was 'uncertain' and that efforts were therefore needed to,

"...increase food production in a sustainable way and enhance food security."

These concerns and issues remain key features of UN policy recommendations and have been incorporated into SDG 2 of the 2030

Agenda, as indicated in the previous section, especially in target 4 of SDG 2 that aims to,

"By 2030, ensure sustainable food production systems and implement resilient agricultural practices that increase productivity and production..."

This target is clearly an attempt to address the problem of 'world hunger'. As discussed in the previous section, millions of people around the world live in a state of 'hunger'; but they do so despite the fact that food production levels are more than adequate to feed everyone. This fact is confirmed by a WFP web page entitled *11 Myths About Global Hunger* that states,

"There is enough food in the world today for everyone to have the nourishment necessary for a healthy and productive life."

There are a number of reasons that 'world hunger' persists despite an ample supply of food, one of which is because 'hungry' people are almost invariably those who are also trapped in a state of 'extreme poverty'; a situation that is exacerbated by static incomes that are unable to absorb rising food prices. But these circumstances are not exclusive to people who live in 'developing' countries, they are also a common feature of life for increasing numbers of people in 'developed' countries.

Two other reasons for the persistence of hunger are suggested by the previously cited *Food Security* report, which refers to conflicts and 'climate change' as the main drivers of worsening world hunger and claims that,

"The food security situation has worsened in particular in parts of sub-Saharan Africa, South-Eastern Asia and Western Asia..."

The term 'Western Asia' refers to the region of the world more commonly known as the Middle East, a region that, in the past few decades, has experienced numerous conflicts, all of which would certainly have had adverse effects not only on the production of food but also its distribution. In these circumstances, the 'food security' situation can only be improved by the resolution of the conflicts and the restoration of peace, rather than the implementation of 'resilient' and 'sustainable' agricultural practices.

During the many thousands of years of human existence, farmers in all regions of the world have domesticated animals and cultivated plants for the express purpose of producing food. Over the course of time, they also developed techniques to improve the quality and quantity of the food crops they could produce and the health of the animals they reared. In respect of plant crops, these techniques included crop rotation, soil fertility maintenance, seed collection, seed variety creation, crop resilience, pest control and irrigation systems, amongst others. Farmers have also had to learn to contend with the vicissitudes of nature and a variety of weather conditions. In the distant past, farms were generally small-scale enterprises; in remote areas, they often comprised a tiny plot of land on which a family would eke out a meagre living from the few foods they were able to grow. Although far less common, subsistence farming of this nature still exists in some regions of the world.

The nature of farming changed dramatically after the development of large plantations, each of which was, and many still are, devoted to the cultivation of a single export crop. These plantations proliferated almost exclusively in colonised countries, in which many colonisers became plantation owners, who, according to the authors of the previously cited book entitled *Food First*,

"...expropriated the best land for continuous cultivation of crops for export."

These large single-crop plantations, or monocultures, caused many problems for the indigenous peoples, one of which was that their forced removal from fertile land onto marginal, and invariably less fertile land, reduced both the quantity and the quality of the food they were able to produce. Furthermore, although the export of plantation crops provided a good source of income, the benefits of that prosperity were only enjoyed by plantation owners. The indigenous population would invariably endure harsh living conditions; a situation that persisted into the 20th century, as discussed by Eduardo Galeano in *Open Veins of Latin America*, in which he states that,

"Subordinated to foreign needs and often financed from abroad, the colonial plantation evolved directly into the present-day latifundio, one of the bottlenecks that choke economic development and condemn the masses to poverty and a marginal existence in Latin America today."

This situation continues into the 21st century, but it is not unique to Latin America; as the authors state in *Food First*,

"To the colonizers of Africa, Asia and Latin America, agriculture became a means to extract wealth..."

The primary purpose of agriculture is to produce food, not wealth; it should therefore be a requirement of agricultural production systems to prioritise domestic consumption needs, and only after these needs have been met should surpluses be made available for export. This idea is, however, anathema to organisations, such as the World Bank and IMF, that regard the ability of a nation to earn income from exports as more important than its ability to provide sufficient food for the population. Nevertheless, the cultivation of cash crops, such as coffee, tea, tobacco and sugar for example, all of which are grown almost exclusively for export purposes, remains a key feature of 'agriculture' in many 'developing' countries within Latin America, Asia and Africa.

Although large monoculture farms first appeared long before the 20th century, they have proliferated since the introduction in the 1960s of the 'Green Revolution', which required the use of large quantities of chemicals on the basis that they would improve agricultural outputs. One of the main effects of large monoculture farms is the depletion of soil fertility, a problem that traditional small-scale farmers had generally avoided through techniques such as crop rotation and mixed crop planting. The 'Green Revolution' solution to the problem inevitably entailed the use of synthetic chemical fertilisers, the first type of which was developed from nitrate compounds that had been produced by the war industry, but had become surplus to requirements at the end of WWII.

Other types of chemical fertiliser contain potassium and phosphorus in addition to nitrates. These are commonly referred to as NPK fertilisers in reference to the chemical symbols for each element; N for nitrogen; P for phosphorus and K for potassium. Although these chemicals are required for soil fertility, they are not the only nutrients necessary for a healthy and fertile soil. The application of N, P and K alone, therefore causes an imbalance in the natural chemical constitution of the soil and consequently affects the nutritional quality of the food crops grown in that soil.

Furthermore, a healthy soil requires more than just chemicals, even if they are in the correct balance; it also requires an abundance of healthy soil organisms, the functions of which include the decomposition of dead organic matter in order to return the released nutrients back into the soil. The synthetic chemical products utilised by 'Green Revolution' methods do not nourish the soil or its community of soil organisms. Most, if not all of the chemical products used are toxic; which means that they are poisonous to the soil organisms essential for a healthy, fertile soil.

Although Latin America was the first region into which the 'Green Revolution' was introduced, India was the first country in Asia to 'benefit' from this new agricultural system. Indian farmers were led to believe that the 'Green Revolution' would lead to greater prosperity; they would not only reduce their costs, as less fertiliser would be needed, but they would also increase their income, because of the greater crop yields they would achieve. Unfortunately for the farmers, the reality, as they soon discovered, was the complete opposite; the Food First 'primer' document entitled *Green Revolution* explains,

> "In Punjab, India, an early Green Revolution showcase, farmers now apply three times the amount of fertilizers to maintain the same yields."

The farmers who adopted the 'Green Revolution' have discovered that this chemical-based system does not increase crop yields, but does require increased quantities of fertiliser and pesticides; the reason that this system failed is succinctly explained by Vandana Shiva PhD, who states in her July 2017 article entitled *The Farmers' Crisis* that,

> "The Green revolution works against the Earth. It is based on war chemicals, and manifests as a war against the earth..."

Another serious consequence of this system of agriculture has been that farmers are required to purchase 'Green Revolution' seeds, as the primer states,

> "By the 1990s around 40 percent of all farmers in the Third World were using Green Revolution seeds."

Prior to the implementation of 'Green Revolution' agriculture, farmers traditionally collected their own seeds, not only for the purposes of planting the next crop, but also for the purposes of developing new varieties and improving seed properties, such as resilience to damage from drought and flood as well as from pests. The requirement for farmers to purchase rather than collect their own seeds has had profound consequences, two of which, according to the primer, are that,

> "The world lost an estimated 75 percent of its agro-biodiversity, and control over seeds shifted from farmers to a handful of corporations, such as Monsanto, DuPont and Syngenta."

The most insidious aspect of the 'Green Revolution', also referred to as

'Industrial Agriculture', is that it has enabled large agribusiness corporations, whose priority is profit not food production, to gain an inordinate level of influence and control over a significant proportion of the world's food supply. Their dominance over agricultural production methods and inputs also enables these huge conglomerates to exert influence over the nature and content of policy recommendations issued by international organisations, including those within the UN system. The reason that they can exert this level of influence is mainly due to cooperation at the highest levels between corporate owners, bankers, financiers, politicians and others; as will be discussed in chapter nine.

Financial aid provided by the IMF and World Bank is, as discussed, always subject to conditions that include policies that must be agreed to and implemented by the recipient country often prior to obtaining the funds. These policies invariably include the imposition of drastic measures that are claimed to be able to improve a country's economic situation and 'income', or GNI as calculated by the World Bank. In her April 2013 article entitled *The Seeds of Suicide: How Monsanto Destroys Farming*, Vandana Shiva discusses the influence of agribusiness corporations over international organisations and explains that,

"The entry of Monsanto in the Indian seed sector was made possible with a 1988 Seed Policy imposed by the World Bank requiring the Government of India to deregulate the seed sector."

The effects of corporate control over seeds can be devastating, as she explains,

"Control over seed is the first link in the food chain, because seed is the source of life. When a corporation controls seed, it controls life, especially the life of farmers."

Agribusiness corporations have gained even greater control through genetic engineering techniques that are claimed to create entirely new types of seed. These techniques have enabled the biotech industry to claim ownership of these seeds on the basis that they are new 'creations' for which they have been granted patents. The consequences of the virtual control of seeds through the issue of patents to biotech corporations are discussed by Vandana Shiva, who states in her article that,

"Through patents on seed, Monsanto has become the 'Life Lord' of our planet, collecting rents for life's renewal from farmers, the original breeders."

The conditions attached to financial assistance provided by the IMF and World Bank often include the requirement for farmers to grow 'cash crops' for export purposes, in order to boost the country's economy. But farmers rarely benefit from any boost to the economy because their incomes are subject to the vagaries of the 'markets' for their produce. Market forces generally mean that the farmers who sell their crops after the harvest in order to earn their income will all do so at the same time, which produces a market glut that forces prices down and reduces the income that farmers can earn. Vandana Shiva states in her previously cited *Farmers Crisis* article, that,

"Farmers are growing monocultures and are dependent on a single buyer – the government or a corporation – to buy what they grow, as a commodity for trading posts."

Alternatively, crops may be stored after the harvest for the purposes of 'food security' and to provide against a possible future harvest failure; however, stocks of this nature can also provide opportunities for market traders to manipulate prices in ways that are beneficial to them, but are almost invariably detrimental to the farmers.

Another difficulty for farmers is that this type of agriculture requires a large capital outlay for the purchase of seeds, fertilisers and other necessities, but this is often beyond their means. To meet these costs, farmers are encouraged to accept credit terms, usually in the form of a loan, which increases their costs. But the agricultural system the farmers have been enticed to adopt does not fulfil the promises of increased prosperity; in virtually all instances, this system leaves farmers in a far worse financial situation and traps them in a cycle of indebtedness from which they are unable to escape. This 'debt trap' has helped to push farmers in all parts of the world into poverty; in India, it has also pushed large numbers of farmers into such a state of desperate helplessness that many have committed suicide; Vandana Shiva explains,

"Debt for purchase of costly non renewable seeds and unnecessary toxic inputs is the primary reason for farmers suicides and farmers protests."

In her article, she reports that the number of farmers who had committed suicide had exceeded 300,000 and that,

"The suicides are concentrated in regions where the Green Revolution has invaded agriculture – destroying diversity, destroying indigenous agriculture, destroying farmers self reliance, destroying soil and water."

She adds the further comment that,

"Suicides are taking place where globalisation policies have destroyed the diversity of crops and diversity of markets."

As previously discussed, globalisation has encouraged food prices to be brought up to their global market levels; a situation that is devastating for people in 'developing' countries in two ways. The first is that people who live in poverty with a static income are unable to absorb increases in the price of any of their basic needs, especially food. The second is that farmers do not gain the benefit from increases in the prices paid by consumers. Vandana Shiva explains this second point in her article and states that,

"Food prices are rising in the Third World, as food subsidies are removed, and the *polarisation*, between prices farmers receive and prices consumers pay, increases."

This situation continues to persist, despite the claim that the UN is committed to addressing the issue of hunger by helping small farmers, as indicated by SDG 2.3 that states the aim to,

"By 2030, double the agricultural productivity and incomes of small-scale food producers..."

The expansion of globalisation and industrial agriculture means that huge agribusiness conglomerates will not readily relinquish their control over food production as it is far too lucrative for them. No matter how impressive the goals of the 2030 Agenda may sound, or how committed the UN Member States are to realising these goals, it is the actions they take that will determine whether the goals can be achieved, or not. The evidence strongly indicates that the actions that have been taken are woefully inadequate; as 'Industrial Agriculture' continues to expand for the benefit of corporations, but to the detriment of small-scale farmers.

One of the main reasons that 'Industrial Agriculture' persists is because it is claimed to be necessary to solve the problem of 'world hunger'; but this claim is refuted by the Food First web page entitled *World Hunger: Ten Myths*, which refers to increased corporate control and states that,

> "The industrial model also ends up accelerating the concentration of control over land and other resources."

The Food First 'primer' document entitled *Land and Resources*, discusses the importance of land in the context of food production and states that,

> "A global wave of land and water grabs is concentrating farmland and other food producing resources in the hands of a few, with serious consequences for both rural and urban communities..."

Land grabs are not a recent phenomenon; they have been a feature of colonialism and other systems of control for many centuries. The justification for grabbing land in colony countries was based on the concept of *Terra Nullius*, which means that the lands were perceived as empty and thus available for use and exploitation by those who merely 'claimed' it. The belief held by colonisers that land could be claimed, and therefore 'owned', was in complete contrast to the beliefs of most indigenous peoples; as indicated by Vandana Shiva in her November 2015 article entitled *Corporate Imperialism – The only reason for GMOs*, in which she states that,

> "Cultures around the world saw people as belonging to the land, not the land belonging to 'one'."

Land grabs have also been instigated to take advantage of tragic events, such as the Bangladesh famine for example, as explained by the authors in *Food First*,

> "During the 1974 famine, rich landholders stood in line all night at land registry offices in order to buy land that hungry, mortgaged small farmers were selling as a last resort."

As the value of land continues to rise, it becomes impossible for lost farms to ever be recovered by their former owners. Increased land values do, however, favour 'investors' who purchase land purely for investment purposes; as discussed in a November 2010 article entitled *The new farm owners: Corporate investors lead the rush for control over overseas farmland*. The article refers to the 2008 global economic crisis that has resulted in large scale purchases of farmland, particularly in 'developing' countries, and states that,

> "For the past two years, investors have been scrambling to take control of farmland in Asia, Africa and Latin America."

One reason claimed to justify 'land-grabs' in these regions is that they are necessary to help solve the world's food production problems; but investors are not farmers. Whilst farmers will utilise land for the production of food, which will help people who are hungry, investors will simply hold land merely as an 'investment', often leaving it entirely unused. The 'scramble' for farmland by corporate investors is in direct contradiction to the aim of SDG 2.3; yet UN Member States have failed to implement policies to rectify this situation, even though the problem of 'world hunger' is recognised to have worsened.

On the website of the FAO, another UN 'specialised agency', is an article entitled *Trends and impacts of foreign investment in developing country agriculture – Evidence from case studies* that refers to a 2012 FAO report with the same title and states that,

"Investors today are keen to capitalize on current high international food prices, and actually seek investment opportunities in developing countries, notably where natural resources abound."

The article refers to some case studies discussed in the report that involved large-scale land acquisitions, about which the article states that the report found,

"...some evidence of negative impacts on the stock of natural resources including land, water, forests and biodiversity."

These large-scale agricultural schemes are clearly detrimental to the environment. The Food First land 'primer' document highlights a main part of the problem, which is that,

"Global institutional investors view agricultural land as an $8.4 trillion market..."

The contemplation of land, especially agricultural land, as a source of investment rather than food production, is also in direct contradiction to concerns about 'food security' and the need to increase food production. Yet these concerns about 'food security' are raised by exactly the same international organisations within the UN system that support the implementation of structural adjustment programmes that require 'cash crops' to be grown for export, instead of food crops for domestic consumption. In *The Globalization of Poverty*, Professor Chossudovsky provides examples of countries, especially in Africa, that have been affected by the onerous policies of the IMF and World Bank. One of the examples he refers to is Rwanda, about which he states,

"It was the restructuring of the agricultural system under IMF-World Bank supervision which precipitated the population into abject poverty and destitution."

The main plantation 'cash crop' in Rwanda was coffee, but when coffee prices plummeted in the 1980s, the country's economy entered a period of severe crisis that was exacerbated by famine. The assistance provided to Rwanda by the IMF was, as usual in these cases, subject to certain conditions; Professor Chossudovsky explains,

"The IMF had demanded the 'opening up' of the domestic market to the dumping of US and European grain surpluses."

The demands to 'open' up domestic markets and to receive 'dumped' surpluses are also common features of the conditions imposed by the IMF and World Bank; a situation that demonstrates their preference for providing support to large corporate enterprises, rather than local food producers who are unable to compete with such cheap imports. But there is a further detrimental aspect to these 'dumped' surpluses, one that is largely hidden but is explained by Professor Chossudovsky who, with reference to the US, states that,

"...they have been peddling the adoption of their own genetically modified seeds under the disguise of emergency aid and famine relief."

Another example he refers to is Ethiopia, a country that has suffered many famines over the past few decades, for which it has received emergency aid and famine relief, as Professor Chossudovsky explains,

"Some 500,000 tons of maize and maize products were 'donated' in 1999-2000 by USAID to relief agencies including the World Food Programme (WFP) which, in turn, collaborates closely with the US Department of Agriculture."

He also reports that almost a third of the foods included in this humanitarian 'aid' were genetically modified. It is clear therefore, that the organisations within the UN system are fully supportive of GM foods; this is further demonstrated by Vandana Shiva in her previously cited *Corporate Imperialism* article, in which she states,

"It is through the WTO that legal structures of entire countries were undermined and GMOs forced upon them."

The WTO is one of the 'related organisations' within the UN system, which, as its name implies, is concerned with world trade. The main function of the WTO, according to the website, is,

"...to ensure that trade flows smoothly, predictably and freely as possible."

The WTO is therefore another organisation that prioritises the needs of trade in preference to the needs of people. The policies of the WTO that force countries to accept GM foods are usually claimed to be justified on the grounds of ensuring 'food security', and the ability to feed the ever-growing world population. The previously cited *GMO Myths and Truths* report describes this argument as a 'myth' and states the 'truth' to be that,

"GM crops are irrelevant to feeding the world."

In support of this argument, the *GMO Myths* report refers to a 1998 statement to the FAO by 24 delegates from 18 African countries, in which they refer to GM technology as,

"...neither safe, environmentally friendly nor economically beneficial to us."

These delegates were clearly aware at an early date that there were many problems associated with GM; they added in their statement that they did not believe that GM technologies,

"...will help our farmers to produce the food that is needed in the 21st century. On the contrary, we think it will destroy the diversity, the local knowledge and the sustainable agricultural systems that our farmers have developed for millennia, and that it will thus undermine our capacity to feed ourselves."

This is a powerful statement; it is also significant that it was made by people from African countries, because they are increasingly the targets of efforts by agribusiness corporations keen to introduce GM crops into Africa, on the basis of the claim that they will 'solve' the problem of hunger within that vast continent. This claim has been proven to be false, as recognised by the African delegates in their statement to the FAO. The continuing pressure on African countries is discussed in a November 2014 article entitled *GMOs in Africa: Capturing frontier markets in the name of food security*, which states that,

"African nations clearly represent the new frontier market for biotech firms."

The efforts of the agribusiness industry to enter the African agricultural market are conducted largely under the auspices of AGRA (Alliance for a Green Revolution in Africa). On a web page entitled *Developing Africa's Seed Systems* is the claim that the performance of African food staples is not as good as those of the rest of the world, and that African crop harvests are substantially below their potential. The AGRA 'solution' to this problem was to create PASS (Program for Africa's Seed Systems), on the basis of,

"The desire to give African farmers a wider range of seed choices – including access to seeds of highly productive crop varieties known as hybrids..."

Although AGRA describes these seeds as 'hybrids', this is disingenuous, as they are far more likely to be GM varieties, which have not been proven to be 'highly productive'. The real purpose of programmes such as PASS is for agribusiness corporations to not only boost sales of their products and amass even greater profits for their owners, but to also gain even greater control over the world's food supply.

The urgency of the desire to increase food production to feed the expanding world population suggests that current production levels are barely able to meet existing needs; however, this is a mistaken idea and needs to be put into the correct perspective. According to the FAO web page entitled *Food Wastage: key facts and figures*, in 2011, the estimated global food wastage was in excess of 1 billion tonnes, which is said to represent more than a quarter of the total amount of food produced globally. The fact that such an immense volume of food wastage occurs in a world where millions live in hunger highlights the existence of severe inequities and inequalities with respect to the distribution of food. It also demonstrates the appalling nature of policies that demand 'cash crops' to be grown for export in preference to food crops grown for domestic consumption. Yet these policies are created by the same organisations that claim to be committed to providing 'food security' by implementing 'sustainable' agriculture methods that are able to increase food production levels.

The FAO web page entitled *Key facts on food loss and waste you should know!* provides a revealing comparison,

"Every year, consumers in rich countries waste almost as much food (222 million tonnes) as the entire net food production of sub-Saharan Africa (230 million tonnes)."

The problem of food wastage has been recognised by the UN and is incorporated into SDG 12.3 that states the aim to,

"By 2030, halve the per capita global food waste at the retail and consumer levels and reduce food losses along production and supply chains, including post-harvest losses."

It is abundantly clear from the discussion in this section that there are many problems with 'Industrial Agriculture'; a system that relies on toxic chemicals, huge monoculture farms, genetic engineering, patents and corporate ownership of all agricultural resources. These problems are discussed by Colin Todhunter in his November 2015 article entitled *The tremendous success of Agroecology in Africa*, in which he states that,

"It is essential that we get off the chemical treadmill that the modern industrial urban-centric food and agricultural system is based on."

As indicated by the title of his article, there are solutions to these problems, but they require an entirely different approach to agriculture; one that places the production of nutritious food as its prime concern. These solutions involve agricultural systems that have been proven to be successful; they include, but are not restricted to, organic systems and agroecology. The *Failure to Yield* report, previously cited in chapter six, refers to the need to increase food production in 'developing' countries and, with reference to organic systems, states that,

"Several recent studies have shown that low-external-input methods such as organic can improve yield by over 100 percent in these countries, along with other benefits."

The GMO Myths and Truths report also refers to organic systems and states that,

"A 2008 United Nations report looked at 114 farming projects in 24 African countries and found that organic or near-organic practices resulted in yield increases averaging over 100%."

These successes from organic agricultural methods alone provide a clear refutation of the AGRA claim that Africa needs access to 'hybrid' seeds to boost their harvests.

Agroecology is defined in the Food First 'primer' document entitled *Agroecology* as the 'science of sustainable agriculture', which suggests that it ought to be recognised and embraced by the UN in its efforts to implement 'sustainable' food production. However, this is unlikely to be the case, because agroecology does not utilise the methods favoured by corporate agriculture, as the primer states,

"In sharp contrast to the proposal to industrialize all of the world's production systems with GMOs and monocultures, Agroecology demands diversification, small and medium land holdings and an emphasis on farming as a livelihood."

Furthermore, the primer also explains that,

"Instead of a steady concentration of wealth and monopoly power, agroecology works to decentralize and equitably distribute the power and wealth in our food systems."

Organic agriculture, agroecology and all similarly ecologically-sound agricultural food production systems are eminently preferable to that of 'Industrial Agriculture'. The page entitled *Organic Movement* on the Navdanya website refers to the reasons that these methods are preferable and should be adopted by all farmers in all regions of the world, in the statement that,

"Our research has proved that contrary to the dominant assumptions, ecological agriculture is highly productive and is the only lasting solution to hunger and poverty."

It is only through agricultural systems of this type that genuinely nutritious foods can be successfully grown; the importance of nutrient-rich foods cannot be over-emphasised, especially in the context of health.

Clean Water & Sanitation

Water is one of the most vital of all 'basic human needs'; without it no human is able to survive for more than a few days. The cellular processes that support virtually all of the functions of the human body require the presence of water; which means that water intended for human consumption should be 'clean'. But this is not the term used by the UN and WHO; instead they use the term 'safe' when referring to water quality.

Although included in the discussions in chapter six, the following statements are repeated for ease of reference in this discussion.

The February 2018 WHO fact sheet entitled *Drinking-water* states that,

"Safe and readily available water is important for public health..."

Target 1 of SDG 6 states the aim to,

"By 2030, achieve universal and equitable access to safe and affordable drinking water for all."

Target 2 of SDG 6 states the aim to,

"By 2030, achieve access to adequate and equitable sanitation and hygiene for all..."

These references to 'safe' water are, however, misleading. The discussions in chapter six demonstrate that the word 'safe', when used with reference to both water and food, has become a relative term to mean 'as safe as possible' rather than absolutely harmless, which is its real meaning. Consequently, the less stringent criterion of 'as safe as possible' permits water intended for human consumption to contain contaminants, provided they remain below the level deemed to pose a 'risk' to human health. The erroneous nature of the idea that 'poisons' only become harmful beyond a certain 'dose' or exposure level has been discussed; but this idea and its consequences for human health are of particular relevance to the populations of 'developing' countries, as this discussion will demonstrate.

The rigid adherence to the 'germ theory' perpetuates the idea that certain 'germs', which are claimed to breed in unhygienic conditions, are the most significant contaminants of water and the main causes of 'water-borne' illnesses. This erroneous idea is contained within the WHO report entitled *Water Quality and Health Strategy 2013-2020*, which will be referred to as the *Water Quality* report. Although the report recognises that water 'of poor quality' can adversely affect health, the effects are claimed to take the form of 'infectious diseases'; as indicated by the statement that,

"Contaminated water serves as a mechanism to transmit communicable diseases such as diarrhoea, cholera, dysentery, typhoid and guinea worm infection."

The February 2018 WHO fact sheet entitled *Sanitation* refers to a similar group of diseases that are associated with poor sanitation and states that,

"Poor sanitation is linked to transmission of diseases such as cholera, diarrhoea, dysentery, hepatitis A, typhoid and polio."

Cholera, which is one of the diseases common to both groups, is defined by the establishment as,

"an acute infection of the small intestine by the bacterium *Vibrio cholera*, which causes severe vomiting and diarrhoea…"

Cholera is not exclusive to 'developing' countries, it can occur anywhere that clean water and sanitation facilities are inadequate or absent. Conditions of this nature are increasingly common within 'inner city slums' in 'developed' countries, and are invariably experienced by people who live in a state of poverty. Although recognised to be associated with insanitary conditions, cholera, like other 'diarrhoeal diseases', is claimed to result from an 'infection' that may also induce vomiting. But this claim is misleading, diarrhoea and vomiting are not caused by 'infections' nor are they 'diseases'; they are both natural mechanisms by which the body expels substances it recognises to be 'toxic'.

The January 2019 WHO fact sheet entitled *Cholera* claims that cholera can be fatal if left untreated, but makes the surprising statement that,

"Most people infected with *V. cholerae* do not develop any symptoms…"

The fact sheet also states that,

"Among people who develop symptoms, the majority have mild or moderate symptoms, while a minority develop acute watery diarrhoea with severe dehydration. This can lead to death if left untreated."

Unlike most other diseases claimed to be caused by bacteria, cholera is not treated with antibiotics; the fact sheet explains the reason in the surprising statement that,

"Mass administration of antibiotics is not recommended as it has no proven effect on the spread of cholera…"

The main 'treatment' for cholera involves rehydration, as the fact sheet states,

"The majority of people can be treated successfully through prompt administration of oral rehydration solution (ORS)."

Rehydration is clearly of vital importance when the body has undergone a significant loss of fluid due to severe bouts of vomiting and diarrhoea, but the claim that rehydration is sufficient treatment for a disease claimed to be bacterial is inconsistent with the theory that cholera is caused by bacteria. In addition, the statement that 'infection' with *V. cholerae* may not produce any symptoms violates Koch's first Postulate.

Although cholera is said to be 'easily treatable', the pharmaceutical industry has developed an oral cholera vaccine that the WHO recommends for use in areas that are cholera endemic, most of which are within 'developing' countries. Previous discussions have indicated that this vaccine will not be able to prevent cholera, but instead, like all other vaccines, will exacerbate existing ill-health problems.

The unhealthy living conditions in which cholera often occurs are the result of various factors; these include wars and conflicts that destroy not only basic infrastructure, but also peoples' homes from which they are forced to flee in order to save their lives. Unfortunately, this 'flight to safety' may force people to endure temporary living accommodation in camps that invariably lack most, if not all, basic facilities, especially clean water and sanitation. The cholera fact sheet recognises that temporary camps set up for refugees and displaced persons generate 'risks' for disease and states that,

> "The consequences of a humanitarian crisis – such as disruption of water and sanitation systems, or the displacement of populations to inadequate and overcrowded camps – can increase the risk of cholera transmission, should the bacteria be present or introduced."

Although it may seem that diseases spread between people through the transmission of 'germs', this is a deceptive appearance, as has been discussed. It does not require the presence of bacteria, or any other so-called 'germ', for severe ill-health to exist amongst large numbers of people who are simultaneously deprived of access to clean water and basic sanitation facilities. The ingestion of water contaminated with human wastes, rotting food and other refuse is more than sufficient to cause 'outbreaks' of vomiting and diarrhoea. The lack of access to clean drinking water for rehydration will exacerbate the situation; persistent dehydration will worsen existing illness and can even lead to death.

Human wastes are clearly a major source of water contamination; the UN web page entitled *Progress of Goal 6 in 2016* claims that almost a billion people practise open defecation, and that almost two billion people are exposed to water sources contaminated by faecal matter. Although the page indicates that the proportion of the world population with access to sanitation facilities continues to increase, it states that,

> "Nevertheless, the unsafe management of faecal waste and wastewater continues to present a major risk to public health and the environment."

Faeces are waste materials produced by the human body; if ingested, they will invariably cause an immediate attack of vomiting. It should be clear, therefore, that it is not due to the presence of 'germs' that water contaminated with human faecal wastes will induce vomiting, diarrhoea or both. As discussed in chapter six, faecal matter is not eliminated from water through treatments that utilise disinfectants for the specific purpose of killing 'germs'. The chemicals used as 'disinfectants', which are mainly chlorine-based compounds, do not purify water. On the contrary, these chemicals pose an additional and significant hazard not only to human health but also to the environment. The problems of 'unsafe water' are clearly not due to 'unsafe management'; they are largely the result of the erroneous belief that 'germs' are a major source of water contamination and therefore need to be killed.

Unfortunately, water disinfection processes in 'developing' countries utilise the same types of chemicals as those used in 'developed' countries; as indicated by the previously cited *Water Guidelines* report, that states,

> "Disinfection of household drinking-water in developing countries is done primarily with free chlorine..."

The hazards to human health from the use of chlorine-based compounds to 'disinfect' water to make it 'safe' for human consumption have been discussed.

Water can be contaminated from numerous other sources, a significant proportion of which are attributable to industrial activities, such as mining, oil and gas extraction, chemical manufacturing, textile manufacturing and agriculture, to name just a few. Most of these industries produce toxic wastes, some of which may be discharged as effluent into bodies of fresh water, such as rivers, that may be used in some areas by the local population as their main source of water, especially for drinking. Liquid wastes discharged by industrial facilities do not just affect surface waters, they can also seep into the soil and, if they permeate deeply into the ground, these toxic substances can eventually reach and thereby poison groundwater, another vital source of fresh water that frequently serves a wider area in addition to local communities.

The contamination of water due to industrial activities has been recognised, albeit to a limited extent, by the 2030 Agenda; as indicated by SDG 6.3 that states the aim to,

> "By 2030, improve water quality by reducing pollution, eliminating dumping and minimising release of hazardous chemicals and materials…"

Unfortunately, merely minimising the release of hazardous chemicals and materials is a woefully inadequate method to improve water quality; at best, this method only permits water to be described as 'less polluted' as it allows the continuing discharge of hazardous materials, even if at a reduced level. It should be clear that 'less polluted' is not synonymous with 'safe' and certainly not with clean. Furthermore, in addition to the fact that few chemicals have been tested for their safety or the full extent of their effects, is the fact that no tests have been conducted to determine the effects of exposures to the countless combinations of the 100,000 or more chemical compounds that have been produced and released onto the market and into the environment.

The industrial pollution of water is of particular concern for the 'developing' countries chosen by industries of 'developed' countries for relocation of their manufacturing facilities. These relocations frequently occur with the specific intention of taking advantage of low costs, especially wages, and less restrictive or even totally absent regulatory systems. The absence of measures that would otherwise protect the integrity of fresh water sources enables industries to discharge toxic substances into local bodies of water, almost with impunity; an extremely hazardous situation that contributes to worsening morbidity and mortality in regions that already suffer disproportionately from severe health problems.

There are numerous industrial chemicals that contaminate water and are present in differing concentrations; a situation with which scientists would seem to be familiar, as indicated by the *Water Guidelines* report that states,

> "In most countries, whether developing or industrialized, water sector professionals are likely to be aware of chemicals that are present in significant concentrations in some drinking-water supplies."

The concentration in which a toxic chemical is present in water does not affect its inherent toxicity; a poison is a poison whatever its concentration.

The concentration does however, determine the severity of the effects the substance is able to cause.

One of the major chemicals of concern referred to in the report is arsenic, which is found in the groundwater of a number of regions of the world, especially, but not solely in 'developing' countries; as indicated by the *Water Quality* report, which states that,

> "Inorganic arsenic is present at high levels in the groundwater of a number of countries, including Argentina, Chile, China, India (West Bengal), Mexico, the United States of America, and particularly Bangladesh..."

Although arsenic is 'naturally-occurring', it is also used by many industrial processes; which means that it may be present in discharged wastes. It is interesting to note the symptoms associated with acute arsenic poisoning, which are described by the February 2018 WHO fact sheet entitled *Arsenic* that states,

> "The immediate symptoms of acute arsenic poisoning include vomiting, abdominal pain and diarrhoea."

Arsenic is only one of many thousands of toxic substances capable of adversely affecting human health; although highly toxic, it is not the most dangerous substance; many of the compounds created by the chemical industry, the family of dioxins for example, are just as hazardous, if not more so.

Another major source of water contamination is 'Industrial Agriculture', which, as discussed in the previous section, utilises a variety of chemical-based products, especially pesticides, which are intentionally toxic. One of the problems that result from the use of toxic compounds for agricultural purposes is chemical 'run-off'; which means that unabsorbed excesses seep into the ground and poison, not only the soil in which plant crops are grown, but also the soil organisms essential for the maintenance of soil fertility and for good crop yields, in terms of both quantity and quality. These toxic chemicals are able to seep into and poison groundwater, which is a matter of great importance for farmers in many 'developing' countries, where water is a scarce resource; this is an extremely compelling reason for farmers to avoid 'Industrial Agriculture'.

Although some pesticides are used to protect crops from 'pests', others are used to eliminate insect pests, such as mosquitoes, that are claimed to be the carriers of parasites, said to be the causes of diseases such as malaria. These 'carriers', or 'vectors', often live and breed in or near water, which is where pesticides are most frequently applied. Pesticides are, however, toxic to all living organisms.

People who obtain water for drinking, as well as other purposes, from fresh water sources where pesticides have been applied, will also be poisoned, although the nature and extent of the effects they experience will vary according to the nature of the chemicals used in the pesticide. As discussed, the mechanisms of action of different chemicals vary; which means that the symptoms they induce will also vary. However, it is likely that, in 'developing' countries, symptoms caused by exposures to pesticides will be attributed to a 'water-borne disease' caused by a 'pathogen' of some description; whether a bacterium, virus, fungus or parasite. Interestingly, the drinking-water fact sheet states that 'vectors' breed in clean rather than dirty water.

The drinking-water fact sheet recognises that industrial activities and agriculture both contribute to water contamination, but claims that 'poor management' is largely to blame; as indicated by the previously cited statement that deserves repetition,

"Inadequate management of urban, industrial, and agricultural wastewater means the drinking-water of hundreds of millions of people is dangerously contaminated or chemically polluted."

This clearly applies to 'developed' as well as 'developing' countries.

Unfortunately, however, good management practices, according to the WHO, include the use of disinfectants to kill 'germs'; which means that they contribute to the contamination of water, not to its purification.

The *Water Guidelines* report is an extensive document of more than 600 pages; one chapter, entitled *Chemical Aspects* provides 'guideline values' for a wide variety of chemicals, but these values are based on the Paracelsus fallacy that a 'safe' exposure level to a toxic substance can be ascertained. However, some of the chemicals referred to in the report have not been assessed, because, according to the report, the chemical,

"Occurs in drinking-water at concentrations below those of health concern."

Alarmingly, this phrase is used for some of the most highly toxic substances, including pesticides that have been banned in certain countries due to their extreme toxicity. It should be noted that a number of these pesticides have remained in use in some 'developing' countries; the continuing use of DDT in India, for example, as well as its re-introduction into some African countries, have been discussed.

The pharmaceutical industry is another major source of water pollution; this is also a matter of particular concern for 'developing' countries, especially those that have established, or have been encouraged to establish, their own pharmaceutical manufacturing facilities. The discharge of pharmaceutical waste effluent into local bodies of water has been shown to produce a significant level of contamination; a situation of serious concern for drought-prone regions where water is a scarce resource and access to fresh water is therefore crucial for survival. The problem of water contamination in 'developing' countries due to the discharge of pharmaceutical industry wastes is discussed in a 2013 article entitled *Global risk of pharmaceutical contamination from highly populated developing countries* that refers to Bangladesh, China, India and Pakistan where,

"...most of their industrial units discharge wastewater into domestic sewage network without any treatment."

The article raises the genuine concern that pharmaceutical contamination of water poses serious risks to health. These health hazards are due to the manufacturing processes and the chemical composition of the wastes discharged; as demonstrated by a 2007 article entitled *Effluent from drug manufacturers contain extremely high levels of pharmaceuticals* that reports on the analysis of,

> "...pharmaceuticals in the effluent from a wastewater treatment plant serving about 90 bulk drug manufacturers in Patancheru, near Hyderabad, India – a major production site of generic drugs for the world market."

The article refers to the results of the analyses, which showed that,

> "The samples contained by far the highest levels of pharmaceuticals in any effluent."

The Blacksmith Institute report entitled *Pharmaceutical Waste Analysis*, previously cited in chapter one, has identified a number of highly toxic chemicals that are used in pharmaceuticals,

> "Priority pollutants, including methylene chloride, toluene, chloroform, 1,2-dichloroethane and phenol were identified as being used in the manufacturing of extractive pharmaceuticals."

Although these are clearly highly toxic compounds, the WHO minimises the health hazards posed by the chemicals used in the manufacture of pharmaceuticals, in a section of the *Water Guidelines* report entitled *Pharmaceuticals in Drinking Water*, which states that,

> "Concerns over pharmaceuticals should not divert the attention and valuable resources of water suppliers and regulators from the various bacterial, viral and protozoan waterborne pathogens and other chemical priorities, such as lead and arsenic."

This is disingenuous; the misplaced concerns are those that relate to so-called 'pathogens'. Concerns about pharmaceuticals are not misplaced; but the harm caused by 'medicines' does not receive the level of attention it should, despite the existence of the phenomenon of iatrogenesis. However, as 'developing' countries seek to establish their own pharmaceutical industries on the basis of the erroneous idea that chemical compounds are 'medicines' that can cure disease, their sources of fresh water will inevitably become increasingly polluted.

Furthermore, the drive to promote the 2030 Agenda goal of 'medicines and vaccines for all' will have a significant impact on the quality of fresh water throughout the world; not only through the discharge of increased volumes of industrial wastes but also through increased human wastes that contain metabolised drug chemicals. The presence in water of pharmaceuticals, their metabolites and active ingredients poses serious hazards to human health, as most existing wastewater treatment plants are unable to remove the vast majority of these compounds; as indicated by the *Water Guidelines* report that states,

> "...wastewater and drinking-water treatment processes are not designed specifically to remove pharmaceuticals..."

It is widely acknowledged that most water treatment processes are unable to remove a significant proportion of all chemicals, not just pharmaceuticals. But the erroneous idea that contaminants do not cause harm if they are present at concentrations below a certain level, means that most water supplies contain combinations of a wide variety of chemicals, the health impacts of which are virtually unknown, because untested; a situation that is totally unacceptable.

All people in all countries of the world should have access to water that is truly 'safe'; but this requires attention to be paid to the real causes of 'unsafe' water. Previous discussions have demonstrated that the implementation of sanitation measures that remove 'wastes' of all types played a significant role in improving the health of the population. Measures that improve the quality of water are also essential; however, these should not involve reference to the removal of 'germs'. The quality of water can only be improved when the integrity of all sources of fresh water are protected from all activities that pollute it. Measures that merely minimise water pollution are no longer adequate; industrial activities, and all other sources of water pollution, must be prohibited entirely from discharging toxic wastes into water.

The only 'safe' water to drink is water that is truly clean; this topic is discussed in more detail in chapter ten.

Chapter Nine

Vested Interests & The Agenda for Control

"We are governed, our minds are molded, our tastes formed, our ideas suggested, largely by men we have never heard of."

Edward Bernays

The United Nations (UN) is an intergovernmental organisation empowered by Charter to undertake all actions deemed necessary to fulfil the purposes contained within that Charter, as detailed in Article 1, which, in addition to the maintenance of peace, refers to,

"...international cooperation in solving international problems of an economic, social, cultural, or humanitarian character..."

In chapter IX of the Charter, entitled *International Economic and Social Cooperation*, Article 55 expands on these purposes with reference to,

"...the creation of conditions of stability and well-being necessary for peaceful and friendly relations..."

In order to create these conditions of peace, stability and well-being, Article 55 states that the UN will promote higher standards of living; solutions to international economic, social, health and related problems; and human rights and fundamental freedoms. The overarching aim of the UN would therefore seem to be to create a better world with a better standard of living for everyone; a noble aim indeed!

By virtue of their membership of the UN, all Member States are committed to the provisions of the Charter, which means they are obliged to undertake the required actions to fulfil the stated purposes, as indicated by Article 56 that states,

"All Members pledge themselves to take joint and separate action in cooperation with the Organization for the achievement of the purposes set forth in Article 55."

Although the United Nations organisation was not created until 1945, the *United Nations Monetary and Financial Conference* was held a year earlier at Bretton Woods in the US. A major outcome of this conference was the creation of two international financial institutions; namely, the IMF and the International Bank for Reconstruction and Development, later renamed the World Bank.

Since 1945, many other international organisations have been created that together form the 'UN system'. Each of these organisations has been designated as the 'authoritative' body responsible for matters pertaining to a specific issue. The WHO, founded in 1948, is responsible for matters relating to health; UNDP, founded in 1965, for matters relating to development; and UNEP, founded in 1972, for matters relating to the environment, to name three important examples.

On the basis that the UN is an intergovernmental organisation and that governments are the elected representatives of 'the people', it may be assumed that the international organisations within the UN system only have the best interests of 'the people' in mind when they develop policies to implement measures intended to maintain peace and solve the issues that confront humanity. It may also be assumed that these international organisations are immune to influences that may divert them from their stated goals.

Unfortunately, these would be mistaken assumptions.

Britain was one of the major 'world powers' prior to the 20th century, but, by the early 1900s, the dominance of the British Empire had begun to diminish, as eventually happens to all empires. Inevitably, there were other countries vying to take Britain's place and create the next 'empire', and none more so than the United States of America, especially after WWI had diminished the power of all of their main rivals. The early decades of the 20th century, which had witnessed the demise of the Ottoman Empire, the revolution in Russia and the defeat of Germany, had also seen the increase in American influence; but it was not until the 1940s that the US would emerge as the world's foremost 'power'.

The financial system created at the 1944 Bretton Woods conference elevated the US dollar to the position of the dominant world currency and the only one to be backed by gold; all other currencies were to be valued against the US dollar; William Engdahl explains in *Gods of Money* that,

> "The dollar became the world's reserve currency, required by all trading nations to conduct trade with one another after 1945."

This was a crucial step in the process of promoting the US to the position of the dominant 'world power'.

In his February 1941 essay entitled *The American Century* published in Life magazine, Henry Luce, who was regarded as one of the most influential Americans of that era, had referred to America as 'the most powerful nation in the world' and asserted that it was the duty of that nation to,

> "...exert upon the world the full impact of our influence, for such purposes as we see fit and by such means as we see fit."

This view of America's power was not unique to Henry Luce, it was an opinion that had been held for many decades by a number of influential Americans, who form part of the group referred to in these discussions as 'vested interests'. The manner in which America was to exert its influence was not to be through an 'empire' as such, as it was not to involve the occupation of other countries; however, as William Engdahl explains,

"It was every bit an empire, albeit a less visible one, based on the role of the United States in international finance with the dollar as the pillar of the postwar system, backed up by overwhelming military superiority."

That 'overwhelming military superiority' was displayed for the whole world to witness when the US dropped two nuclear bombs onto Japan in 1945; an unprecedented course of action that demonstrated the US had not only developed weapons of mass destruction, but was also prepared to unleash them onto their 'enemies'.

Based on the belief that it was the 'duty' of America to lead the world, the 'vested interests' behind US policy decisions were to undertake various actions to create and maintain a dominating influence over all the world's systems and the organisations created to manage those systems; as William Engdahl further explains,

"The American domination of the world after 1945 would be accomplished via a new organization, the United Nations..."

He adds that this American domination was also extended to,

"...the new Bretton Woods institutions of the International Monetary Fund and World Bank..."

The domination of these financial institutions by 'vested interests' based mainly, although not exclusively, in the US has been amply documented. In his June 2018 article entitled *From Global Poverty to Exclusion and Despair: Reversing the Tide of War and Globalization*, which will be referred to as the *Global Poverty* article, Professor Michel Chossudovsky states that,

"The Bretton Woods institutions are instruments of Wall Street and the corporate establishment."

The existence of a group of 'vested interests' that sought to gain control over the world financial system for their own private gain was recorded in the work of historian Carroll Quigley, a highly respected professor at Georgetown University. His study of the documents and papers of a particular group of 'vested interests' resulted in his 1966 magnum opus entitled *Tragedy and Hope*, in which he refers to the 'far-reaching aim' of this group, which was,

"...nothing less than to create a world system of financial control in private hands able to dominate the political system of each country and the economy of the world as a whole."

Professor Quigley was not opposed to the objectives of this group, only to their methods; his main criticism was that they operated in secret; as he states,

"This system was to be controlled in a feudalist fashion by the central banks of the world acting in concert, by secret agreements arrived at in frequent private meetings and conferences."

Although the individual members of the various groups of 'vested interests' have changed over the course of time, the overall objective of controlling the world economy has been retained and continues to be implemented. The financial system that operates within most countries of the world is largely under the control of a group of 'vested interests' that formulate their policies at secret meetings, and therefore operate outside of any democratic processes. In another book, the aptly-titled *The Anglo-American Establishment*, Professor Quigley discusses the composition of the group he had studied in detail and expresses some of his concerns about them, which include,

> "...their tendency to place power and influence into hands chosen by friendship rather than merit, their oblivion to the consequences of their actions..."

These are valid concerns; although they are by no means the only concerns that should be raised about the actions of groups, including international organisations like those within the UN system, that claim to have the 'authority' to generate the policies in respect of the various issues that affect the lives of everyone, everywhere.

All UN organisations hold conferences, whether separately or jointly, to discuss existing problems and to propose measures to resolve them; their proceedings are documented in published reports and made available to the public. Although not held in secret, these meetings are nevertheless influenced by 'vested interests'. One particularly significant conference was the UNCED conference held in 1992 in Rio de Janeiro, Brazil. It was at this conference, known as the Earth Summit, that the attendees adopted the first 'global plan', known as Agenda 21, the *Preamble* to which, as previously cited, states that,

> "We are confronted with a perpetuation of disparities between and within nations, a worsening of poverty, hunger, ill-health and illiteracy, and the continuing deterioration of the ecosystem on which we depend for our well-being."

The next 'global plan' was the Millennium Declaration, which was adopted by UN Member States a few years later at the Millennium Summit held in September 2000; this Declaration states that,

> "We believe that the central challenge we face today is to ensure that globalization becomes a positive force for all the world's people."

The Millennium Declaration committed all UN Member States to certain objectives codified into eight goals, known as the Millennium Development Goals (MDGs), which were intended to address the problems that predominantly affected 'developing' countries and countries with 'economies in transition'. These problems included poverty, hunger, disease, illiteracy and inequalities; in other words, the same problems that had been previously identified by Agenda 21. In addition, MDG 7 referred to 'environmental sustainability' and MDG 8 to the need for a 'global partnership' to enable countries to develop. These subjects had also been incorporated into Agenda 21.

On the expiration of the MDGs in 2015, the UN held the United Nations Sustainable Development Summit that generated the next 'global plan', known as the 2030 Agenda, the main objective of which is claimed to be to address all of the issues that confront humanity in the 21st century through the full implementation of all 17 goals and 169 targets within a period of 15 years. This objective is justifiably claimed to be both ambitious and far-reaching, especially as some of the problems, particularly poverty and ill-health, have existed to varying degrees throughout human history. Nevertheless, the 2030 Agenda document makes the bold statement that,

> "If we realize our ambitions across the full extent of the Agenda, the lives of all will be profoundly improved and our world will be transformed for the better."

This is clearly an extension of the purposes expressed in the UN Charter. However, despite the determination declared within the 2030 Agenda document, some of the SDG targets will not be attained, no matter how fully the proposed measures are implemented or how strictly they are followed. The main reason for the inevitable failure of these targets is because their proposed solutions are based on flawed theories. One pertinent example is SDG 3.8 that aims to improve health through better access to 'medicines and vaccines for all', but, as previously discussed, pharmaceutical products are inimical to health, not supportive of it. Nevertheless, the agenda is to involve all UN Member countries, as the document states,

> "All countries and all stakeholders, acting in collaborative partnerships, will implement this plan."

These 'collaborative partnerships' are to include a wide variety of organisations and 'stakeholders', including 'the people'; as the document also states,

> "Our journey will involve Governments as well as Parliaments, the UN system and other international institutions, local authorities, indigenous peoples, civil society, business and the private sector, the scientific and academic community – and all people."

This is effectively the same idea as the 'global partnerships' referred to in both Agenda 21 and MDG 8; it also clearly reveals the insidious encroachment of 'globalisation' into all aspects of life.

The involvement of a wide variety of 'stakeholders' in the implementation of the 'global plans' and the required measures to ostensibly address humanity's problems, has required some fundamental changes to be made to the way that various 'systems' operate. In the 'health system' for example, the necessary changes are described in a 2009 article entitled *The Global Role of the World Health Organisation*, which will be referred to as the *Global Role* article; the article states that,

> "In the midst of an increasingly globalizing world, however, a new international health framework is emerging; one that is no longer dominated by a few organizations, but that consists of numerous global health actors."

The identification of certain 'global health actors', as well as their role in and influence over the medical establishment system, are discussed later in this chapter.

Many of humanity's problems are genuinely interrelated; the co-existence of poverty and ill-health has been discussed. However, some of these problems are claimed to be interrelated on the basis of some rather tenuous and, in some instances, flawed ideas. For example, the *Overview* of the *World Bank Development Report 1993: Investing in Health*, refers to an 'interplay' between health policies and development that is based on the idea that,

> "Because good health increases the economic productivity of individuals and the economic growth rate of countries, investing in health is one means of accelerating development."

The purpose of the report, which closely followed Agenda 21 in both timing and content, was to provide advice for the governments of 'developing' countries about the nature of the health policies they should implement. One of the recommendations included in the World Bank report is that government spending should be directed towards,

> "...low-cost and highly effective activities such as immunization, programs to combat micronutrient deficiencies, and control and treatment of infectious diseases."

As previously discussed, these activities are not effective as they do not improve human health; their only 'effectiveness' is in their ability to serve the purposes of certain 'vested interests', especially, but not exclusively, those of the pharmaceutical and vaccine industries.

A key feature of globalisation is that it facilitates increased cooperation between various 'stakeholders'. As the 2030 Agenda document indicates, these 'stakeholders' include the 'private sector'; in other words, corporations whose main objective is to generate profits for their shareholders. But pursuing the 'profit-motive' is rarely compatible with the objective of solving humanity's problems; measures that are beneficial for corporate interests are almost always prejudicial to the interests of the general public.

Another key feature of 'globalisation' is that it requires 'harmonisation' of the rules, regulations and standards that govern all systems, which is one of the reasons that these systems are undergoing changes. The inevitable consequence, if the 'agenda' is fully and successfully implemented, will be a full 'harmonisation' of all systems, and their eventual merger into a single 'global' system controlled by a single central 'authority' that can be influenced or even controlled by 'vested interests'.

The idea that there are 'vested interests' whose aim is to gain control over the systems that govern virtually all aspects of life may seem highly controversial, but that does not invalidate the idea. It is, however, an idea that is gaining acceptance by an ever-larger number of people, as they become increasingly aware that the 'systems' that control most aspects of their lives do not function in the manner in which they are reported to function; this is patently obvious from the evidence that most problems are worsening, not improving as they are claimed to be.

The main reason that these problems are worsening is because, as indicated by the Edward Bernays' quote that opens this chapter, the public is 'governed' largely by people who are entirely unknown to them. These unknown and unelected people, together with people who may be known to the public, comprise the 'vested interests' that are in control of most of the systems that affect the lives of the entire world population; but these 'vested interests' have an entirely different 'agenda' from that of solving all of humanity's problems.

Problems can only be resolved if their causes have been fully identified. For some of the problems documented in the various agendas, the causes are attributed to factors that do not contribute significantly, if at all, to the problem; for others, the alleged causes are entirely irrelevant. The most notable example of the misattribution of a problem to an irrelevant cause is the idea that certain diseases are caused by 'germs'.

The reasons that the causes of some of the most crucial problems are attributed to the wrong factors owe their origin almost entirely to the influence of 'vested interests'; as the discussions in this chapter will demonstrate.

Wealth, Power & Influence

The popular saying that 'money is the root of all evil' is a modification of a biblical saying that claims it is the love of money that is the 'evil'. Nevertheless, the idea remains that money, which has been used as a medium of exchange for goods and services for many centuries, is evil; but this is a false notion, because 'money' is inanimate and therefore has no inherent attributes. However, what can be subjected to critical assessment and assigned labels such as 'evil', are the methods by which money is acquired and the purposes for which it is used.

In the midst of the many hundreds of millions of people around the world who live in a perpetual state of abject poverty, is a very small group of extremely wealthy people who are often referred to as the 'one per cent', although in reality, this group of the 'super-rich' represents a much smaller percentage of the total world population. The March 2018 Forbes article entitled *Forbes Billionaires 2018: Meet The Richest People On The Planet* states that there were 2,208 individual billionaires at the beginning of 2018; that their combined worth was approximately $9.1 trillion; and that the combined worth of the 20 richest people was $1.2 trillion. It should be noted that they are not all Americans. This immense wealth is put into perspective by a January 2017 Oxfam press release entitled *Eight people own same wealth as half the world*. The purpose of this press release is to draw attention to the 2016 Oxfam report entitled *An Economy for the 99%*. With reference to the findings of the report, the press release states that,

> "...in 2015 the world's richest one percent retained their share of global wealth and still own more than the other 99 percent combined."

This group of extremely wealthy people has continued to expand in number, as indicated by the January 2018 Oxfam report entitled *Reward Work, Not Wealth*, which states that,

> "Last year saw the biggest increase in billionaires in history..."

According to the report, which corroborates the above cited Forbes article, billionaires not only experienced an increase in their numbers, they also experienced an increase in their combined wealth. The press release web page that highlights the publication of the Oxfam report is entitled *Richest*

1 percent bagged 82 percent of wealth created last year – poorest half of humanity got nothing. The title is self-explanatory, but it demonstrates unequivocally that, contrary to the claims of the World Bank and others, extreme poverty is not being successfully reduced.

It is a commonly-held belief that the wealth created by industrialists and corporate owners through their business acumen and skill is beneficial for the rest of humanity. It is claimed that corporate wealth will 'trickle down' to the rest of society, because it will be used to generate employment opportunities, which, in turn, will generate prosperity for the workers. The findings of the two Oxfam reports referred to above provide a clear demonstration that this theory has not been put into practice; none of the increased wealth generated by the 'one per cent' during 2017, had 'trickled down' to the almost four billion people who comprise the poorest half of humanity, none of whom experienced any increased prosperity.

It is evident that there are vast inequalities, which, together with the ever-widening 'wealth gap', provide demonstrable proof that the 'global agendas' have failed to end or even reduce 'world poverty'. On the contrary, the policies of international agencies, especially the IMF and World Bank, contribute not only to the perpetuation, but to the worsening of poverty; they do not contribute to its eradication. As Professor Chossudovsky states in his *Global Poverty* article,

> "The 'globalization of poverty' in the post-colonial era is the direct result of the imposition of deadly macroeconomic reforms under IMF-World Bank jurisdiction."

The purpose of this discussion is not to criticise wealth per se; the intention is to expose the use of wealth for the purposes of exploitation, whether of people or resources. For example, the purpose of the 'conquest' of America in 1492 was mainly to find and exploit new territories, but it could not have occurred without the large funds made available by the king and queen of Spain. Nor could it have been 'successful' had it not been accompanied by the brute force and violence used by the Spaniards, in combination with deadly weapons superior to those possessed by the peoples they 'conquered'.

The most common application of wealth combined with brute force, violence and deadly weapons has the seemingly respectable label of 'war'. The need for funds to prosecute wars has precipitated many monarchs, governments and other leaders in the past, to become deeply indebted to the bankers and financiers that provided the necessary funds, usually in the form of interest-bearing loans. The funds required to finance the debt repayments to the bankers have almost invariably been raised through taxes levied on the population; a practice that persists to the present day.

Although the methods by which wars are funded have changed little, the nature of war has changed dramatically. The belief that it is appropriate to wage war in order to ensure peace, a complete contradiction in terms, has encouraged the 'war industry' to continue to develop ever more sophisticated weapons that are purchased by governments and used by the military. War has become a highly lucrative enterprise in terms of industrial output, but it is an extremely costly enterprise in terms of human life; as acknowledged by Major General Smedley Butler, who, in his book entitled *War is a Racket*, refers to the 'war racket' and states poignantly that,

> "It is the only one in which the profits are reckoned in dollars and the losses in lives."

In his description of the WWI 'war racket', Major Butler details the huge profits made by certain industries, and explains that the provision of supplies to the military enabled some industrialists to become millionaires. In a succinct summary, he states that war,

> "...is conducted for the benefit of the very few, at the expense of the very many."

Towards the end of WWII, however, the 'war industry' took weapons development to an unprecedented level with the creation of the atomic bomb, the first real weapon of mass destruction. Devastating though the first bombs were, as attested to by the people of Hiroshima and Nagasaki, the 'war industry' has continued to develop nuclear technology and produce weapons that are so powerful that, were only a fraction of the total to be deployed, they could not only annihilate all life on Earth, they could potentially destroy the entire planet in the process.

Although there has not been a 'world war' since 1945, numerous conflicts have been waged throughout many parts of the world in the intervening decades. These wars have enabled the 'war industry' to continue to produce enormous quantities of nuclear and non-nuclear weapons, as well as a wide variety of other military equipment that generate huge revenues and profits; as indicated by a March 2015 article entitled *Blood Money: These Companies and People Make Billions of Dollars from War*. The article claims that the 'top' position in this industry is held by Lockheed Martin, a US company, whose profits for 2013 are quoted to have been $3 billion, which was earned from sales of $35.5 billion. War clearly remains an extremely profitable 'racket'.

The corporations that benefit from war are not restricted to those directly involved in the 'war industry' and the supply of weapons and other military equipment; the chemical and vaccine industries are also assured a substantial boost to their revenues and profits, as indicated by the discussion about GWS in chapter seven.

War is by no means the only enterprise that is highly profitable for many different corporations. Although they normally conduct their activities within the fields of 'trade' and 'commerce', some corporations have extended their activities to matters that would normally be expected to fall within the purview of 'government'; as explained by Ralph Nader, who states in his book entitled *In Pursuit Of Justice* that,

> "Unfortunately, the modern corporation has come to infiltrate, and dominate, spheres of society once considered off-limits to commerce: elections, schools, health-care systems, media, prisons and much more."

It may be assumed that, despite the involvement of corporations in these activities, governments nevertheless remain the primary drivers of all relevant policies, and that any financial benefits that corporations gain as the result of such policies are purely incidental; but this would be a mistaken assumption. Through the utilisation of their immense wealth, the owners and decision-makers behind most large corporations have become capable of exerting a significant degree of influence in many spheres of society, including politics; as indicated by Ralph Nader, who, with reference to the US, states that,

"Corporations dominate our political process."

The American political system is one that permits corporations to make contributions to political campaigns, but these donations are not purely philanthropic; as Ralph Nader further explains,

"After they make their contributions, corporations expect their money to buy access, and it does."

To this statement he adds the comment that,

"They expect this access to yield influence, and it does."

Political and other systems invariably differ throughout the world; however, the gradual encroachment of 'globalisation', which requires the 'harmonisation' of rules and systems, will, if fully implemented, completely eradicate all existing differences. Furthermore, the dominance of US 'interests' will ensure that all other rules and systems will be 'harmonised' in line with those that operate within the US; a situation that would be disastrous for many reasons, as discussed in this chapter.

The emergence of the US as the dominant 'world power' after WWII is often claimed to be a demonstration of America's 'right' to lead the world. In his June 2014 article entitled *What Obama Told Us at West Point*, Dr Paul Craig Roberts discusses 'American exceptionalism' and refers to a speech by Barack Obama, who, when US President, had stated that,

"America must always lead on the world stage..."

The claim that the US 'must always lead' has fostered the belief that US corporate interests also have the 'right' to dominate all other 'interests'.

It is commonly believed that US 'influence' is solely exerted by the President and government officials, but this is not necessarily the case. US-based corporations in particular, have gained such a significant degree of 'influence' that they claim the 'right' to intervene in the affairs of other countries in order to protect their own interests.

An illustrative example of such an intervention, in which US corporate interests sought preference over the interests of a democratically elected government in a sovereign country, is the overthrow of Jacobo Árbenz Guzmán from his position as President of Guatemala during a coup d'état in 1954. The reason for his ousting from office was claimed to be that his government had been 'infiltrated' by communists, the sworn enemies of 'Western democracy'. The real reason was that President Árbenz had implemented agrarian reforms that, amongst other things, granted land to landless peasants; but these reforms posed a threat to the Guatemalan operations of the US-based United Fruit Company, whose officers lobbied the US administration for their assistance to remove this threat. The resulting coup, which is officially acknowledged to have been carried out by the CIA (Central Intelligence Agency), precipitated the resignation of Jacobo Árbenz, whose successor reversed the land reforms to the benefit of the United Fruit Company, but to the detriment of the Guatemalan people.

The creation of international organisations has expanded rapidly since the establishment of the World Bank and IMF in 1944 and the United Nations in 1945. Another international body is the WTO, a *Related Organisation* of the UN that was formed in 1995 to govern 'world trade' and, according to the WTO website, is,

> "...the only international organization dealing with the global rules of trade between nations."

Like the World Bank and IMF, the WTO is perceived to operate entirely independently, but it too, is heavily influenced by US 'vested interests'. In his November 2015 article entitled *Corporate Parasites and Economic Plunder: We Need a Genuine Green Revolution*, Colin Todhunter refers to US influence over all three organisations and states that,

> "With its control and manipulation of the World Bank, IMF and WTO, the US has been able to lever the trade and financial system to its advantage by various means..."

The Industrial Revolution facilitated the manufacture of goods on a far larger scale than had previously been possible; a situation that increased trade and enabled a relatively small number of industrialists to become extremely wealthy. In addition, advances in technology have facilitated the production of an ever-increasing variety of goods in even larger quantities; but these goods need to be sold to increasing numbers of consumers in order for business owners to increase their wealth. This objective can be accomplished through gaining unrestricted access to 'foreign markets'; an activity that is often referred to as 'free trade'.

The US Department of Commerce acknowledges that foreign markets may be 'opened' for the express purpose of benefitting American corporations; as indicated by the web page entitled *Free Trade Agreements*, which states that,

> "Free Trade Agreements (FTAs) have proved to be one of the best ways to open up foreign markets to US exporters."

Despite the seemingly innocuous nature of this term, 'free trade' is often accompanied by aggressive corporate policies to maximise profits through the reduction of costs, especially wage costs, as indicated by Professor Michel Chossudovsky who explains in *The Globalization of Poverty* that,

> "...'free market' reforms have contributed ruthlessly to opening up new economic frontiers, while ensuring 'profitability' through the imposition of abysmally low wages and the deregulation of the labor market."

The WTO supports the promotion of 'free trade' within a 'free market', but this support is not equitably applied across all sectors of 'trade'. On the contrary, the WTO favours corporate interests rather than those of small local producers, as Professor Chossudovsky further explains,

> "Derogating the rights of citizens, 'free trade' under the World Trade Organization (WTO) grants 'entrenched rights' to the world's largest banks and global corporations."

The WTO, free trade and trade agreements are discussed in detail in the next section.

A list of the world's largest corporations and the wealth they generate is compiled annually by Fortune magazine, which states, on the web page entitled *Global 500*, that,

"The world's 500 largest companies generated $27.7 trillion in revenues and $1.5 trillion in profits in 2016."

Interestingly, it is reported that the combined 2016 revenue of the top 500 companies in the world substantially exceeded the 2016 GDP of the US, the world's largest economy in that year.

A proportion of this immense wealth was generated from the exploitation of workers through the payment of 'abysmally low wages' that kept them in a state of poverty, despite their employment. Had these people been paid a decent wage, they could have been genuinely lifted out of poverty.

Although many are privately-owned, some of the 500 largest companies are state-owned enterprises; for example, the largest petroleum companies are owned by the Chinese state. In fact, of the ten largest companies in 2016, four belong to the oil and gas industry, an extremely profitable and powerful industry. The power of this industry has been gained, not only through its virtual monopoly of a major source of energy, but also through the perpetuation of a myth. As briefly mentioned in chapter six, it is commonly believed that oil is a 'fossil fuel'; but this is not the case. The belief is based on an idea that oil is produced from the compression of fossilised plant and animal remains over the course of hundreds of millions of years. The fact that only a finite quantity of fossilised remains can exist, has been used as the basis for the idea that only a finite quantity of oil can exist.

One of the main theories associated with the idea that oil is a 'fossil fuel' was posited in the 1970s; this theory, which became known as 'Peak Oil' claimed that, if extraction continued at the prevailing rate, the earth would soon 'run out' of oil. However, not only has the oil industry continued to extract oil in huge volumes throughout the entire period since the 1970s, it has continued to discover new oil fields; all of which strongly suggests that the world is not about to 'run out' of oil and that oil exists in far greater abundance than has previously been estimated, or admitted.

The existence of vast, and possibly unlimited, quantities of oil does not, however, justify its continued extraction, nor does it justify the use of chemicals derived from oil, known as petrochemicals, in the manufacture of the majority of everyday products. It certainly does not justify the use of petrochemical-derived compounds, most of which are toxic, in 'medicines' or as ingredients of 'food products'.

The interesting 'alternative' theory about the origin of oil first emerged in the mid-20th century. This theory claims that oil is not a 'fossil fuel' but is 'abiotic' in nature; which means that it does not originate from any form of biological matter. In his September 2007 article entitled *Confessions of an 'ex' Peak Oil Believer*, William Engdahl explains that, in the late 1940s, Russian scientists had begun to conduct investigations into the nature of oil and 'natural gas' and concluded in 1956 that,

"Crude oil and natural petroleum gas have no intrinsic connection with biological matter originating near the surface of the earth."

This theory is highly controversial, at least as far as most members of the oil and gas industry are concerned, but there is ample evidence to support it. This evidence, which is almost exclusively restricted to Russian science journals, demonstrates that oil originates under the ground at levels that are far deeper than those at which any fossilised animal or plant remains are possible. One of the few scientific papers that is available in English is entitled *An introduction to the modern petroleum science, and to the Russian-Ukrainian theory of deep, abiotic petroleum origins*. This paper was written by J F Kenney PhD, a geophysicist of the Russian Academy of Sciences and the Joint Institute of the Physics of the Earth, who states that,

> "The modern Russian-Ukrainian theory of deep, abiotic petroleum origins recognizes that petroleum is a primordial material of deep origin which has been erupted into the crust of the Earth."

This is not merely a 'theory'; its principles have been implemented with success by the Russian oil industry, which, it should be noted, is one of the world's largest producers of oil and gas.

Furthermore, recent discoveries by NASA (National Aeronautics and Space Administration) provide additional corroborative evidence for the assertion by Russian scientists that oil is derived from mineral deposits, rather than compressed animal and plant remains. A November 2014 article entitled *Russians and NASA Discredit 'Fossil Fuel' Theory* details NASA's discoveries of the existence of hydrocarbons in other parts of the solar system. The scientific interpretation of these findings is that 'oil' is mineral in nature and must therefore be a renewable resource, not a finite one.

The most significant consequence of this discovery is that high prices are no longer justifiable on the basis of a claim that oil is a 'scarce resource'. However, it should be noted that some of the most powerful 'vested interests' involve the members of families that have been involved in and even controlled the oil industry for decades. The level of control by these people and their associates over the oil and banking industries have enabled them at various times to manipulate oil prices to serve their own interests.

In *Gods of Money*, William Engdahl explains that the huge oil price increases that occurred during the early 1970s were not 'natural', but the result of price manipulations by US-based 'vested interests' to serve their own purposes. One of the main purposes was to save the US economy, because all oil was traded in US dollars; another purpose was to maintain the US position as 'world leader'. US 'vested interests' also needed to ensure that the dollar would retain its position as the world's reserve currency after it had been taken off the 'gold standard' in 1971.

Although the huge oil price increases benefitted US 'vested interests', they were disastrous for people, whose energy costs had risen by 400 per cent within a very short period of time. These rising energy costs contributed significantly to the ensuing economic crises experienced within many countries, especially those referred to as 'developing'. But these crises were again used for exploitative purposes, because they facilitated interventions through the imposition of programmes by the IMF and World Bank, known as SAPs, that were claimed to provide assistance but, in reality, led to further impoverishment.

The oil industry is by no means the only one in which there are highly influential 'vested interests'; but it is a particularly illustrative example of the influence that can be brought to bear, in order to deceive the public through the suppression of an extremely important scientific discovery and the perpetuation of a myth.

The use of wealth to gain influence is encapsulated in the saying that 'he who pays the piper calls the tune'. The extent to which wealth can be used to exert influence, and the manner in which wealthy 'vested interests' can gain influence over major international organisations, is explained by Professor James Petras in his October 2017 article entitled *How Billionaires Become Billionaires*, in which he states that,

"Billionaires buy political elites who appoint the World Bank and IMF officials..."

Corporate wealth is used to exert influence in a variety of ways to ensure that policies are enacted that will favour business interests; the 'purchase of influence' is a practice that is better known by the more respectable label of 'lobbying'. Unlike public relations, which aims to influence the public, lobbying aims to influence decision-makers, particularly politicians, policy-makers and law-makers; Ralph Nader explains in *In Pursuit of Justice* that,

"...a swarm of lobbyists meet privately with politicians and their minions to present public officials with corporate wish lists..."

Although the presentation of a corporate wish list to a politician does not guarantee a successful outcome, lobbying is sufficiently successful to warrant the large sums of money corporations are willing to invest in this activity, otherwise the practice would have ceased long ago. It should be obvious, however, that the fulfilment of corporate wishes by public officials undermines the democratic process; politicians are the elected representatives of 'the people' and should therefore serve the interests of the people who elected them, rather than corporate interests. Public interests and corporate interests rarely overlap; they are often mutually exclusive.

Nevertheless, the successful outcomes achieved by lobbyists for their corporate clients have enabled lobbying to become a highly profitable industry that functions in a number of countries, especially the US. The influence of lobbyists in America is described by Lee Drutman PhD in his April 2015 article entitled *How Corporate Lobbyists Conquered American Democracy*, in which he states that,

"Of the 100 organizations that spend the most on lobbying, 95 consistently represent business."

In the article, he explains that, during the 1960s, lobbyists were more frequently engaged by public interest groups and labour unions than by corporations. But, as indicated by the above statement, corporations and corporate interests now dominate lobbying; a situation that is partly the result of the increasingly closer cooperation between corporations and governments. These 'public-private partnerships' generate a strong system of mutual support that can be extremely effective in presenting a 'consensus' view, whether or not it is correct. The mutual support that each partner offers to the other partners can also be an extremely effective method to counter public opposition to government policies that favour corporate interests over those of the public; as Lee Drutman explains,

> "...the self-reinforcing quality of corporate lobbying has increasingly come to overwhelm every other potentially countervailing force."

Another mechanism by which corporations can exert influence is the 'revolving door' through which government officials and business executives can pass to enter each other's world; as Ralph Nader states,

> "Revolving doors, through which corporate executives glide effortlessly between private sector employment and government jobs and back again, seem to be a fixture of every national administration."

The previously cited *Blood Money* article not only provides details of campaign contributions by leading military supply corporations to US political parties and of the millions of dollars spent on lobbying, it also discusses the participation of lobbyists in 'revolving door' activity, an example of which is that,

> "69 out of 109 Lockheed Martin lobbyists in 2013-14 have previously held government jobs."

The fundamental problem is that corporations have wrested control out of the hands of elected officials in charge of most of the issues that affect people's lives, as Ralph Nader states,

> "Corporate decision-making determines many of the key questions that affect our lives."

He emphasises that these decisions,

> "...are not made through the democratic process..."

A country in which corporate 'vested interests' rather than politicians determine the content of policies can no longer be correctly described as a 'democracy'; it would be more accurate to describe such a country as a 'plutocracy', which means 'rule by the richest'. A plutocracy is a system that totally excludes the public from involvement in the 'political process' and denies them a voice in any of the decision-making processes.

The increasingly close working relationships that exist between governments and corporations, as well as the support that the former provides to the latter, means that virtually all 'rules' favour corporate interests through 'corporate-friendly' legislation and regulations, as Ralph Nader explains,

> "...legislators enact pro-corporate laws which ensure continued growth of corporations' mega-wealth."

The main consequence of this is that, as Ralph Nader poignantly indicates,

> "...the public pays the price."

It is for this reason that people urgently need to become aware of the increasing degree of control exerted by 'vested interests' over most, if not yet all, of the systems that govern the most important aspects of their lives.

Globalisation & The Control Agenda

The term 'globalisation' refers in a general context to the

interconnectedness between people and nations around the globe through improved travel and communications systems. More specifically, 'globalisation' is the term used to refer to the interconnectedness between nations in order to facilitate 'global trade'.

The interconnectedness between people forms the basis of claims that the 'issues that confront humanity' affect everyone, everywhere, and that all of these issues can be resolved through the implementation of a single set of policy measures incorporated into a 'global plan', the most recent of which is the 2030 Agenda. This 'global plan' promotes the formation of a 'global partnership' to facilitate the implementation of all 17 goals and 169 targets; as indicated by SDG 17 that aims to,

> "Strengthen the means of implementation and revitalize the global partnership for sustainable development."

The 2030 Agenda document states that each country has primary responsibility for their own development, but adds the statement that,

> "At the same time, national development efforts need to be supported by an enabling international economic environment, including coherent and mutually supporting world trade, monetary and financial systems, and strengthened and enhanced global economic governance."

One of the aims of 'globalisation' is the complete harmonisation of all of the rules that operate within all 'systems', not just trade, monetary and financial ones; a significant consequence of this would be that countries would only be able to implement policy measures that complied with those of the 'global systems'.

It may be assumed that the UN would ensure that these 'global systems' would operate for the benefit of everyone, everywhere in order to fulfil the stated purposes of the UN Charter. But this would be a mistaken assumption, because, as discussed, the international organisations of the UN system are heavily influenced by 'vested interests' based mainly in the US. It has also been demonstrated that these 'US interests' have asserted the 'right' to lead the world, or, more accurately, to dominate the world. These 'US interests' often promote their 'leadership' as being for the benefit of humanity, but this is not the case; their domination is for the benefit of their own interests.

In addition to the UN organisations established for the purpose of solving humanity's problems, are a number of US organisations established ostensibly for the same purpose. For example, in addition to UNDP, the UN 'development agency', is a US 'development agency' namely, USAID (United States Agency for International Development), which claims, on the web page entitled *What We Do*, that,

> "USAID is the world's premier international development agency..."

It is not clear why the world needs two 'international development agencies' or which of them is the leading agency, but the existence of both raises a number of questions, not least of which is whether they have the same 'agenda'. The answer to this question would seem to be 'no', on the basis that USAID readily admits to primarily serving US interests, as demonstrated by the statement on the same page that,

"USAID's work advances US national security and economic prosperity..."

In addition, on the USAID page entitled *Where We Work* is the statement that,

"Through our assistance programs, USAID plays an active and critical role in the promotion of US foreign policy interests."

These 'assistance programmes' usually provide financial and other 'aid', ostensibly for the purposes of helping other countries to manage certain 'problems', population growth, for example. Although the issue of rapid population growth in 'developing' countries was discussed by the UN in Agenda 21, it had been discussed almost two decades earlier by the US in a 1974 report entitled *Implications of Worldwide Population Growth for US Security and Overseas Threats*. This report, which remained classified until 1980, will be referred to as the *NSSM 200* (National Security Study Memorandum); the document can be accessed from the USAID website. As indicated by its full title, the *NSSM 200* expressed concern about population growth purely from the perspective of 'US interests' and with respect to the potential impact it may have for 'US security'. Furthermore, although the *NSSM 200* discusses possible strategies to address the perceived 'problem', it suggests that these efforts should focus only on certain key countries and states that,

"Assistance for population moderation should give primary emphasis to the largest and fastest growing developing countries where there is special US political and strategic interest."

The *NSSM 200* indicates that this 'assistance' would be provided through USAID programmes, including education programmes for women in 'developing' countries to inform them about various issues, such as limiting their family size through different methods of birth control. However, the *NSSM 200* makes the revealing comment that,

"Bilateral population assistance is the largest and most invisible 'instrument' for carrying out US policy in this area."

The main purpose of the aid provided by USAID is to further US policy rather than further 'international development'; as indicated by the *NSSM 200*, which, under the sub-heading *Political Effects of Population Factors*, states that,

"The political consequences of current population factors in the LDCs ... are damaging to the internal stability and international relations of countries in whose advancement the US is interested, thus creating political or even national security problems for the US."

The US was only concerned about certain countries, which were mainly those with the resources required by US interests, as the *NSSM 200* explicitly states,

"The United States has become increasingly dependent on mineral imports from developing countries in recent decades, and this trend is likely to continue."

It should be noted that most 'developing' countries, including many African countries, are rich in a wide variety of minerals and other resources that are extremely valuable for US corporate interests.

Many of the concerns about the rate of population growth and its consequences that are expressed in the *NSSM 200* were carried forward and incorporated into Agenda 21, Chapter 5 of which states that,

"The growth of world population and production combined with unsustainable consumption patterns places increasingly severe stress on the life-supporting capacities of our planet."

Concerns about the growing world population are also expressed within the 2030 Agenda, although not described as such. Instead the problem is expressed in terms of equality, women's reproductive rights and the 'empowerment' of women; as indicated by SDG 5, the main aim of which is to,

"Achieve gender equality and empower all women and girls."

The recommendation in the *NSSM 200* for women in 'developing' countries to be 'educated' about topics such as reproduction, the ideal family size and birth control methods, remains at the heart of the 'agenda'; as indicated by SDG 5.6, which states the aim to,

"Ensure universal access to sexual and reproductive health and reproductive rights..."

The discussion about 'reproductive health' in chapter eight referred to efforts to encourage pregnant women, especially in 'developing' countries, to visit antenatal clinics to receive 'health care'. These visits also provide opportunities for women to be 'educated' about their reproductive 'rights' and to be subjected to 'HIV tests'. Previous discussions have referred to the fact that pregnancy is one of the main conditions known to produce a false-positive 'HIV test' result, and to the fact that 'HIV tests' only detect 'antibodies'; they do not detect the presence of any virus. Nevertheless, on the basis of this spurious test, the medical establishment claims that millions of people have been 'infected' with HIV. Although the erroneous nature of this claim has been discussed, the reasons for the perpetuation of fear about 'HIV', or any other allegedly pathogenic 'virus', are discussed later in this chapter.

Concerns about 'population growth' are most frequently expressed in terms of the ability to grow sufficient food to feed ever-larger numbers of people, as has been previously discussed. This concern was discussed by the *NSSM 200* in the statement that,

"Growing populations will have a serious impact on the need for food especially in the poorest, fastest growing LDCs."

However, although the *NSSM 200* refers to the continuing need for adequate levels of food to be produced, which is certainly a matter of importance, the underlying concern about the large number of hungry people in 'developing' countries was not for their welfare, but for the potential unrest and political instability that these hungry people may cause in countries where the US had an 'interest'.

As discussed in chapter eight, 'food scarcity' is a myth; virtually all 'developing' countries are eminently capable of growing sufficient food without using the detrimental agricultural practices that agribusiness corporations attempt to impose on them. 'Modern agriculture', as practised by the giant biotechnology and agribusiness conglomerates, utilises toxic synthetic chemicals as pesticides and fertilisers and promotes GM technologies; it also favours huge plantations in which single crops can be grown for the export market. This form of agriculture is promoted for 'developing' countries on the basis that increased exports facilitate 'economic growth' and enable 'development'. This idea is promoted by USAID on the web page entitled *Economic Growth and Trade* that states economic growth is an important factor for development, and refers to one of the areas in which USAID works, which is,

> "Giving people access to markets, where they can sell their goods and services and play a productive role in their economies."

These are false promises; small businesses do not have the same access to these markets as large businesses. In reality, most markets are controlled by corporate interests, including the markets for agricultural products. The consequences of globalisation and the increasing corporate takeover of agriculture is demonstrated by the example of India, as explained by Vandana Shiva in her previously cited article entitled *The Farmers' Crisis*,

> "The corporate takeover of Indian agriculture has been facilitated by the globalisation of agriculture, through the imposition of Structural Adjustment by the World Bank and IMF, and the trade rules of WTO..."

The benefits gained by multinational corporations from the takeover of Indian agriculture, have cost the lives of more than 300,000 Indian farmers who have committed suicide due to their unbearable debt burden. As previously discussed, these huge debts accrued as the result of the failure of the 'Green Revolution' to fulfil its promises of larger crop yields and increased prosperity for the farmers who adopted it. The 'Green Revolution' clearly serves corporate interests in preference to those of farmers; for example, the oil industry is a major beneficiary of agricultural practices that require petrochemical-based pesticides and fertilisers. But the problem is far worse than mere corporate greed.

Although promoted as necessary for 'economic growth' and 'development', the production of single crops for the export market destroys local agriculture and therefore, the ability to produce sufficient food for domestic consumption, the result of which is the exacerbation of hunger, poverty and ill-health; this point is discussed in a June 2017 article entitled *Challenging Neoliberal Dogma: Pushing Indian Farmers into Bankruptcy Isn't 'Development'!* The title is self-explanatory, but the article makes the salient point that,

> "The future of our food is being decided by unregulated global markets, financial speculators and global monopolies."

This situation is an intentional part of the 'agenda' for US domination; as Professor Chossudovsky explains in his *Global Poverty* article, in which he states that,

> "This US hegemonic project largely consists in transforming sovereign countries into open territories, controlled by dominant economic and financial interests."

These dominant interests control many aspects of the 'world trade, monetary and financial systems' that form part of the 'enabling economic environment' to ostensibly facilitate 'development'. But these 'systems' operate for the benefit of 'vested interests'; they do not operate for the benefit of 'the people', as the example of Indian agriculture demonstrates, nor do they facilitate genuine 'development'. In his previously cited article entitled *Corporate Parasites and Economic Plunder*, Colin Todhunter identifies some of the 'vested interests' and states,

> "The current economic system and model of globalisation and development serves the interests of Western oil companies and financial institutions (including land and commodity speculators), global agribusiness and the major arms companies."

The 2030 Agenda document indicates that the preferential treatment afforded to 'business interests' has a purpose because,

> "Private business activity, investment and innovation are major drivers of productivity, inclusive economic growth and job creation."

This statement is clearly an attempt to promote the theory that corporate wealth 'trickles down' to benefit 'the people' through the creation of employment opportunities. But this theory does not operate in the real world, as indicated by Professor Chossudovsky in his June 2016 article entitled *Neoliberalism and The Globalization of War: America's Hegemonic Project*. In this article, which will be referred to as the *Neoliberalism* article, he explains that the American 'project' involves 'economic warfare' that includes,

> "...the imposition of deadly macro-economic reforms on indebted countries as well as the manipulation of financial markets, the engineered collapse of national currencies, the privatization of state property, the imposition of economic sanctions, the triggering of inflation and black markets."

The imposition of 'reforms' on indebted 'developing' countries, especially in Africa, began in the late 1970s and has since been extended into most other countries, including European countries. People in almost every country have been forced to suffer the adverse effects of severe austerity measures that have been imposed on them by the IMF and World Bank; measures that are claimed to be able to assist countries to 'better manage their economies'. However, as Professor Chossudovsky explains, the real purpose of these policies is to enable the 'dominant economic and financial interests' to control the economies of all sovereign countries. In his *Neoliberalism* article, he explains that the nature of these 'reforms' has changed, although not for the better, and states that, since 1997,

> "...the IMF-World Bank structural adjustment program (SAP) has evolved towards a broader framework which consists in ultimately undermining national governments' ability to formulate and implement national economic and social policies."

As previously discussed, the IMF and World Bank have effectively been under the control of 'US interests' since their formation in 1944, despite claims that the main purpose of these two institutions is to provide financial assistance to countries to help end poverty. The controlling 'vested interests', which are not solely US-based, are described by Professor Chossudovsky in his *Global Poverty* article as a 'New World Order', about which he states,

"What we are dealing with is an imperial project broadly serving global economic and financial interests including Wall Street, the Military Industrial Complex, Big Oil, the Biotech Conglomerates, Big Pharma, the Global Narcotics Economy, the Media Conglomerates and the Information and Communication Technology Giants."

The 'vested interests' referred to in these discussions include people who control these huge corporate conglomerates; they are therefore the major beneficiaries of 'world trade', the promotion of which is a key aspect of 'globalisation' and a major component of the 'global agenda', as indicated by the 2030 Agenda document that states,

"We will continue to promote a universal, rules-based, open, transparent, predictable, inclusive, non-discriminatory and equitable multilateral trading system under the World Trade Organization (WTO), as well as meaningful trade liberalization."

Trade liberalisation is another term for 'free trade', which means trade that operates without restrictions. Under normal circumstances, 'free trade' could operate in ways that are 'non-discriminatory and equitable', except that the current circumstances are not 'normal'. The existing trading system, which is the one promoted by the WTO and other international organisations, is not 'free', nor is it 'non-discriminatory' or 'equitable'. As discussed, the mantra of 'free trade' is used in order to 'open' foreign markets and facilitate access to them for large multinational corporations, not small businesses.

Although a *Related Organisation* of the UN, the WTO has nevertheless been granted a role in the trading system promoted by the 2030 Agenda. The WTO web page entitled *The WTO and the Sustainable Development Goals* refers to the incorporation of the 1995 WTO TRIPS (Trade-Related Aspects of Intellectual Property Rights) agreement into SDG 3; the page claims that this agreement will,

"...make it easier for developing countries to have a secure legal pathway to access affordable medicines..."

This agreement clearly favours the interests of 'Big Pharma'.

The domination of corporate interests over the global trading system has been achieved through a variety of means, not least of which involves trade treaties and agreements. The creation of some of these trade agreements has involved the participation of certain 'interested parties', that have therefore been able to exert influence over the content to ensure that the agreements will favour their interests.

Although there are many trade agreements currently in operation, two proposed treaties require further examination; these are TTIP (Transatlantic Trade and Investment Partnership), an agreement between the US and EU, and CETA (Comprehensive Economic and Trade Agreement), an agreement between the EU and Canada. At the time of writing, the implementation of TTIP has been halted, however CETA has been in force 'provisionally' since September 2017. Although not yet fully implemented, these treaties require further discussion because of the excessive and totally inappropriate 'rights' they would confer on corporate entities.

One of the most significant aspects of these treaties is that they will impose the 'harmonisation' of rules, the purpose of which is to ensure that the least restrictive rules will apply to all parties of the agreements. STOP TTIP is a 'European Initiative Against TTIP and CETA'; the web page entitled *TTIP and CETA in detail* provides more information about these treaties and states that,

"The main objective of the TTIP is to harmonise to the greatest extent possible transatlantic rules, regulations and standards..."

Contrary to a commonly-held belief, the US does not operate the most restrictive regulatory systems and practices; it is reported that the US operates some of the least restrictive standards. This is a matter of crucial importance because, although the implementation of TTIP was halted in 2016, many provisions of CETA, to which Canada is a major party, are currently applicable. Canadian standards, however, commonly follow those of the US, as explained by William Engdahl in his May 2018 article entitled *Austria's New Coalition Betrays on CETA Trade Agreement*,

"The Canadian government has largely followed US loose corporate regulations in recent years..."

CETA therefore could be devastating for European countries because the less restrictive Canadian standards will be imposed on them. One of the potentially devastating impacts for European countries relates to agriculture, as William Engdahl explains in his article with reference to a joint study by the Institute for Agriculture and Trade Policy and Greenpeace-Holland that is quoted to state,

"Canada has weaker food safety and labelling standards than the EU, and industrial agriculture more heavily dependent on pesticides and GMO crops."

The full implementation of the provisions of CETA therefore has the potential to override existing GMO bans and undermine organic agriculture in EU countries.

The consequences of corporate influence over the drafting of trade treaties and agreements, such as TTIP and CETA, are not restricted to the effects on agriculture, they also have the potential to extract huge sums of money from governments, and therefore from taxpayers; Colin Todhunter explains,

"The consequences include proposals for excessive investor rights, which mean corporations could sue governments for implementing regulations that affect profits, potentially leading to multibillion euro taxpayer payouts in compensation."

Through a system called ISDS (Investor-state dispute settlement), the proposals within trade agreements, such as CETA, permit an 'investor' to bring a case before an arbitration tribunal, if they consider that their investment has been adversely affected by decisions made by the government of a country in which they have invested. The ISDS system is being replaced in the EU by a system referred to as ICS (Investment Court System), which is claimed to offer better protection for investors. Currently, the ICS only applies to bilateral agreements between the EU and other countries; however, it is proposed that ICS should be extended to apply to all agreements and become a 'multilateral institution'; in other words, it is intended to be applicable globally to all trade agreements. This system is likely to make governments reluctant to enact legislation that may potentially be interpreted by an investor as posing a threat to their investment in that country. The implications of such a system are immense!

The WTO Trade Facilitation Agreement (TFA), which came into force in February 2017, promotes 'free trade' and claims to 'reduce trade costs' in order to 'boost global trade'. According to the web page entitled *Trade facilitation*,

"Bureaucratic delays and 'red tape' pose a burden for moving goods across borders for traders."

This trade agreement is discussed in more detail by James Corbett in his article entitled *The Globalist Trade Agreement You Didn't Hear About*, in which he explains that,

"Under cover of 'development' and 'trade' ... this agreement in fact does little but penalize the poorest countries by forcing them to adopt standards and practices that are as expensive and difficult to implement as they are useless to local industries, farmers and laborers."

The TFA is yet another effort to enforce the 'harmonisation' of all processes connected to 'trade'; which means that, as James Corbett states, all countries are forced to,

"...adopt the same standards and regulations on imports and exports."

The justification for the harmonisation of all rules, standards, regulations and processes related to all systems is articulated in the UNDP Annual Report for 2007 entitled *Making Globalization Work for All*, which refers to the need for all UN organisations to 'deliver as one'. The report unsurprisingly claims that development is a key aspect of 'moving forward', but because nations are not all developing at the same pace, there remain many inequalities, about which the report states,

"Addressing these inequalities is our era's most important development challenge, and underscores why inclusive development is central to the mission of the UN and UNDP."

Development, trade and economic growth are all central to the globalisation agenda, but the idea of continual economic growth is highly problematic, as Colin Todhunter explains in his *Corporate Parasites* article,

"The model of 'development' based on endless GDP growth being sold to the world via the neoliberal globalisation agenda is a cynical unattainable con-trick..."

GDP (gross domestic product) is an economic measure calculated by reference to the value of goods and services produced. As previously discussed, the World Bank assesses the income status of each country by reference to its GNI, an economic measure that is calculated from the combination of GDP and certain other income factors.

The existence within a country of economic activities, such as the production of goods, forms the basis of the idea that these activities can be consolidated into a distinct entity that can be referred to as a 'national economy'. This concept has been extrapolated to apply to the consolidation of all economic activities of all nations around the globe into a distinct entity that is referred to as the 'global economy'. Although certain activities, such as exports for example, can be consolidated and measured, the concept of a 'global economy' is highly problematic, not only because it is a concept that has been contrived solely for the purposes of supporting globalisation, but also because it facilitates the notion that this entity called the 'global economy' can be, and even ought to be managed.

There are many competing economic theories, but it is beyond the intended scope of this discussion to examine any of them. The purpose of this discussion is to highlight the fundamental problem common to most, if not all of them, which is the belief in the existence of a distinct entity that can be identified as a 'global economy'. The reason that this belief is problematic is because its acceptance permits the 'global economy' to be under the full control of institutions that claim to provide 'sound economic governance', but instead implement policies that serve the 'vested interests' that have long held the goal to control the world's financial system. In other words, through their control of the policies of international institutions, 'vested interests' seek to consolidate their control over what is referred to as the 'global economy'; a situation that facilitates their control over all of the financial and monetary aspects of life for everyone, everywhere.

The mistaken notion that there is an entity that can be identified as a 'global economy', or even a 'national economy', is discussed by economist Friedrich Hayek in the second of his 3-volume work entitled *Law, Legislation and Liberty*. In that second volume, entitled *The Mirage of Social Justice*, he describes an 'economy' and states that,

> "An economy, in the strict sense of the word…consists of a complex of activities by which a given set of means is allocated in accordance with a unitary plan among the competing ends according to their relative importance."

People are different and therefore have different priorities; this means that people will invariably allocate resources in different ways according to their relative importance to them as individuals; Friedrich Hayek further explains the highly complex nature of an 'economy' and states that,

> "What is commonly called a social or national economy is in this sense not a single economy but a network of many interlaced economies."

The simplification of the complex network of activities that operate within any country into a single entity that can be easily expressed by an economic theory, and therefore managed, is fraught with many problems; it is virtually an impossible task. Although this is part of the reason for the failure of most economic policies, another and more pertinent part of the reason is because most 'national economies' are managed for the benefit of certain 'vested interests', which are usually the 'global economic and financial interests' that control the monetary systems.

Nevertheless, international organisations continue to promote a belief in the existence of 'the global economy'; as indicated by the previously cited 2007 UNDP Annual Report, which, under the heading *Inclusive Globalization* states that,

> "The global economy has been especially strong in recent years, with average worldwide per capita income growing as rapidly as ever before."

Statistics about 'averages' are highly misleading as they fail to disclose the situation at each end of the range, thereby avoiding exposure of extreme wealth as well as extreme poverty. Furthermore, the UNDP statement that the economy was strong is rather surprising considering that the 'global economy' in 2007 was in the early stages of a financial crisis that has been described as the worst since the depression of the 1930s.

Harmonisation is also to be applied to regulations and regulatory systems, including those that govern foods, chemicals management, product safety and the environment, to name just a few examples. However, in common with all other organisations, regulatory agencies are not immune to the influence of 'vested interests'; as indicated by Dr Peter Breggin, who explains in *Toxic Psychiatry* that,

> "Regulatory agencies are notorious for coming under the control of the industries they regulate because the giant corporations have the power and money with which to buy influence and to obtain favours from government bureaucrats and politicians."

At the time that Dr Barry Commoner wrote *Making Peace With the Planet*, environmental organisations were seriously concerned about environmental pollution caused by industrial activities; as indicated by his statement that,

> "The battle lines are predictable: the environmental organizations call for stricter standards, the corporate lobbyists for weaker ones, with the EPA reflecting whatever position seems politically expedient at the moment."

The 'politically expedient' position taken by the EPA, and virtually all other regulatory agencies, has been one that favours corporate 'vested interests' for reasons that ought to be increasingly obvious. However, a matter of great concern is the fact that most environmental organisations have been taken over by factions that promote 'climate change' as the major environmental challenge, and deflect attention away from environmental pollution due to industrial activities; the reasons for this are less obvious, but mainly owe their origins to the influence of other 'vested interests', as explained later in this chapter.

Although not the only industry responsible for environmental degradation, the chemical industry does bear a significant proportion of the blame for the problem; however, public attention has been diverted away from the health hazards of chemicals through the promotion of the idea that chemicals are essential for life; as explained by Sheldon Rampton and John Stauber, in *Trust Us, We're Experts*,

> "As evidence began to mount in the 1970s about the harmful effects of chemicals such as DDT, PCBs, vinyl chloride and benzene, companies – including Mobil Oil, Monsanto and Union Carbide – launched multiple massive advertising and public relations campaigns, using slogans like Monsanto's 'without chemicals, life itself would be impossible'."

Public relations campaigns are tools commonly used for the purposes of manipulating public perception about a variety of issues; as also discussed later in this chapter.

The EPA mainly functions within the US; but, in common with other US agencies, it also intervenes in other countries. The reference to EPA's programmes on the web page entitled *Where EPA Works Around the World* was cited in chapter six, but deserves repetition; it states that these programmes,

"...allow other countries – especially developing countries and countries with economies in transition – to benefit from US experience in developing appropriate and effective environmental programs."

This work would seem to duplicate that of UNEP, the UN's 'global environmental authority'; which yet again, raises the question of why two agencies are necessary for the work of protecting the global environment. However, despite claims to the contrary, the EPA's environmental programme is not 'effective', as it permits industrial activities that are highly detrimental to the environment. One example is hydraulic fracturing, which is proven to be environmentally destructive, but continues to be conducted throughout the US. It would seem therefore, that the EPA prefers to protect US corporate interests rather than the US environment.

It is commonly believed that 'developed' countries, especially the US, maintain strict regulatory systems; which is cited as a key reason that industries choose to relocate their manufacturing facilities to 'developing' countries; but this is not the case. As previously stated, the US does not operate the most restrictive standards; the main reason for relocating manufacturing facilities is to take advantage of the lower costs of production that can usually be achieved in 'developing' countries.

A further problem with US environmental regulations is explained by Barry Commoner in *Making Peace With the Planet*, in which he states that,

"There is a basic flaw embedded in the US environmental laws: they activate the regulatory system only after a pollutant has contaminated the environment – when it is too late."

The inability of the laws to prevent the release of hazardous materials into the environment means that any adverse effects they produce can only be identified by epidemiological studies after the event. Epidemiology is defined by the establishment as,

"the study of the distribution of diseases and determinants of disease in populations."

Although epidemiological studies are clearly based on the 'official', but flawed, theories of disease causation, they were nevertheless able to discover the association between smoking and lung cancer. But epidemiology is not immune to the influence of 'vested interests', especially those of the industry responsible for an environmental hazard; as Dr Devra Davis explains in *The Secret History of the War on Cancer*,

"The foundations of epidemiology as a science can't easily be separated from the industrial forces that decided what information got released and what questions were asked and answered."

The influence of 'industrial forces' over the information provided by epidemiological studies is unsurprising considering the extent of the hazards caused by their activities, as Dr Davis also states,

"The result is that what began as an earnest effort to understand the dangers of the real world has often turned into a way of covering them up."

No matter how thorough epidemiological studies may be, they are virtually incapable of detecting the health effects of a single substance amidst the innumerable combinations of substances that now permeate the environment.

Existing environmental regulations permit pollutants to be released into the environment if exposure levels are maintained below the level deemed to be 'safe'; but, as discussed, the underlying theory on which these regulations are based is fundamentally flawed. Nevertheless, human health and the environment are claimed to be protected by regulatory measures that claim exposures to toxic substances are not harmful if they do not exceed the appropriate threshold. Joe Thornton explains the problem with the idea of 'safe thresholds' in *Pandora's Poison*, in which he states that,

> "...thresholds provide the intellectual justification for a system of environmental decision making that benefits toxicologists as a professional group and the industries that support much of their research."

The 'vested interests' that benefit from the denial of environmental hazards from industrial activities clearly include the leaders and owners of the industries responsible; but they also include the scientists whose careers and salaries depend on their ability to determine the 'safe' level of any substance or influence that may be hazardous to health, whether chemical or electromagnetic in nature.

It is clear that 'globalisation' serves a variety of 'vested interest' groups that have seized control over many of the systems that govern most aspects of life, including health, as discussed in the next sections.

Control of the Medical System

The core aim of the WHO, as stated on the website, is to achieve,

> "Better health for everyone, everywhere."

In common with all other issues that confront humanity in the 21st century, ill-health is claimed to be a 'global problem' that requires 'global action' to implement 'global solutions'. But problems can only be resolved if they are fully understood and their causes correctly identified so that the appropriate solutions can be implemented.

To assist with the identification of the various conditions of ill-health, known as 'diseases', the WHO has continued to produce updated versions of the ICD, which, as previously cited in chapter seven, is referred to as,

> "...the diagnostic classification standard for all clinical and research purposes."

The currently applicable version of this standard is ICD-10, which, according to the WHO web page entitled *Classification of Diseases*,

> "...is cited in more than 20,000 scientific articles and used by more than 100 countries around the world."

This standard is clearly intended to be the definitive 'global' reference guide for the identification of all diseases by all agencies and personnel involved in the 'medical system', referred to in this book as the 'medical establishment'.

Within the ICD classification system, each 'disease' is allocated a unique 3-character code; for example, rabies is identified by the code A82.

However, some conditions have multiple sets of codes; for example, 'HIV disease' is allocated 5 sets of codes, namely B20 to B24. In addition, subsets of codes are used to identify variations of the disease; for example, B20.0 refers to 'HIV disease resulting in mycobacterial infection'. Therefore, although there are many thousands of different codes, there is not an equal number of unique diseases. But, whatever the number of diseases that are claimed to exist, they are all categorised as either communicable, if caused by 'germs', or noncommunicable, if caused by factors other than 'germs', and they are each treated by a 'medicine' deemed to be the appropriate remedy.

It is entirely reasonable to suggest therefore, that, if the medical establishment had correctly identified the causes of all forms of disease and was treating each one with the appropriate 'medicine', the incidence of 'disease' would be in rapid decline, and people everywhere would experience improving health; but this is not the case. On the contrary, the incidence of 'disease' is rapidly rising, and the majority of people everywhere experience worsening health.

The logical conclusion to be drawn from this is that the causes of diseases have not been correctly identified; this conclusion is supported by the discussions in chapter seven that revealed the medical establishment's poor level of knowledge about the causes of noncommunicable diseases. This logical conclusion is also supported by the discussions in chapter three that revealed the erroneous nature of the theories that claim 'germs' to be the causes of communicable diseases.

The failure of the medical establishment to correctly identify the real causes of disease means that the methods used to treat and prevent them, namely medicines and vaccines, are inappropriate 'solutions' to the problem. But this raises the question of why 'medical science' does not acknowledge the full extent of the problem, and instigate a complete re-evaluation of the prevailing theories about diseases and their causes. It should be clear from the discussions in this chapter, however, that these theories are retained almost entirely due to the influence of 'vested interests'.

As previous chapters have discussed, there are many reports and articles that have documented the serious adverse health effects, referred to as 'side effects', that can be produced by a wide variety of pharmaceuticals. One article, entitled *The Epidemic of Sickness and Death from Prescription Drugs*, which was cited in chapter eight, highlights one of the problems, which is that,

> "Many people, even doctors, assume that if the FDA approves a new drug, it must be safe, effective, and better; but this is far from actual practice."

The reason that 'even doctors' are guilty of this mistaken assumption is due to their medical education, as discussed in the next section.

The CDER (Center for Drug Evaluation and Research) is the division of the FDA that, as its name indicates, evaluates drugs as part of the approval process. The FDA web page entitled *Development & Approval Process (Drugs)* states that an evaluation by CDER 'prevents quackery', which is clearly intended to suggest that only FDA-approved drugs are suitable 'medicines'; but this is misleading. The FDA does not conduct tests to confirm the safety and efficacy of any drug prior to its approval; instead, pharmaceutical companies are required to perform their own studies of a drug's 'safety and efficacy' and send the study data to the CDER for evaluation and review. The FDA page states that,

"If this independent and unbiased review establishes that a drug's health benefits outweigh its known risks, the drug is approved for sale."

It is a contradiction in terms to suggest that a substance can simultaneously confer health benefits and pose health risks.

It is clear that 'FDA approval' does not mean that a pharmaceutical drug has been proven to be either safe or effective. This can be demonstrated by the many reports about drugs that had received FDA approval, but were subsequently withdrawn from use when found to cause serious adverse health effects, and even death; the example of Vioxx was referred to in chapter seven.

The idea that drugs are appropriate for the treatment of disease, even though it is contradicted by the admission that they simultaneously pose risks to health, is perpetuated largely by the pharmaceutical industry that has a clear 'vested interest' in the continuing existence of a medical system that relies on its products. This problem is discussed in a June 2013 article entitled *Institutional Corruption of Pharmaceuticals and the Myth of Safe and Effective Drugs* that refers to 'heavy commercial influence' in the US. However, the pharmaceutical industry has gained a substantial level of influence that extends beyond the US and into many aspects of the entire medical system; the article states that,

"The pharmaceutical industry has corrupted the practice of medicine through its influence over what drugs are developed, how they are tested, and how medical knowledge is created."

This last point is extremely important; the medical establishment will not be able to reach a true understanding about 'disease' or about human health whilst it remains under the influence of the pharmaceutical industry, although the industry is not the only 'vested interest' group that has corrupted 'healthcare' and gained a significant level of control over the creation of 'medical knowledge'.

There are some differences between the drug approval procedures that operate in different countries, but these remaining differences will be eradicated should 'globalisation' and its accompanying 'harmonisation' be fully implemented. It should be noted that the harmonisation of drug approval procedures is already in progress. The organisation responsible for accomplishing this is ICH (International Council for Harmonisation of Technical Requirements for Pharmaceuticals for Human Use), which was founded in 1990. The home page of the ICH website states that,

"ICH's mission is to achieve greater harmonisation worldwide to ensure that safe, effective and high quality medicines are developed..."

The ICH is another international organisation that fully supports the belief that pharmaceuticals are safe and effective, but fails to acknowledge the seriousness of the 'risks'. This bias is almost entirely due to the involvement of the pharmaceutical industry in the harmonisation process; the ICH web page entitled *Harmonisation for Better Health* states that,

"Harmonisation is achieved through the development of ICH Guidelines via a process of scientific consensus with regulatory and industry experts working side-by-side."

The phrase 'scientific consensus' is an oxymoron; as has been discussed, consensus stifles science, which is of particular concern with respect to health matters, because consensus will ensure the retention of the prevailing theories about disease, virtually all of which are fundamentally flawed.

The ICH is supportive of both the medical establishment system and the pharmaceutical industry; this can be demonstrated by the organisations involved in ICH, which is funded through annual membership fees. One ICH member is PhRMA, which is the representative body of America's leading pharmaceutical and biotechnology companies. Another ICH member is BIO (Biotechnology Innovation Organization); the *About BIO* web page states that,

"BIO is the world's largest trade organization representing biotechnology companies, academic institutions, state biotechnology centers and related organizations across the United States and in more than 30 other nations."

Although PhRMA and BIO mainly represent pharmaceutical companies, especially US companies, it is interesting to note that BIO also represents academic institutions, which constitute another group with a 'vested interest' in the prevailing medical system; an interest that arises mainly from the financial rewards that can be gained through medical research funding, as discussed later in this chapter.

The provision of funds, as previously discussed, almost invariably enables the provider to exert influence over the activities of the recipient. The organisations within the UN system are mainly funded by the contributions of Member States that are assessed according to each country's GNI. As the country with the largest GNI, the US contributes the most to UN agencies, a position that the US has exploited. A January 2006 article entitled *The World Health Organization and the Transition From 'International' to 'Global' Public Health* explains that, in 1985, the US took a decision to,

"...withhold its contribution to WHO's regular budget, in part as a protest against WHO's 'Essential Drug Program' which was opposed by leading US-based pharmaceutical companies."

This 'programme' is now the Essential Medicines List (EML), which, according to the web page entitled *WHO Model List of Essential Medicines*,

"...serves as a guide for the development of national and institutional essential medicine lists..."

The inclusion of their products in the 433 drugs listed on the 2017 EML, and referred to by the WHO as 'essential', is of immense benefit for the drug companies that produce them; sales of these products will inevitably boost the companies' revenues and profits. However, pharmaceutical companies are not the only 'vested interests' that benefit from the perpetuation of the prevailing 'medical system'.

The general meaning of the term 'vested interest' refers to someone with a personal interest in the outcome of an event. In the context of the medical system, every person employed within that system has a vested interest in its perpetuation, and will therefore be extremely reluctant to acknowledge the existence of any flaws. Their reluctance can be a direct result of their dependence on the 'medical system' for their careers and salaries; this loyalty can be illustrated by a saying attributed to Upton Sinclair that,

> "It is difficult to get a man to understand something when his salary depends on his not understanding it."

The protection of careers and salaries can, to a certain extent, explain why the majority of scientists accept the 'consensus' view in their field of science and fail to challenge it; as Professor Duesberg indicates in *Inventing the AIDS Virus*,

> "Few scientists are any longer willing to question, even privately, the consensus views held in any field whatsoever."

This is an extremely worrying situation, as it will prevent any progress in the field of true 'healthcare'.

Although every person who works in the medical system has an obvious 'vested interest' in its continuing existence, and would be affected by its demise, the vast majority of these people only have a very limited 'interest', which does not permit them any real influence over its activities, nor does it permit them to initiate substantive changes. The real 'vested interests' are clearly those who do have the ability to influence the activities of, and instigate changes to the 'medical system'; but they do so purely to serve their own interests. They also benefit from 'globalisation' that facilitates the concentration of power into a single entity or a coordinated central group.

Not only is the WHO the 'governing body' of the medical establishment, it is also the 'coordinating body'; a position that requires collaboration with a variety of organisations; as the WHO web page entitled *Collaborations and partnerships* states,

> "One of our core functions is to direct and coordinate international health work by promoting collaboration, mobilizing partnerships and galvanizing efforts of different health actors to respond to national and global health challenges."

One of these 'health actors' is the CDC, the US health agency that also operates beyond the US borders; the CDC page entitled *Global Health* states that,

> "CDC helps other countries increase their ability to prevent, detect and respond to health threats..."

This statement would seem to indicate that the CDC is another US organisation whose work overlaps that of a UN organisation, in this instance the WHO. The CDC justifies its interventions into other countries on the basis that 'health threats' elsewhere in the world pose risks to the health of Americans. Although this is a mistaken notion, the CDC page asserts that,

> "The US cannot protect its borders and the health of its citizens without addressing diseases elsewhere in the world."

The CDC claims that serious threats to 'global health' are mainly posed by 'infectious diseases' that are able to spread rapidly throughout the world. The 1918 Flu and Black Death are often cited as examples of the devastation such 'epidemics' can cause, and used to create fear in the minds of the public. This fear is also used to justify continual surveillance around the world to detect any new and potentially dangerous 'outbreaks'. On the basis of the claim that an 'infectious disease' outbreak threatens 'global health', the CDC collaborates with various organisations in the promotion of 'global health security', which is discussed on a series of CDC web pages entitled *Global Health Security Agenda*, one of which states that,

> "In partnership with US government sister agencies, other nations, international organizations, and public and private stakeholders, CDC seeks to accelerate progress towards a world safe and secure from infectious disease threats and to promote global health security as an international security priority..."

One of the core aims of the 2030 Agenda is to ensure that everyone, everywhere has access to 'life-saving' vaccines. Another 'plan' with the same goal is called the Global Vaccine Agenda Plan (GVAP), which, according to the WHO web page entitled *Global Vaccine Action Plan 2011-2020*,

> "...is a framework to prevent millions of deaths by 2020 through more equitable access to existing vaccines for people in all communities."

Previous discussions have demonstrated that vaccines confer no 'benefits', but have been proven to cause serious harm to health, and even death; they certainly do not save lives. Unsurprisingly, the CDC is also involved with GVAP through GID (Global Immunization Division), which is part of the CDC and,

> "...works closely with a wide variety of partners to protect global citizens against contagious and life-threatening vaccine-preventable disease..."

The CDC certainly serves the interests of the vaccine industry.

The term 'global citizen' is, however, disingenuous; its use is an insidious attempt to foster the notion that everyone has a duty to be vaccinated to achieve 'herd immunity', which can protect the whole world population. The erroneous nature of the concept of 'herd immunity', as well as the flawed nature of the claims that any disease can be prevented by vaccines, have been discussed.

The promotion of 'global health threats' does however, permit 'non-health actors' to also be involved in matters pertaining to 'global health'; one of these 'actors' is USAID, whose work in this area is explained on the USAID web page entitled *Promoting Global Health*, which makes a similar claim to the CDC and states,

> "Epidemics don't adhere to international borders."

The intervention of USAID into other countries is justified on the basis of the claim that epidemics are,

> "...invisible threats to our national security."

The purpose of USAID is, however, to promote 'US foreign policy interests'; this agency has been involved in many interventions in other countries with different motives than that of protecting the health of American citizens. The retention of a belief in the 'germ theory' serves purposes that are entirely unrelated to human health, but instead, seem to be more closely related to matters of 'national security'.

The WHO also promotes 'global health' on the basis that diseases pose threats to 'health security', as discussed on the web page entitled *Health security*, which states that,

"...universal health coverage and health security are two sides of the same coin: improved access to health care and strengthened health systems provide a strong defense against emerging health threats, whether natural or man-made."

The WHO explains the meaning of the term 'health security' and states,

"Global public health security is defined as the activities required to minimize the danger and impact of acute public health events that endanger the collective health of populations living across geographical regions and international boundaries."

The concept of 'collective health' is misleading. A person's health is not dependent on the health of others, although it is dependent upon certain factors, including external ones; it is only in this context that the term 'collective health' can be used. The Bhopal tragedy in 1984 is an example of an event that affected, and still affects, the 'collective health' of the local community, as discussed in chapter eight. But this is not the context in which the WHO refers to 'collective health'; instead, the WHO uses the term in reference to the idea that 'infectious diseases' can be transmitted throughout communities and across international boundaries; this idea is erroneous.

The WHO claims that addressing problems related to 'health security' necessitates the implementation of the appropriate 'regulations', namely the IHR, the purpose of which is explained on the web page entitled *International Health Regulations (IHR)* that states,

"Their aim is to help the international community prevent and respond to acute public health risks that have the potential to cross borders and threaten people worldwide."

The claimed interconnection between UHC and 'health security' is used to drive the agenda to achieve both UHC and increased access to 'medicines and vaccines for all'. These core aims of SDG 3.8 have also been incorporated into a 2017 WHO report entitled *Towards Access 2030*, the purpose of which is,

"...to focus and reinforce WHO's ability to help Member States achieve universal access to safe and quality-assured health products and universal health coverage."

The WHO would therefore seem to be oblivious to the overwhelming body of evidence that demonstrates pharmaceutical medicines and vaccines are not 'safe', but are, in reality, responsible for causing a wide variety of adverse health effects, including death. Nevertheless, the report refers to the MDGs, which were in operation between 2000 and 2015, and states that, during this period, the WHO,

"Strengthened pharmaceutical systems in low- and middle-income Member States."

These 'strengthened pharmaceutical systems' have inevitably increased the incidence of ill-health caused by, but rarely attributed to, pharmaceuticals. Instead, these iatrogenic illnesses would have been attributed to the various 'diseases' that are claimed to disproportionately affect the populations of 'developing' countries.

Disturbingly, however, the *Towards Access* report asserts that the WHO needs to 'scale up' efforts to further strengthen pharmaceutical systems during the period that the SDGs are in operation. This can only result in an even greater incidence of iatrogenic ill-health that will predominantly affect the people who already suffer from poor health, but will be mistakenly attributed to 'diseases', for which people will be treated with even more pharmaceuticals. The worsening of human health will encourage further demands for better access to 'medicines and vaccines', and produce an ever-worsening vicious cycle of iatrogenic ill-health and pharmaceutical use that will almost certainly lead to greatly increased mortality.

Nevertheless, the efforts to implement UHC by 2030 persist and have been supported by a newly-formed organisation aptly named UHC2030, which is referred to as a 'global movement' whose purpose is described on the web page entitled *Our Mission*, which states that,

> "UHC2030's mission is to create a movement for accelerating equitable and sustainable progress towards universal health coverage (UHC)."

The web page also provides an explanation about UHC that states,

> "UHC is based on the principle that all individuals and communities should have access to quality essential health services without suffering financial hardships."

The implication of this mission statement is that Big Pharma is greedy, and their prices are too high for the 'poor people' in 'developing' countries who are most in need of affordable 'medicines and vaccines'. It is undeniable that pharmaceutical companies charge high prices to generate large profits for distribution to their shareholders, but even if pharmaceuticals were easily affordable, or even free, they would not confer health benefits; on the contrary, they are inimical to health.

Other groups with which the WHO collaborates are 'non-State actors' that are described on the page entitled *WHO's engagement with non-State actors* that states,

> "WHO engages with non-State actors in view of their significant role in global health for the advancement and promotion of public health and to encourage non-State actors to use their own activities to protect and promote public health."

In addition to NGOs and philanthropic foundations, the term 'non-State actor' also refers to academic institutions. The scientists who conduct research in these institutions are believed to be entirely objective and therefore immune to influence; but this is not necessarily the case. Most research, especially if it is laboratory-based, requires a significant level of funding. Scientists' careers are therefore dependent on their ability to obtain the necessary funds; but this too can depend on whether the scientist accepts or challenges the 'consensus' view that prevails in their field. Paul Craig Roberts states, in his previously cited article entitled *The Oceans Are Dying*, that,

"Corporate and government money has purchased many scientists along with the media and politicians."

The idea that scientists can be 'bought' may seem controversial, but as Sheldon Rampton and John Stauber point out in *Trust Us, We're Experts*, 'scientists' are human and therefore,

"...are not immune from political ideologies or the lure of money."

It is clear therefore that most scientists will conduct research that conforms to the 'consensus' view and facilitates the continuation of their career; but this does not necessarily facilitate scientific progress.

Although a number of 'non-State actors' are discussed later in this chapter, one foundation was particularly influential in the development of the American medical system in the 20th century; as discussed in the previously cited *Global Role* article that states,

"In the first few decades following the creation of the United Nations (UN) and the WHO, there were few major international players with the political and/or financial clout to influence global agendas."

The article identifies the Rockefeller Foundation as one of those 'players' with significant financial 'clout' that, together with the WHO, UNICEF and the World Bank, have,

"...heavily influenced global health priorities for research, policy and investment."

It is important to reiterate that most pharmaceutical products are manufactured from petroleum-derived chemicals. It is similarly important to note that the Rockefeller family played key roles in the development of the oil industry in the US; the wealth generated by the Rockefeller-owned Standard Oil company enabled the family to virtually control the oil industry. The Rockefellers therefore, clearly had a 'vested interest' in the development of a 'medical system' that utilised their products. As discussed in the next two sections, the Rockefellers were not only instrumental in the development of the American medical system, they were also involved in 'medical research', some of which had little to do with facilitating improved health. The use of petroleum as 'medicine' arose from the belief that it had curative properties, although it is now widely recognised to be harmful to health, as indicated by an article entitled *A Look Into the Petrochemical Industry*, which states that petroleum-derived chemicals can be,

"...hazardous and toxic to the health of living beings and the earth's ecosystems."

The article contains an admission that can only be described as astounding in view of the long period during which petrochemical-derived compounds have been used as ingredients of 'medicines'; it states that,

"We are still in the early days of understanding the adverse effects of petrochemicals on our health and environment."

The article is surprisingly honest in its admission of the harm that petrochemicals can cause and further states that,

"...they can accumulate in human tissues and organs such as the brain and liver and cause brain, nerve and liver damage, birth defects, cancer, asthma, hormonal disorders and allergies."

The reason that petrochemicals remain the major ingredients of 'medicines' is due to the erroneous belief that a harmful substance can be beneficial if used in the 'correct dose'; the retention of this belief is clearly of benefit to the 'vested interests' of the oil industry.

As previously discussed, safety tests determine the dose at which there is 'no observable adverse effect'; but this is not the same as 'no effect'. Furthermore, no tests are conducted to determine the adverse effects that arise from the myriad combinations of pharmaceuticals and chemical substances to which people are exposed on a daily basis. The denial of the harm to human health caused by all of these substances clearly benefits all of the relevant industries that utilise, produce and discharge these toxic substances.

It is clear that there is a vast network of organisations that continue to promote the message that everyone, everywhere needs better access to affordable medicines and vaccines that are claimed to save lives. The majority of the people who work within these organisations do so with the best of motives; in other words, they genuinely wish to help people. The problem is that the people who are not medically trained rely on the 'expertise' of those who are; but this does not prevent the promulgation of incorrect information about the nature of 'disease' and flawed theories about their causes, especially those that relate to 'germs'. The reason that flawed information remains at the heart of the 'medical system' is due to the nature of 'medical education', which also operates under the influence of 'vested interests'.

Medical Education

Education is the process of imparting knowledge, although it is equally useful for the dissemination of false information, as Herbert Shelton indicates in *Natural Hygiene: Man's Pristine Way of Life*,

"No man is so confirmed in falsehood as he who has been educated into it..."

Although medical school curricula vary, they inevitably include courses that teach medical students that 'medicines' are appropriate treatments for disease; as described by Dr Russell Blaylock in *Health and Nutrition Secrets*,

"Doctors' entire educations have been based on a belief in pharmaceutical agents to treat disease..."

In courses referred to as microbiology, pathology, pharmacology and immunology, medical students learn about 'germs', diseases, medicines and vaccines. They are also taught that the knowledge they acquire at medical school represents scientific 'truth' and that any other 'knowledge' is to be disparaged; although previously cited, the words of Dr Carolyn Dean yet again, bear repetition,

"In fact, we were told many times that if we didn't learn it in medical school it must be quackery."

The term 'quack' is used to describe a person who claims to have medical knowledge, but does not have the appropriate medical qualification and is therefore not allowed to practise 'medicine'. The term is also used to describe substances that are used as remedies for illness but have not been 'approved' by the appropriate regulatory body. The purpose of this derogatory terminology is to reinforce the ideas that only those people who have received the appropriate 'medical education' have the knowledge to practise 'medicine', and that only those substances that have been approved are suitable 'medicines' for the treatment of 'disease'. However, as the discussions in this book demonstrate, 'approved' is not synonymous with effective.

An approved medicine is a compound that is claimed to have benefits that outweigh its 'known risks'. These 'risks' manifest as adverse health effects, the importance of which is minimised by reference to them as merely 'side effects'; but this label is misleading; all effects are the direct result of the 'medicine'. The main reason that pharmaceuticals cause adverse health effects is because their ingredients include petroleum-derived chemicals, which are acknowledged to be hazardous to human health.

Another problem is that 'modern medicine' focuses on treating the disease, not the patient. This approach is based on a fundamentally flawed understanding about both the nature of 'disease' and the human body; it does however, provide the most compelling explanation for the otherwise inexplicable circumstances in which people with the same 'disease' respond very differently to exactly the same 'treatment'; this is discussed further in chapter ten.

The reason that petrochemicals are used in 'medicines' is, at least partly, based on a long-held belief that 'crude oil', like many other toxic substances, had curative properties. In her two-volume work entitled *The History of Standard Oil*, Ida Tarbell relates that during the 19th century, 'crude oil', also known as 'rock oil', was sold in America as a patent medicine and claimed to be a 'cure-all'; she states that,

> "While it was admitted to be chiefly a liniment it was recommended for cholera morbus, liver complaint, bronchitis and consumption..."

Although petroleum has become far more important as a source of fuel, it remains a key ingredient of 'medicines', as indicated by a September 2011 article entitled *Petroleum and Health Care* that states,

> "...nearly 99% of pharmaceutical feedstock and reagents are derived from petrochemicals..."

Oil had been utilised with little, if any, refining throughout many regions of the world over the course of many centuries, if not millennia. The modern 'oil industry' is, however, a very different phenomenon; its origins in the late 19th century can be almost entirely attributed to the development of technologies that facilitated the extraction of oil in ever-greater quantities from ever-greater depths underground. Progress in the field of chemistry enabled 'crude oil' to be refined and transformed into petroleum, from which useful substances such as petrochemicals were derived. Although oil wells existed in other parts of the world, they had not been drilled and were therefore not deep wells. The drilling technologies developed and used in the US facilitated the rapid growth of the American oil industry to the extent that, in the early 20th century, the US was the largest oil producer in the world; the largest American oil company at the time was the Rockefeller-owned Standard Oil company.

The use of their product as medicine was a practice that certain 'vested interests' within the oil industry were naturally keen to encourage; it is understandable that they would therefore seek ways to ensure that 'medicines' would remain dependent on petroleum. The most effective way, and the one that was implemented, would involve the development of a 'medical system' that only promoted the use of petrochemical-based medicines, in conjunction with a system of 'medical education' that ensured its perpetuation. It should not be surprising therefore, to find that some of the people who were instrumental in the development of the American medical and 'medical education' systems in the early 20th century held 'vested interests' in the American oil industry.

The laboratory-based investigation of diseases and their causes had developed rapidly during the 19th century in European countries, especially Germany. This 'scientific approach' was greatly admired by American physicians, many of whom were inspired to visit Germany for a course of study at a German university that taught this method. On their return to the US, most of these physicians incorporated the information they had gained into their own practices. Others, however, were inspired to develop systems of 'medical education' and 'medical schools' similar to those in Germany. In his book entitled *Rockefeller Medicine Men*, E Richard Brown refers to the example of Johns Hopkins medical school, which was,

> "...modeled after the German university medical schools with a heavy emphasis on research in the basic medical sciences."

He reports that Johns Hopkins was the first medical school to have a laboratory science faculty with full-time teachers and researchers. The growing interest in 'scientific medicine' was to inspire the demand for major changes to the practice of medicine in the US, as he further explains,

> "...the medical profession adopted an effective strategy of reform based on scientific medicine and the developing medical sciences. Their plan was to gain control over medical education for the organized profession representing practitioners in alliance with scientific medical faculty. Their measures involved large expenditures for medical education and required a major change in the financing of medical schools."

The demand for change was not universally supported by physicians and this produced a conflict within the different factions; however, as E Richard Brown states,

> "The conflict over who would rule medical education...was fundamentally a question of whose interests the medical care system would serve."

The large expenditures that were required could not be met by physicians; they did not have the necessary funds to fulfil their plans for a system of laboratory-based 'scientific medicine' and therefore, as he continues,

> "The financing of scientific medical schools required tremendous amounts of capital from outside the medical profession."

The wealthy industrialists and financiers who could provide the necessary capital were themselves provided with a unique opportunity; as E Richard Brown indicates,

"Those who provided the capital had the leverage to impose policy."

Through the provision of the required capital, wealthy industrialists, especially the Rockefellers and Carnegies, would gain the most influence over the direction of the American medical system; this began when Abraham Flexner was commissioned to investigate and report on the condition of American medical schools. During his investigations, Abraham Flexner visited Germany and studied the German laboratory-based system of medical education, which he too admired. An article entitled *The Flexner Report – 100 Years Later* states that the German system was,

> "...a system in which physician scientists were trained in laboratory investigation as a prelude and foundation for clinical training and investigation in university hospitals."

It was laboratory-based research that led Dr Robert Koch to claim that the bacterium, *M. tuberculosis* was the causal agent of tuberculosis. However, as has been discussed, people can be 'infected' by the bacterium but not have symptoms of the disease; these exceptions violate his first Postulate and disprove his theory. Although previously cited in chapter three, the words of Dr Peter Duesberg bear repetition,

> "A single exception would be enough to pronounce the microbe innocent of creating that disease."

Unfortunately, despite the existence of far more than a single exception, the microbe known as *M. tuberculosis* has not been pronounced innocent and remains the alleged causative agent of tuberculosis. This theory, although thoroughly disproven by empirical evidence, is retained in the microbiology courses taught to medical students at medical school, as if it were scientific 'knowledge'.

Nevertheless, the findings of the Flexner Report in 1910 were to inspire a complete transformation of the American medical education system; the *Flexner Report* article states that this transformation was to establish,

> "...the biomedical model as the gold standard of medical training."

Yet again, the US is the acclaimed 'leader' in the field of medicine; the article states that the Flexner Report,

> "...resulted in the science-based foundation of medical training that has made the United States the recognized leader in medical education and medical research today."

This claim is however, unsubstantiated by the evidence; in reality, the American 'medical system' fares poorly when compared to those of other 'developed' countries. A 2017 report prepared by the Commonwealth Fund compared the health systems of 11 'developed' countries and placed the US in the last position in respect of 'health care system performance'. Most notably, the US was placed in the bottom position in the category of 'Health Care Outcomes'; a situation that challenges the CDC claim that their work 'saves lives'. Despite the fact that the US spends the largest amount on health care than any other country, the overall poor performance of the US medical system contrasts significantly with the idea that the US is the 'leader' in medical education and medical research.

The 'medical education' systems in all countries that have adopted the

Western 'scientific approach' continue to require substantial levels of funding, much of which is provided by the pharmaceutical industry; but this has become a contentious issue, because it is recognised that providing the funds means that the industry can exert influence over the content of medical school 'knowledge'. This problem is discussed in a May 2010 article entitled *Funding for Medical Education: Maintaining a Healthy Separation from Industry*, which states that,

> "...in the realm of teaching, whether of medical students, house officers, or practitioners, there is a growing concern that educational activities should not be supported or influenced by companies whose profitability and very existence depend on the sales volume of the products they make."

The funding of education by organisations whose core aim is to make profits, generates conflicts of interest and ethical problems, both of which would seem to be largely ignored, as Dr Carolyn Dean explains,

> "An important ethics question that was never addressed in medical school was whether doctors and medical schools should accept drug company funding."

Despite the failure to address ethical issues or conflicts of interest that arise solely as the result of pharmaceutical industry funding of medical education, medical school curricula remain biased in favour of the use of pharmaceuticals as appropriate for the treatment of disease. Medical students are therefore taught to regard pharmaceuticals as 'essential medicines'; this has been amply demonstrated by the creation of an organisation known as UAEM (Universities Allied for Essential Medicines), which, on the UAEM web page entitled *Who We Are*, states that,

> "We are a global network of university students who believe that our universities have an opportunity and a responsibility to improve global access to public health goods."

The motive of these students would appear to be the desire to help poor people, especially in 'developing' countries, to access affordable 'medicines', as indicated by the same web page, which, under the heading *Our Values*, states that,

> "As committed students from all over the world who passionately believe in social justice and health equity, we find it unacceptable that millions of people do not have access to medicines."

Although highly commendable, their passion is, unfortunately totally misplaced, but it is clearly based on the training they have received in medical school, which teaches them that pharmaceuticals are the most, and indeed the only, suitable method by which diseases should be treated. In addition, these students are promoting the 2030 Agenda goals, whether knowingly or otherwise, although the language used on this website strongly indicates the former.

The UAEM is a movement that began in 2001 when, according to the website, students of Yale University joined with Médecins sans Frontières to influence the University and a major pharmaceutical company in order to convince them,

> "...to permit generic production of a critical Yale-discovered HIV/AIDS drug in sub-Saharan Africa..."

The idea that medical students were able to influence a major pharmaceutical company and gain a concession from them is rather extraordinary, the industry is not noted for philanthropy, especially when their profitability is threatened. Yale University, however, had a clear vested interest in the drug it had discovered and would inevitably benefit from its sales. According to the website, the concession also resulted in price reductions for other drugs, which,

"...enabled a major scale-up of HIV treatment throughout the continent."

The fundamental problems with 'HIV' and 'HIV treatments' have been discussed. The belief that it represents a genuine disease continues to be promoted by well-meaning, but misinformed, people, such as the UAEM students. Meanwhile millions of people continue to be harmed on a daily basis by the toxic ARV 'medicines' with which they are treated. Even more heart-breaking is the fact that the genuine health problems with which these people suffer remain almost entirely unrecognised, and largely ignored by the medical establishment.

Medical education does not, however, cease after students have obtained their qualification. All qualified doctors are required to attend courses for CME (continuing medical education), which also inevitably receives a substantial level of funding from pharmaceutical companies; the above cited May 2010 article about medical education funding states that,

"The most direct form of industry-supported education is through funding for continuing medical education (CME) activities."

An August 2014 article entitled *Industry involvement in continuing medical education*, which mainly discusses the situation in Canada, indicates that the problems arising from industry funding are ubiquitous. The ability to fund CME enables the industry to exert influence over the content of courses in a number of ways, as the article states,

"...CME with industry involvement has a narrower range of topics and more drug-related content than CME without direct industry involvement."

The influence of commercial activities that enable financial gains to be made from pharmaceutical products and medical devices pervades the entire medical education system, as the article indicates,

"Faculty members or their institutions, such as medical schools or teaching hospitals, may also hold shares of patents and thereby derive financial benefit from the use of particular drugs, devices or tests."

It should be clear that all of the people who derive a financial benefit from drugs, tests, patents, or any other commercial product, hold a 'vested interest' in the perpetuation of a 'medical system' that utilises the product.

Although the increasingly sophisticated technical equipment used in laboratory experimentation and medical student training is generally equated with 'medical science', this is a mistaken view. Experiments are not necessarily synonymous with 'science'; as Professor Duesberg explains in *Inventing the AIDS Virus*,

"The transition from small to big to mega-science has created an establishment of skilled technicians but mediocre scientists, who have abandoned real scientific interpretation and who even equate their experiments with science itself."

The limitations of 'scientific experimentation' were discussed in chapter three.

Another form of 'further education' available in the US to medically trained people is a CDC programme called EIS (Epidemic Intelligence Service), a 2-year postgraduate training programme. The CDC web page entitled *What EIS Officers Do* refers to them as 'disease detectives' and explains that,

> "EIS officers serve on the front lines of public health, protecting Americans and the global community..."

EIS officers comprise some of the key personnel that travel to the location of a disease 'outbreak', whether in the US or elsewhere in the world. Their function is to carry out the necessary investigation to identify the cause of the disease and to implement the appropriate solutions to contain the problem. The page entitled *Who We Are* claims that more than 3,600 EIS officers have been trained since the programme was established in 1951. It is interesting to note that EIS officers have been appointed to some rather important and influential positions within the 'medical system'; as the page also states,

> "EIS alumni have gone on to become CDC directors; leading CDC scientists; acting surgeons general; WHO assistant directors-general, regional directors and country directors; public health and medical school faculty and deans; city health commissioners; and state epidemiologists."

Even more significantly, EIS officers have been appointed to important and influential positions outside of the 'medical system'; as the page states,

> "Many others take on leadership roles in industry, foundations, nongovernmental organisations and the news media."

These influential positions ensure the perpetuation of the prevailing 'medical system'.

Medical students are also taught about 'mental health' in order to be able to diagnose 'mental disorders', which are claimed to affect increasing numbers of people around the world. Dr Peter Breggin states that conditions diagnosed as 'mental disorders', especially depression, are far more likely to be a manifestation of 'overwhelming emotions' caused by the stresses and strains of life. Unfortunately, students are taught about the appropriate 'medicines' that can be prescribed for such conditions, but, as Dr Breggin explains on the web page entitled *Empathic therapy: psychotherapy, not psychoactive drugs,*

> "Blunting ourselves with drugs is not the answer to overwhelming emotions."

The failure to recognise that emotions are normal human functions and not indicative of a 'mental disorder' has serious consequences; as he further explains,

> "Unfortunately, when health professionals are taught to rely on the prescription of psychoactive drugs, they are in effect instructed how to suppress the emotional lives of their patients and clients."

Interestingly, medical students and practising doctors are also reported to experience 'mental health problems', as indicated by an April 2019 BMA article entitled *Supporting the mental health of doctors and medical students*, which refers to the situation in the UK and states that,

"At any one time, a proportion of the medical workforce is managing a diagnosed mental health condition of their own."

The symptoms reported to be experienced by people in the medical workforce include depression, anxiety, burnout and stress. The problem with categorising these symptoms as 'mental health problems' is discussed further in chapter ten; however, it is worrying that people who are responsible for the health of their patients can be considered to have 'abnormal thoughts, perceptions, emotions and behaviours'.

It is clear that physicians, psychiatrists and medical students have a particularly strong 'vested interest' in the perpetuation of the prevailing 'medical system'. The many years of study required to attain their qualification will ensure that their beliefs in the 'system' in which they were trained are deep-seated. It can therefore be extremely difficult to overcome this belief system and acknowledge the many flaws inherent within 'modern medicine'. Although the difficulties are understandable, they are not insurmountable; as demonstrated by the many qualified physicians quoted in this book who discovered the problems and have spoken or written about them. The most obvious situation that alerts a physician to the existence of problems within the 'medical system' is the failure of their efforts to improve a patient's health, despite the use of the recommended treatments; this is recognised by Dr Derrick Lonsdale MD who states in his book, *Why I Left Orthodox Medicine*, that,

"...it is sometimes difficult for a physician to observe that his treatment is making things worse."

Another serious criticism that can be levelled at the content of 'medical education' is the failure to include an adequate level of training on the topic of 'nutrition'. The almost total omission of any reference to the importance of nutrition is even more surprising considering that the WHO includes 'unhealthy diet' as one of the key risk factors for NCDs, although, as discussed in chapter seven, the WHO defines 'unhealthy diets' mainly in the context of the dietary intake of salt and sugar; this is woefully inadequate.

Nevertheless, the inclusion of 'unhealthy lifestyles' as risk factors for disease, means that doctors are increasingly advised to inform their patients about adopting a 'healthy lifestyle', but few of them have the necessary knowledge, as medical school training is invariably deficient on the topic. This deficiency has been highlighted in a September 2017 article written by two UK medical students and surprisingly, published on the website of the *BMJ*. The article, entitled *Medical schools should be prioritising nutrition and lifestyle education*, refers to claims that European medical schools provide more courses about 'healthy lifestyles' than those in the US, but states that all medical schools are deficient in this regard.

The article claims that the reason for this deficiency is because 'nutrition science' is subordinated in medical school curricula and that,

"Dietary interventions are considered to be outside of the evidence base, unscientifically 'fluffy' and the domain of dieticians rather than doctors."

This is entirely the wrong approach to nutrition, the importance of which cannot be overstated, as discussed in more detail in chapter ten.

The main problems with the 'medical system' arise from the dependence on flawed 'science' and the use of highly technical laboratory equipment. This is exacerbated by beliefs about the nature of diseases and by ideas that their causes can be discovered by the examination of 'diseased' cells, tissues or molecules. These flawed ideas and beliefs are perpetuated through their inclusion in the curricula of 'medical schools'. The dependence upon science in the field of medicine is accompanied by claims that scientists who made important discoveries are to be regarded as the experts in their field and their work is not to be challenged; but, as Professor Krimsky states in *Science in the Private Interest*,

"...we rarely have the luxury of questioning whether the expertise is trustworthy."

The expertise of certain 'scientists', such as Edward Jenner and Louis Pasteur for example, has been shown in previous discussions to be untrustworthy; yet the medical establishment continues to regard them as some of medicine's greatest heroes; these accolades are undeserved. Unfortunately, too few physicians challenge the medical system in which they were trained, even when their experience demonstrates the existence of serious problems with the methods they were taught to employ.

Education is clearly important, but as EF Schumacher states in *Small is Beautiful: A Study of Economics as if People Mattered*,

"More education can help us only if it produces more wisdom."

Wisdom can never be produced through 'education' that disseminates erroneous information based on flawed theories.

It is clear that the art of healing was lost when transformed into the 'science of medicine' that is only practised by qualified 'medical doctors' who have been educated in an approved 'medical school'. It should be equally clear that 'modern medicine' does not perform 'healing', it only 'treats' disease.

It is ironic that this 'scientific medical system' was created in order to protect people from 'quackery'; yet the practice of 'modern medicine' is based on a number of erroneous beliefs that are not substantiated by the empirical evidence. These beliefs are not only perpetuated through 'medical education' they are sustained through 'medical research'.

Medical Research

Medical research is a core component of the 'medical system'.

The purpose of medical research was discussed in a February 2013 editorial in *The Lancet*; this article, appropriately titled *What is the purpose of medical research?* argues that suitable replies would state,

"...to advance knowledge for the good of society; to improve the health of people worldwide; or to find better ways to treat and prevent disease."

Despite public perception that these are indeed the objectives of medical research, *The Lancet* editorial states that, in reality, the situation is rather different and that instead, research has become an extremely lucrative activity, the scale of which is that,

"About $160 billion is spent every year on biomedical research."

But this huge level of expenditure is far from cost-effective; the editorial refers to a 2009 study article whose authors,

"...estimated that 85% of research is wasteful or inefficient..."

This level of waste and inefficiency ought to be a matter of serious concern to the medical research community, but it would seem to be an ongoing problem. The editorial refers briefly to some of the sources of the problem, one of which is the failure to assess the relevance or importance of a research project prior to its commencement. Other concerns that were raised refer to the failure to assess whether the research was 'unbiased', or even 'clinically meaningful'.

The existence of pharmaceutical industry bias in medical research is undeniable; industry research is conducted almost exclusively for the purpose of developing marketable products, especially medicines and vaccines, from which large profits can be made. Although research costs are high, they are invariably recouped when products reach the marketplace; as indicated by Dr Carolyn Dean in *Death by Modern Medicine*,

"The bias of medical research makes it search for a patentable drug that will eventually pay for the costly studies necessary to bring it to market."

But this industry bias is inappropriate; in her book entitled *The Truth About the Drug Companies*, Dr Marcia Angell MD refers to,

"...a growing pro-industry bias in medical research – exactly where such bias does not belong."

There is another form of bias in medical research, which is that funding grants are almost always allocated to research projects that support the 'consensus' view. Fortunately, there are some scientists who do not follow the 'consensus'; but, unfortunately, as Dr Paul Craig Roberts explains in his previously cited article entitled *The Oceans Are Dying*, those who are able to maintain their independence do so under rather difficult circumstances,

"The independent scientists who remain have great difficulty obtaining funds for their research, but the corporate scientists have unlimited funds with which to lie."

A pertinent example of the difficulties faced by independent scientists who challenge the 'consensus' view, is the loss of funding experienced by Professor Duesberg when his research, which revealed that 'HIV' was not the cause of AIDS, was published, as discussed in chapter four. The preference for only funding research projects that preserve the 'consensus' also exists in the field of 'mental health'; Dr Peter Breggin explains in *Toxic Psychiatry* that,

"The search for biochemical and genetic causes keeps psychiatrists, as medical doctors, in the forefront of well-funded research in the field."

The erroneous nature of the idea that 'mental disorders' are either 'genetic' or 'biochemical' in origin has been discussed.

A key focus of medical research is the investigation of disease; as previously discussed, the ICD is the internationally-recognised 'standard' for the classification of diseases for both clinical and research purposes. The use of this definitive guideline by the research community ensures that diseases are investigated solely in the context of their ICD definition, which inevitably perpetuates the 'consensus' view. But this approach places severe restrictions on the nature of 'medical research', especially investigations of diseases believed to be 'infectious' and the mistaken idea that they are caused by 'germs'. Although medical research invariably facilitates the development of medicines and vaccines for use in a clinical context, this does not mean that the research has therefore been 'clinically meaningful'; as demonstrated throughout this book, pharmaceuticals are inimical to human health, not supportive of it.

It is abundantly obvious that pharmaceutical companies benefit significantly from the revenues generated by the medicines and vaccines developed as the result of medical research, however, medical schools and universities may also benefit financially from such research projects, as Dr David Michaels explains in *Doubt is Their Product*,

"Universities and university scientists have enrolled in joint ventures and profit sharing arrangements with chemical and pharmaceutical manufacturers."

The campaign led by Yale University students to reduce the price of generic 'HIV' drugs, as discussed in the previous section, was the inspiration behind the creation of the UAEM movement that now operates in a number of countries around the world. The website claims that,

"The campaign showed those students that, as major contributors to drug development, universities are well positioned to influence the way medical technologies are developed and distributed, and thus can do much to help alleviate the access-to-medicine crisis."

A lack of access to medicine is not a crisis; on the contrary, the real crisis is the use of 'medicine' in the continuing, but mistaken, belief that pharmaceuticals provide the only solution to the very real problem of 'ill-health'. This mistaken belief is compounded by the continuing failure of the medical establishment to conduct genuine 'medical research' into the nature of 'disease' and discover the real causes. Research projects that would undertake genuine investigations of that nature do not occur for a number of reasons, one of which is that the pharmaceutical industry, which is one of the main funding sources of research, would not benefit financially because those projects would not result in marketable products. It is clear therefore, that the industry has a 'vested interest' in the existing form of 'medical research'.

It is equally clear that the entire medical research community has a similar 'vested interest' because their careers and salaries depend on the continuing existence of the system in which they were trained. A successful career in this system is dependent upon certain factors, as described by Professor Duesberg in *Inventing the AIDS Virus*,

"The successful researcher – the one who receives the biggest grants, the best career positions, the most prestigious prizes, the greatest number of published papers – is the one who generates the most data and the least controversy."

But the generation of data and the avoidance of controversy are not synonymous with 'science'. In a further reference to successful researchers Professor Duesberg states that,

"They pride themselves on molding data to fit popular scientific belief..."

This approach is contrary to genuine 'science', which holds that evidence is primary.

One of the most popular beliefs in the field of medicine is the theory that 'germs' cause disease. Although erroneous, it is a core belief to which medical researchers continue to mould their data. Researchers who study diseases claimed to be 'infectious' do so on the basis of the assumption that 'germs' are the causal agents, despite the complete lack of knowledge about the mechanisms by which microorganisms are able to induce the wide variety of symptoms associated with these diseases.

The main purpose of most 'medical research' is to lead to the development of 'medicine'. Most laboratory-based research studies begin with the 'discovery' that a particular chemical compound produces an effect perceived to be 'beneficial' on a cell, tissue or molecule. When certain tests, usually performed on animals, indicate that the compound may be 'clinically meaningful' for humans, it will be developed into a drug that will be tested in clinical trials. These human trials are conducted in four 'phases', the first three of which, referred to as Phase I, Phase II and Phase III, evaluate the drug's effectiveness and assess its 'side effects'; in all three phases the human test subjects are healthy volunteers.

If a drug proceeds successfully through these three phases and its 'benefits' are deemed to outweigh its 'risks', study data are submitted to the appropriate regulatory agency for approval; different approval procedures may of course apply in different countries. However, if successfully approved, the drug will enter Phase IV, in which it is introduced onto the market and prescribed to the general public; this phase is also referred to as 'post-marketing surveillance'. It is during this stage that the drug is prescribed to people diagnosed with the 'disease' for which it was developed; in other words, by definition these people are not healthy, which is the reason that Phase IV is the most important stage as far as the general public is concerned.

During Phase IV, not only is the drug taken by people who are not healthy, it is often taken for much longer periods of time than the duration of clinical trials. Many drugs are recommended to be taken for many months, years or even for the rest of a person's life, whereas the drug may only have been tested over the course of a few weeks or months. It is, therefore, only during Phase IV that a drug's long-term 'side effects' can be ascertained, by which time it may have harmed many people. If these 'effects' are considered to be sufficiently serious, the drug may be withdrawn from the market, but this is not always the case; thalidomide for example, remains in use as a treatment for a certain type of cancer, although it is no longer prescribed for pregnant women.

Clinical trials are another activity that may be relocated to 'developing' countries to take advantage of cheaper labour and other costs, although minimising costs does not necessarily compromise the quality of the trials.

A matter of more serious concern, however, relates to the ethical nature of clinical trials, wherever they may be conducted. This problem is discussed in a 2008 briefing paper, appropriately titled *Unethical Trials*, that was produced by the Centre for Research on Multinational Corporations (SOMO). According to this paper, ethical norms are contained within the Declaration of Helsinki (DoH) which asserts that,

> "The research is only justified if there is a reasonable likelihood that the populations in which the research is carried out stand to benefit from the results of the research."

The SOMO paper describes a study in which an antihypertensive drug was tested on babies that were acknowledged to be ill, although the nature of their illness is not disclosed. Nevertheless, whether or not the babies had been diagnosed as suffering from hypertension, 49 of them died during the trials; the drug was clearly toxic. With reference to unethical trials in general, the paper makes the sobering comment that,

> "...the scale of the problem is unknown, because it cannot be estimated how many unethical trials escape public attention and therefore remain unnoticed."

The publication of research study papers in a medical journal is regarded as an extremely important aspect of the work of researchers. However, in his April 2016 article entitled *What are medical journals for and how well do they fulfil those functions?* Richard Smith, former editor of the *British Medical Journal*, states that more than a million studies are published each year in more than 20,000 medical journals. Interestingly, he concludes that,

> "Medical journals are now a poor way to publish science..."

Nevertheless, research study papers continue to be published in medical journals after they have passed the peer review process, which is widely promoted as the 'gold standard' of science. In *Trust Us, We're Experts*, authors Sheldon Rampton and John Stauber explain that,

> "In theory, the process of peer review offers protection against scientific errors and bias."

But this is another situation in which the reality differs from the theory due to the influence of 'vested interests', as they further explain,

> "In reality, it has proven incapable of filtering out the influence of government and corporate funders, whose biases often affect research outcomes."

The process of 'peer review' is recognised to be fraught with problems, as Richard Smith explains in his article about medical journals,

> "Quality assuring research is poor as we know that most published findings are false and it's not surprising as peer review is fraught with problems and lacks evidence of effectiveness."

The comment that 'most published findings are false' refers to a 2005 article entitled *Why Most Published Research Findings Are False*, in which the author, Dr John Ioannidis MD, states that,

> "...for many current scientific fields, claimed research findings may often be simply accurate measures of the prevailing bias."

This statement highlights one of the many problems with the 'peer review' process, which is that it relies on and perpetuates the prevailing 'consensus' view and denies the publication of research that challenge this consensus. This is discussed by Dr Breggin in *Toxic Psychiatry*, in which he describes peer review as,

> "...one more old-buddy network guaranteeing that critical viewpoints never see the light of day while badly flawed studies supporting the establishment are rushed into print."

One example of the 'network' closing ranks against a critical viewpoint is the case of Dr Andrew Wakefield, whose work revealed an association between gastrointestinal problems and autism and implicated the MMR vaccine, which posed a serious threat to the vaccine industry. Although his research paper had passed the 'peer review' process and been published by a respected medical journal, it was subsequently retracted and is now reported as 'fraudulent' and 'discredited'.

The influence of the pharmaceutical industry over the publication of medical research study articles is widely recognised to be a problem. In his essay entitled *Medical Journals Are an Extension of the Marketing Arm of Pharmaceutical Companies*, Richard Smith quotes Richard Horton, a former editor of *The Lancet*, who stated in 2004 that,

> "Journals have devolved into information laundering operations for the pharmaceutical industry."

Richard Smith refers in his essay to the publication of studies, which show beneficial results from a new drug or vaccine, as an effective method of publicity and states,

> "For a drug company, a favourable trial is worth thousands of pages of advertising..."

Although it may be assumed that a published research study demonstrates a scientific 'truth', this would be a mistaken assumption; Dr Ioannidis explains in his above cited 2005 article that,

> "Published research findings are sometimes refuted by subsequent evidence..."

Medical journals are also heavily influenced by the pharmaceutical industry, but only partly as the result of the advertising revenue they receive. The industry also employs other, more effective, tactics, one of which is to employ 'ghostwriters'. In *Trust Us, We're Experts*, the authors quote science writer Norman Bauman, who describes ghostwriting, and states that it includes,

> "...hiring freelance writers to write articles for peer-reviewed journals, under the byline of doctors whom they also hire."

It is generally assumed that the named authors listed on a published article are the researchers who conducted the study; but this is not necessarily the case, as ghostwriting would seem to be increasingly commonplace. Professor Sheldon Krimsky explains in *Science in the Private Interest* that,

> "...there is a ghostwriting industry in science and medicine."

But this is not a new industry, as Dr Carolyn Dean explains in *Death by Modern Medicine*,

> "According to Sergio Sismondo, drug companies have been paying ghostwriters

to produce papers for decades..."

In 'medical science', unlike in fiction, ghostwriting does not merely provide assistance for a 'less able' writer, as Dr Leemon McHenry PhD explains in his 2010 article entitled *Of Sophists and Spin-Doctors: Industry Sponsored Ghostwriting and the Crisis of Academic Medicine*,

"This practice, however, goes beyond simple drafting of a manuscript; it provides an academic façade for research..."

The existence of this practice refutes the claim that the peer review and publication process represent a 'gold standard' system. However, although an 'academic façade' is a matter of concern, the implications of the practice of ghostwriting are far more profound, as he states,

"Such camouflaged authorship undermines scientific integrity and jeopardizes public health."

Another, more troubling, tactic used by the pharmaceutical industry is referred to as 'ghost management', which is described by Professor Sergio Sismondo in his September 2007 article entitled *Ghost Management: How Much of the Medical Literature is Shaped Behind the Scenes by the Pharmaceutical Industry*. In his article he explains that 'ghost management' exists when,

"...pharmaceutical companies and their agents control or shape multiple steps in the research, analysis, writing, and publication of articles."

The full extent of this industry is unknown because its activities remain largely hidden from view; its effects are more conspicuous because, as Professor Sismondo states, ghost management permits,

"...the pharmaceutical industry considerable influence on medical research and making that research a vehicle for marketing."

The extent of pharmaceutical industry influence over all aspects of medical research, including the writing and publication of study articles, raises serious concerns. Dr Blaylock explains in *Health and Nutrition Secrets* that,

"...most editorial staff members of these scientific journals, as well as editors-in-chief, also receive research funding from pharmaceutical companies, and even hold stock in the companies from which they take money."

This clearly raises the issue of 'conflicts of interest', a problem that Professor Sheldon Krimsky has investigated in the wider field of science, although his findings are also applicable to 'medical science'. In *Science in the Private Interest*, he explains that,

"Scientific conflicts of interest are taken much less seriously than allegations of fraud or misconduct..."

He cites an example of a conflict of interest that arose from a rotavirus vaccine 'approved' by the FDA in 1998 and states that,

"Within about a year after the vaccine had been licensed, it was removed from the market after more than one hundred cases of severe bowel obstruction were reported in children who had received the vaccine."

Professor Krimsky refers to the conflicts of interest that were discovered during the investigation and showed that,

"...the advisory committees of the FDA and the Centers for Disease Control were filled with members who had ties to the vaccine manufacturers."

This type of 'conflict of interest' is increasingly common and a clear manifestation of the 'revolving door' in action.

Dr Arnold Relman MD, like his wife Dr Marcia Angell, was a former editor of the *New England Journal of Medicine*. In 1980, Dr Relman wrote an editorial expressing his concern about the involvement of physicians with drug companies, which, he states, represents a conflict of interest with the duty physicians owe to their patients. In his book, Professor Krimsky quotes Dr Relman's suggestion that,

> "...practicing physicians should derive no financial benefit from the health-care market except from their own professional services."

The same should also apply to the scientists involved in 'medical research'.

There are clearly many problems with 'medical research', most of which are the direct result of the influence of the pharmaceutical industry that is solely interested in developing marketable 'healthcare' products.

However, other 'vested interests' have instigated 'medical research' projects for purposes that have little, if anything, to do with healthcare. One particular series of projects involved the investigation of methods to reduce fertility in both men and women with a view to solving the alleged problem of 'population growth'. This research was originally incorporated into 'eugenics', which, contrary to popular belief, began in England in the late 19th century when Francis Galton coined the term. However, interest in the topic soon spread to America, where it was turned into a popular movement.

As previously discussed, the *NSSM 200* expressed concerns in the 1970s about the rapid rate of population growth, especially in 'developing' countries; but these concerns were couched in terms of the potential effect on 'US political and foreign policy interests' and on US 'national security'; the document states that,

> "The proposed strategy calls for a coordinated approach to respond to the important US foreign policy interest in the influence of population growth on the world's political, economic and ecological systems."

However, 'research' into effective birth control methods had begun during the early decades of the 20th century. Some of the research was funded by the Rockefeller Foundation and is recorded in the Foundation's annual reports; the 1968 report provides an update on the progress of the research and states that,

> "...several types of drugs are known to diminish male fertility, but those that have been tested have serious problems of toxicity."

This report also states that,

> "Very little work is in progress on immunological methods, such as vaccines, to reduce fertility, and much more research is required if a solution is to be found here."

The report announces that the Foundation would offer funding for further research into 'immunological methods'.

Some decades later, 'medical research' finally discovered a mechanism by which female fertility could be interrupted; as indicated by a November 1993 article entitled *Functional and immunological relevance of the*

COOH-terminal extension of human chorionic gonadotropin beta: implications for the WHO birth control vaccine that states,

"The World Health Organisation (WHO) Task Force on Birth Control Vaccines has selected the pregnancy hormone human chorionic gonadotropin (hCG) as a target molecule for a contraceptive vaccine."

HCG is a female hormone that supports the normal development of an egg in the womb, but can be suppressed by 'anti-hCG antibodies'; this suppression is the mechanism on which the development of a 'birth control vaccine' was based. The vaccine was tested in clinical trials in a number of countries, one of which was India. A 1994 article entitled *A vaccine that prevents pregnancy in women* reports on the trials and states that,

"The present study provides evidence for prevention of pregnancy in women by circulating anti-hCG antibodies."

The vaccine is claimed to be effective when 'antibody titers' reach a certain level, however, this level must be maintained by regular injections or 'boosters'. The article reports that, in the trials, it was discovered that when booster injections were no longer applied, the 'titers' declined and fertility eventually returned, although often after a period of many months. It should be noted that one of the funding supporters of this clinical trial was the Rockefeller Foundation.

Another ongoing research programme with immense and potentially disastrous implications for human health, and therefore a matter of serious concern, involves the topic referred to as 'gene editing', which is described on the Genetics Home Reference web page entitled *What are genome editing and CRISPR-Cas9?* that states,

"Genome editing (also called gene editing) is a group of technologies that give scientists the ability to change an organism's DNA."

The ultimate goal of this research is to use these technologies to alter human DNA; the page also states that,

"These technologies allow genetic material to be added, removed, or altered at particular locations in the genome."

The discussion about GMOs in chapter six referred to the problems that have arisen from the genetic engineering of plant seeds. It also referred to the fact that the underlying assumption of genetic engineering, which is that each gene encodes for a unique protein, was proven by the Human Genome Project to be entirely unfounded. Nevertheless, the GHR page states that,

"Genome editing is of great interest in the prevention and treatment of human disease."

The diseases of most interest to these researchers are those considered to be 'genetic' in origin; the page states that,

"It also holds promise for the treatment and prevention of more complex diseases, such as cancer, heart disease, mental illness and human immunodeficiency virus (HIV) infection."

These diseases have all been discussed and shown not to be caused by faulty genes.

The manipulation of human genes, even if claimed to be for the purpose of treating 'disease', clearly has immense ethical implications. The Nuffield

Council on Bioethics began an enquiry into the ethical issues of gene editing in September 2016 and published a report in July 2018. The key findings of this report, entitled *Genome editing and human reproduction: Social and ethical issues*, are that,

> "We conclude that the potential use of heritable genome editing interventions to influence the characteristics of future generations could be ethically acceptable in some circumstances..."

This can only be described as outrageous; it is especially so because, as discussed, diseases are not 'genetic'; they cannot therefore, be treated by the manipulation of a person's genes. There is, however, a more sinister aspect to this research. In his July 2018 article, aptly-titled *Son of Frankenstein? UK Body Backs Human Embryo Gene Editing*, William Engdahl correctly asserts that gene editing,

> "...belongs in the category of eugenics."

On the basis that fertility-reducing vaccines also belong in the same category, it is not surprising to find the same 'vested interests' involved in both projects. William Engdahl states that the supporters of gene editing research include the Rockefeller Foundation, the Bill and Melinda Gates Foundation, major pharmaceutical companies and GMO seed companies; he also states that,

> "The methodology of manipulating a specific part of a DNA chain to change human embryos is based on flawed scientific reductionism, which ignores the complexity of biophysical reality and of the fundamental laws of nature."

Although the European Court of Justice ruled in July 2018 that gene editing is to be treated as GM and to be subjected to the same regulations, the existence of regulations will not deter 'vested interests' from continuing such research.

Promulgating Deceptions

The 2030 Agenda represents the most recent version of the efforts of the international community to solve the problems that confront humanity in the 21st century. The *Transforming Our World* document claims that 'the public' was included in the preparation of the goals and targets of the Agenda; as indicated by the statement that,

> "The Goals and targets are the result of over two years of intensive public consultation and engagement with civil society and other stakeholders around the world..."

The 'public' involved in the consultation processes would only have been small representative groups; implementation of all of the 2030 Agenda goals and targets, by comparison, requires engagement with most, if not all of the people.

The strategies to increase public awareness of the Agenda and gain support for the implementation of the solutions have included the creation of organisations such as Global Goals, which claims, on the web page entitled *The 17 Goals*, that,

> "These goals have the power to end poverty, fight inequality and stop climate change."

The prominence of these three aims suggests that they are the most important goals; this is, however, part of the deception.

The organisation behind Global Goals is Project Everyone, whose mission is described on the Global Goals web page entitled *Project Everyone*, which states that,

"Our mission is to ensure that everyone on the planet knows what the Global Goals are so that they stand the greatest chance of being achieved."

The Project Everyone website claims that,

"Project Everyone seeks to put the power of communications behind the Sustainable Development Goals, also known as the Global Goals."

In addition to utilising the 'power of communications' to increase public awareness, Project Everyone employs highly emotive language to persuade people of the importance of these goals; as can be seen by the statement that urges campaign supporters to,

"Be the first generation to end extreme poverty, the most determined generation to end inequality and injustice and the last generation to be threatened by climate change."

It is clear that many of the 'Global Goals' identify genuine problems that affect large numbers of people around the world; demands that these problems are solved are therefore laudable. Unfortunately, most of the people involved in these projects and campaigns unquestioningly believe and support the establishment narrative, and are completely oblivious of the flawed nature of the theories on which a number of the goals have been based.

It is important to reiterate that problems can only be solved if they have been fully understood and their causes have been correctly identified.

The information the public receives about the issues contained within these 'Global Goals' is almost invariably promulgated by 'experts', who are perceived to understand the problems and therefore should not be challenged or even questioned. Yet, in many cases there are equally qualified 'experts' who do challenge those 'experts', but are increasingly marginalised or even prevented from promulgating their views through mainstream media channels. A pertinent example of this situation can be seen in the promotion of the idea that 'climate change' poses one of the greatest threats to humanity and the accompanying vilification of those who refute this idea.

This does, however, raise the question of how 'vested interests' are able to influence scientific 'experts' and ensure that they support the consensus relating to 'climate change', or any other aspect of the agenda. The response to this question requires reference to the fact that most fields of 'science' have been manipulated to the extent that 'science' no longer performs its intended purpose; but instead, has become a dogmatic discipline that demands strict obedience to the 'consensus' view and thwarts any view that challenges that 'consensus'. This is recognised in a February 2001 article entitled *The New Thought Police Suppressing Dissent in Science*, which explains that,

"Science has seldom lived up to its ideal as an open, disinterested enquiry into nature, as any scientist who has ever tried to publish genuinely new ideas or findings in the 'peer-reviewed' scientific journals will know too well."

If 'science' had remained open and disinterested, a number of the issues that are said to confront humanity would be less severe and many would not even exist.

The reason that the 2030 Agenda goals are based on flawed theories is not solely due to the failure of 'experts' to fully understand the nature and causes of the problems, it is also due to the influence of 'vested interests' that seek to dominate and control the actions to be taken to resolve these problems. The presence of these 'vested interests' can be seen by the reference to 'other stakeholders' in the *Transforming Our World* document, which provides no further details about this group of 'interested parties'.

It should be noted that the influence of 'vested interests' is not exclusive to science; it has permeated virtually all fields of enquiry.

The influence of 'vested interests' and the promulgation of deceptions to the public about the 'Global Goals' can certainly be seen in SDG 3, which relates to 'health', the main topic of this book. The flawed nature of the theories relating to 'infectious diseases', especially 'HIV', malaria and tuberculosis, which are referred to as 'epidemics' that need to be ended, has been discussed. Although ill-health is a genuine problem that needs to be resolved, the proposed solution that includes increasing access to affordable medicines and vaccines will exacerbate the problem, not solve it, as has been demonstrated throughout this book.

Another flawed Global Goal is SDG 2 which refers to solving the problem of hunger, but contains erroneous ideas about nutrition. The reason that the medical establishment fails to fully understand 'nutrition' is mainly because it is claimed to be 'unscientific', 'fluffy' and to belong in the domain of dieticians not doctors. This flawed perception of nutrition is the justification for the existence of few, if any, nutrition courses in medical school curricula. This is also deceptive, because 'good nutrition' is central to 'good health'. The Global Goals web page entitled *Healthy Not Hungry* recognises the connection between hunger and ill-health and states that,

"Achieving zero hunger and good health go hand in hand..."

The *Healthy Not Hungry* campaign involved Project Everyone, WFP and UNICEF and was intended to increase awareness of and make progress towards achieving both SDG 2 and SDG 3; surprisingly, however, this campaign did not involve the WHO or any other 'health' organisation.

IMPACT 2030 is another effort to promote greater awareness of the 2030 Agenda; the website explains that,

"IMPACT 2030 is a private sector-led initiative, in collaboration with the United Nations, social and public sectors, and academia, with the unique mission to activate human capital investments through employee volunteer programs to advance the achievement of the Sustainable Development Goals (SDGs)."

It is interesting to note that the Founding Partners of this 'private sector-led initiative' include GlaxoSmithKline, Dow Chemical and Pfizer. An IMPACT2030 document entitled *Human Capital Investment for*

Sustainable Development states that,

"We believe that corporations are a valuable resource uniquely poised to help respond to the needs of a rapidly changing world."

This would seem to suggest that corporations can and will help to address humanity's problems, but this is yet another deception. A corporation's core purpose is to provide shareholders with a return on their investment; this means that making profits is a far more important priority for them than solving humanity's problems. The response of corporations, especially those within industries that contribute to the problems, is to provide solutions that benefit their interests. The pharmaceutical industry, for example, which is responsible for contributing to human health problems, has a clear 'vested interest' in promulgating the deception that medicines and vaccines will achieve Goal 3. The chemical industry, for another example, which is responsible for contributing to environmental pollution, has a clear 'vested interest' in promulgating the deception that chemicals can solve many problems, such as increasing food production through 'Industrial Agriculture' that will help to feed the hungry people of the world.

Another interesting international organisation is the World Economic Forum (WEF), a not-for-profit foundation based in Switzerland which states on the web page entitled *Our Mission* that,

"The Forum engages the foremost political, business and other leaders of society to shape global, regional and industry agendas."

The WEF would seem to duplicate the work of the UN; this can be seen more clearly in the statement on the web page entitled *Improving the state of the world*, that,

"The Forum creates impact by gathering leaders from business, government, international organisations, academia, civil society and youth to work together to drive positive change."

The engagement of business leaders in an international 'think tank' that shapes the global agenda, is another method by which 'vested interests' are able to exert their influence, and ensure that the 'agenda' conforms to their preferred 'consensus' views that serve their interests. Although not part of the UN system, the WEF nevertheless supports the 2030 Agenda; the web page entitled *Sustainable Development Impact Summit* refers to the summit held in September 2018 and states that,

"Accelerating progress on the Sustainable Development Goals and Paris Agreement commitment requires global dialogue, deeper public-private cooperation and wider application of Fourth Industrial Revolution technologies."

The reference to the Paris Agreement demonstrates that the WEF is a firm supporter of the 'consensus' view about climate change. The claim that progress on the 2030 Agenda requires 'wider application' of technologies is of extreme importance. A January 2016 WEF article entitled *The Fourth Industrial Revolution: What it means, how to respond* explains that,

"The First Industrial Revolution used water and steam power to mechanize production. The Second used electric power to create mass production. The Third used electronics and information technology to automate production."

The page claims that the Fourth builds on the Third and that,

> "It is characterized by a fusion of technologies that is blurring the lines between the physical, digital, and biological spheres."

There are profound and very disturbing implications of the fusion of technologies with biology; the notion that this represents 'progress' is based on fundamentally flawed ideas that the human body is essentially a 'machine' and that the brain is little more than a 'processor' that can be likened to a computer.

Yet again, nothing could be further from the truth.

Developments in technology have certainly enabled people to be interconnected in ways that have never been previously possible; the article refers to a number of innovations such as,

> "...emerging technology breakthroughs in fields such as artificial intelligence, robotics, the Internet of Things, autonomous vehicles, 3-D printing. Nanotechnology, biotechnology, materials science, energy storage, and quantum computing."

The article claims that, like the three previous Industrial Revolutions, the technologies of the Fourth Industrial Revolution have,

> "...the potential to raise global income levels and improve the quality of life for populations around the world."

As previously discussed, the first Industrial Revolution, which introduced mechanisation into factories, only increased the income level and improved the quality of life for a very small group of people, mainly the industrialists and financiers; whereas 'the people', in stark contrast, fared rather poorly and inequalities increased. The same occurred as the result of the Second and Third Revolutions. The Fourth Revolution has the potential to do likewise, as the article admits,

> "In addition to being a key economic concern, inequality represents the greatest societal concern associated with the Fourth Industrial Revolution."

Technologies that lead to greater inequalities are incompatible with the core aim of the 2030 Agenda to reduce inequalities; they cannot therefore be regarded as a means by which the goals of the Agenda can be attained. This is yet another example of a proposed solution that will exacerbate an existing problem rather than resolve it. Nevertheless, the 'vested interests' within technology companies associated with the WEF will inevitably be fully supportive of the idea that 'Fourth Industrial Revolution technologies' are essential to accelerate progress on the 2030 Agenda.

One of the many strategies employed by 'vested interests' to maintain their influence and control, is to ensure that the theories that favour their interests are firmly embedded into the establishment consensus, even if the consequences are damaging to human health and the environment; David Michaels explains in *Doubt is their Product* that,

> "Polluters and manufacturers of dangerous products also fund think tanks and other front groups that are well known for their antagonism toward regulation and devotion to 'free enterprise' and 'free markets'. There are dozens of these organizations working on behalf of just about every significant industry in this country."

These strategies involve a variety of activities; Andrew Rowell explains in *Green Backlash* that,

"Overtly and covertly, by stealth and by design, big business has perverted the democratic process by buying politicians, by bribing them, by funding 'independent' think tanks, by forming 'corporate front groups', by bullying citizens, by lobbying and by lying – all in the name of profit."

It is clear that 'vested interests' employ a large range of activities to influence and control the information promulgated to the public, who remain largely unaware that they have been, and continue to be, deceived about almost all aspects of their daily lives.

PR & Propaganda

Public relations (PR) is a marketing tool used by many businesses to provide the public with information about their products and services. This information, often in the form of a press release, is intended to generate interest in, and therefore purchase of, the organisation's products and services. Press releases are also used by non-commercial entities; the WHO, for example, issues news releases to notify the public about matters such as the latest 'disease outbreak'. The Chartered Institute of Public Relations web page entitled *What is PR* defines PR as,

"...the discipline which looks after reputation, with the aim of earning understanding and support and influencing opinion and behaviour."

In *Toxic Beauty*, Dr Samuel Epstein refers to some of the organisations that have used PR to protect their 'reputations',

"The FDA, NCI and ACS spend millions of dollars on public relations in attempts to reassure the public they are doing a good job, despite their lack of progress."

PR is clearly intended to inform the public, but it can also be used to misinform them; an example is the April 1984 press conference at which it was claimed that the probable cause of 'HIV' had been found; the deceptive nature of this claim has been discussed.

Propaganda, which is said to differ from PR, is defined by the Oxford Dictionary as,

"false or exaggerated information, used to win support for a political cause or point of view."

The function of propaganda is therefore to inform the public, but to do so for the purposes of promoting a cause or an 'agenda' of some description.

The main difference between PR and propaganda would seem to be that the latter involves the deliberate use of false or misleading information; in other words, propaganda is intended to be deceptive. Nevertheless, PR and propaganda have a similar underlying function, which is to influence people in order to achieve a specific objective. This similarity can be largely attributed to Edward Bernays, often referred to as the 'father of public relations' who wrote a book entitled *Propaganda* in which he states that,

"The conscious and intelligent manipulation of the organized habits and opinions of the masses is an important element in democratic society. Those who manipulate this unseen mechanism of society constitute an invisible government which is the true ruling power of our country."

He continues with the statement quoted at the beginning of this chapter,

> "We are governed, our minds are molded, our tastes formed, our ideas suggested, largely by men we have never heard of."

A simple interpretation of these statements would be that they refer to the unknown people who are the heads of major corporate entities and employ PR to manipulate public tastes and ideas to generate consumer demand for their organisation's products and services. However, the idea that consumers are the driving force behind the production of goods is misleading; Barry Commoner explains in *Making Peace With the Planet* that,

> "There is a popular myth that in America 'the consumer is king', issuing commands for new products that are obediently met by producers."

This seemingly innocuous 'myth', although a successful marketing ploy, is deceptive because it obscures the reality that manufacturers serve their own interests, not those of consumers. This means therefore, that consumers have little influence over the products that most industries produce, as he further states,

> "...the change in production technology ...is initiated by the producer and is governed by the producer's interests."

One of the major changes in production technology was the manufacture of synthetic chemicals, often derived from petroleum, and their use as ingredients of the vast majority of consumer products. This change cannot be attributed to consumer demand, as people would not knowingly have commanded manufacturers to create products using inherently toxic substances that are harmful to their health and the environment. This is clearly a process that has been initiated by producers, as the vast majority of consumers are completely oblivious of the hazards posed by many of the everyday household products they use, and the processed food products and drinks they consume.

The lack of public awareness of these hazards can be partly attributed to a general assumption that these products would not be on the market if they were unsafe. Most efforts to convince the public about product safety involve reference to 'risk assessments' and scientific evidence that are claimed to demonstrate that the product and its ingredients are 'safe' when used as recommended. But it has been shown that the vast majority of chemicals have not been tested for their safety or for the full extent of any potential health hazards they pose; these claims must therefore be seen as PR rather than 'science'; as John Stauber and Sheldon Rampton explain in *Trust Us, We're Experts*,

> "In order to understand the manipulations that are practiced today in the name of science, it is necessary to understand the particular habits and practices of a particular class of experts who specialize in the manipulation of perception itself – namely, the public relations industry."

Commercial entities, especially large corporations, certainly seek to influence and manipulate public tastes and opinions in order to promote their products; but this is not the only valid interpretation of Edward Bernays' previously cited statements. The 'true ruling power' of which he writes is held by those referred to in this book as 'vested interests', whose power extends beyond the borders of the US and into many countries around the world. Although the individuals that comprise this 'ruling power' are invisible to the public, the effects of their influence are discernible in the increased level of power wielded by 'global' organisations that collaborate with corporations and governments, and in the decreased level of power and independent action permitted to 'the people'.

It has been established that opinions and beliefs can be relatively easy to manipulate by people perceived to be an 'authority figure' or 'expert'; this is further explained in *Trust Us, We're Experts*,

"When psychologists have explored the relationship between individuals and authority figures, they have found that it can be disturbingly easy for false experts to manipulate the thinking and behaviour of others."

A well-known example of an investigation of this nature is the series of experiments conducted by psychologist Stanley Milgram in the 1960s. The purpose of his experiments was to determine the extent to which study participants would obey instructions given by an 'authority figure', even though their actions appeared to inflict harm on other people; it must be noted that nobody was actually harmed. These experiments revealed a disturbingly high level of public trust by the participants in the 'authority figure', who was merely playing a role for the purposes of the experiments.

The fact that the majority of people will trust an 'authority figure' has been exploited by 'vested interests' in various ways, not least of which is by ensuring that information they wish the public to believe is promulgated by 'experts' that represent an 'authoritative body'. The WHO and the World Bank are both perceived as 'authoritative', therefore the public will almost certainly believe reports issued by these organisations and not realise that this information forms part of the 'agenda'. An example of this can be seen in a June 2015 joint WHO/World Bank press release entitled *New report shows that 400 million do not have access to essential health services* that claims,

"...6% of people in low- and middle-income countries are tipped into or pushed further into extreme poverty because of health spending."

The purpose of this joint press release is to promote the idea that there is an urgent need for people who live in poverty to have Universal Health Coverage and better access to 'essential health services'; in other words, this press release anticipates the 2030 Agenda that was agreed to by the UN later that same year. The 'essential health services' the press release refers to include: child immunisation; antiretroviral therapy; tuberculosis treatment; and 'family planning'. None of these 'services' are essential for human health, but they are all essential for the profitability and even the survival of the pharmaceutical industry. Interestingly, the Rockefeller Foundation is included as one of the supporters of the report referred to in this press release.

It is not disputed that many people who live in poverty face the dilemma of whether to spend their meagre income on food or 'medicines'. Unfortunately, however, all too many of them choose the latter instead of the former under the mistaken belief that 'medicines' will improve their health. The claim that many people have been further impoverished by their 'health spending' contradicts the previously cited World Bank claim that the number of people living in extreme poverty has declined. Furthermore, as has been discussed, loans issued by the World Bank and IMF to 'developing' countries are subjected to certain conditions that invariably involve reductions to government spending in order to meet interest and loan payments. These spending reductions affect the country's health budget and diminish any existing health services; it is clear therefore that the World Bank is responsible for reducing, not improving health services.

It must be noted that the joint press release does state that 'health services' should include better access to clean water and sanitation, which would certainly promote better health. However, water is not made 'clean' or 'safe' by treatment with chlorine or any other toxic disinfectant chemical.

Another effective method by which public opinion can be manipulated is through fear. This strategy is often used by the medical establishment, in conjunction with their reliance on the public's trust in 'authority', to perpetuate deceptive ideas that 'infectious diseases' are caused by dangerous 'pathogens' and pose serious threats to health, but can be prevented by vaccines. Although most people continue to believe these ideas, there is a growing awareness that vaccines are not as safe as they are claimed to be, which clearly poses a threat to the vaccine industry. The increasing number of people who refuse to be vaccinated or have their children vaccinated has provoked recommendations within the medical establishment to introduce mandatory vaccination programmes, but this has been met with some resistance; as indicated by a July 2017 article entitled *UK doctors re-examine case for mandatory vaccination* on the website of the *BMJ*, that states,

"Mandating childhood immunisation continues to be contentious in the UK..."

One of the responses to this article was written by Jackie Fletcher, the mother of a child she claims was damaged by the MMR vaccine and the founder of JABS, a support group for the parents of vaccine-damaged children. In her response, she reports that the JABS group includes parents who are also part of the medical establishment; however, when asked to speak out about the dangers of vaccines, she states that they,

"...have told us of their fears for their reputations, promotion prospects, even their final pension plans."

These fears are likely to have resulted, at least in part, from the campaign that has successfully discredited Dr Andrew Wakefield and his work; it is therefore unsurprising that medical doctors and researchers are reluctant to be subjected to the same disgraceful treatment. Although their response is understandable, there is a more important issue at stake, which is that their reluctance prevents greater awareness of the reality of the problem. This leads to the painful but urgent question of how many more children have to suffer vaccine-damage before members of the medical establishment who are aware of the problem, but fearful for their reputations, careers and pensions, end their silence and speak out.

It should be noted that not only is there a *Vaccine Damage Payment* system in the UK, but the MMR vaccine is included in the list of vaccines for which a payment may be made, subject, of course, to certain conditions.

It may be argued that, because only a very tiny percentage of children are 'damaged', it is reasonable to refer to vaccines as 'safe'. The suitable response to such an argument should include reference to two important points; firstly, that the existence of a single exception is sufficient to refute a rule; but there are far more than a single exception, as many people, especially children, have been damaged by vaccines. Secondly, vaccines are acknowledged to produce 'side effects', which are reactions that result from the administration of the vaccine, they are therefore 'direct effects'. If all of these 'side effects' were recognised as 'vaccine-caused damage', which is what they truly are, the deceptive nature of the claim that vaccines are 'safe' would soon become apparent to everyone.

The idea that vaccines are effective is also proven to be deceptive by the acknowledged existence of 'vaccine failures'. According to a January 2016 article entitled *Primary vaccine failure to routine vaccines: Why and what to do*, 'non-responsiveness' to a vaccine,

"...is currently described by the inability of the host/vaccine to mount sufficient protective antibody responses after primary or booster vaccination."

This 'problem' is claimed to only affect between two and ten per cent of healthy individuals; but again, this is a clear demonstration of exceptions that refute 'the rule'. Although this is the proportion of healthy people who may not respond to vaccine, the situation is rather different with respect to people who are not healthy. The article claims that certain factors, such as age, chronic diseases, allergies and obesity, affect the immune system and therefore affect the way people with these conditions respond to vaccines. According to the article, these 'human-related factors' for non-responsiveness to vaccines,

"...are more difficult to define and underlying mechanisms of vaccine failure are largely unexamined or unknown."

This is yet another huge 'knowledge gap' that would seem to be ignored by the medical establishment, which continues to promote the claim that vaccines are one of the greatest 'achievements' of modern medicine; this claim, which has been proven to be erroneous, must therefore be viewed as propaganda, not information.

Another strategy used by some PR companies involves diverting public attention from the real causes of certain problems, especially environmental pollution, as Andrew Rowell indicates in *Green Backlash*,

"It is also the job of the PR companies to shift the blame of pollution from their corporate clients onto the public at large."

A more egregious PR or, more accurately, propaganda strategy involves the creation of a campaign that includes reports by 'experts' to vilify anyone who challenges the 'consensus' view and discredit their work. This tactic has been used to discredit scientists and others who are also 'experts' in their field. Dr Epstein states in *Toxic Beauty* that,

"A more subtle layer of public deception that shields dangerous chemicals from scrutiny is the result of the intimidation tactics sometimes used against experts who go public about health hazards."

A prime example of this strategy are the actions taken by the chemical industry to discredit Rachel Carson after the publication of *Silent Spring*. In *Green Backlash*, Andrew Rowell quotes extracts from his interview with John Stauber, the founder of the Center for Media and Democracy and co-author of *Trust Us, We're Experts*. In the interview, John Stauber describes one of the disgraceful tactics used against Rachel Carson's work,

> "The National Agricultural Association doubled its PR budget and distributed thousands of book reviews trashing *Silent Spring*."

Mark Purdey, who revealed the real cause of BSE and stated that it resulted from a toxic organophosphate 'wash' used to protect cattle from warble flies, was also subjected to abusive campaigns to discredit him and his work; in the *Foreword* to *Animal Pharm*, his brother writes that,

> "Those who criticised the official orthodoxy were cruelly derided and dismissed as being 'unscientific' and lacking in objectivity."

Mark Purdey also explains that,

> "Despite publication in a variety of scientific journals, the authorities and their key advisors are ignoring these findings and are doing their utmost to marginalise those of us who are trying to pursue this line of research."

Those with a vested interest in preventing certain information from reaching the public will use a variety of tactics against any form of opposition to their 'consensus' view, even if this involves a government department; as demonstrated by the chemical industry's fight against the EPA after the *Dioxin Reassessment* report was published in 1994. Joe Thornton writes in *Pandora's Poison* that the fight by the industry was to,

> "...aggressively defend the industry's credibility through the use of third party sources ...ostensibly to debunk what they referred to as 'EPA's misleading claims'."

In this instance, EPA's claims were not misleading; dioxins are recognised to be some of the most toxic substances known to science. Yet, despite this recognition, the chemical industry denied that dioxins are extremely hazardous because it was incompatible with their 'interests'. The toxicity of dioxins is no longer disputed.

It is clear therefore, that PR campaigns are often used to discredit the work of those who dare to challenge the 'consensus' view in almost any field; but the inclusion of deceptive information in those PR campaigns indicates that they are, in reality, propaganda campaigns that intentionally misinform the public about issues that increasingly affect the lives and health of everyone, everywhere.

Philanthropy, Charity & The Third Sector

Society is said to be comprised of three 'sectors', the first of which is the private or business sector and the second is the public or government sector. The third sector, also referred to as 'civil society', is comprised of non-profit, non-governmental organisations, the main function of which is to 'help people in need', in other words, to performs acts of charity and philanthropy.

It is claimed that charity and philanthropy are different; the former is said to be reactive and short-term and the latter proactive and long-term, although in practice these differences are not always apparent. A more significant difference relates to their sources of finance; philanthropy is funded mainly by wealthy individuals, families and corporations, often through foundations, whereas charity is funded mainly by the general public.

According to the page entitled *Recent charity register statistics: Charity Commission*, in 2018 there were 167,972 charities in the UK that had a combined annual income of £76 billion. The income of individual charities, however, varies widely; at one extreme, 65,448 are reported to have had an income of £10,000 or less, whereas at the other extreme, 2,251 are reported to have had an income of £5 million or more.

The situation in the US is reported in two articles; the first is a March 2010 article entitled *Number of Charities and Foundations Passes 1.2 Million*. The second is a June 2018 press release entitled *Giving USA 2018: Americans Gave $410.02 Billion to Charity in 2017, Crossing the $400 Billion Mark for the First Time*. The titles are self-explanatory.

It is clear that non-profit organisations are collectively able to raise huge sums of money for a large number and wide variety of 'good causes'. But it is equally clear that certain causes are far better funded than others; a situation for which there are a number of explanations, not least of which is that some causes, such as cancer for example, receive a great deal of publicity. Other explanations are less obvious but significant, one of which is that the increasingly close cooperation between organisations within all three sectors of society enables 'vested interests' to promote the 'causes' that best serve their interests.

The expansion of civil society has led to the formation of various organisations for the purposes of managing and assisting third sector organisations, such as the Charities Aid Foundation (CAF) for example. CAF, a UK-based non-profit organisation that operates 'globally', claims, on the page entitled *What We Do*, to 'help donors' and states that,

"We do this by working globally to increase the flow of funds to the charity and non-profit sectors through the provision of philanthropy products and services, whilst providing fundraising solutions and support for charities internationally."

One of the organisations that manage internet-based charitable donations is Just Giving, which is described on the website as,

"...the world's most trusted platform for online giving."

On the *About Us* web page is the statement that,

"We are enormously proud to have helped people in 164 countries raise over $4.5 billion for good causes since we were founded in 2001."

Another organisation that 'manages' charitable donations is the UK-based Charities Trust, which is described on the website as,

"...a leading donations management organisation committed to growing charitable giving since 1987."

One of the ways in which 'charitable giving' has increased in recent years is through donations via employers' schemes, as indicated by an August 2018 article entitled *New global partnership to boost employee giving in the UK* on the Charities Trust website. This article refers to a new partnership between Charities Trust and YourCause; the latter is described as,

> "...the US-based leader in enterprise philanthropic technology..."

The purpose of this partnership is to enable businesses to set up 'schemes' to increase charitable donations, including schemes whereby employees can donate to charities through the payroll. Business-led schemes of this nature are claimed to be part of 'corporate social responsibility' (CSR), a term that refers to a variety of corporate responsibilities that include their obligations to society as well as to shareholders. CSR also involves 'sustainable practices'; which means that corporations are increasingly obliged to follow the 2030 Agenda, especially SDGs 8 and 9. The aim of SDG 8 is to,

> "Promote sustained, inclusive and sustainable economic growth, full and productive employment and decent work for all."

The aim of SDG 9 is to,

> "Build resilient infrastructure, promote inclusive and sustainable industrialization and foster innovation."

As previously discussed, the mission of IMPACT2030 is to increase financial support for the 2030 Agenda goals through 'volunteer employee programmes'; as indicated by the web page entitled *Employees Teach the Global Goals*, which refers to,

> "Mobilizing employee volunteers to educate and inspire millions of young students around the world about the Global Goals."

In addition to educating and inspiring people, these organisations also seek to raise money through organisations such as YourCause, which promotes IMPACT2030 and provides a platform for organisations to support the SDGs of their choice; as indicated by the page entitled *The Global Goals Gateway* which states that,

> "Our first step in promoting IMPACT2030 to our partners is a tool for nonprofits called The Global Goals Gateway."

SDG Watch Europe is another organisation that is fully supportive of the 2030 Agenda; it describes itself as an alliance of civil society organisations whose goal, according to the website is,

> "...to hold governments to account for the implementation of the 2030 Agenda..."

A leaflet produced by SDG Watch states that,

> "Civil society plays an essential role in pointing out the contradictions between goals and in advocating for the full participation of civil society in all Agenda 2030 implementation and monitoring mechanisms."

Another organisation that promotes the 2030 Agenda, but is mainly aimed at young people, is SDSN (Sustainable Development Solutions Network) Youth, which, according to the website, aims to 'educate' young people about the SDGs and,

> "...provides opportunities for them to pioneer innovative solutions to address the

world's biggest challenges."

The 'education' provided to these young people will inevitably include erroneous ideas about 'climate change' and 'infectious disease', to name just two, as well as the inappropriate solutions claimed to be able to address these problems.

Another organisation that is fully supportive of the 2030 Agenda is the UN Foundation, which, despite its title, was not created by the UN, but by billionaire Ted Turner, who, in 1997, donated an initial 'gift' of 1 billion US dollars. On the web page entitled *What We Do* is the statement that,

"We are an advocate for the United Nations and a platform for connecting people, ideas and resources to help the UN solve global problems."

It is clear that there is a concerted effort by many 'interested parties' to promote the 2030 Agenda goals through charitable and philanthropic organisations in order to increase public awareness and enlist their support.

One of the world's biggest challenges is poverty, the topic of SDG 1 and a 'cause' that has received a huge level of support from the campaigns of many civil society organisations. The anti-poverty campaign known as *Make Poverty History* was launched in 2005 in the UK, but developed into a worldwide phenomenon. A May 2013 Oxfam press release entitled *Make Poverty History, and G8 promises – was it worth it?* states that this campaign became,

"...a worldwide alliance of anti-poverty organisations and individuals from over 70 countries organised under the umbrella of the 'Global Call to Action against Poverty'."

This worldwide alliance is described on the GCAP (Global Call to Action against Poverty) website as,

"...the world's largest civil society movement calling for an end to poverty and inequality."

On the website is a 2018 statement signed by GCAP that urges action on the SDGs; this statement claims that little progress has been made since the 2030 Agenda was adopted and that the world remains 'unequal', despite the aim of SDG 10 to,

"Reduce inequality within and among countries."

It would seem that the response to the question raised by the above cited Oxfam press release must be an emphatic 'no'; poverty has not been 'made history'. Instead, it has continued to worsen, as demonstrated by the 2017 and 2018 Oxfam reports cited earlier in this chapter.

One of the main reasons that the anti-poverty movement has failed to eradicate poverty is because it has failed to tackle the underlying causes of poverty, which are the result of a variety of factors, including the economic policies of the IMF and World Bank.

War on Want (WoW), a UK-based organisation that also claims to be 'fighting global poverty', states on the website that they are different from other charities and justifies this claim on the page entitled *What We Do*, which states that,

"We believe poverty is caused by the political choices made by powerful elites: governments, wealthy corporations and others."

It would seem that WoW recognises some of the key problems; as indicated by the statement on the same page, under the heading *Economic justice and corporate accountability*, that,

"War on Want actively opposes trade deals and practices that promote the domination of markets over people's livelihoods, welfare and rights."

The web page also identifies some of the other problems, such as those caused by corporate ownership and exploitation of land and resources and by the corporate ownership and control of food and agriculture. These are some of the underlying causes of the problems that were also identified by Professor Chossudovsky and described in *The Globalization of Poverty*, as previously discussed in chapter eight.

The solution to 'poverty' cannot involve a continuation of the existing programmes, because none of them has been able to make any significant impact to reduce the scale of the problem. It is clear therefore that a different approach is required; an approach that correctly identifies and removes the causes of the problem. Oscar Wilde suggests in his book *The Soul of Man Under Socialism* that,

"The proper aim is to try and reconstruct society on such a basis that poverty will be impossible."

The purpose of citing this quote is not to advocate 'socialism', as that is not the solution. Instead, its purpose is to highlight that the only approach that will succeed in eradicating poverty is one that will remove its causes, so that poverty will cease to exist. Most of the causes of existing poverty owe their origin to the manner in which society, especially the 'money system', has been constructed and continues to operate, which is largely under the control of 'vested interests' that do not operate for the benefit of 'the people'.

Another of the world's biggest challenges is 'health', or more correctly 'ill-health', for which a large number of charities have been established to raise funds for increased research into a specific disease or type of disease. Public support for these charities is all too often generated by raising fear in people's minds with claims that anyone can be affected by the disease in question; Dr Carolyn Dean explains in *Death by Modern Medicine* that,

"Each charity would first build on the fear of getting their dread disease and convince people that money was the cure."

One of the most feared diseases is cancer, for which there are several charities that raise funds for research to find the 'cure'. Cancer Research UK, which was originally founded in 1902 as the Imperial Cancer Research fund, makes the claim on their website that,

"Together we will beat cancer."

This claim is misleading; like virtually all other cancer charities, Cancer Research UK supports the traditional 'treatments' for cancer, which include surgery, chemotherapy, radiation, hormone therapy, targeted drug therapy and immunotherapy, amongst others. The problems with these 'treatments' have been discussed; the main reason they are unsuitable is because they do not address the real causes of cancer.

The web page entitled *Causes of cancer and reducing your risk* claims that 4 in 10 of UK cancer cases 'can be prevented', and that the 'risk' of cancer depends on genes, as well as environmental and lifestyle factors that can be controlled. The page does, however, recognise that one of the controllable lifestyle factors that play a role in cancer is a 'healthy diet'; the web page entitled *Diet and cancer* states that,

"A healthy balanced diet with plenty of fibre, fruit and vegetables and less red and processed meat and salt can help cut cancer risk."

Although not incorrect, this information is inadequate. Unfortunately, this charity also promulgates erroneous information; such as the page entitled *Food controversies*, which states, under the heading *Pesticides and organic foods*, that,

"High doses of some pesticides can cause cancer in animals, but the levels found in foods are tightly regulated to make sure they are well below this dose."

The page makes the further claim that,

"There is also evidence that eating organic food – which usually doesn't use pesticides – doesn't affect cancer risk."

Further claims are made on the page entitled *Cancer controversies*, one of which relates to personal care products about which the page states that,

"...there is no good scientific evidence to show that these products affect the risk of cancer."

These claims about diet, pesticides, organic foods and personal care products are erroneous, as demonstrated by the discussions throughout this book.

Dr Samuel Epstein spent decades exposing the flawed nature of the information promulgated by the 'cancer establishment'; he states in *Toxic Beauty* that,

"The cancer establishments worldwide still rely on questionable data and biased claims from publicly funded institutional apologists for the status quo and academics working for the very industries they should be exposing."

The ACS page entitled *Does This Cause Cancer?* makes the interesting statement that,

"Some people might be surprised to learn that there's no single, comprehensive list of all chemicals that cause cancer."

It is shocking rather than merely surprising that no single organisation maintains a comprehensive and regularly updated database of all substances shown to be potentially, if not actually carcinogenic. This is even more shocking considering that the WHO has predicted that the incidence of cancer will continue to rise into the foreseeable future. Part of the reason for this situation is because the vast majority of chemicals remain untested; a fact that is acknowledged by the ACS in the statement that,

"...it's not possible to study the millions of chemicals (natural and man-made) people can be exposed to."

The justification for the failure to study all chemicals is that,

"It would simply be too expensive, would take too long, and in many cases, it wouldn't be necessary."

The question that ought to be raised is whose interests these cancer organisations represent; a question that Dr Epstein addresses in *Toxic*

Beauty in his statement that,

> "The US cancer establishment's professional mindset and politically misshapen priorities are compounded by disturbing conflicts of interest, particularly for the ACS, because of its relationship with the cancer drug industry, as well as with the petrochemical and other polluting industries..."

Dr Epstein maintains that most cancers are preventable and that the war against cancer is winnable, but reveals the influence of 'vested interests' in the statement that,

> "The worldwide cancer establishments share major responsibility for losing the winnable war against cancer, a fact that is all the more serious in view of the strong influence that US cancer establishment policies continue to exert on other nations worldwide."

He also reveals that the NCI, the US cancer research agency, has spent more than $50 billion since the 'War on Cancer' was declared in 1971, but that,

> "...less than 2 percent of its budget has gone to cancer prevention."

The discussion in chapter seven revealed that cancer does not need to be 'fought'; it does not require a war to defeat the disease, but it does require an understanding of the real causes.

The Cancer Research UK web page about 'cancer controversies' also refers to *Mobile phones, wifi and power lines*; in other words, non-ionising radiation. Although the page acknowledges that the IARC classified mobile phones as Group 2B, in other words, as 'possibly' carcinogenic to humans, it also claims that,

> "...the scientific evidence shows it is unlikely that mobile phones could increase the risk of brain tumours..."

Nothing could be further from the truth.

The discussions in chapters six and seven demonstrate that there is an abundance of evidence that shows a statistically significant increased risk of developing brain tumours due to mobile phones, especially when they are held in very close proximity to the head for extended periods of time. These risks are shown to be even greater for young children whose heads are still growing.

The page also claims that evidence shows that wi-fi and smart meters do not pose a risk to health; this too is erroneous. Chapter six revealed the existence of a large and growing body of evidence that demonstrates the adverse health effects, including cancers, due to exposures to non-ionising radiation. The imminent introduction of millimetre waves to facilitate 5G and SMART technologies will only exacerbate the problem, unless the public is made aware that this will endanger the health of everyone, everywhere and takes action to halt its implementation.

Although foundations are established ostensibly for philanthropic purposes, some of the activities for which they have been, and in some cases still are used cannot be described as being for the benefit of 'people in need'. The funding of research into 'fertility reduction' as a method of reducing the growing world population by the Rockefeller Foundation has been discussed. However, research of this nature is ongoing and would seem to receive support from other 'philanthropists', most notably, Bill Gates. At a TED2010 conference, Bill Gates presented a talk entitled *Innovating to Zero*, in which he discussed ideas to reduce manmade CO_2 emissions to zero. He also referred to continuing population growth and claimed that the world population would soon reach 9 billion. In his March 2010 article entitled *Bill Gates talks about 'vaccines to reduce population'*, William Engdahl reports that in this talk, Bill Gates refers to the size of the population and states that,

> "Now if we do a really great job on new vaccines, health care, reproductive services, we lower that by perhaps 10 or 15 percent."

Although he does not refer to vaccines as the sole method by which the world population can be reduced, he clearly considers it to be one of the approaches. However, the Bill and Melinda Gates Foundation (BMGF) is well-known for its extraordinary efforts to deliver vaccines to all children, especially in 'developing' countries and particularly in countries within Africa. In his article, William Engdahl also reports that, in 2010, Bill Gates,

> "...announced his foundation would give $10 billion (circa €7.5 billion) over the next decade to develop and deliver new vaccines in the developing world."

The BMGF is involved in many vaccine-promoting organisations, one of which is GAVI, which, on a web page entitled *Working together for healthy vaccine markets*, emphasises the commercial rather than the 'philanthropic' aspect of the market. Nevertheless, the page also promotes the standard establishment view that vaccines are essential in the statement that,

> "A proactive effort to make vaccine markets work better for lower-income countries is essential to reach all children with life-saving vaccines..."

Although this statement may be interpreted as simply PR, in reality, it should be seen as propaganda; vaccines are not 'life-saving'. The claim that they save lives is refuted by the many thousands of people, and especially children, who have been damaged by them and by the huge sums of money that have been paid by vaccine damage compensation funds. It is interesting, but unsurprising, that UHC2030, the movement to accelerate access to Universal Health Care and to 'medicines and vaccines' is funded by a number of 'global partners' that include: UNAIDS, the World Bank, GAVI Alliance and the Global Fund to Fight AIDS TB & Malaria, as well as the Rockefeller Foundation and the Bill and Melinda Gates Foundation.

Another of the world's major issues is hunger, which is perceived to be caused by an inadequate production of food. Although this claim has been shown to be erroneous, philanthropic organisations have also become involved in efforts to introduce 'industrial agriculture', especially into Africa through AGRA. BMGF is one of the funders of AGRA that continues its efforts to introduce the 'Green Revolution' into African countries, despite the strong resistance of many African people who are perfectly aware of the hazards with which this method is associated.

Another organisation involved with efforts to introduce 'industrial agriculture' around the world is CGIAR (Consultative Groups on International Agricultural Research), which states on the website that,

"Towards a world free of poverty, hunger and environmental degradation, CGIAR is the world's largest global agricultural innovations network."

CGIAR is certainly a large organisation; it claims to have a research fund of almost a billion dollars. However, although the stated objective sounds highly 'philanthropic', the organisations that provide the funds reveal a very different underlying objective. In addition to the BMGF, the list of CGIAR funders includes: USAID, World Bank Group, the Rockefeller Foundation, FAO, OPEC (Organization of Petroleum Exporting Countries), UNDP and Syngenta Foundation, to name just a few. It is clear that CGIAR supports the 2030 Agenda; as indicated by the web page entitled *Health*, on which it is stated that more than 800 million people are chronically undernourished, but that,

"CGIAR research to improve nutrition and health contributes strongly to the United Nation's Sustainable Development Goals and targets for the 2030 agenda..."

Syngenta, another funder of CGIAR, is a global agribusiness company based in Switzerland that produces agrichemicals and GM crops. On the web page entitled *Who We Are* is the claim that,

"Our business – and the world's food security – depend on sustainable natural resources, healthy ecosystems and thriving rural communities."

The discussions in chapters six and eight demonstrate that the consequences of agribusiness practices are detrimental to the ecosystem, as well as unhealthy and unsustainable. Yet Syngenta supports the 2030 Agenda, which claims to be able to solve hunger and illness; this further substantiates the assertion that the underlying purpose of the 'agenda' is not to make the world a better place for everyone, everywhere, but only to make it better for 'vested interests'.

It is clearly of the utmost importance that people become aware that a significant proportion of the 'information' they receive about the 'good causes' they are encouraged to support, especially those related to the 2030 Agenda, is, in reality, little more than PR and propaganda.

The Media

The website of 'Oxford Dictionaries' defines the term 'media' as,

"The main means of mass communication (broadcasting, publishing and the Internet) regarded collectively."

The conventional view of 'the media' is that the information, or news, they provide is factual because the sources are deemed to be trustworthy; as indicated by the previously cited ACS page entitled *Does This Cause Cancer*, which claims that,

"Major news sources generally try to provide accurate, unbiased information."

This view is, however, grossly misleading.

The media sources deemed to be 'trustworthy', often referred to as the mainstream media (MSM), have been shown to be increasingly responsible for reporting inaccurate and biased information. The main reason for this is due to the influence of 'vested interests' that own or otherwise control the major media corporations; their ownership enables them to ensure that the information promulgated to the public as 'news' conforms to their 'agenda'.

Although it is commonly believed that the journalists who report the 'news' have conducted a full investigation of the 'stories' about which they write, this is now rarely the case; in his 2008 book entitled *Flat Earth News*, Nick Davies refers to,

"...journalists who are no longer out gathering news but who are reduced instead to passive processors of whatever material comes their way, churning out stories, whether real event or PR artifice, important or trivial, true or false."

He explains that a substantial proportion of the 'material' made available to journalists is sourced from newswires or PR agencies, and that journalists no longer have any time to investigate this material in any depth to determine whether it is 'real' or merely PR. As previously discussed, information provided by a PR agency in the form of a press release will be biased by intention. It is therefore possible for a press release promoting an 'agenda' to be mistaken for a news story containing genuine information. The comment by Nick Davies that 'news stories' may not even be true is corroborated by Professor Chossudovsky who asserts in *The Globalization of Poverty* that,

"The global media fabricates the news and overtly distorts the course of world events."

Although 'vested interests' are able to influence a significant proportion of the information available on the internet, mainly through their influence over social media websites and the most commonly used 'search engine', they do not actually control the internet.

However, although the internet remains a valuable resource and a source of genuine information, people who wish to utilise this resource for the study of a particular subject must be aware that it is also a source of misinformation and disinformation. The internet is increasingly used to vilify anyone who challenges the 'consensus' view and to discredit them and their work with the use of derogatory labels; for example, anyone who challenges the consensus view on 'climate change' is likely to be labelled a 'climate change denier', a 'conspiracy theorist' or possibly worse.

The fact that the internet remains a source of information that challenges the establishment narrative and exposes the deceptions promulgated by the mainstream media, poses a threat to 'vested interests', whose determination to retain control of the narrative on virtually all topics has led to the implementation of different strategies designed to combat this threat. One of these strategies has been to employ the phrase 'fake news' and apply it to all information that does not conform to the 'mainstream narrative'; it is most commonly applied to non-mainstream media sources, usually referred to as the 'alternative media'. Although some 'alternative media' sources provide accurate and unbiased information, others do not; some even promulgate disinformation. More importantly, however, some sources have been found to disseminate a mixture of genuine and misleading information, all of which makes internet research extremely complex and fraught with many difficulties.

The strategy of applying the label 'fake news' to any and all information that challenges the 'establishment narrative' promulgated by the MSM, can be demonstrated by the initiation of an enquiry into 'fake news' by the UK government; as indicated by the January 2017 web page entitled *Fake news' inquiry launched* that states,

"The Culture, Media and Sport Committee launches an inquiry into 'fake news': the growing phenomenon of widespread dissemination, through social media and the internet, and acceptance as fact stories of uncertain provenance or accuracy."

The interim report produced by this enquiry recommends the use of 'fact checking' organisations, of which there is an increasing number. However, this raises the question of who is to be responsible for determining what are the 'facts'. One 'fact checking' organisation is called Full Fact, which is described on the website as,

"...the UK's independent factchecking charity."

The website claims that, not only is Full Fact independent, it is also neutral and does not support any view; the objective of Full Fact is stated to be,

"...to make sure that there are systems in place so that only valid and validated claims are put into the public domain..."

It should be noted, however, that one of the funders of Full Fact is the Open Society Foundations (OSF), the creation of billionaire George Soros. On the OSF website is a page entitled *Access to Medicines* that states,

"The Open Society Foundations support efforts to increase access to essential medicines for people in low-resource countries, especially for poor and marginalized populations."

It is therefore extremely unlikely that OSF would permit Full Fact to acknowledge that medicines are harmful and to recognise the previously cited July 2000 article by Dr Barbara Starfield, in which she revealed statistics about the adverse health events due to correctly prescribed medicines. Her findings were recognised to have been 'valid and validated' and fully supported by scientific evidence; yet they remain unknown to the vast majority of the general public.

However, OSF is not the only influence over Full Fact; one of the main sources of their information is Public Health England (PHE), which, as a department of the UK government, inevitably adheres to the 'medical establishment' narrative on topics relating to 'medicines'; which means that it is extremely unlikely that Full Fact would expose the true extent of the hazards of pharmaceuticals.

It is clear that 'fact checking' organisations provide opportunities for the mainstream narrative on a particular topic to be asserted as representing 'truth', even though ample evidence exists to refute that claim and prove the narrative to be deceptive. Although most MSM journalists no longer conduct in-depth investigations, it does not necessarily require a great deal of effort to discover information that refutes the false nature of certain 'news stories'; as the following three examples will demonstrate.

The first example relates to 'news stories' about measles, which, until relatively recently, was considered to be a mild illness, but is now reported to be highly contagious and potentially fatal; as indicated by the May 2019

WHO *Measles* fact sheet that states,

"Even though a safe and cost effective vaccine is available, in 2017 there were 110,000 measles deaths globally..."

This claim is misleading; these deaths are not directly attributable to measles but to 'complications', as the fact sheet acknowledges,

"Most measles-related deaths are caused by complications associated with the disease."

Interestingly, however, the fact sheet claims that,

"Severe complications from measles can be reduced through supportive care that ensures good nutrition, adequate fluid intake and treatment of dehydration..."

The complications of measles are admitted to be mainly suffered by 'poorly nourished' young children in 'developing' countries. Nevertheless, the fact sheet insists that measles is caused by a 'virus' and asserts that,

"The virus remains active and contagious in the air or on infected surfaces for up to 2 hours."

It would seem that the WHO has failed to consult standard microbiology textbooks that do not describe viruses as 'alive', but invariably refer to them as being 'inert outside the host cell'; the word 'inert' is defined on the Oxford Dictionaries website as,

"Lacking the ability or strength to move. Chemically inactive."

Despite the fact that some microbiology textbooks can be accessed and read online for free, few, if any, journalists have utilised these valuable resources to investigate the real nature of viruses and discover that they are not 'living organisms' and are inert outside of a cell; which means that they cannot 'remain active' either in the air or on any surface. Unfortunately, journalists invariably write reports that conform to the consensus view that 'viruses' are dangerous pathogens that 'infect' people and cause 'disease'. A pertinent example is an August 2018 article entitled *Measles cases hit record high in Europe*, which states that,

"More than 41,000 have been infected in the first six months of 2018, leading to 37 deaths."

This article was sourced from the WHO news release entitled *Measles cases hit record high in the European Region* that states,

"To prevent outbreaks, at least 95% immunization coverage with 2 doses of measles-containing vaccine is needed every year in every community..."

However, the author of the 2018 article ought to have contrasted this WHO release with a 1987 article entitled *Measles outbreak in a vaccinated school population: epidemiology, chains of transmission and the role of vaccine failures*. This peer-reviewed article, which was published in the *American Journal of Public Health*, states that,

"An outbreak of measles occurred in a high school with a documented vaccination level of 98 per cent."

The article also states that 70 per cent of the measles cases occurred in vaccinated students and are therefore to be regarded as 'vaccine failures', the existence of which challenges the claim that vaccines are effective. Nevertheless, the website of the UK NHS promotes the idea that vaccines prevent measles, which is,

"...now uncommon in the UK because of the effectiveness of vaccination."

Yet a June 2018 article entitled *Measles outbreak in Bristol prompts public health warning*, reports that,

"People shunning vaccination is part of the problem, say experts."

The article also made the statement that,

"Although research published 20 years ago about a possible link between the MMR vaccine and autism has been discredited, the scare it created damaged some people's trust of the vaccine."

This is clearly a reference to the work of Dr Andrew Wakefield that is claimed to have been 'discredited'; but it fails to explain the contradiction between the NHS claim that measles is uncommon due to vaccination and the claim of unnamed 'experts' that people have shunned the vaccination.

However, conspicuous by its absence is any reference to the work of Dr Stefan Lanka who established in a court of law in Germany that the scientific papers claimed to demonstrate the existence of a 'measles virus' do no such thing; there is no definitive evidence that 'measles' is caused by a 'virus', as previously discussed. The real cause of the ill-health referred to as 'measles' is explained by Dr John Tilden in a statement previously cited in chapter four that bears repetition,

"Measles is the manner in which a child's body throws off toxemia."

The second example relates to 'news stories' about 'Ebola', which the May 2019 WHO fact sheet entitled *Ebola virus disease* refers to as,

"...a rare but severe, often fatal illness in humans."

It is claimed that this 'disease' has a case fatality rate that varies between 25 and 90 per cent, but is, on average, approximately 50 per cent; it is therefore an extremely serious health problem. The fact sheet states that,

"It is thought that fruit bats of the Pteropodidae family are natural Ebola virus hosts."

The phrase 'it is thought' indicates that these bats have not been proven to be the 'natural' hosts of the so-called 'virus'. The fact sheet reports that the first signs of 'Ebola' include common symptoms such as fever, headache and muscle pain; but later symptoms are more significant and are reported to include vomiting and diarrhoea as well as,

"...symptoms of impaired kidney and liver function..."

In early 2018, an outbreak of Ebola was reported to have occurred in the Democratic Republic of Congo (DRC). One of the efforts by the WHO and others to contain this 'outbreak' involved the administration of a newly developed vaccine, as indicated by a May 2018 GAVI article entitled *Ebola vaccine to help tackle DRC outbreak*, which referred to 'vaccination teams' in the area to administer the vaccine to those considered to be 'at risk'. This vaccine was very quickly reported to have been successful; as indicated by a July 2018 GAVI article entitled *Ebola vaccine praised as Congo outbreak declared over*, which states that,

"A total of 3,300 people received investigational doses of the vaccine as part of a ring vaccination protocol..."

The outbreak was declared to be 'over' when no new cases had been reported for a 42-day period. However, praise for the vaccine was premature because, as reported by a WHO *Ebola situation report*, on 1st August 2018 the Minister of Health for the DRC announced a new 'outbreak'; a situation that led to an expansion of the vaccination programme.

It is clear from the symptoms that the causes of the condition referred to as 'Ebola virus disease' involve toxins of some description. Unfortunately, the focus of health organisations, especially the WHO, on an alleged viral cause means that no toxicological tests are likely to have been conducted to determine the real causes of this serious condition; however, there are some clues to potential candidates. The Democratic Republic of Congo is known to be a country that has significant quantities of valuable minerals, not least of which are cobalt, copper, diamond, tantalum, tin and gold. It is widely reported that many international mining companies operate in the DRC including in North Kivu, the region in which the August 2018 'outbreak' occurred. Previous discussions have indicated that mining is a particularly hazardous occupation; but ill-health caused by exposures to and inhalation of various substances during mining rarely features in any reports by the MSM.

The third and final example to be discussed relates to 'news stories' about Lyme disease, for which there is no WHO fact sheet. A CDC web page entitled *Lyme Disease* states that,

"Lyme disease is caused by the bacterium *Borrelia burgdorferi* and is transmitted to humans through the bite of infected blacklegged ticks."

Like mosquitoes, newly emerged ticks are said to be uninfected, but can become 'infected' through the ingestion of bacteria if they bite an 'infected' animal. The web page claims that fever, headache and fatigue, as well as a distinctive rash, are the most common symptoms associated with Lyme disease, but other, more serious symptoms can develop in the absence of treatment; the page states that,

"If left untreated, infection can spread to joints, the heart and the nervous system."

The recommended treatments for Lyme disease are antibiotics, of which the most commonly used are doxycycline, amoxicillin, and cefuroxime, all of which are intentionally toxic, as their purpose is to kill bacteria. In common with all pharmaceuticals, these antibiotics produce 'effects', some of which are similar to the symptoms associated with the disease, such as fever and headache. Other 'effects' of these antibiotics are vomiting and diarrhoea, both of which are indicative of the body's efforts to eliminate 'poisons', including the toxic 'medicines'.

The belief that Lyme disease is caused by bacteria has prevented investigation of any potential toxicological causes; however, again there are some clues as to potential candidates. One of the likely causal factors are insect repellents, especially those produced from synthetic pyrethroid compounds. Whilst permethrin is commonly used as an insect-repellent treatment for clothing, bifenthrin is commonly used as an outdoor spray for gardens. Interestingly, insect repellents have been shown not to be an effective method of reducing the incidence of Lyme disease. An August 2013 article entitled *CDC Study Finds Pesticide Ineffective at Stopping the Spread of Lyme Disease*, published on the website of Beyond Pesticides, refers to the study and states that,

> "...spraying lawns with the insecticide bifenthrin does not reduce the incidence of tick-borne diseases."

According to the NPIC (National Pesticide Information Center), both permethrin and bifenthrin interfere with the insects' nervous system; but these synthetic pyrethroids are also neurotoxic to humans. The claim that 'untreated' Lyme disease can affect the nervous system, raises the question of whether those people whose nervous system has been affected had been exposed to a pyrethroid-based insect-repellent, or to some other neurotoxic substance.

It is clear from these three examples that the public is not only ill-informed, but often misinformed about many topics, especially those that relate to health matters. Although many non-mainstream media sources challenge the mainstream view on a wide variety of topics, very few, if any of them challenge the theories about the causes of 'disease' that have been shown throughout this book to be fundamentally flawed.

It would seem appropriate to close this chapter with the saying attributed to Mahatma Gandhi that was quoted at the beginning of chapter two,

> "An error does not become truth by reason of multiplied propagation, nor does truth become error because nobody sees it."

Chapter Ten

The Real Nature and Causes of Illness

"The belief in diseases and cures stands as an effective
barrier to a true education in healthful living."

Herbert Shelton

Modern medicine is based on the core assertion that impaired health can be remedied through the use of medicines that fight diseases and vaccines that prevent them. Furthermore, modern medicine is claimed to be the only healthcare system capable of defeating and preventing disease because it is the only one that is firmly grounded in evidence-based science.

However, as demonstrated by the discussions throughout this book, and especially in this final chapter, nothing could be further from the truth.

It is generally claimed that modern medicine emerged as the result of scientific advances made during the 17th and 18th centuries, although it was not until the late 19th century that some of the most significant medical 'breakthroughs' occurred. The most important of these include: the identification of different bacteria, the formulation of the 'germ theory' and the development and use of a number of vaccines.

The pace at which modern medicine progressed began to accelerate through the early decades of the 20th century, mainly as the result of technological innovations. The invention of the electron microscope in the 1930s, for example, enabled scientists to view smaller structures than had previously been possible, which led them to discover the particles that became known as 'viruses'. The development of advanced technologies progressed at an increasingly faster pace during the latter part of the 20th century and has continued to do so into the early 21st century. These technologies have been utilised by modern medicine and have facilitated the development of increasingly sophisticated medical devices and equipment for purposes such as diagnostics, treatments and laboratory-based research.

Yet modern medicine can only boast a single victory over diseases that affect humans, namely, the eradication of smallpox; but, as previously discussed, this is an invalid boast. It is clear therefore, that, despite the passage of more than two centuries and the expenditure of unimaginably huge sums of money, the successful defeat of 'human disease' remains elusive to the medical establishment.

Although claimed to be thoroughly scientific, modern medicine adopted an approach towards disease and its treatment that was based on two long-held beliefs that substantially predate the era of modern science. One of these beliefs claims that each disease is a distinct entity that attacks the human body; the other claims that each disease can be defeated through the use of the appropriate medicine. The acceptance of the 'germ theory' led to the adoption of a third belief, which claims that diseases caused by 'germs' can be prevented by vaccines. These beliefs are, however, fundamentally flawed; they do not accurately represent the nature of disease or the means by which diseases should be treated or can be prevented. The failure of modern medicine to defeat disease is entirely attributable to the rigid adherence to these flawed beliefs.

Unfortunately, virtually all forms of 'healthcare' operate from the basis of the same flawed theories about the nature of disease. The reason for the focus on 'modern medicine', or the medical establishment as it is referred to in this book, is because it is the healthcare system that is to be implemented by all WHO Member States in order to achieve the aims of the 2030 Agenda, which include the introduction of universal health coverage and increased access to 'medicines and vaccines for all'. It is therefore imperative to expose the erroneous nature of the theories that underpin the practices of this healthcare system; such exposure is a core purpose of this book.

It is important to reiterate that the failings of the medical establishment system, as described throughout this book, refer solely to the approach to 'disease', they do not apply to emergency procedures or the use of surgical operations for physical injuries. Herbert Shelton explains this distinction in the statement that,

> "Only those materials and influences which are useful in the preservation of health are useful in the restoration of health. To this principle Hygienists make but one exception: namely, constructive surgery, as employed in wounds, broken bones, accidents, dislocations, etc."

All quotes by Herbert Shelton included in this chapter are from his book entitled *Natural Hygiene: Man's Pristine Way of Life*, unless otherwise stated.

It should be noted that the materials used by the medical establishment for the treatment and prevention of disease are not conducive to the preservation or restoration of health. All medicines and vaccines produced by the pharmaceutical industry are acknowledged to induce unintended effects in addition to their intended effects. But these additional effects are usually referred to as 'side effects' as if they are of little importance, but this is grossly misleading. Although unintended, these effects are, in reality, direct effects; their occurrence after the administration of a medicine or vaccine provides clear confirmation that these products are inimical to health, not supportive of it. Evidence of the harm they can cause is also confirmed by the phenomenon known as iatrogenesis, the incidence of which continues to rise.

It may be argued that the occurrence of adverse effects after the administration of a medicine or vaccine may indicate a correlation but should not be interpreted as evidence of causation. This argument is, however unjustified and unjustifiable; it can be refuted by the counter argument that all pharmaceutical medicines and vaccines are acknowledged to produce 'side effects'; they are therefore the direct causes of these effects. Furthermore, the majority of the chemical ingredients of pharmaceuticals, both medicines and vaccines, are inherently toxic to the human body. Many medicines are intentionally toxic; for example, the purpose of antibiotics and antivirals is to kill 'germs' and the purpose of cancer treatments is to kill cancerous cells. However, although treatments of this nature are known to be harmful to the patient, they are believed to be able to kill the causal agents of disease and therefore restore the patient to health.

The notion that poisons can preserve or restore health is entirely unfounded; it is impossible to poison a body back to health.

The inherently toxic nature of pharmaceuticals means that their effects are always harmful, as Herbert Shelton explains,

> "The only legitimate study of drugs in their relation to the body is that of toxicology. The local, general, synergistic, antagonistic, therapeutic and physiological 'actions' of drugs are myths, equally with their 'empiric actions'. That they accumulate in the body, that they occasion 'side actions', that they poison and injure, we do not deny. We only deny that they ever do anything else."

It is clear therefore, that the idea that pharmaceuticals can have a 'beneficial' effect on health is grossly mistaken. The reason they may appear to be beneficial is due to a complete misunderstanding of the nature and functions of the human body. As discussed in more detail later in this chapter, the human body is not mechanistic in nature; it is not an inert, albeit living, machine. On the contrary, it is a complex, self-regulating organism that is the only 'agent' with the ability to defeat disease; it is only the body that is able to restore and maintain health, which is the body's natural state.

A problem can only be solved when the nature of the problem has been fully understood and its root cause or causes have been correctly identified. Once this knowledge has been gained, it is possible to devise and implement the appropriate measures that have the ability to address the causes and thereby resolve the problem, which will eventually cease to exist.

It is clear that the problem of disease remains unresolved by the medical establishment; unfortunately, it is a problem that is not even in the process of being resolved. On the contrary, it is a continually worsening problem; the health of the vast majority of the people around the world is deteriorating not improving.

One of the main contributory factors to this problem is the fact that the medical establishment, which has assumed responsibility for the health of the entire world population, operates from the basis of fundamentally flawed beliefs about diseases and their causes as well, as the methods by which they should be treated and prevented. The rigid adherence to these erroneous beliefs perpetuates the existence of a serious obstacle to the medical establishment's ability to gain a full understanding of the real nature of disease, and thereby solve the problem.

The failure of modern medicine to solve this problem does not mean that it cannot be solved; as the discussions in this chapter will demonstrate.

The Nature of 'Disease'

The establishment defines a 'disease' as,

> "a disorder with a specific cause (which may or may not be known) and recognizable signs and symptoms..."

It is a core assertion of this book that the medical establishment has a poor level of understanding of the real nature of 'disease'. Whilst this assertion will no doubt be considered highly controversial; it is nevertheless corroborated by many of the medical establishment's own statements. The discussions in chapter seven, for example, reveal admissions that not only are the exact causes of a number of major NCDs unknown, but that many aspects of these diseases remain poorly understood. In addition, although infectious diseases are claimed to be understood, the discussions in chapter three reveal the existence of many anomalies and contradictions that seriously challenge this claim, and show that many aspects of these diseases also remain poorly understood.

In addition to the three beliefs discussed in the previous section, modern medicine has also adopted two philosophical doctrines; namely, mechanism, which posits the view that the human body is little more than a complex, albeit living, machine, and determinism, which posits the view that events are largely governed by pre-determining factors. In the context of disease, these doctrines mean that the human organism, which is considered to be essentially 'inert', can be attacked by any disease 'entity' as the result of certain pre-determining factors, especially genes, and that the battle against these disease entities, especially 'germs', can be successfully fought by the methods and practices of modern medicine. This is discussed in a 1977 article entitled *Modern Medicine's Shortcomings: Can We Really Conquer Disease?* that states,

> "Modern medicine holds to an essentially deterministic and mechanistic view of disease, in which the individual has no control over his disease and consequently must submit himself to the intervention of an external agent."

Although this view of disease is in accordance with the beliefs that underpin the practices of modern medicine, it too is fundamentally flawed.

It is clear therefore, that there are many genuine gaps in the knowledge the medical establishment claims to possess about disease, whether infectious or noncommunicable; however, it is generally believed that these knowledge gaps will be closed when sufficient information has accumulated as the result of medical research. But this is a mistaken belief; these gaps will not be closed by research conducted within a medical system that operates from the basis of an inadequate understanding of the fundamental nature of the problem it is studying.

Diseases are claimed to be identifiable by their signs and symptoms, but a number of diseases, especially those referred to as 'infectious', are associated with the same symptoms; fever, cough, fatigue and diarrhoea, for example, are common to many of them. The treatment of these conditions involves the use of medicines to alleviate the patient's symptoms, on the basis that the cessation of symptoms means that the disease has been defeated. If their symptoms fail to respond to this initial treatment, it may be suggested that the patient should undergo certain tests that will enable a more accurate diagnosis of the disease and lead to more effective treatment. The fact that such tests may need to be conducted in order to correctly identify a patient's disease, would seem to contradict the claim that diseases have recognisable signs and symptoms; many of them clearly do not.

The study of disease is conducted within the scientific field of pathology, the establishment definition of which is,

"the study of disease processes with the aim of understanding their nature and causes."

This is, however, rather misleading; a process involves actions, but pathology is the study of effects, not actions; as indicated by the definition, which continues with the statement that,

"This is achieved by observing samples of blood, urine, faeces and diseased tissue obtained from the living patient or at autopsy by the use of X-rays and many other techniques."

The study of samples of this nature involves a variety of preparation procedures to facilitate their observation under a microscope. The nature of these procedures is described by Dr Harold Hillman in his previously cited 2011 article entitled *Cell Biology at the Beginning of the 21st Century is in Dire Straits*, which bears repetition,

"When a tissue is prepared for histology, histochemistry, electron microscopy, or immunochemistry, an animal is killed; the tissue is excised; it is fixed or frozen; it is embedded; it is sectioned; it is rehydrated; it is stained; it is mounted; it is radiated by light, or bombarded by electron beams."

Although this refers to the study of animal tissue, the same, or very similar, procedures are employed in the study of diseased tissue obtained from a human patient, but these procedures, as well as the chemicals used as stains and fixatives, directly affect the tissue samples, which are clearly no longer alive when observed. Furthermore, the laboratory apparatus and the laboratory itself are sterile environments that bear no resemblance whatsoever to the natural environment of the tissue samples within the human body, from which they have been removed. Unfortunately, as discussed in chapter three, researchers are mostly oblivious of the extent to which their preparation procedures affect the samples they study.

It is acknowledged by some researchers that there are certain limitations to laboratory studies of this nature and to the conclusions that can be drawn from them with respect to their relevance to human disease; this is, however, a gross understatement. The changes to tissue samples produced by both the environment in which they are studied and the procedures to which they are subjected, are of such a profound nature that they raise serious questions about the ability of such studies to ascertain any useful information about the nature or causes of human disease.

This problem is compounded by the fact that the medical establishment operates according to a mechanistic view, on the basis of which it is believed that each disease is unique and identifiable by the specific effects it produces within the human body, which is also claimed to function mechanistically. If the mechanistic view were correct, the effects of each disease would be uniform and predictable, and all patients diagnosed with the same disease would exhibit exactly the same symptoms. Similarly, patients with the same disease would all respond in exactly the same manner to the same treatments, whether medicines or vaccines. But this does not reflect reality; in the real world, there is a great deal of variability, not only in the nature and severity of the symptoms exhibited by people diagnosed with the same disease, but also in people's responses to the same medicines; there is also a wide variability in people's reactions to vaccines. It is clear therefore, that the mechanistic view completely fails to represent an accurate description of the nature of disease or the functions of the human body.

Although the vast majority of disease research studies have been conducted with non-living samples, a few have been conducted with living specimens and these have generated some useful insights. The most significant insight, which has been gained from the study of cells and bacteria in particular, is the extent to which these living specimens can be affected by their environment.

As previously discussed, bacteria have demonstrated the ability to change their form in response to changes in their environment; a phenomenon known as pleomorphism. Living cells also respond to the condition of the environment in which they are placed, as demonstrated by Dr Bruce Lipton who describes his experiments with living cells in his book entitled *The Biology of Belief* and states that,

> "When I provided a healthy environment for my cells they thrived; when the environment was less than optimal, the cells faltered. When I adjusted the environment, these 'sick' cells revitalized."

The effect of the environment on human health has also been recognised by the medical establishment in the previously cited *Healthy Environments* report.

The 'environment' referred to is clearly the 'external' environment; but the health of living organisms is also affected by the condition of their 'internal' environment. All substances and influences that have the ability to adversely affect any aspect of the environment, whether internal or external, will adversely affect the health of the living organisms exposed to them. It is clear therefore, that harmful substances and influences not only contribute to ill-health, but, in reality, are some of the main causes of disease.

It is not the purpose of this section to discuss the causes of diseases, which are discussed later in the chapter; the ensuing discussion examines the real nature of the phenomenon known as 'disease'.

The philosophical principle known as Ockham's razor proposes that, when faced with different explanations about a phenomenon, the simplest one that contains the least number of assumptions is the one that is most likely to be correct. This principle will therefore be applied to the different explanations of 'disease', to determine which of them is the most appropriate to this phenomenon.

The first explanation to be examined in more detail is that of 'modern medicine', which, according to the establishment definition, describes 'disease' as,

"any bodily abnormality or failure to function properly..."

Although seemingly simple, this description is based upon the underlying belief that each bodily abnormality or malfunction is indicative of a unique disease entity that has attacked the body, and produced the signs and symptoms by which it can be identified. But, although claimed to be true, this belief represents a collection of assumptions including the notion that there are many hundreds, if not thousands, of different diseases that each affect the body in a specific manner and produce recognisable signs and symptoms.

It is indisputable that people can and do experience varying combinations of symptoms, but the existence of different symptom-complexes, together with the fact that each has been assigned a specific label, do not constitute irrefutable evidence of the existence of unique disease entities. As previously discussed, there is a great deal of variability in the nature and severity of the symptoms that people diagnosed with the same disease can experience; this variability poses a serious challenge to the assumption that each disease produces distinct and easily recognisable symptoms.

The medical establishment claims that disease exists in two forms; that they can be either infectious or non-infectious, although the latter are usually referred to as noncommunicable. The idea that certain diseases are infectious is based on the theory that pathogenic microorganisms invade and infect the body thereby causing disease; this theory also claims that 'germs' are transmissible between people. It is generally asserted by proponents of modern medicine that this theory has been established beyond any doubt, but this is not the case. As previously discussed, the explanations about infectious diseases contain many anomalies, one of which is that 'infection' is not always accompanied by symptoms; another is that 'infection' is not always followed by disease. Yet another anomaly is that infected people do not always transmit their 'germs' to others. These anomalies remain unexplained; they therefore challenge the underlying assumptions of the theories pertaining to 'infectious diseases'.

In addition, many other aspects of these diseases also remain unexplained; for example, the medical establishment provides no explanations of the mechanisms by which microorganisms are able to cause disease, or the mechanisms by which they are able to induce a range of symptoms that vary widely in severity, and can even cause death. The failure to explain these mechanisms poses yet another direct challenge to the veracity of the claim that microorganisms cause disease.

These challenges, as well as the discussions in chapter three, provide a clear refutation of the 'germ theory' and repudiate the existence of the phenomenon referred to as an 'infectious disease'.

The explanations about noncommunicable diseases (NCDs) are acknowledged to contain many unknown and poorly understood aspects, but they too, contain a number of assumptions. One of these assumptions is that 'genetic factors' play a major role in increasing the risk that a person will develop or die from an NCD; in other words, it is claimed as a fact that people with certain genes have a 'genetic predisposition' to develop a specific disease such as cancer, for example. But this is not a fact; the idea that genes are determining factors has, as previously discussed, been proven to be unfounded by the Human Genome Project.

The idea that genetic factors determine a person's state of health has also been disproven by research in the field of epigenetics, which Dr Lipton discusses in *The Biology of Belief*. He explains that genes do not control biology, which means that people do not have a 'genetic predisposition' to any disease, and states that,

> "In the last decade, epigenetic research has established that DNA blueprints passed down through genes are not set in concrete at birth. Genes are not destiny."

Despite the importance of these new research findings, the WHO has failed to amend the fact sheet about NCDs, the June 2018 version of which continues to claim that these diseases can result from a combination of factors that include 'genetic factors'.

Although individual NCDs were discussed in chapter seven, it is possible for people to be affected by more than one of these chronic conditions. The co-occurrence of two or more chronic conditions in the same patient is a phenomenon known as multimorbidity, which is acknowledged to be increasing in incidence, as indicated by a 2016 article entitled *Multimorbidity: What do we know? What should we do?* that states,

> "The number of people affected by multiple chronic diseases (multimorbidity) is increasing dramatically around the world..."

The growing prevalence of multimorbidity has also been recognised in a 2016 WHO report entitled *Multimorbidity* that states,

> "People living with a long-term condition often have multiple rather than a single condition. Such multimorbidity is common and has been rising in prevalence over recent years."

This statement is highly significant as it contradicts the most recent Global Burden of Disease (GBD) report of 2017, which asserts that people around the world have been experiencing improved health. A November 2018 editorial in *The Lancet* entitled *GBD 2017: a fragile world* claims that the GBD reports for the previous ten years have,

> "...portrayed an ever-healthier world."

The explanation in the 2016 WHO report for the increased incidence of multimorbidity is that it is related to increased life-expectancy, because it is a phenomenon that occurs more frequently in people over the age of 65; yet the report also states that,

"...the absolute number of people with multimorbidity has been found to be higher in those younger than 65 years..."

However, although it may be more common in people of advanced years, multimorbidity is not an inevitable consequence of ageing.

The medical establishment admits to the existence of knowledge gaps with respect to individual chronic conditions; it is therefore unsurprising that there are gaps in their knowledge about multimorbidity. These gaps are recognised by The Academy of Medical Sciences in a 2018 report entitled *Multimorbidity: a priority for global health research*, which will be referred to as the AMS report, that states,

"While it is generally accepted that multimorbidity is an increasing global health challenge, there remain massive gaps in our knowledge."

Part of the reason for the existence of these knowledge gaps is claimed to be due to insufficient research, as the report also states,

"Research into multimorbidity in younger adults and those living in low- and middle-income countries is particularly lacking."

Whilst a lack of research certainly hinders an understanding about the extent of the problem, increased research will not help to explain the reason for its existence, nor will it help to solve the problem, mainly because it will not result in the medical establishment altering its typical approach towards the treatment of disease.

Patients diagnosed with a single chronic condition are prescribed the medicine deemed to be the appropriate treatment for that condition. Patients diagnosed with multiple chronic conditions are therefore prescribed multiple medicines, each of which is deemed to be the appropriate treatment for each of their diseases; the use of multiple medicines to treat multiple conditions is referred to as polypharmacy. However, as previously discussed, all medicines are known to produce unintended adverse effects; this means that patients who take multiple medicines will invariably experience multiple adverse effects; a fact that is acknowledged in a March 2015 *BMJ* editorial entitled *Guidelines, polypharmacy and drug-drug interactions with multimorbidity* that states,

"One common consequence of polypharmacy is the high rate of adverse drug reactions..."

Furthermore, people diagnosed with multimorbidity can suffer from varying combinations of different chronic conditions, as the AMS report states,

"While there are limited data about the most commonly occurring clusters of conditions, it is accepted that multimorbidity is highly heterogenous and patients can experience a wide array of different combinations of conditions."

Patients with multimorbidity are treated with varying combinations of different medicines, each of which is claimed to have the ability to target, and therefore correct, the bodily abnormality or malfunction associated with each disease. But this claim is unfounded; the effects that a medicine

674

can induce can occur in many different parts of the body, they are not restricted to the specified target site. The use of multiple medicines can therefore result in multiple effects in multiple parts of the body; as the previously cited 2015 *BMJ* article states,

"Drugs have a network of effects that go well beyond a specific drug target, particularly in patients with multimorbidity."

The main problem is that pharmaceuticals are almost entirely untested for their efficacy, safety or potential adverse effects in the multiple combinations that may be prescribed to patients with multiple chronic conditions, as the AMS report explains,

"Although all medicines are rigorously tested, clinical trials for particular medical conditions don't usually include patients suffering from other conditions – which means there isn't a bank of good evidence showing how different medicines work together in patients suffering from multimorbidity."

One of the reasons that the vast majority of drug combinations remain untested is suggested by a 2018 article entitled *Artificial intelligence helps Stanford computer scientists predict the side effects of millions of drug combinations*, which admits that,

"Millions of people take upward of five medications a day, but testing the side effects of such combinations is impractical."

The 'impracticability' of conducting such extensive tests means that patients diagnosed with multimorbidity will have little, if any, information about the full range of potential 'side effects' they may experience, as the result of the particular combination of multiple medicines they have been prescribed as treatment for their particular combination of multiple chronic conditions.

Multiple medicines are also used in the treatment of a single disease; the recommended treatment of TB for example, involves the use of multiple antibiotics. This phenomenon, referred to as 'polypharmacology', is also increasingly common. The reason that multiple drugs are deemed to be necessary for the treatment of a single condition is explained by a 2014 article entitled *Systematic prediction of drug combinations based on clinical side-effects*, which states that a single drug,

"...sometimes shows limited efficacy, especially for complex diseases..."

Some of the most common diseases for which multiple drugs are used, because a single drug shows 'limited efficacy', are those said to be caused by bacteria. The reason that a single antibiotic drug is not effective is claimed to be because the bacteria have developed 'resistance' to it; but the use of multiple antibiotics is not necessarily more effective, as indicated by the phenomenon of MDR-TB (multidrug-resistant TB). However, bacteria are not the only microorganisms claimed to have developed 'drug resistance', which is perceived to pose a dire threat to health; as indicated by the February 2018 WHO fact sheet entitled *Antimicrobial resistance* that claims this to be,

"...an increasingly serious threat to global public health..."

This claim is misleading for reasons discussed in chapter three. The discussions presented within this book show that the explanations of disease promulgated by the medical establishment are fraught with problems of such a profound nature, that they challenge the veracity of the underlying theories, and raise doubts as to whether these explanations can be considered to fulfil the criteria of Ockham's razor as the most likely to be correct. These problems inevitably raise the further question of whether another explanation of disease exists that is better able to fulfil these criteria.

The forms of healthcare that operate outside of the 'mainstream' are commonly referred to as 'complementary and alternative medicine' (CAM), but proponents of 'modern medicine' invariably dismiss these as 'unorthodox', and refer to them using such derogatory terms as unscientific, pseudo-science, pseudo-medicine or quackery.

These CAM healthcare systems incorporate a wide variety of different practices, but often adopt a similar approach; for example, many employ the use of 'natural' substances as medicines and treat the patient rather than the disease. Whilst this approach may be considered preferable to that of the medical establishment, it is nevertheless dependent upon the same underlying theories, which are: that there are many distinctly different diseases; that certain diseases are caused by 'germs'; and that people affected by disease can only recover their health through treatment with some form of medicine. But these theories are flawed; any healthcare system that adopts an approach based on them will clearly be subject to the same, or at least very similar, problems as those encountered by the medical establishment. These systems are therefore, unable to furnish a more credible explanation of 'disease' than that of the medical establishment.

There are, however, 'non-mainstream' healthcare systems that operate from the basis of a different approach towards disease, its causes and treatment. The most notable of these is Natural Hygiene, which was developed during the 19th century. Although some of the early practitioners were qualified medical doctors, the pioneers of Natural Hygiene rejected the approach adopted by modern medicine, especially with respect to the use of 'medicines', which they recognised to be toxic, and with respect to the study of disease within the confines of the laboratory, as Herbert Shelton, a lifelong practitioner of Natural Hygiene, explains,

> "Its modern pioneers were brilliant men who were not afraid to depart from the ruts of orthodoxy and search for truth in despised places, but they were not men of the cloistered laboratory."

In their search to understand the real nature of disease, these men studied the 'laws of nature' and the application of these laws to human health. The studies these pioneers conducted over the course of many years, led them, and many who followed them, to the understanding that 'disease' is not an entity that attacks the body and needs to be fought and destroyed through the use of toxic 'medicines'. Their departure from orthodoxy, although earning derision from their contemporaries engaged in 'modern medicine', enabled them to develop a very different understanding of the nature of the human body, which they recognised to be a living organism that functions holistically in accordance with 'laws of nature'. They also discovered that anything that disrupts the body's functions will have a detrimental impact on health, as Herbert Shelton explains,

"The human organism is an indivisible whole and anything that tends to interfere with the unity of its structure or the unity of its function becomes a factor in the causation of disease."

The explanation of disease presented by Natural Hygiene can therefore be articulated as follows: 'disease' represents disruptions to the body's ability to function properly, and 'symptoms' are the manifestation of the body's responses to the presence of harmful substances and influences that include actions to expel toxins, repair damage and restore the body to its natural state of health.

The credibility of this new explanation can be demonstrated by reference to two symptoms, namely vomiting and diarrhoea. According to the medical establishment view, these symptoms are indicative of a 'disease' that is often, but erroneously, attributed to 'germs'. Yet no explanation is offered for the mechanism by which pathogens are able to cause these symptoms, the severity of which can vary widely. Such symptoms are however, perfectly explicable within the context of the new explanation of disease, as the body's responses to the presence in the digestive system of harmful substances and its efforts to expel them, as Herbert Shelton explains,

"A poison is taken into the stomach; the organism senses the presence of a non-usable and harmful substance and prepares to act accordingly. It is sent out by vomiting, or it is sent along the digestive tract into the colon and is expelled by means of a violent diarrhea."

The digestive system is clearly not the only part of the body that can be affected by harmful substances that need to be expelled; toxic materials can also enter the body through inhalation, absorption through the skin or injection, both intradermal and intramuscular. The route by which toxins enter the body will determine the tissues and organs that will be affected, and the nature of the responses the body will produce to expel them. Air pollutants, for example, which are inhaled, will have a greater impact on the respiratory system. The body's efforts to expel inhaled toxins will include symptoms such as sneezing and coughing, which are amongst the symptoms typical of respiratory 'diseases' such as asthma; the association between the inhalation of toxic irritants and asthma was discussed in chapter seven.

As the discussions in chapter six made perfectly clear, there are a huge number and wide variety of harmful substances and influences to which people are exposed in varying combinations on a daily basis; but these 'poisons' are not always or immediately expelled in such a simple manner as those that enter the digestive system. Some toxic substances, such as dioxins for example, bioaccumulate and are therefore more difficult to expel. But this does not mean that the body is powerless to expel toxins of this nature; on the contrary, the body possesses many self-protective mechanisms, as Herbert Shelton explains,

"When poisonous matter has accumulated in the system to the point where it becomes a menace to life, the body makes a violent effort to cast it out and we have pain, inflammations, fevers, and the whole train of acute diseases."

The use of the term 'acute diseases' in the above statement should not be construed as confirmation of the existence of distinctly different types of disease, for this is not his intended meaning. Instead, this term is used to represent short-lived conditions that are accompanied by self-limiting symptoms such as fever, sneezing, coughing, vomiting and diarrhoea, all of which are clearly indicative of the body's response to the presence of harmful substances and influences, and its efforts to expel them. As Herbert Shelton explains, the term 'acute disease' refers to,

"...vital action in some one or all of the living tissues or organs in resisting and expelling injurious substances and influences and in repairing damages."

When the body has expelled the 'injurious substances', these vital actions, or symptoms, will subside and then cease; but the cessation of symptoms should not be interpreted to indicate that all toxic materials have been eliminated from the body. The body constantly seeks to attain and maintain itself in the state of 'health', the vital actions necessary to expel toxins, repair damage and restore health are therefore ongoing processes that continue throughout life, as Herbert Shelton explains,

"The struggle of the system to cast out its accumulated toxins continues so long as the organism remains alive."

It should be clear therefore, that the greater the level of accumulated toxins in the body, the greater the effort required to eliminate them; toxins and their elimination are discussed in more detail later in this chapter.

Unfortunately, the body's vital actions in resisting and expelling harmful substances are interpreted as symptoms that need to be 'cured' through the use of medicine. However, pharmaceuticals, as well as a number of 'natural' medicines, contain substances that the body recognises as harmful and therefore need to be expelled through the appropriate vital actions; but these actions are then interpreted as symptoms of yet another disease that needs to be cured. This inevitably leads to a vicious cycle of diseases and 'cures'; a cycle that results in a progression from a series of 'acute diseases' to more serious conditions, usually referred to as 'chronic diseases', as Herbert Shelton explains,

"A child frequently develops colds. It develops sore throat, tonsillitis, bronchitis, pneumonia, all of which are cured, and soon followed by another cold, another tonsillitis, another bronchitis, and this process continues until chronic disease of the lungs evolves."

Chronic diseases are invariably of a longer duration and indicative of a far more serious health problem than acute diseases; they are therefore associated with very different symptoms, most of which do not represent obvious efforts to expel toxins, but they do represent the body's efforts to protect itself, repair damage and restore health. This means that the 'new' explanation of disease is equally applicable to chronic conditions, the symptoms of which are indicative of disruptions to the body's ability to function properly; cardiovascular diseases, for example, are a group of chronic conditions that represent dysfunctions within the cardiovascular system.

The real functions of the symptoms associated with chronic conditions can be demonstrated by the example of inflammation, which is acknowledged to be the body's response to injury, but is erroneously claimed by the medical establishment to be a main cause of many chronic conditions, including major NCDs. Inflammation is claimed to be a serious symptom that needs to be suppressed with anti-inflammatory drugs such as NSAIDs; but this course of action is based on a mistaken understanding of the role of inflammation. In addition to being the body's response to injuries and wounds, inflammation is also one of the mechanisms by which the body repairs damage; it is described by Herbert Shelton as 'remedial action'. The purpose of inflammation in both injury and disease is to provide the affected area with an increased supply of repair materials through an increased supply of blood. When the damage has been repaired, the blood supply returns to normal and inflammation ceases; the continuing presence of inflammation indicates that the damage has not been fully repaired, but it can be prolonged for other reasons, as discussed later in this section.

It has been demonstrated in many of the discussions in this book that pharmaceuticals are inherently toxic due to the nature of some, if not all of their ingredients; but this toxicity is virtually always intentional, the main purpose of the 'active' chemical ingredients of pharmaceuticals is to defeat disease or kill germs. Nevertheless, despite their toxicity, pharmaceuticals are credited with the ability to restore health. It should be noted that many 'natural' medicines, which are similarly credited with the ability to restore health, also contain toxic ingredients.

One of the main reasons that medicines, whether pharmaceutical or natural, are claimed to successfully achieve their intended purpose, is because people report that their symptoms reduced in severity, and even ceased entirely after they had taken the 'medicine'. They therefore attribute their 'recovery' from illness to the actions of the medicine; but this attribution is misplaced. No medicine possesses the ability to heal the body; the only 'agent' that does possess this ability is the body itself. The recovery from illness is solely due to the body's innate self-healing mechanisms, as Herbert Shelton explains,

"It is these processes of resistance and expulsion and the processes by which damages are repaired that are mistaken for the actions of drugs."

The most significant departure from orthodoxy of the early practitioners of Natural Hygiene was the rejection of the foundational beliefs on which 'modern medicine' is based, especially the belief that medicines cure disease. It is particularly notable that many of these practitioners were medical doctors who had obtained their qualification through the mainstream medical system, but rejected that system when they recognised its failings. Their studies led them to discover that obedience to the 'laws of nature' was the only effective method by which health could be attained, and they therefore incorporated this approach into their treatment of patients. In his book *Toxemia Explained*, Dr John Tilden MD refers to his experiences of using and then eschewing the use of 'medicines'; his words, which were cited in chapter one, bear repetition,

"Twenty-five years in which I used drugs, and thirty-three in which I have not used drugs, should make my belief that drugs are unnecessary and in most cases injurious, worth something to those who care to know the truth."

It is appropriate to therefore examine the explanation of disease presented by Natural Hygiene in the context of the criteria of Ockham's razor. As stated earlier, this 'new' explanation states that 'disease' represents disruptions to the body's ability to function properly, and that 'symptoms' are the manifestation of the body's responses to the presence of harmful substances and influences that include actions to expel toxins, repair damage and restore the body to its natural state of health.

In addition to its simplicity and lack of assumptions, this 'new' explanation dispels the many anomalies raised by the medical establishment explanation; for example, the varying nature and severity of the symptoms experienced by people alleged to have the same disease is no longer an anomaly because people do not have the same disease. Each person experiences differing symptoms that are manifestations of their body's response to the conditions within their 'inner environment'; as discussed in the later sections about the causes of 'disease'. Furthermore, this 'new' explanation of disease does not depend on assumptions about unknown processes, such as the mechanisms by which 'germs' are able to induce a wide variety of symptoms.

It is clear that this 'new' explanation of disease is the simplest and the one with the least number of assumptions; it therefore qualifies, in accordance with Ockham's razor, to be the one that is most likely to be correct. The veracity of this explanation is not only 'likely', but can be shown to be fully in accordance with a large and growing body of scientific evidence, as will be demonstrated.

It should be noted that, although the 'new' explanation of disease presented by Natural Hygiene forms the basis of the discussions in this chapter, this book presents a few differences with respect to some of the details. For example, the discussions in this book have demonstrated that 'germs' play no role whatsoever in disease, whereas the proponents of Natural Hygiene suggest that they may play a secondary, albeit minor role. In addition, the discussions in this final chapter provide a fuller explanation of the nature of disease, as well as the processes involved; they also include reference to all of the factors that contribute to the development of disease.

This 'new' explanation of disease, although highly controversial because of its divergence from orthodoxy, is corroborated by the findings of scientific research into the processes involved in virtually all diseases. One of its main assertions is that individual disease entities do not exist; that what have traditionally been referred to as different 'diseases' are, in reality, different expressions of an underlying disruption to the body's normal functions that manifest as a variety of different symptoms. Although the idea that there are no distinct disease entities may also be regarded as controversial, it is nevertheless corroborated by a growing body of evidence that demonstrates all 'diseases' share a common underlying mechanism. This common mechanism is oxidative stress; as indicated by a June 2000 article entitled *The Evolution of Free Radicals and Oxidative Stress*, which states that,

"Perhaps the most noteworthy observation concerning the role of oxidative stress in human disease is the commonality of it."

Free radicals are produced by the body's normal processes, including cell metabolism; but these molecules have unpaired electrons, which makes them highly reactive and potentially dangerous because, if not reduced by antioxidants, they can cause serious damage to the surrounding cells. The existence in the body of oxidative stress indicates the presence of an excessive level of free radicals that have begun the process of damaging the body's cells; it should be noted that cellular damage is also a common feature of 'disease'.

The growing body of research that has found oxidative stress to be the common underlying mechanism, although with different manifestations, of most, if not all noncommunicable diseases, is demonstrated by a 2014 article entitled *Introduction: oxidation and inflammation, a molecular link between non-communicable diseases*, which states that,

"Recent investigations show that many of these diseases share common pathophysiological mechanisms and are, at least in part, different manifestations in different organs of similar molecular alterations."

Pathophysiology is the study of functional changes that occur as the result of disease.

The article also states that,

"Mitochondrial alterations, oxidative stress and inflammation are inextricably linked and play major roles in the onset and development of non-communicable diseases."

It should be noted that mitochondrial alterations, or dysfunctions, can occur as the result of oxidative stress and the ensuing free radical damage.

Inflammation is a significant aspect of many major NCDs, but it is not a causal factor as the medical establishment suggests. Instead, it is oxidative stress, which is the underlying mechanism common to virtually all NCDs, that causes inflammation; as indicated by a 2014 article entitled *The role of oxidative stress during inflammatory processes* that states,

"In recent years, evidence has emerged that oxidative stress plays a crucial role in the development and perpetuation of inflammation."

As stated earlier in this section, inflammation may persist, especially within certain organs and tissues of the body where damage has occurred; but the reason that inflammation persists is because of the persistence of its underlying cause, namely oxidative stress.

The commonality of oxidative stress and free radical damage in NCDs also applies to cancer, as indicated by a 2014 article entitled *Inflammation, Free Radical Damage, Oxidative Stress and Cancer* that states,

"Tumor cells usually have an imbalanced redox status..."

Redox is the abbreviation of reduction-oxidation. Redox status is described as the balance between oxidants and antioxidants.

The discussion about cancer in chapter seven refers to the link between aneuploidy and cancer, in addition to which is a substantial volume of evidence that links aneuploidy and cancer to oxidative stress. This provides yet more evidence of the commonality of the processes and mechanisms involved in all conditions of ill-health, and further demonstrates the veracity of the 'new' explanation of disease.

Although oxidative stress is mainly associated with noncommunicable diseases, it has been recognised for more than two decades to also be associated with 'infectious diseases'; as indicated by a 1995 article entitled *The role of oxidative stress in HIV disease*, which states that,

"Indications of oxidative stress are observed in asymptomatic HIV-infected patients early in the course of the disease."

The medical establishment claims that one of the functions of free radicals is to defend the body against an attack by 'pathogenic microorganisms'; but this claim is clearly erroneous. If it were correct, the co-existence of oxidative stress and 'infection' with HIV, or any other so-called 'germ', would not be possible, because the invading pathogen should have been destroyed by the free radicals. This is yet another anomaly within the context of the 'germ theory' of disease. This anomaly is, however, removed by reference to the 'new' explanation of disease, which excludes any reference to 'germs', but fully recognises the role of oxidative stress and free radical damage.

Oxidative stress has also been observed to occur in cases of infections alleged to be caused by parasites, as indicated by a 2012 article entitled *Involvement of free radicals in parasitic infestations* that states,

"Several studies have reported the presence of oxidative stress in humans and animals infected with parasites..."

These 'infestations' include the parasites alleged to be the cause of malaria, as indicated by a 2012 article entitled *Oxidative Stress in Malaria*, which admits to the existence of yet another knowledge gap in the statement that,

"Despite the significant effort to eradicate this dangerous disease, lack of complete knowledge of its physiopathology compromises the success in this enterprise."

Both of these articles claim that oxidative stress is caused by the 'infections', but this is clearly a complete contradiction of the claim that the purpose of free radicals is to defend the body against 'infection'. Furthermore, despite the assertion that 'infections' cause oxidative stress, the medical establishment does not understand the mechanisms involved, as indicated by a 2017 article entitled *Oxidative stress in infection and consequent disease*, which refers to 'overwhelming evidence' of the existence of oxidative stress in many 'infectious diseases' but states that,

"...the impact of the majority of infectious agents on the host redux systems is not sufficiently characterized, with published data plagued by controversies."

Unfortunately, these controversies will persist whilst the medical establishment continues to believe that microorganisms are pathogenic.

Another particularly significant discovery is that oxidative stress, with the resulting free radical damage, is the common mechanism by which all of the 'substances and influences' that cause disease produce their harmful effects. The association between toxic substances and oxidative stress was recognised more than two decades ago, as indicated by a 1995 article, entitled *The role of free radicals in toxicity and disease*, which explains that,

"The toxicity of many xenobiotics is associated with the metabolic activation of foreign compounds to form free radicals..."

Xenobiotics are substances that are foreign to the body; a term that is commonly used to refer to synthetic chemicals, including pharmaceuticals.

The inclusion of pharmaceuticals in the category of 'xenobiotics' provides further corroboration of the assertion that the body recognises 'medicines' as 'foreign compounds' that are toxic and therefore need to be expelled. The assertion that pharmaceuticals are damaging rather than health-promoting is also substantiated by the acknowledgement that they produce the same mechanism by which all toxins cause damage. In other words, pharmaceuticals also increase the generation of free radicals; as indicated by the above cited article about malaria, which states that the drugs used in the treatment of the disease,

"...are inducers of free radical production."

Although free radicals are produced by normal metabolic functions, the body has innate mechanisms to protect itself against free radical damage; as indicated by a 2008 article entitled *Free Radicals, Antioxidants in Disease and Health* that states,

"The human body has several mechanisms to counteract oxidative stress by producing antioxidants..."

However, in order for these protective mechanisms to function properly, the body must be provided with all of the materials these mechanisms require. Although many antioxidants are obtained from the diet, some are also produced endogenously; but they are both necessary to protect the body from free radical damage, as the article states,

"Endogenous and exogenous antioxidants act as 'free radical scavengers' by preventing and repairing damages caused by ROS and RNS..."

ROS are reactive oxygen species and RNS are reactive nitrogen species.

The discussion in this section has demonstrated that 'disease' is not an entity that attacks the body, but represents dysfunctions within the body that have the same underlying mechanism. This unity of 'disease' can therefore be shown to be fully consistent with what has been referred to as the 'new' explanation of disease, but, in reality, should now be recognised to represent the real nature of disease, and therefore be the only explanation.

However, although the body is perfectly capable of maintaining itself in a state of health, the innate self-protective and self-healing mechanisms it employs can only be fully effective when they are supported by observing the 'laws of nature'. These 'laws' require that, where possible, exposures to harmful substances and influences should be avoided or minimised if complete avoidance is not possible. In addition, these 'laws' require that attention is paid to the substances consumed as food; the importance of 'nutrition' cannot be overstated.

The laws of nature can only be followed with sufficient knowledge about the factors that support health, so that they can be increased, and the factors that impede health, so that they can be avoided. These factors are the topics of the remaining sections of this chapter, after a brief discussion about the role of 'physical activity'.

Fitness & Exercise

The February 2018 WHO fact sheet entitled *Physical activity* states that,

"Insufficient physical activity is one of the leading risk factors for death worldwide."

In addition, one of the 'key facts' is claimed to be that,

"Globally, 1 in 4 adults is not active enough."

These are extremely bold claims, especially in view of the fact that the vast majority of the world population live in countries that are acknowledged to have poor health data collection systems.

The concern of the WHO about the low level of physical activity amongst the adult population, is based on the idea that 'physical inactivity' increases the risk of developing and dying from an NCD, as the fact sheet states,

"Insufficient physical activity is a key risk factor for noncommunicable diseases (NCDs) such as cardiovascular diseases, cancer and diabetes."

Whilst a low level of physical activity may have been observed to correlate with a diagnosis of an NCD, this does not prove the existence of a causal relationship. The discussion in the previous section showed that oxidative stress is the underlying mechanism of all types of disease, especially chronic diseases.

Despite the attempt to promote the idea that a causal link exists, there is no evidence that physical inactivity alone produces oxidative stress or causes any NCD. Nevertheless, on the basis of the claim that a causal relationship does exist, the medical establishment has increased its efforts to promote the health benefits of increased physical activity. A major part of this effort is the launch of a WHO-led initiative called *The Global action plan on physical activity 2018-2030* that includes a June 2018 report entitled *More Active People for a Healthier World*, which expands on the information in the fact sheet and states that,

"All forms of physical activity can provide health benefits if undertaken regularly and of sufficient duration and intensity."

It is not disputed that there are benefits to be gained from a certain level of physical activity; these benefits include increased mobility, flexibility and stamina, all of which are aspects of 'fitness' that can improve overall well-being. But the WHO erroneously equates physical activity with health, as indicated by the fact sheet that claims,

"Physical activity has significant health benefits and contributes to prevent NCDs."

The misleading nature of this claim can be demonstrated by the numerous examples of athletes who have tragically succumbed to, and even died from CVDs and cancers, the two major noncommunicable diseases. Most significantly, a substantial number of these athletes died at a very young age, often in their 20s or 30s; their high level of physical activity clearly failed to provide them with significant health benefits or prevent their premature death.

The sudden and unexpected death of an adult is a recognised phenomenon known as 'sudden cardiac death' (SCD), which is defined by a December 2016 article entitled *A Clinical Perspective on Sudden Cardiac Death* as,

"...death due to cardiac causes occurring within 1 hour of the onset of symptoms."

The article discusses the rate of 'sports-related death' in the general population, but adds the comment that,

"The sports-related sudden death rate is higher in elite athletes..."

Unfortunately, the article fails to explain why elite athletes experience a higher rate of sudden death from cardiac problems than the general population; but this finding directly contradicts the WHO claim that physical inactivity, rather than physical activity, increases the risk of dying due to a cardiac problem.

Although previously discussed, it is important to reiterate that the heart functions electrically, as acknowledged by the NHLBI (National Heart, Lung, and Blood Institute) web page entitled *Sudden Cardiac Arrest*, which states that,

"The heart has an electrical system that controls the rate and rhythm of the heartbeat. Problems with the heart's electrical system can cause irregular heartbeats called arrhythmias."

Interestingly, the above cited December 2016 article about Sudden Cardiac Death states that,

"SCD with negative pathological and toxicological assessment is termed 'sudden arrhythmic death syndrome'."

As previously discussed, 'sudden death' is not a syndrome.

The adverse health effects of the 'unnatural' EM radiation produced by all electrical devices, electronic equipment and wireless communications have been discussed, and will be further discussed later in this chapter; but it is important to emphasise the failure of the medical establishment to acknowledge the serious health hazards of exposures to electromagnetic radiation at levels far below that at which heating occurs.

The NHLBI web page makes an extremely interesting comment that there is no requirement for a pre-existing condition in cases of sudden cardiac arrest (SCA), which, it states,

"...can happen in people who appear healthy and have no known heart disease or other risk factors for SCA."

The absence of a pre-existing heart condition raises the inevitable question of what is the real cause of these sudden cardiac problems and sudden deaths.

It is obvious that there remain many significant knowledge gaps in the understanding the medical establishment claims to possess about 'sudden' cardiac problems, and in particular, the phenomenon of sudden death in otherwise healthy young adults; especially athletes who were obviously extremely 'physically active'. This phenomenon is however, entirely explicable from the perspective of the 'new' explanation of disease and an understanding of human biology with particular reference to the body's normal processes. One of the body's key processes is metabolism, which the establishment defines as,

"the sum of all the chemical and physical changes that take place within the body and enable its continued growth and functioning."

As previously discussed, normal metabolic processes involve the generation of free radicals; however, as Dr Russell Blaylock explains in *Health and Nutrition Secrets*, physical activity increases the rate of metabolism, which, in turn, increases the generation of free radicals and, as he states,

"...the number of free radicals generated during exercise depends on the intensity of the exercise and its duration."

He also explains the consequences of substantially raising the duration and intensity of physical activity,

"It is now known that intense exercise dramatically increases free-radical production and lipid peroxidation."

A dramatic increase in the production of free radicals can lead to oxidative stress and cause free radical damage, the underlying mechanism that is recognised to be common to virtually all types of 'disease', including those that affect the cardiac system.

Free radical damage is not an inevitable consequence of all forms of physical activity; it will only occur in the absence of an adequate level of antioxidants that can neutralise them. Unfortunately, most people, including elite athletes, are unaware that increased physical activity should be accompanied by an increased intake of antioxidants. As Dr Blaylock explains, this lack of awareness means that, when they increase their level of physical activity,

"...most people do not correspondingly increase their antioxidant intake."

Antioxidants are extremely important for providing protection against free radical damage, but they are not the only group of nutrients essential for health. Another extremely important nutrient is magnesium, a deficiency of which is also linked to cardiac problems, as Dr Carolyn Dean explains in *The Magnesium Miracle*,

"Magnesium deficiency may cause sudden cardiac death in healthy adults."

It is clear therefore, that 'fitness' is not synonymous with 'health'. Physical activity is beneficial, but it is vital that the body is in a state of 'good health' prior to an increase in the level of physical activity, otherwise, as this discussion has shown, it may be accompanied by serious health problems. Although an increased intake of nutrients, especially antioxidants, is an important aspect of 'good health', it is not the only factor to which people need to pay attention; as discussed in the remaining sections of this book.

The Four Factors

It has been asserted in previous discussions that conditions of ill-health are always the result of multiple factors; an assertion that is recognised, albeit to a limited extent, in the *Healthy Environments* report, which acknowledges that,

"...the root causes of ill health are multifactorial..."

The factors referred to in the report include many that cannot be described as 'causes'; whereas those discussed in the remaining sections of this chapter have been proven to be causal factors, because they induce the underlying mechanism common to all diseases.

The medical establishment erroneously claims that the conditions of ill-health referred to as infectious diseases are caused by 'biological factors'; in other words, pathogenic microorganisms. The conditions of ill-health referred to as noncommunicable diseases are, however, claimed to result from a combination of 'risk factors', which, according to the WHO fact sheet about NCDs, are genetic, physiological, behavioural and environmental.

A 'risk' refers to the possibility that an effect may occur, whereas a 'cause' is something that produces an effect; these terms are clearly not synonymous. The term 'risk factor' is defined on the WHO web page entitled *Risk factors* that states,

> "A risk factor is any attribute, characteristic or exposure of an individual that increases the likelihood of developing a disease or injury."

The reason that the medical establishment refers to 'risk factors' rather than causes is due to their lack of knowledge about the exact causes of NCDs; but this 'knowledge gap' is due entirely to their lack of understanding about the nature of 'disease' and the functions of the human body. The lack of understanding about the latter can be demonstrated by the idea that 'genetic factors' pose a significant risk to health; as Dr Bruce Lipton explains in his February 2012 article entitled *Epigenetics*,

> "Conventional medicine is operating from an archaic view that we're controlled by genes. This misunderstands the nature of how biology works."

The claim that 'environmental factors' contribute to ill-health cannot be disputed, although the medical establishment fails to acknowledge all of the relevant factors.

The subtitle of the *Healthy Environments* report is: *A global assessment of the burden of disease from environmental risks*. The purpose of the report is to identify the environmental factors associated with disease that are 'modifiable', so that interventions can be implemented to reduce the overall burden of disease. Unfortunately, many of the interventions used for the purpose of reducing disease exacerbate rather than solve the problem. One particularly pertinent example is the use of highly toxic pesticides for the purpose of eradicating vectors, especially mosquitoes, which are claimed to transmit parasites that are said to cause various diseases, such as malaria.

On the basis of the erroneous belief that 'diseases' are individual entities, the *Healthy Environments* report presents the results of its 'assessment' by reference to a number of diseases, each of which is considered separately in the effort to identify the specific 'environmental risks' with which that disease is associated. One of the listed diseases is 'asthma', a major determinant of which is erroneously claimed to involve 'genetic predisposition'. Although the report correctly attributes a role to air pollution, it is only in the context that air pollution provokes and exacerbates asthma; which indicates that the condition already exists. It should be noted however, that many components of air pollution are known to cause oxidative stress and that a recognised association exists between oxidative stress and asthma.

Whilst the report acknowledges many 'environmental risk factors' that have been associated with various 'diseases', it fails to recognise the full range of hazardous substances and influences or the full extent of their adverse effects on the environment. One of the reasons that the report fails to include all of the relevant 'environmental factors' is claimed to be because their 'risk' has not been fully assessed; as indicated by the statement that,

"There are many examples of risks that have not been adequately evaluated, including the effects of emerging risks (e.g. more intensive agricultural practices and zoonoses), the effects of many longterm chemical exposures on cancers or endocrine disorders, and the impact of electromagnetic and other exposures from new technologies."

This statement is disingenuous; many of the risks associated with chemical and electromagnetic exposures have been evaluated and are known, as will be further discussed in this chapter; the main reasons that the medical establishment denies that they pose serious risks to health were discussed in chapter nine.

The 'new' explanation of the nature of 'disease' states that disruptions to the body's ability to function properly are caused by exposures to 'harmful substances and influences', although the body has innate mechanisms by which it can protect itself. However, the ability of these mechanisms to function properly and protect the body, can be compromised if exposures to 'harmful substances and influences' reach a substantially high level; which is precisely the predicament now faced by the vast majority of the world population.

It is, however, possible to improve this situation, but it requires people to have the necessary information to enable them to take the appropriate actions; these actions involve reducing exposures to harmful substances and influences, and require attention to be paid to everything that is supportive of health. All of the substances and influences that affect human health, whether beneficially or otherwise, can be identified as belonging to one of four categories, which are referred to in the remaining sections of this chapter as 'the four factors'; these are nutrition, toxic exposures, EM radiation exposures and stress.

Nutrition

The medical establishment acknowledges that 'nutrition' is important, but has a poor understanding of the full meaning of the term and of its importance to health. The WHO web page entitled *Nutrition* defines the term as,

"...the intake of food, considered in relation to the body's dietary needs."

The real meaning of nutrition refers to far more than is included in this definition, as this discussion will demonstrate.

Although the Oxford Concise Medical Dictionary defines 'nutrition' with reference to the intake of nutrients, it defines a nutrient as,

"a substance that must be consumed as part of the diet to provide a source of energy, material for growth or substances that regulate growth or energy production."

This definition highlights one of the major, but erroneous, ideas promulgated by the medical establishment about nutrition, which is that the main purpose of food is to provide the body with 'energy'; as also demonstrated by the WHO *Nutrition* web page, which defines 'good nutrition' as,

"...an adequate, well-balanced diet combined with regular physical activity..."

Physical activity is not a component of 'good nutrition'. The reason for its inclusion in the definition is to promote the idea that an 'adequate' diet is one that provides sufficient calories to meet, but not exceed, the body's requirement for energy to be expended in physical activity; as indicated by the WHO October 2018 *Healthy diet* fact sheet which claims that,

"Energy intake (calories) should be in balance with energy expenditure."

A diet that is focused on the energy value of foods is not synonymous with a 'healthy diet', nor does it represent 'good nutrition'. The claim that energy intake should balance energy expenditure is based on the notion that an intake of calories that exceeds those expended in physical activity is the main cause of overweight and obesity; as indicated by the February 2018 WHO fact sheet entitled *Obesity and overweight* that states,

"The fundamental cause of obesity and overweight is an energy imbalance between calories consumed and calories expended."

Overweight and obesity are defined in the fact sheet by reference to the accumulation of body fat. But body fat does not accumulate solely as the result of an excess intake of calories; it is far more closely and causally related to the quality of the foods consumed. The fact sheet explains that overweight and obesity are determined by reference to a measurement known as BMI (body mass index). For adults, overweight is defined as a BMI between 25 and 30, whereas obesity is defined as a BMI of 30 or higher; the criteria for children are different and dependent on their age.

The most significant aspect of a high BMI is that it is associated with an increased 'risk' of developing an NCD; as indicated by the fact sheet that claims,

"Raised BMI is a major risk factor for noncommunicable diseases..."

The main NCDs associated with a high BMI are cardiovascular disease, diabetes and certain cancers, but these conditions are not caused by an excess intake of calories. In accordance with the 'new' explanation of disease, these conditions represent different manifestations of dysfunctions within the body, due to exposures to 'harmful substances and influences' that increase the generation of free radicals, induce oxidative stress and result in damage to the body's cells and tissues.

The emphasis by the medical establishment on the energy value of foods is largely based on the mechanistic view of the body that promotes the idea that the human requirement for food is analogous to a vehicle's requirement for fuel. But this is a false analogy; the human body is not mechanistic in nature. Although there is a need to consume foods that provide the necessary materials for conversion into energy, the human body is a living organism whose complex life-sustaining processes bear no resemblance whatsoever to the purely mechanical functions of machines, including those produced using the most advanced technologies.

The fundamental purpose of eating is to provide the body with the necessary materials to support all of its processes, not merely those that involve the production of energy. Substances consumed as food should therefore contain those necessary materials, more commonly referred to as nutrients. This means that 'nutrition' should be more correctly defined as the intake of nutrients and their transformation into materials for utilisation in the body's biochemical processes that promote health and sustain life; as summarised by Herbert Shelton who explains that,

> "To serve in any proper sense as food a substance must be capable of assimilation by the tissues; this is to say, the cells must be able to take it up from the blood stream and incorporate it into themselves and make it a normal constituent of cell substance and use it in the processes of life."

Any substance that cannot be transformed into materials that the body can utilise is not a nutrient; a substance that is unusable by the body will be antagonistic to it and must therefore be regarded as a 'poison', as he also explains,

> "Any substance that cannot be so appropriated by the cells and organized into living structure, this is to say, any substance that cannot be metabolized, is a poison."

Although the WHO refers to good nutrition as 'a cornerstone of good health', it nevertheless fails to recommend policies that would make nutrition a cornerstone of healthcare. One of the reasons for this failure is due to the influence of vested interests, especially of the chemical, pharmaceutical and food industries, whose profitability would be threatened by increased public awareness of the true meaning of nutrition.

Furthermore, most members of the medical establishment are reluctant to improve their knowledge about 'nutrition' because, as previously discussed, the topic is considered to be 'unscientific', 'fluffy' and the 'realm of dieticians not doctors'. The perpetuation of this disparaging attitude is largely due to the virtual absence of nutrition courses in the curricula of most medical schools. This is, however a serious omission; understanding nutrition is fundamental to an understanding of human health, which, according to the medical establishment, is the indisputable 'realm of doctors'. However, medical researchers do not understand health because they study 'disease', or more accurately, they study the effects of disease; but their investigations are based on an erroneous understanding of the nature of the phenomenon that they study.

Another reason for the perpetuation of such a disparaging attitude towards the topic is because a genuine study of nutrition involves a different approach from that employed by 'modern medicine'; as indicated by Dr T Colin Campbell PhD who, in his 2017 article entitled *Nutritional Renaissance and Public Health Policy*, states that,

> "Nutrition is a wholistic science whereas medical practice is reductionist, a serious mismatch that causes biased judgement of nutrition."

This reductionist approach is widespread throughout modern medicine; this can be seen by the fact that there are many different specialist fields that each focus on a separate part of the body or on a single disease. It is therefore unsurprising that the medical establishment studies individual nutrients on the basis of the idea that they each function independently; but this too is a serious error.

The development of microscopes with increased lens magnification that enabled scientists to discover the fundamental components of 'matter', also facilitated the study of foods, which were discovered to be comprised of the substances known as nutrients, of which there are two main categories. Nutrients that are required by the body in relatively large amounts are referred to as macronutrients, of which there are three types; namely, carbohydrates, fats and proteins. Nutrients that are required in comparatively small amounts are called micronutrients, of which there are two types; namely, vitamins and minerals.

Carbohydrates, a group that comprises starches, sugars and fibre, are found in a wide variety of foods. They are referred to as the body's main source of energy, because most carbohydrates are broken down during the digestive processes and converted into sugars, the main type of which is glucose, also known as blood sugar, that is used or stored according to the body's energy needs. Although sugars are a form of carbohydrate, they are not all the same nor are they all processed by the body in the same way, as discussed in chapter six. However, it is important to emphasise that the processes that convert carbohydrates into glucose and release glucose into the bloodstream are tightly controlled by the body's self-regulating mechanisms; but these mechanisms can be disrupted by the consumption of certain carbohydrates, especially refined carbohydrates and sugars.

Sucrose, or refined sugar, is a manufactured substance that is a common ingredient of processed food products and has been associated with many conditions of ill-health, including diabetes. The consumption of sucrose disrupts the body's normal control mechanisms and causes a surge in the level of sugar released into the bloodstream. It is widely acknowledged that this 'sugar surge' increases the generation of free radicals that can lead to oxidative stress and free radical damage, the underlying mechanism common to most, if not all, chronic health problems, including diabetes.

The problems with refined sugars were discussed in chapter six, but it is important to reiterate that the recommendation to reduce the intake of 'free sugars' does not apply to the natural fructose found in fresh foods, especially fruits and vegetables.

Starches are found in some vegetables but mostly in grains; they are the carbohydrates common to most staple foods, such as bread, pasta, rice, corn and potatoes. They are also the main form of carbohydrates that are converted into glucose and therefore constitute a major source of calorie intake. It is for this reason that starch-based foods are usually minimised, or even avoided, by people who wish to lose weight by reducing their calorie intake.

This is yet another example of the misplaced focus on the calorific value of foods rather than their nutritional value. A far more important quality of starch-based foods that should be considered is whether they have been refined or not. In common with all forms of processing, the 'refining' of grains substantially reduces their nutritional content to the extent that most have little, if any, remaining nutritional content. Rice, for example, is refined by the removal of the husk, bran and germ, but these are the parts that contain virtually all of the nutrients; refined rice is therefore almost entirely devoid of any nutritional value.

Many refined grains, such as wheat, and the products with which they are made, such as breads, are then 'fortified' to replace the nutrients lost in processing; but, for reasons discussed later in this section, the nutritional content is not improved through fortification with individual nutrients. Most refining processes also deplete grains of their fibre, which is another extremely important component as it provides the roughage necessary for proper digestion. There is, however, an increasing acknowledgement that whole grains are healthier than refined grains; even the WHO *Healthy diet* fact sheet refers to the inclusion of whole grains as part of a healthy diet.

Proteins, the second category of macronutrients, are comprised of amino acids, some of which are synthesised by the body, although others, referred to as essential amino acids, are not and must therefore be obtained from the diet. Animal-based foods, such as meat and dairy products, are rich sources of protein and believed to be the body's main, if not only, source of protein. On the basis of the erroneous belief that humans are 'natural' meat-eaters, a topic that will be discussed later in this section, it is claimed that diets that exclude animal foods will be protein deficient. This is, however, an erroneous claim; as indicated by a 2013 article entitled *Nutritional Update for Physicians: Plant-Based Diets*, which states that,

"Generally, patients on a plant-based diet are not at risk for protein deficiency."

Although the article defines a 'plant-based diet' as one that minimises rather than avoids the consumption of animal foods, it nevertheless, recommends that physicians encourage their patients to increase their consumption of plant foods.

It is important to note that a fully plant-based diet, in other words, one that totally excludes animal foods, is perfectly capable of fulfilling the human requirement for protein. Furthermore, in his book entitled *The China Study*, T Colin Campbell refers to a significant volume of compelling research which shows that,

"...plant protein, which allows for slow but steady synthesis of new proteins, is the healthiest type of protein."

Fats, the third category of macronutrients, are important components of the diet, even though they are notoriously high in calories. However, like the other macronutrients, fats have also been the subject of misleading information, the most significant of which relates to the association between the intake of fats, raised cholesterol levels and increased 'risks' to health. Although the mistaken ideas about 'good' and 'bad' cholesterol were discussed in chapter one, it must be reiterated that cholesterol is essential for many of the body's functions, and that most of the body's cholesterol is produced by the liver. It is also important to repeat that the health problems claimed to be associated with high cholesterol levels are not caused by 'bad' cholesterol, but by oxidised cholesterol. In his 2006 book, *Health and Nutrition Secrets*, Dr Russell Blaylock states that,

"More than fifteen years ago it was discovered that cholesterol is not dangerous unless it is oxidised..."

The reason that LDL cholesterol has been designated as the 'bad' form is because it is easier to oxidise than HDL cholesterol. As discussed in chapter seven, Dr Blaylock explains that cholesterol is oxidised by free radicals and that,

"...oxidized HDL cholesterol is just as dangerous as oxidised LDL cholesterol."

The most unhealthy types of fat are hydrogenated fats and industrially-produced trans-fats; as indicated by the WHO *Healthy diet* fact sheet which states that these fats,

"...are not part of a healthy diet and should be avoided."

It should be noted that these fats are only found in industrially-produced processed food products; they are therefore easy to avoid.

The fact sheet also recommends that the intake of saturated fats, which are almost exclusively found in animal foods, is reduced. The suggested ways to achieve this reduction include the replacement of full-fat dairy foods with reduced-fat versions; but these are not necessarily healthier options because the removal of the fat content requires additional processing, which further reduces the overall nutritional content.

Another suggested method by which the intake of saturated fats can be reduced is the replacement of fats such as butter, lard and ghee, with polyunsaturated fats, such as soybean, canola, safflower and sunflower oils, on the basis that they are healthier; but this too is not necessarily the case. Some of these oils are produced from GM crops; this is particularly the case with respect to oils made from soybeans, which are one of the most common GM crops. Furthermore, these oils, which are often described as 'refined', are usually produced by industrial processes that subject the crops to harmful chemicals in the extraction of the oil.

Oils can be produced by methods that do not involve GM crops or harmful chemicals and are therefore healthier; cold pressing, for example, is the method commonly used to produce oils such as olive and coconut oils. Although there are recommendations that even these oils should be avoided because of their fat content, this advice is based on the erroneous idea that all forms of 'fat' raise cholesterol to a dangerous level.

It is clear from the foregoing that plant foods are excellent sources of all three macronutrients; but they are also vital sources of micronutrients, which the WHO web page entitled *Micronutrients* refers to as,

"...the 'magic wands' that enable the body to produce enzymes, hormones and other substances essential for proper growth and development."

One of the essential roles of micronutrients, with particular reference to the underlying mechanism of all forms of 'disease', is to act as antioxidants and therefore protect the body from oxidative stress and the resulting free radical damage; as Dr Russell Blaylock explains in *Health and Nutrition*

Secrets,

"... most of us are familiar with vitamin antioxidants such as vitamin A, beta-carotene, vitamin C, and vitamin E. All are powerful antioxidants that neutralize a significant number of free-radicals. Less well-known antioxidants are vitamins D and K, magnesium, zinc and manganese. Also, there are over forty carotenoids and five thousand flavonoids from plants in the human diet that act as antioxidants."

He explains that all of these antioxidants are important for the body because,

"Each antioxidant acts in a different place in the cells and tissues."

Although the identification of different micronutrients has facilitated a certain level of understanding of nutrition, the study of individual nutrients and their functions is a perfect example of the reductionist approach that prevails within the medical establishment and, to a certain extent, the 'alternative health' community, many of whom also promote the health benefits of individual nutrients. The main consequence of this approach has been to ignore the wholeness of foods and to only consider their individual fragmented components. This is, however, a serious mistake; in the case of food, the whole is definitely far greater than the sum of its parts.

Nevertheless, the study of the individual nutrient components of foods has led to ideas that a deficiency in a single nutrient can lead to specific health problems; the WHO, for example, claims on the web page entitled *Micronutrient deficiencies* that,

"Vitamin A deficiency (VAD) is the leading cause of preventable blindness in children..."

Other 'diseases' have also been associated with specific nutrient deficiencies; scurvy, for example, is claimed to be caused by a severe vitamin C deficiency. However, the 'new' explanation of disease demonstrates that scurvy can be more accurately described as a condition that results from oxidative stress and free radical damage due to a severe antioxidant deficiency. This can be seen by the fact that scurvy can be resolved by the addition of citrus fruits such as limes or lemons to the diet. As discussed below, foods contain complex mixtures of nutrients; which means that deficiency diseases can never be due to a deficiency of only one single type of nutrient.

It is increasingly recognised that the 'modern diet', meaning one comprised mainly, if not entirely of manufactured processed food products and drinks, is unable to supply all of the micronutrients essential for health. However, it is believed that this problem can be solved through the use of dietary supplements that supply 'missing' nutrients. But this is an erroneous belief for many reasons, one of which is that it is virtually impossible to test for individual nutritional deficiencies. But even if a deficiency of a particular nutrient could be ascertained, the problem cannot be solved by chemical compounds synthesised in a laboratory. Although the dietary supplements industry justifies the use of synthetic chemicals on the basis that they are 'chemically identical' to the nutrients that occur naturally in foods, this is grossly misleading. The problem with vitamin supplements is explained by Dr Robert Thiel PhD in his article entitled *The Truth About Vitamins in Supplements*, in which he states that,

> "The truth is that most vitamins in supplements are made or processed with petroleum derivatives or hydrogenated sugars."

In his article entitled *Food Antioxidants are Superior to Isolated Antioxidants*, he further explains that, even if they were chemically similar, the vitamins in manufactured supplements are structurally different from those found in foods. An even more important fact is that the vitamins in foods are always accompanied by 'other elements' that are necessary for the absorption of the nutrients into the body's cells, but are entirely absent from supplements. The vitamins in supplements are therefore incomplete nutrients, as Dr Thiel explains,

> "Isolated, non-food vitamins, even when not chemically different are only fractionated nutrients."

Although certain vitamin supplements are claimed to be 'food-based', these too lack all of the 'other elements' that occur naturally in foods and are essential for the proper functioning of nutrients. The importance of these 'other elements' cannot be overstated; their absence is a major obstacle that prevents supplements from being able to confer any significant health benefits. It is for this reason that research studies, which investigate the effects of individual nutrients by conducting experiments with synthetic chemical compounds, invariably report few, if any beneficial health effects.

These problems are not exclusive to vitamin supplements; they also apply to mineral supplements, as Dr Thiel explains in his article entitled *The Truth About Minerals in Nutritional Supplements*,

> "The truth about nearly all minerals in supplements is that they are really industrial chemicals made from processing rocks with one or more acids."

The human body is unable to digest rock minerals, which are rejected as unusable and expelled from the body; supplements of this nature are therefore entirely useless. Plants, by comparison, are perfectly able to absorb natural rock minerals and convert them into a form that is suitable for digestion, absorption and assimilation by the human body when plants are consumed. It is for this reason that plants are the only sources of minerals that the human body can absorb, as Herbert Shelton states,

> "We have to draw our mineral nutrients exclusively from the plant kingdom and not from the soil."

In order to function effectively, minerals also require the presence of 'other elements', including other minerals that must be in the right form and in the right balance with respect to each other. The importance of this relative balance can be demonstrated by reference to the relationship between calcium and magnesium. Calcium is known to be essential for healthy bones, but its effectiveness also requires the presence of vitamin D, as indicated by the NHS web page entitled *Food for strong bones* that states,

> "You need sufficient calcium to strengthen your bones and vitamin D to help your body absorb calcium."

On the basis of this need for adequate calcium, people are advised to ensure their diet includes a good supply of calcium-rich foods, especially milk and dairy products. But a high intake of calcium alone is unable to strengthen bones, even in the presence of adequate levels of vitamin D. The reason is that the absorption of calcium into the bone also requires adequate levels of magnesium, which the NHS web page clearly fails to mention. Nevertheless, Dr Carolyn Dean explains in *The Magnesium Miracle* that,

"Adequate levels of magnesium are essential for the absorption and metabolism of calcium."

Most diets provide a sufficient intake of calcium, but rarely provide sufficient magnesium. The inevitable result of the regular consumption of a magnesium-deficient diet will be an imbalance between the relative levels of calcium and magnesium; an imbalance that can have many potentially harmful consequences for health. A high level of calcium that is not readily absorbed into bone due to insufficient magnesium can result in a build-up of calcium in the blood, which can cause kidney stones. If the level of calcium becomes very high, it can lead to a condition known as hypercalcemia, which, although rare, can impair the normal functions of the brain and heart.

Magnesium is therefore an extremely important mineral, but its functions are not limited to assisting the absorption of calcium into bone; it is also associated with many other functions, as Dr Dean states,

"Magnesium regulates more than 325 enzymes in the body..."

One of the main reasons that most diets are magnesium deficient is because this essential mineral is depleted by all forms of processing; processed food products will therefore be particularly low in magnesium. This deficiency can, however, be rectified by the consumption of magnesium-rich foods, as Dr Dean advises,

"To enrich your diet with magnesium, increase your consumption of green vegetables, nuts, seeds, legumes and unprocessed grains."

A similar relationship exists between sodium and potassium, both of which are important for the healthy functioning of cells, especially those of the heart. The WHO *Healthy diet* fact sheet recommends that the intake of salt is reduced in order to lower the body's sodium levels. But this is misleading; the body cannot metabolise rock minerals and therefore does not absorb sodium from 'table salt'. As discussed in chapter one, one of the main causes of elevated sodium levels is a deficiency of potassium. The medical establishment has, however, begun to recognise the importance of potassium in balancing the level of sodium; as indicated by the October 2018 WHO *Healthy diet* fact sheet which states that,

"Potassium can mitigate the negative effects of elevated sodium consumption on blood pressure. Intake of potassium can be increased by consuming fresh fruit and vegetables."

It is clear that an increased intake of fresh fruits, vegetables and other plant foods will mitigate many health problems.

Soil nutrient levels have unfortunately declined substantially over the past few decades in many parts of the world and this has inevitably reduced the nutritional content of the foods grown in such nutrient-poor soils; but this problem cannot be solved through the use of nutritional supplements or the fortification of foods. The only solution is to replenish the soil with nutrients. It is claimed that fertilisers perform the important task of replacing lost nutrients; but the products used by most industrial agricultural practices are NPK fertilisers, which means they only contain nitrogen, potassium and phosphorus, and are therefore deficient in all of the other important minerals, especially magnesium. However, the fact that they lack many essential nutrients is not the only problem associated with these fertiliser products; the discussion in chapter six referred to the sources of the phosphorus and nitrogen used by the fertiliser industry.

In addition to the major minerals, are others that are required in such tiny amounts that they are referred to as 'trace elements'. In 1996, the WHO produced a report entitled *Trace elements in human nutrition and health*, which, according to a web page with the same title, provides authoritative recommendations about nineteen trace elements divided into three categories. The page states that,

"These include essential elements, such as iodine and zinc, probably essential elements, such as manganese and silicon, and potentially toxic elements, such as fluoride, lead, cadmium and mercury, which may also have some essential functions at low levels."

This report appears to be the most recent WHO publication on the topic of 'trace elements' but it is in urgent need of revision. An abundance of evidence has accumulated since 1996 that demonstrates unequivocally that fluoride, lead, cadmium and mercury are all definite rather than merely 'potential' toxins; there is also ample evidence that demonstrates none of them has any 'essential function' in the human body at any level.

It should be clear that a reductionist approach to nutrition is entirely wrong because the focus on individual nutrients ignores the importance of the wholeness of foods; as indicated by Herbert Shelton who states in his book entitled *The Science and Fine Art of Natural Hygiene* that,

"All of this modern attention to separate food factors—proteins, carbohydrates, fats, minerals, vitamins, etc.—amounts to fragmentation of what should be something whole and sound, accessible to us without our having to take thought."

The nutrients contained in different foods, although in varying amounts and combinations, are always accompanied by all of the necessary 'other elements' that enable them to perform their function, which is to support the body's processes that maintain health as well as sustain life, as Dr Blaylock explains,

"There is growing evidence that it is the combined effects of these complex nutrients – not single nutrients – that provide us with such memorable health benefits."

The reason that foods provide such health benefits is because the nutrients they contain function synergistically, as indicated by Dr Campbell who, in his previously cited *Nutritional Renaissance* article, states that,

"The wholeness of food illustrates how nutrients working collectively and dynamically, create health."

Another misleading idea, which is based on the exhortation by Hippocrates to 'let thy food be thy medicine', is that certain foods have 'medicinal properties'. Some foods, for example, are claimed to be 'natural antibiotics'; but this is an erroneous claim. The human body is the natural home of trillions of bacteria, most of which reside in the digestive system where they assist the digestive processes. This not only means that real foods do not kill bacteria, but that substances that do kill bacteria cannot be referred to as 'foods'. Although some are claimed to be particularly beneficial for health, foods do not act as 'medicine'; as Herbert Shelton states,

"...in no sense can foods be regarded as medicinal. Foods are nutritive substances..."

Foods therefore, do not kill germs, 'heal' the body or 'cure' any disease. Healing is a biological process that is solely performed by the body, whose innate self-healing mechanisms are supported by the nutrients obtained from foods.

One of the consequences of the reductionist approach to nutrition, together with the belief that 'everything is made from chemicals', has been that the food industry has been permitted to use synthetic chemicals as ingredients of their products, and as food additives to perform certain 'technological functions'. However, despite the claim that they are 'chemically identical' to the elements found in a food, no industrially-produced compound can reproduce a product of nature in exactly the same form as that provided by nature; as Herbert Shelton explains,

"It is possible to analyze an apple and ascertain its chemical constituents; but all the chemists in the world cannot make an apple, nor anything that can substitute for it."

Nevertheless, the WHO approves the use of chemical substances in food products on the proviso that they meet the standards set by the Codex Alimentarius Commission. Although previously cited in chapter six, the definition of a 'food additive', according to Codex standard STAN 192-1995, deserves repetition; it states,

"Food additive means any substance not normally consumed as a food by itself and not normally used as a typical ingredient of the food, whether or not it has nutritive value..."

A substance that is not normally consumed as a food or has no nutritive value cannot be described as a 'food'. As stated earlier in this discussion, a substance that is not a nutrient will be antagonistic to the body and should, more accurately, be described as a 'poison'. Nevertheless, the WHO, which claims to be the authority for public health, permits the use of 'poisons' on the basis that they are deemed 'safe' according to JECFA. However, as discussed in chapter six, 'safe' is a relative term that means the substance is regarded as safe provided it does not exceed the recommended usage level.

Real foods are inherently safe; their safety can only be compromised if they have been contaminated by toxic substances. However, even if uncontaminated, real foods may cause digestive discomfort, but this will only occur if an excessive amount has been consumed, as Herbert Shelton explains,

"The overconsumption of the best foods will produce trouble."

This 'trouble' may include pain and discomfort, which are the body's signals to cease eating so that the over-extended digestive system can process the food already consumed. It is inappropriate to interpret these symptoms to mean that the food has become a 'poison' due to the consumption of a large dose.

Food additives, by comparison, are inherently toxic due to the nature of their ingredients, but the consumption of foods that contain additives may not immediately produce an effect, because the additive may be at a sufficiently low level that the body is able to process and expel it. However, the ability to tolerate toxins will differ according to each individual and their state of health.

The body's reactions to the consumption of foods containing toxic substances may be dramatic and involve symptoms such as vomiting and diarrhoea, or they may involve symptoms that are commonly associated with 'allergies'; the problems with the attribution of symptoms to a 'food allergy' were discussed in chapter seven. However, it is not insignificant that there is an increased incidence of allergies that correlates with the increased use of toxic chemicals in agriculture and food production. It may be argued that this correlation is not proof of causation, but this is an inappropriate argument, because there is an abundance of evidence that undeniably shows direct links between allergies, exposures to toxic substances, oxidative stress and illness. The problems with toxins are discussed in more detail later in the chapter.

In addition to the acknowledgement by the WHO on the *Nutrition* web page that 'good nutrition' is an important component of 'good health', is the acknowledgement that 'poor nutrition' is related to 'poor health'; as indicated by the statement that,

"Poor nutrition can lead to reduced immunity, increased susceptibility to disease, impaired physical and mental development, and reduced productivity."

Although 'poor nutrition' is often equated to 'underfed', these terms are not synonymous; as previously discussed, people who are well-fed can also suffer from 'poor nutrition', or 'malnutrition' as it is also called. This is particularly the case when the diet is one that is almost entirely comprised of processed food products and drinks that are low in nutrients, even though they may be high in calories. The WHO recognises that 'malnutrition' can be caused by nutrient deficiencies; as indicated by the previously cited WHO *Malnutrition* fact sheet that states,

"Malnutrition refers to deficiencies, excesses, or imbalances in a person's intake of energy and/or nutrients."

This statement is however, misleading with reference to excesses in the intake of nutrients; as the discussions about carbohydrates, proteins and fats have demonstrated, it is not the quantity but the quality of these macronutrients that is most important to health. Furthermore, the claim that malnutrition can occur due to an insufficient intake of 'energy', meaning calories, is erroneous; 'calories' are not nutrients.

People who consume large quantities of processed foods that are high in calories but low in nutrients may, however, continue to feel hungry, but this is not because the body craves 'more food'; instead, the feeling of 'hunger' is more likely to indicate a craving for nutrients; as Dr Carolyn Dean explains,

"Food craving and overeating can be simply a desire to continue eating past fullness because the body is, in fact, craving nutrients that are missing from processed food."

According to the *Malnutrition* fact sheet, one of the forms of malnutrition is 'undernutrition', which is claimed to have four sub-forms, namely, wasting, stunting, underweight and deficiencies in vitamins and minerals. But 'undernutrition' by definition refers to an inadequate intake of nutrients; which means that wasting, stunting and underweight are the result of 'undernutrition', not different sub-forms of it.

Another 'form' of malnutrition is referred to as 'protein-energy malnutrition', which is described in a WHO document entitled *Global burden of protein-energy malnutrition in the year 2000* that states,

"Protein-energy malnutrition is a nutritional deficiency resulting from either inadequate energy (caloric) or protein intake and manifesting in either marasmus or kwashiorkor."

Protein is especially important for growth and development and is therefore essential for the diets of young children. However, 'malnutrition' cannot be attributed to a single nutrient deficiency; as discussed earlier in this section, foods provide a wide variety of different nutrients, both micronutrients as well as macronutrients, all of which are essential, not only for growth and development but for other functions. Unfortunately, the interventions provided by the WHO and other aid agencies in order to help solve the interrelated problems of hunger and undernutrition, involve the distribution of certain pre-packaged 'food products'. As discussed in chapter eight, one of these products is called RUTF (ready-to-use therapeutic food). The UNICEF web page entitled *Ready-to-Use Therapeutic Food for Children With Severe Acute Malnutrition* describes RUTF as energy-dense pastes that have been enriched with micronutrients and states that,

"Typical primary ingredients for RUTF include peanuts, oil, sugar, milk powder, and vitamin and mineral supplements."

Although products like RUTF may provide temporary relief from acute starvation, they do not provide the solution to 'undernutrition'. The description of these products as 'energy-dense' means that they are high in calories, but that does not mean that they are nutrient-dense. The typical primary ingredients of RUTF, as listed above, do not contain the wide range of essential micronutrients, especially antioxidants, that are necessary to protect the body from free radical damage. The increased susceptibility to disease that is recognised to be associated with malnutrition, can only be addressed by providing people suffering from malnutrition with real foods that are rich in all of the nutrients, not just those that provide energy. Furthermore, the addition of supplements to these products will not resolve the nutritional deficiencies of their primary ingredients.

Nutritional supplements are frequently taken in the absence of any test to determine the nature of the deficiency or even if any deficiency actually exists; it should be noted that no test can determine the body's nutritional status, as many nutrients are retained in organs and tissues that cannot be tested. One of the main reasons that people take supplements is to boost their intake of vitamins and minerals on the basis of the health benefits they are claimed to confer. Yet rarely do people realise that their nutritional intake would receive a far greater boost if they improved their diet; the main reason that many people are reluctant to make fundamental changes to their diet is suggested by Dr Campbell, who, in his previously cited 2017 article, states that,

"A major reason why isolated nutrients, as supplements, are still used by the public is the false assumption (or excuse?) that we can retain the desired health while continuing to eat our favorite foods, however unhealthy they may be."

It should be clear from this discussion that the only real source of the nutrients required by the body is food, especially fresh, whole, plant-based foods that have not been subjected to toxic chemicals, such as pesticides, or unnatural processes, such as genetic modification. These are the types of foods that comprise a healthy diet. However, although referred to as a 'diet', the regular consumption of nutrient-rich foods should not be regarded as a temporary measure to attain a particular goal, but as a new and healthy way of living, as Dr Henry Bieler explains in *Food is Your Best Medicine*,

"For proper food is not just for the health faddist but is, when you are aware of the facts, truly a way of life."

The ubiquitous use of synthetic chemicals means that it is almost impossible to ensure that foods are entirely chemical-free, but it is possible to minimise exposures by choosing to consume produce that has been grown organically. Exposures to toxic substances can also be reduced by avoiding processed food products and drinks that almost inevitably contain chemical additives. The increased demand for healthy foods has led some manufacturers to produce foods that contain fewer unhealthy ingredients; it is therefore important to read product labels to make healthy choices.

The healthiest diet is, however, one that is comprised of fresh, whole, unprocessed, organic plant-based foods, as Dr Blaylock suggests,

"In truth, the only way to protect yourself and your family is to eat only fresh foods that have no additives."

As briefly mentioned earlier in this section, it is widely believed and commonly argued that humans are natural omnivores; the main justification for this argument is the existence of prehistoric hunter-gatherer societies in many parts of the world. This argument can, however, be refuted by three counter-arguments.

Firstly, the fact that prehistoric peoples ate meat only proves the existence of a behaviour that has become a habit, it does not prove that the behaviour is natural. Secondly, many societies around the world have an equally long-established habit of abstaining from eating animal foods, in addition to which are the many millions of people today who continue to not only survive, but thrive on a meat-free diet; which demonstrates unequivocally that meat is not an essential component of the human diet. The third, and most compelling, refutation of the idea that humans are natural meat-eaters argues from the perspective of human anatomy and physiology, rather than human behaviours and habits.

A comparison of certain aspects of human anatomy and physiology with those of carnivores, omnivores and herbivores demonstrates a number of differences, the most significant of which occur within the digestive system. Whilst similarities exist between the digestive systems of carnivores and omnivores, they are both significantly different from the human digestive system. The only reason for these differences must be related to the foods the digestive system is capable of processing.

It is clear that, despite the passage of many hundreds of thousands of years, humans have not 'evolved' to become natural meat-eaters, because the human digestive system has not adapted to become more like that of carnivores and omnivores that can easily process meat.

Although it is sometimes suggested that humans are more akin to herbivores, this too is incorrect, as the human digestive system cannot process the cellulose found in many of the plants, especially grasses, that are consumed by herbivores. The diet most suited to humans, because it is most suited to human anatomy and physiology, is a frugivorous one; as indicated by Herbert Shelton, who states in his book entitled *The Hygienic System: Vol II Orthotrophy* that,

"The number and structure of his teeth, the length and structure of his digestive tract, the position of his eyes, the character of his nails, the functions of his skin, the character of his saliva, the relative size of his liver, the number and position of the milk glands, the position and structure of the sexual organs, the character of the human placenta and many other factors all bear witness to the fact that man is constitutionally a frugivore."

The term 'frugivore' aptly describes a diet comprised of fruits, vegetables, nuts and seeds; however, it also includes other parts of plants, as he further explains,

"As there are no pure frugivores, all frugivores eating freely of green leaves and other parts of plants, man may, also, without violating his constitutional nature, partake of green plants. These parts of plants possess certain advantages, as has been previously pointed out, in which fruits are deficient. Actual tests have shown that the addition of green vegetables to the fruit and nut diet improves the diet."

The term frugivore has not however, been widely adopted, except by people who follow the practices of Natural Hygiene. People who eat neither meat nor fish but do eat dairy foods are vegetarians, whereas people who abstain entirely from animal and dairy foods are vegans. However, vegetarian and vegan diets are not necessarily 'healthy' because they do not automatically preclude the consumption of processed food products. The term 'whole food plant-based' may also be used to describe this type of diet. Whatever label may be chosen to best describe it, the healthiest type of diet is one that includes a wide variety of fresh, whole, unprocessed, plant-based foods that have not been genetically modified or exposed to toxic chemicals.

Also important is that foods should be minimally processed, if at all, because all forms of processing, including cooking, reduce their nutritional content; this means that, where possible, foods should be consumed raw, as Herbert Shelton indicates,

"It is almost axiomatic that fruits, nuts and vegetables are the only foods that can be relished raw."

It is also axiomatic that a diet that contains a variety of these foods will be one that provides the human body with the nutrition required to ensure optimal functioning, and thereby ensure good health. But the attainment of good health also requires attention to be paid to the fluids consumed.

Water is an essential component of the body's cells; its presence in the body in adequate amounts is therefore vital, not only for health but for survival.

The body loses fluids throughout the day due to normal bodily functions such as respiration and excretion. If lost fluids are not replaced, the body's cells and tissues will soon become dehydrated, which, if prolonged, will lead to impaired functioning of many vital organs, especially the kidneys, and can eventually lead to death.

In his book entitled *Your Body's Many Cries for Water*, Dr F Batmanghelidj MD refers to chronic cellular dehydration and claims that it is the main cause of most chronic health conditions. However, although dehydration may be a contributory factor, it cannot be regarded as the main cause of chronic conditions, which are always the result of a combination of some, if not all, of the 'four factors' discussed in this chapter. Significantly, from the perspective of the 'new' explanation of disease, dehydration causes the body to become 'stressed', which increases the generation of free radicals that can induce oxidative stress and lead to free radical damage, the underlying mechanism common to virtually all conditions of ill-health, especially chronic conditions.

It is generally asserted that the human body requires a daily intake of approximately 6 to 8 glasses of fluids; there are, however, differing opinions about which beverages can be included in those fluids. Dr Batmanghelidj, for example, advises that the daily intake should be comprised solely of water in order to ensure that the body is fully hydrated.

By contrast, the British Nutrition Foundation (BNF) states that consuming water is a 'good choice', but that it is not necessary to only consume water because,

"Other drinks such as squash, fruit juice, fizzy drinks, tea and coffee contribute to our daily requirements too."

This statement is highly misleading, but illustrative of the poor level of knowledge about nutrition promulgated by organisations that claim to be in a position to educate the public on the subject. On the BNF web page entitled *Healthy hydration guide*, it is acknowledged that fizzy drinks and squashes contain sugar and that their consumption should be minimised, but it is nevertheless claimed that these sugary drinks can be replaced by 'diet' versions; the problems with the artificial sweeteners used to replace sugar in foods and drinks have been discussed. Furthermore, although tea and coffee contain water, they both have a diuretic effect, which increases the volume of fluids lost to excretion and therefore increases the body's fluid intake requirement.

It would therefore seem preferable that water is the main, if not the only, liquid consumed each day, as Dr Batmanghelidj advises; unfortunately, virtually all of the water made available for drinking is not as 'clean' as it ought to be.

According to the claims of the medical establishment, the main problem that affects the cleanliness of drinking water is the presence of 'germs' that are said to cause a number of diseases that can be transmitted through contaminated water; as indicated by the February 2018 WHO fact sheet entitled *Drinking-water* that states,

> "Contaminated water can transmit diseases such as diarrhoea, cholera, dysentery, typhoid, and polio."

Although the WHO recognises faecal matter to be the main contaminant, it is claimed that these 'diseases' are caused by 'germs' that infect people via the faecal-oral route, and that it is the 'germs' that cause the symptoms associated with these diseases; it should be emphasised that diarrhoea is a symptom not a disease. These claims are however, disingenuous. Symptoms such as vomiting and diarrhoea are not caused by any 'germ'; instead, they are the body's reactions to toxic substances, such as faecally-contaminated water, and represent its efforts to expel those toxins. The WHO claims that diarrhoeal diseases, which are said to be mainly prevalent in 'developing' countries, are largely the result of the inadequate management of water; as indicated by the statement in the fact sheet that was cited in chapter six, but deserves repetition,

> "Inadequate management of urban, industrial and agricultural wastewater means the drinking-water of hundreds of millions of people is dangerously contaminated or chemically polluted."

Yet water management systems that are claimed to be 'adequate' also supply hundreds of millions of people with water that is contaminated and chemically polluted; some of the chemical pollutants are the substances used to 'treat' water to make it 'safe', but again, safe is only a relative term. As discussed in chapters six and eight, most of the water made available for human consumption, especially through municipal water supplies, cannot be referred to as either safe or clean.

The chemicals used to 'purify' water are claimed to be present in concentrations that are within the levels deemed to be safe; but these chemicals are inherently toxic as their purpose is to kill bacteria, which are living organisms. The Paracelsus fallacy that claims a substance is only a poison when it reaches a certain 'dose' therefore permits water to be poisoned. In addition to the toxic substances used to 'purify' water, are the many chemical contaminants, especially those produced by industrial and agricultural activities and discharged as effluent, that remain in water, because water treatment systems are unable to remove them.

It is clear that the quality of water supplied as 'drinking water' is extremely poor, as discussed in chapter six, despite claims that it is 'safe'. There are however, solutions to the problem of the poor quality of drinking water that can be applied in the home or workplace. These solutions involve the use of filters or filtering systems that are able to remove some or even most of the contaminants in water. This inevitably raises the question of why these filters are not applied before the water is delivered to the public.

One type of water filtering systems involves the use of reverse osmosis, which is claimed to remove virtually all contaminants, including fluoride and pharmaceuticals, but also removes minerals from the water, which has led to some controversy about whether these systems can be considered beneficial or not.

Water is represented by the chemical symbol H_2O. Although this 'pure' form of water may be consumed for a short period of time to assist with detoxification, it is considered by many to be unsuitable for consumption for extended periods of time or on a regular basis; however, in *Orthotrophy* Herbert Shelton states that,

"Fresh rain water and distilled water are best. Distilled water is not dead, as some foolishly say it is. Pure water from a rock spring is excellent drink."

The increasing level of air pollution means that rain water is no longer a good source of truly clean fresh water. The reason that 'pure' or distilled water is claimed to be unsuitable for drinking is because it is devoid of minerals; however, Herbert Shelton refutes this claim in *Orthotrophy* in which he states that,

"It is said that the body needs the minerals dissolved in the water. That the body needs minerals is certain, but it needs them, as previously shown, in the form of organic salts and derives these from foods."

Although most information about fluid intake refers solely to liquids, some recognise that many foods, especially fruits and vegetables, contain a significant volume of water that contributes to the daily intake of fluids, as Herbert Shelton also states in *Orthotrophy*,

"Most green vegetables and fresh fruits contain a higher percentage of water than the adult body. If the diet contains an abundance of these foods little or no additional water will be required."

He adds that,

"Dr Alcott and others of the vegetarian school proved by direct experiments that those who adopt an exclusively vegetable regimen and make a large proportion of their diet consist of juicy fruits and succulent vegetables can be healthfully sustained and nourished without water-drinking."

A frugivorous diet therefore not only provides the body with water, but the water it provides is of a far superior quality to 'treated' water; as Dr Henry Bieler states in *Food is Your Best Medicine*,

"The quality of water found in melons, papayas, raw carrots, cucumbers and celery is distinctly more beneficial to the body than the chlorinated, chemically processed and irritating fluid that too often comes from the faucet."

However, unless people consume a wholly frugivorous diet, it will be necessary to consume some additional fluids; but these fluids can be provided by healthy drinks, especially freshly-prepared, home-made fruit and vegetable juices. There are many different machines available that are able to extract juice from a wide variety of fruits and vegetables; it should be obvious from the discussion in the previous section that, where possible, the fruits and vegetables to be juiced should be organically grown to ensure that they have been minimally exposed to toxic chemicals and have not been genetically modified.

It should be clear that freshly-prepared juices from clean, organically-grown fruits and vegetables are far healthier than manufactured juices and juice drinks, especially those that have been made from concentrates and contain high levels of sugars or artificial sweeteners. It should be noted that packaged juices and juice drinks will invariably have been pasteurised, a process that further reduces their nutritional content. Freshly-prepared home-made juices will not only boost the body's intake of fluids, they will also increase the intake of nutrients; fresh juices should, however, be consumed in addition to whole fruits and vegetables; they are not to be considered as substitutes for these whole foods.

Toxic Exposures

The word 'toxin' is derived from the Greek word for poison, but its meaning has been altered so that it only refers to a specific type of poison; as indicated by the previously cited establishment definition that describes a toxin as,

"a poison produced by a living organism, especially by a bacterium."

There are a number of living organisms that can produce poison, the purpose of which is either defensive, to protect themselves against predators, or offensive, to incapacitate or kill their prey. Bacterial toxins, by contrast, are claimed to have an entirely different purpose, which is to cause disease; as indicated by a January 2019 article entitled *Evolutionary Features in the Structure and Function of Bacterial Toxins*, which states that,

"Bacterial toxigenesis is a major mechanism by which pathogenic bacteria produce diseases."

The article acknowledges that toxins are only produced by some bacteria, but exposes yet another 'knowledge gap' in the statement that,

"It is still a mystery, however, as to why certain bacteria produce such potent molecules while others do not."

This mystery will not, however, be solved whilst the medical research community continues to adhere to the erroneous idea that any bacterium produces a 'poison' with the sole purpose of causing disease, especially within the human body.

The original Latin word for poison or poisonous substance is 'virus', the definition of which has been so completely altered that it now refers exclusively to an 'infectious agent'. However, as previously discussed, the particles referred to as 'viruses' are pieces of genetic material in a protein coating that possess none of the properties required to justify their description as either 'alive' or 'infectious'.

The theories that claim bacteria, viruses, or any other 'germs' to be responsible for causing disease have been shown to contain many knowledge gaps, as well as a number of anomalies and contradictions. Yet, although the medical establishment acknowledges the existence of these gaps, anomalies and contradictions, it fails to recognise that their combined effect is to pose a challenge to the veracity of those theories, and that this challenge is of such a serious and fundamental nature that it completely undermines the existence of the phenomenon referred to as an 'infectious disease'.

One of the main reasons that the medical establishment continues to adhere to the 'germ theory' involves the influence of vested interests, especially those that control the industries that produce, use and discharge 'toxic substances'. The attribution of blame for a large number of diseases to so-called 'pathogenic microorganisms' is clearly of immense benefit to these industries, as it deflects attention away from their hazardous activities and products. But, in reality, it is the continual exposure to these hazards that not only poses the real threat to human health, but also endangers the lives of all living organisms.

Although previously cited, it is useful to repeat that the establishment definition of a poison refers to,

"any substance that irritates, damages, or impairs activity of the body's tissues."

It is also useful to compare this to the establishment definition of a 'disease', which refers to,

"any bodily abnormality or failure to function properly..."

It is clear that these establishment definitions highlight a striking resemblance between the effects of a poison and 'disease'. Unfortunately, the significance of this similarity is invariably obfuscated by reference to the Paracelsus fallacy, which claims that everything is a poison in the appropriate dose; as indicated by the establishment definition of a 'poison' that also states,

"In large enough doses almost any substance acts as a poison, but the term is usually reserved for substances such as arsenic, cyanide and strychnine, that are harmful in relatively small amounts."

The idea that the dose determines whether a substance acts as a poison or not is grossly mistaken; the dose of a substance cannot determine its fundamental nature, as Herbert Shelton indicates in his 1968 article entitled *What is a Poison?* in which he states that,

"Poisons are such qualitatively and not merely quantitatively."

The dose of a poison does, however, determine the degree of harm it will cause. Although a low dose of a toxic substance may not appear to cause harm, this does not mean that no harm has occurred. One reason for an apparent absence of harm at a low dose is due to the body's ability to expel toxins and repair damage; but this does not mean that the substance can be considered 'safe' at that low dose. The degree of harm caused by a toxic substance also depends on the health status of the individual person exposed to that substance; a circumstance that is ignored by the medical establishment that operates according to the mechanistic view of the human body. But this view is fatally flawed, as it fails to acknowledge the existence of the body's innate self-protective and self-healing mechanisms; it also ignores the uniqueness of each individual person with respect to their health status and their existing body burden of toxins.

Furthermore, the idea that 'almost any substance' can act as a poison fails to differentiate between substances that are inherently toxic, and therefore harmful to all living organisms, and those that are not inherently toxic, but may nevertheless adversely affect some organisms. The importance of this distinction cannot be overstated. It can, however, be illustrated by reference to a comparison between arsenic and citrus fruits.

Arsenic, a naturally-occurring substance, is inherently toxic and will therefore harm all living organisms, including cats, dogs, rabbits and humans. The degree of harm arsenic will cause to each type of organism, whether cat, dog, rabbit or human, will differ according to the exposure level and to the existence of innate abilities within each species to expel this particular toxin and repair the resulting damage. The degree of harm caused by arsenic will also depend on the unique health status and the unique body burden of toxins of each individual cat, dog, rabbit and human.

Citrus fruits are not inherently toxic; they are eminently suitable foods for humans, but are poorly tolerated by, and even considered 'toxic' to cats, dogs and rabbits. However, cats are carnivores, dogs are omnivores and rabbits are herbivores; they therefore have different dietary requirements from humans, who, as discussed in the previous section, are frugivores. The reason they all have different dietary requirements is due to anatomical and physiological differences, especially within the digestive system; it is these differences that determine which substances are recognised by the body as 'food' and which are recognised as 'non-food'. Nevertheless, the over-consumption of foods may produce unpleasant effects, but this discomfort should not be interpreted to suggest that the food has become a poison. The main purpose of such discomfort is to prevent any further intake of food as this would impede the digestive system's ability to process the food that has already been consumed.

Another reason that substances that are not inherently toxic, but may cause adverse effects, involves a disturbance to homeostasis, which is described in chapter 26 of the book entitled *Anatomy and Physiology*,

"Homeostasis, or the maintenance of constant conditions in the body, is a fundamental property of all living things."

Homeostasis requires that all of the substances necessary for the body to function properly are present in the 'right' amount; substances that are present in the 'wrong' amount will disturb homeostasis and therefore disrupt the body's ability to function properly, as the book also states,

"In the human body, the substances that participate in chemical reactions must remain within narrow ranges of concentration. Too much or too little of a single substance can disrupt your bodily functions."

The disruption to bodily functions caused by the 'wrong' amount or concentration of essential substances, can be demonstrated by reference to the adverse health effects caused by a combination of excess calcium and insufficient magnesium, as discussed in the previous section. It should be obvious that calcium and magnesium do not become 'poisons' simply as the result of their presence in the body in the 'wrong' amounts; this is clearly the case with respect to insufficient magnesium; a substance cannot become a 'poison' by virtue of its presence at an inadequate level.

The plethora of substances that are inherently toxic include, not only the vast majority of the chemicals and compounds synthesised in the laboratories of the chemical industry, but also a number of naturally-occurring substances that have been exposed or brought to the surface from deep underground by the activities of various industries, as discussed in chapter six. Their inherently toxic nature means that these substances are incompatible with the human body's biochemical processes that sustain life; which means that they should not be ingested, inhaled, injected or otherwise absorbed into the body at any dose or exposure level.

Although different substances may cause different degrees of harm, they all cause damage at the cellular level, because the mechanism by which most, if not all toxic substances cause harm, is through the generation of free radicals that induce oxidative stress and lead to damage to the body's cells and consequently to tissues and organs. The growing body of evidence that recognises oxidative stress to be the underlying mechanism common to most chronic health problems further demonstrates that the relationship between 'toxic substances' and 'disease' is direct and causal.

The mechanism by which toxic substances produce their adverse effects was first recognised more than three decades ago; as indicated by a 1986 article entitled *Free radicals and environmental toxins*, which states that,

"Some chemicals that contaminate our environment exert their toxic effects by virtue of their ability to form free radicals."

Research studies in the 1990s discovered that the ability to form free radicals was not merely restricted to 'some' chemicals, but was found to be the mechanism common to increasing numbers of them; as indicated by a 1993 article entitled *Free radicals in toxicology*, which states that,

"Free radicals are recognized more and more frequently as being involved in the mechanism of toxicity of chemicals."

The human body is not defenceless against the plethora of toxic substances to which it is regularly exposed; on the contrary, the body possesses a number of organs and systems that facilitate the removal of toxins from the body, otherwise known as detoxification. The most important organ that plays a vital role in detoxification is the liver, the establishment definition of which states that,

"It has an important role in the detoxification of poisonous substances..."

The definition also states that,

"The liver is the site of many important diseases..."

The 'diseases' referred to include hepatitis, cirrhosis and dysentery, all of which represent the efforts of the body to expel 'poisonous substances', as indicated by their common symptoms, especially vomiting and diarrhoea.

Although toxic substances can damage the liver, the body also possesses the ability to regenerate this important organ, as indicated by a 2007 article entitled *Liver Regeneration*, which states that,

"Liver manages to restore any lost mass and adjust its size to that of the organism, while at the same time providing full support for body homeostasis during the entire regenerative process."

The ability to expel toxins and regenerate the liver are two of the reasons that the human body is able to withstand certain levels of exposures to toxic substances. The body's self-protective and self-healing mechanisms can, however, be compromised, by a single dose of or exposure to an extremely toxic substance, such as cyanide for example, that is potentially life-threatening. These mechanisms can also be compromised by continual exposures to toxic substances, which, although not life-threatening in a single dose or exposure, will nevertheless continue to cause damage at the cellular level and reduce the body's ability to function properly. These persistent exposures will also compromise the liver's ability to function properly and can even damage this vital organ.

Unfortunately, one class of 'toxic substances' that are known to cause damage to the liver are the pharmaceutical products used as 'medicines' to treat diseases, including diseases that affect the liver. The ability of commonly-used drugs to harm the liver is discussed in a 1986 article entitled *The Spectrum of Hepatotoxicity Due to Drugs*, which states that,

"Drugs in common use can cause toxic effects on the liver which can mimic almost every naturally occurring liver disease in man."

Disease does not occur naturally; as the 'new' explanation states, disease represents disruptions to the body's functions due to exposures to harmful substances and influences. The claim that the toxic effects of drugs 'mimic' disease is therefore disingenuous; their inherently toxic nature means that drugs are the cause of damage to the liver; in other words, they are the direct cause of 'liver disease'. This phenomenon is recognised by a 2010 article entitled *Drug-induced Liver Injury*, which states that,

"Drug-induced liver injury (DILI) is common and nearly all classes of medications can cause liver disease."

Although paracetamol (acetaminophen) is the drug most commonly associated with liver damage, the article refers to some of the other classes of 'medications' known to damage the liver,

"...a broad range of different pharmacological agents can induce liver damage, including anasthetics, anticancer drugs, antibiotics, antituberculosis agents, antiretrovirals, and cardiac medications."

This statement is an unambiguous admission that the substances used as 'medicines' to treat disease in the name of 'healthcare' are inherently toxic, and that, instead of restoring health, these 'medicines' cause damage to the liver, and thereby impair the activity of the main organ that processes toxins and expels them from the body.

Although the medical establishment claims that medicines 'work' by actions that are intended to stimulate, block, depress, stabilise or otherwise correct bodily dysfunctions, it is clear that it is these 'medicines' that are the cause of dysfunctions, which the body's self-healing mechanisms need to rectify. Unfortunately, however, the body's ability to expel toxins, repair damage and restore health is almost invariably, albeit mistakenly, attributed to the drugs, as Herbert Shelton explains,

"It is these processes of resistance and expulsion and the processes by which damages are repaired that are mistaken for the actions of drugs."

The only actions that drugs are capable of performing, involve the mechanism by which virtually all toxic substances are known to cause harm to the body at the cellular level, namely the generation of free radicals that induce oxidative stress; as indicated by a 2012 article entitled *Drug-Induced Oxidative Stress and Toxicity*, which states that,

"Drug-induced oxidative stress is implicated as a mechanism of toxicity in numerous tissues and organ systems..."

One of the organs known to be adversely affected by drug-induced oxidative stress is the liver, as demonstrated by the acknowledged presence of oxidative stress in 'liver diseases', such as hepatitis, cirrhosis and dysentery.

Furthermore, as indicated by the above cited 2010 article about DILI, antituberculosis agents are one of the classes of drugs recognised to induce liver damage; in other words, the drugs used to treat tuberculosis are known to be hepatotoxic. A 2018 article entitled *Oxidative Stress and First Line Antituberculosis Drug-Induced Hepatotoxicity* refers to the hepatotoxicity resulting from antituberculosis drugs as a 'serious adverse reaction' and states that,

"The association of oxidative stress with isoniazid-induced hepatotoxicity appears to be reasonably well understood."

The failure of a patient to respond to first line TB drugs such as isoniazid is often interpreted to mean that the 'bacteria' have developed 'resistance'; but, as previously discussed, this is an erroneous interpretation. The article states unequivocally that isoniazid induces hepatotoxicity and that this toxicity involves the mechanism of oxidative stress. This means that a patient's continuing, and often worsening, ill-health after treatment with isoniazid is due to hepatotoxicity and a reduction in the liver's ability to adequately process and eliminate this toxin. The problem of liver damage due to all types of pharmaceutical drugs is demonstrated by the 2010 article about DILI, which admits that,

"Indeed, drug-induced hepatotoxicity is the most frequent cause of acute liver failure in US."

The reasons that drug-induced hepatotoxicity has become such a serious problem in the US are highlighted by an August 2017 article entitled *Too May Meds? America's Love Affair With Prescription Medication*. This article refers to a study, which had shown that more than half of all Americans take at least one prescription medication, and states that Americans take far more 'pills' than the people of any other country. In addition, prescription drug use in America has risen dramatically in the past few years, as indicated by another August 2017 article entitled *Americans taking more prescription drugs than ever: a survey*, which states that, according to one 'health research firm',

"The number of prescriptions filled for American adults and children rose 85 percent between 1997 and 2016, from 2.4 billion to 4.5 billion per year..."

If pharmaceutical drugs were safe and effective, as the medical establishment claims them to be, then Americans ought to be the healthiest people in the world, but this is not the case; the discussion in chapter one referred to reports that show Americans to be some of the least healthy population of a 'developed' country. Furthermore, the harm caused by pharmaceuticals is also recognised by 'establishment' organisations, as indicated by the previously cited *Too Many Meds* article, which states that, according to estimates based on data from the CDC and FDA,

"Almost 1.3 million people went to U.S. emergency rooms due to adverse drug effects in 2014, and about 124,000 died from those events."

The scale of adverse drug effects is a matter of serious concern. It is particularly significant with respect to the 2030 Agenda goal to ensure that everyone, everywhere has access to universal health coverage, and receives healthcare that includes the provision of 'essential' medicines and vaccines. Unfortunately, the toxic nature of these products will inevitably exacerbate health problems, not solve them.

Another group of 'harmful substances' to which people are commonly exposed are those collectively referred to as pesticides, the intended purpose of which is to destroy a wide variety of living organisms considered to be pests. Pesticides are therefore toxic by intent, but they are also toxic by definition; the origin of the suffix '-cide' is the Latin term that means to kill. The best-known types of pesticide are insecticides, herbicides, rodenticides and fungicides, but there are many others, which, according to the EPA web page entitled *Types of Pesticide Ingredients*, include antimicrobials, biocides, disinfectants and microbial pesticides, all of which are used to kill 'pathogenic microorganisms', especially bacteria and viruses. But viruses should not be referred to as 'organisms' as they are not alive, which means they cannot be 'killed'.

The EPA web page entitled *Basic Information about Pesticide Ingredients* states that pesticides contain both active ingredients, which disable or destroy the target pest, and inert ingredients, which perform other functions, such as extending the product's shelf-life, for example. Although the EPA evaluates the active ingredients and the overall product, inert ingredients only require EPA 'approval', because, as the page also states,

"Under federal law, the identity of inert ingredients is confidential business information."

Of particular note is the statement on the EPA web page that,

"The name 'inert' does not mean non-toxic."

Furthermore, inert ingredients are not required by US law to be identified on product labels; a situation that impedes independent scientific analysis of these ingredients to determine their potential adverse health effects either individually, or in combination with any other chemicals. Although these are US laws, it must be emphasised that the largest chemical companies are multinational corporations and that, as discussed in chapter nine, most regulatory agencies are heavily influenced by corporate vested interests.

A variety of different pesticides are used in industrial agricultural practices, which is one of the most compelling reasons for choosing organically grown foods; however, pesticides are also used in the name of 'healthcare' to control, but mainly to kill, a number of different 'vectors' claimed to cause various diseases by transmitting the parasites they are said to carry. These vectors, many of which are insects, are described in the October 2017 WHO fact sheet entitled *Vector-borne diseases*, which states that,

"Vector-borne diseases are human illnesses caused by parasites, viruses and bacteria that are transmitted by mosquitoes, sandflies, triatomine bugs, blackflies, ticks, tsetse flies, mites, snails and lice."

The diseases referred to include malaria, schistosomiasis, human African trypanosomiasis, leishmaniasis and Chagas disease, all of which were discussed in chapter eight. Although the WHO's response to these diseases involves the implementation of treatment and vaccination programmes, it also involves strategies to control the vectors, such as insecticide-treated nets and indoor residual spraying techniques. It is claimed that the problem of vector-borne diseases is worsening; as indicated by the 2017 WHO report entitled *Global Vector Control Response 2017-2030*, which states that,

"In recent years, vector-borne diseases have moved into new territory: many diseases once limited to tropical and subtropical zones are now increasingly seen in temperate zones."

One of the stated goals of this report, which will be referred to as the *Vector Control* report, is to prevent epidemics of vector-borne diseases in all countries by 2030; this clearly aligns with the 2030 Agenda, the problems with which have been discussed.

The 'public health measures' claimed to prevent the spread of these vector-borne diseases include 'aircraft disinsection', which entails the use of insecticides to kill any insects that may have inadvertently entered an aircraft and prevent them from being introduced into other countries. Aircraft disinsection was first introduced in the 1940s to prevent the spread of malaria, although it was restricted to countries most affected by this disease. The *Vector Control* report claims that 'increased global travel' is one of the factors that has enabled insect vectors to move into new territories and cause increased outbreaks of these diseases. Interestingly, however, a web page entitled *Aircraft Disinsection* on the EPA website states that,

"According to the Centers for Disease Control and Prevention (CDC), there is no evidence to show that using insecticide to kill mosquitoes inside aircraft cabins is effective in preventing introduction and spread of mosquito-borne disease."

There is, however, a fundamental problem with the basic idea that aircraft carry these insects into 'new territories' where they cause disease. The discussion about malaria in chapter eight demonstrated that *Anopheles* mosquitoes, as well as the *Plasmodium* parasites they are claimed to carry, are ubiquitous; they inhabit every continent on the planet, with the sole exception of Antarctica.

Nevertheless, the 2030 Agenda goal to end the epidemic of malaria, in conjunction with the increasing focus on many other neglected tropical diseases, has encouraged the expansion of 'aircraft disinsection' programmes. The insecticides recommended by the WHO for use in these programmes are cited in the 2013 IPCS report entitled *Aircraft Disinsection Insecticides*, which states that,

"For aircraft disinsection, WHO currently recommends *d*-phenothrin (2%) for space spraying and permethrin (2%) for residual disinsection."

Permethrin and phenothrin are synthetic pyrethroids that are claimed to be of 'low toxicity' to humans, but this does not mean that they are safe; however, the WHO web page entitled *Aircraft disinsection* states that,

"...WHO has found no evidence that the specified insecticide sprays are harmful to health when used as recommended."

This statement is disingenuous, especially in view of the 2013 IPCS report that states,

"To date, no widely-accepted, peer-reviewed human health risk assessment model for aircraft disinsection insecticides has been available."

It is clear that the information promulgated by the WHO contains many contradictions; the claims that there are no human health risks and that the risks have not been assessed, differ substantially from those of the *Healthy Environments* report, which acknowledges the toxicity of the insecticides used to 'manage' vectors and states that,

"The use of chemicals raises issues of human and animal toxicity, environmental pollution and sustainability as resistance remains a constant threat."

The contradictory nature of the information promulgated by the WHO is further demonstrated by a comparison between the denial that insecticides are harmful to human health and the findings of a WHO-led consultation in July 2018, which were published in a report entitled *Methods and operating procedures for aircraft disinsection*. The report refers to concerns raised by some of the participants about the active ingredients in the insecticides used, and states that,

"...some can be detrimental to human health when applied in cabins."

Despite the obfuscation by the WHO about the adverse health effects of the ingredients of 'aircraft disinsection' insecticides, there is a growing body of evidence that demonstrates their active ingredients, especially permethrin, to be harmful to human health; as indicated by a 2016 article entitled *Permethrin-induced oxidative stress and toxicity and metabolism. A review*, which states that it was originally believed that permethrin (PER) had 'low mammalian toxicity', but adds the comment that,

"However, as its use became more extensive worldwide, increasing evidence suggested that PER might have a variety of toxic effects on animals and humans alike..."

It would seem that the WHO website requires an urgent update to include this scientific evidence.

In common with all other toxic substances, the mechanism of action of permethrin's toxicity involves oxidative stress, as the article also states,

"A growing number of studies indicate that oxidative stress played critical roles in the various toxicities associated with PER."

The article further states that the toxic effects of permethrin include neurotoxicity and reproductive effects. Permethrin-based insecticides are used for aircraft disinsection on flights involving countries said to be 'at risk' from the Zika virus, which is claimed to be transmitted by mosquitoes. It should be noted that the health problems claimed to be caused by this virus include 'neurological disorders' and 'neonatal malformations'; in other words, the Zika virus is claimed to cause exactly the same health problems that have been demonstrated to be caused by permethrin.

Previous discussions, especially those in chapter eight, demonstrate that so-called 'vector-borne' diseases are not caused by parasites transmitted by mosquitoes, or any other vector; instead, as the 'new' explanation states, disease is the result of exposures to 'harmful substances'.

Pharmaceuticals and pesticides are clearly not the only 'harmful substances' to which people are exposed, but the purpose of the foregoing discussions is to highlight the inappropriate use of products that contain toxic ingredients in the name of healthcare.

Despite the incessant media reports which erroneously claim that climate change due to high atmospheric levels of carbon dioxide poses the most serious threat to humanity, there is a small, but growing level of public awareness that the very real and far more serious threat to humanity is posed by environmental pollution caused by the toxic substances produced, used and discharged by many different industries. There is also a growing level of awareness amongst the research community that environmental pollutants are a significant contributory factor to human health problems; as indicated by a 2017 article entitled *Impact of nutrition on pollutant toxicity: an update with new insights into epigenetic regulation*, which states that,

"Exposure to environmental pollutants is a global health problem and is associated with the development of many chronic diseases..."

The only environmental pollutants specifically referred to in the article are POPs, heavy metals and air pollution, but there are many others. The article does however, refer to oxidative stress as the mechanism by which these pollutants exert their harmful effects.

The hazardous nature of the chemical ingredients of a wide variety of products commonly used in the home and workplace was discussed in chapter six, which also revealed that, although some have been tested individually and deemed 'safe', the vast majority of chemicals remain untested. More importantly, none of the combinations of chemicals to which people are regularly exposed has ever been tested for their safety or to determine their potential adverse health effects.

It may seem that the health hazards due to environmental pollution are of such a magnitude that it must be virtually impossible for anyone to be able to become and remain healthy; but this is not necessarily the case. As previously discussed, the body possesses innate mechanisms to expel toxins, repair damage and restore health. Although these mechanisms and the processes they regulate will be damaged and their effectiveness weakened by continual exposure to toxic substances, this damage can be mitigated, but it requires ongoing efforts to minimise exposures to toxic substances. It also requires ongoing efforts to maximise the intake of nutrients, especially antioxidants to counteract free radicals and prevent them from causing damage within the body.

Informed decisions can only be made when people are in possession of all the necessary information; therefore, in order to minimise and even avoid exposures to toxic substances, it is essential to know about all types of applications that utilise products that contain ingredients made from harmful substances. Whilst it may not be possible to completely avoid all toxins, it is certainly possible to avoid a significant proportion of them, especially those that are ingredients of products to which the body is directly exposed; these include products that are ingested and inhaled as well as those applied directly onto the body.

One group of products that are introduced directly into the body are those consumed as foods and drinks, although medicines and vaccines also fall into this category. The discussion about nutrition and water in the previous section demonstrates that a diet comprised of fresh, whole, organically-grown, plant-based foods is one that will maximise the intake of nutrients. This type of diet will also help to minimise the intake of toxins, as it will preclude the intake of the toxic chemicals commonly used by industrial agricultural practices. Furthermore, in addition to boosting the intake of nutrients, a diet of this nature will also assist with detoxification; as explained by Dr Blaylock in *Health and Nutrition Secrets*,

"...numerous pesticides, herbicides, foreign organic chemicals, fluoride, mercury, aluminium, and other toxic substances are assaulting our bodies. All of these compounds must be detoxified, putting a heavy demand on our detoxification systems – all of which are dependent on nutrition."

It must be noted that, in the same way that toxins accumulate in the body over the course of time, their elimination from the body will also require time; detoxification is therefore an ongoing process. In addition, it must be emphasised that the processes that expel toxins from the body often involve 'symptoms' that are commonly associated with 'disease'; but, in accordance with the 'new' explanation, these symptoms must now be recognised as normal bodily processes, which means that they should not be 'treated' with pharmaceuticals.

Although certain programmes are promoted as methods to accelerate detoxification, they are not recommended, except in cases of acute poisoning with a highly toxic substance. One of the reasons to avoid such programmes is because the body's detoxification organs are likely to have been compromised, which means that the elimination processes may not function as efficiently as they should. It is preferable, and safer, to allow the body to perform its detoxification processes naturally and to support these innate self-healing mechanisms by minimising the intake of toxins and maximising the intake of nutrients.

The main group of products that are regularly applied directly onto the body are cosmetics and personal care products, many of which, as previously discussed, contain toxic ingredients. But they are a source of toxic exposures that can be minimised and even avoided; as Dr Epstein explains in *Toxic Beauty*,

"Cosmetics and personal-care products today constitute our single largest but generally unrecognised class of avoidable exposure to toxic ingredients and their health dangers."

The health dangers of the toxic ingredients used in many cosmetics and personal care products are no longer 'generally unrecognised'; instead, the problem has received sufficient attention that it has raised public awareness of and concern about these toxic chemicals. The adverse publicity this has generated has also been of such concern to the manufacturers of these products, that some have changed their formulations and replaced toxic ingredients, such as phthalates, parabens, SLS and SLES, with 'new' chemicals. But this has not always resulted in 'safer' products; some of the replacement chemicals have been found to be equally if not more toxic.

Fortunately, there are many new companies that are producing their own ranges of cosmetics and personal care products without toxic ingredients; information about these companies and their products can be found throughout the internet. The website of the Environmental Working Group (EWG), a US-based organisation, is one example of a useful resource with information about the toxic chemical ingredients of cosmetics and personal care products and about safer alternatives.

The Good Trade website is another example of a useful resource; as indicated by the information provided in the article entitled *10 Natural & Organic Makeup Brands Your Face Will Love You For*. People must, however, investigate for themselves the ingredients of the products they intend to purchase, especially as terms such as 'natural' may be used as marketing ploys, as indicated by the article that states,

"Many makeup brands marketed as 'natural' or 'green' are often not actually either of these things..."

One of the most powerful actions that people can take is to 'vote with your wallet'; to reject toxic products and support the manufacturers of safer, non-toxic products.

It is important to emphasise that the references in this section to websites that feature safer alternatives should not be construed as recommendations or as endorsements of any of the listed products, as this is not the case. These websites are included solely for the purpose of illustrating the kind of information that is available for people who wish to reduce their toxic exposures, and to enable them to make informed decisions about the products they wish to purchase.

One of the myths listed on the EWG web page entitled *Myths on cosmetics safety* is the idea that chemicals are generally absorbed in only negligible amounts into the body. The EWG response to this myth includes reference to studies in which many toxic chemicals, such as phthalates, parabens and triclosan, have been found in significant amounts within the bodies of men, women and children. Furthermore, the discussion about 'poisoned bodies' in chapter six refers to the 2014 IPCS *Dermal Exposure* report, which admits that substances can cross the skin barrier and cause 'systemic effects', and exposes yet another medical establishment 'knowledge gap' in the statement that,

"For most chemicals, however, the relationship between dermal uptake and health effects observed elsewhere in the body is still poorly understood."

It should be noted that, not only have many chemicals been recognised to penetrate the skin and enter the bloodstream, but that phthalates, parabens and triclosan are all associated with oxidative stress. This clearly provides a full explanation for the relationship between toxic chemicals applied to the skin and adverse health effects, despite the lack of understanding exhibited in the IPCS report.

Another large group of products that constitute a major source of toxic exposures are those utilised for tasks such as cleaning and general maintenance, whether in the home or workplace. Although these products contain a variety of different chemical ingredients, a significant proportion of them contain volatile organic compounds (VOCs), which are substances that are released as gases that can be inhaled; it is for this reason that some of the most common health effects of VOCs involve the respiratory system, although other important organs and systems can also be adversely affected.

The EPA web page entitled *Volatile Organic Compounds' Impact on Indoor Air Quality* states that the adverse health effects of VOCs include damage to the liver, kidneys and central nervous system, which is a clear demonstration of their hazardous nature. Two well-known VOCs are benzene and formaldehyde, both of which are highly toxic chemicals that are known to exert their toxic effects through oxidative stress and the resulting cellular damage by free radicals. The types of products that may contain VOCs are listed on the EPA web page and include: paints, paint strippers and other solvents; cleansers and disinfectants; building materials and furnishings; and graphics and craft materials. Perchloroethylene, which is commonly used in dry-cleaning operations, is also a VOC.

Exposures to VOCs and many other toxic chemicals can, however, be minimised and even prevented as many safer products with less toxic or even non-toxic ingredients are available. The EWG web page entitled *Guide to Healthy Cleaning* for example, provides information about safer cleaning products available in the US. The Good Trade website also provides information about safer cleaning products, such as the article entitled *11 Natural & Eco-Friendly Cleaning Products For The Conscious Home*, for example. Many cleaning tasks can be performed using entirely natural materials; as indicated by the Organic Consumers Association article entitled *How Toxic Are Your Household Cleaning Supplies?* which states that,

"A few safe, simple ingredients like soap, water, baking soda, vinegar, lemon juice and borax, aided by a little elbow grease and a coarse brush for scrubbing, can take care of most household cleaning needs."

Clothes are another group of products that are often manufactured using toxic materials and processes, as discussed in chapter six. Although some well-known clothing manufacturers have agreed to reduce the amount of toxic chemicals they use, there are many new companies that manufacture clothes using non-toxic materials, such as organic cotton, and safer processes using azo-free dyes, for example. The Good Trade web page entitled *35 Fair Trade and Ethical Clothing Brands Betting Against Fast Fashion* lists a number of these new clothing companies, most, but not all, of which are based in the US. A number of clothing companies based in Europe are listed on the Ecocult web page entitled *The Best Sustainable and Ethical European Fashion Brands*. There are also safer alternatives for soft furnishings and bedding; as indicated by The Good Trade web page entitled *10 Organic Sheets and Bedding Sources To Help You Sleep Sweetly*.

Plastics are another group of toxic materials that are widely used to make a huge variety of products, containers and wrapping materials; the hazardous nature of plastics and their lack of biodegradability were discussed in chapter six. There is, however, a growing level of public awareness of the problem of environmental pollution due to plastics. There is also an increasing variety of products that are made without plastics; the Life Without Plastics website, for example, features a number of plastic-free products. The Recycling website also features a variety of plastic-free products available in the US on a page entitled *Kickstart Your Zero Waste Lifestyle*. Plastic-free products available in the UK are featured on the website of The Plastic Free Shop.

It is abundantly clear from the discussion in this section that toxic chemicals are entirely unnecessary for the manufacture of a huge variety of products and that there are safer, less toxic alternatives for many of the products people use on a regular, if not daily basis. It is equally clear that choosing safer alternatives will contribute to a significant reduction in each person's level of toxic exposures.

EM Radiation Exposures

Electromagnetic radiation is a form of energy that extends over a range of frequencies and wavelengths collectively known as the electromagnetic spectrum. Although different sections of the spectrum have been given different labels, such as visible light and microwaves, for example, all forms of electromagnetic radiation are categorised as either ionising or non-ionising according to the intensity of the energy they possess.

As previously discussed, the Earth has always existed in the presence of a low level of ionising radiation, known as 'natural background radiation', that occurs as the result of a combination of the radioactivity emitted by naturally-occurring radioactive materials, within or beneath the Earth's crust, and the presence in the atmosphere of cosmic radiation emitted by the sun and stars. Although the background level had been gradually augmented due to radioactive materials released by activities such as mining, it was profoundly altered in the mid-20th century as the result of the development, testing and use of nuclear weapons. Environmental levels of ionising radiation have continued to rise mainly as the result of the ongoing operations of the nuclear industry, especially nuclear power plants. There are other applications of ionising radiation that have contributed to the increased level of exposure; as indicated by the April 2016 WHO fact sheet entitled *Ionizing radiation, health effects and protective measures* that states,

"Ionizing radiation has many beneficial applications, including uses in medicine, industry, agriculture and research."

The natural electromagnetic environment has also been altered by 'unnatural' non-ionising radiation, the level of which began to increase after the introduction of AC (alternating current) electricity as the main power source for virtually all machines and equipment, both domestic and industrial. As previously discussed, all electrical equipment and appliances that utilise electricity produce electromagnetic fields (EMFs). Environmental concentrations of EM radiation have further increased, and more rapidly, since the latter part of the 20th century as the result of the new technologies developed by the telecommunications industry, such as mobile phones and wireless communications, that utilise electromagnetic frequencies in the RF and ELF ranges.

It is clear that the Earth's electromagnetic environment has been irrevocably altered at an incredibly rapid pace and over the course of an incredibly short period of time. Dr Robert Becker MD describes the situation in his 1990 book *Cross Currents*,

"Today, we swim in a sea of energy that is almost totally man-made."

The problem with this man-made sea of energy is that it interferes with the functioning of the natural electrical systems of living organisms, especially humans. In their book entitled *Earthing: The Most Important Health Discovery Ever!* co-authors Clinton Ober, Martin Zucker and Stephen Sinatra MD explain that,

"We all live and function electrically on an electrical planet."

Interestingly, there is a growing body of compelling evidence that indicates the entire universe is fundamentally electrical in nature.

Human health can be adversely affected by exposures to 'harmful influences', such as 'man-made' electromagnetic radiation, as well as 'harmful substances', such as 'man-made' chemicals. Although the chemical industry justifies the production and use of synthetic chemicals on the basis of the claim that 'everything is made of chemicals', this claim is misleading because 'matter' is also electrical in nature.

All matter is composed of atoms and each atom is composed of a combination of three main subatomic particles, namely, protons, neutrons and electrons. The nature of each chemical element is determined by its atomic structure; a hydrogen atom, for example, contains one proton and one electron, whereas a carbon atom contains six protons and six electrons. The electrical aspects of matter are, however, primary because all subatomic particles have electrical properties; protons have a positive electrical charge and electrons a negative charge. Neutrons are said to have equal negative and positive charges which balance each other to produce an overall neutral charge. In most atoms, the number of protons equals the number of electrons, which means there will be no overall electrical charge; but if proton and electron numbers are not equal, the atom will have a charge. An electrically charged atom or molecule is known as an ion.

Ions are produced by different processes, one of which, known as 'dissociation', refers to the separation of chemical compounds into smaller particles, including ions, when dissolved in a liquid. Sodium chloride, for example, will dissolve in water and separate into positive sodium ions and negative chloride ions. Within the body, however, ions, or electrolytes as they are also called, perform important functions that include transmitting an electrical current across the cell membrane. A number of important minerals, especially sodium, potassium, calcium and magnesium, are also electrolytes, which means that they are of extreme importance to the maintenance of electrical homeostasis as well as chemical homeostasis.

It is clear that, although electrical properties are primary, the electrical and chemical aspects of matter are intimately interconnected; it is therefore more accurate to state that 'everything', including the human body, is electro-chemical in nature.

Ions are also produced by ionising radiation, which involves a very different process from dissociation; as previously discussed, ionising radiation possesses sufficient energy to break molecular bonds and release free electrons. However, although 'free electrons' are also known as 'free radicals', those produced by ionising radiation are far more dangerous to living cells. In his 1997 article entitled *The Free-Radical Fallacy about Ionizing Radiation*, Dr John Gofman MD explains that,

"Ionizing radiation instantly unloads biologically abnormal amounts of energy at random in an irradiated cell."

It is the release of 'abnormal amounts' of energy in a very short period of time that results in adverse effects that occur almost immediately; as indicated by the previously cited WHO *Ionizing radiation* fact sheet, which states that,

"Acute health effects such as skin burns or acute radiation syndrome can occur when doses of radiation exceed certain levels."

The CDC web page entitled *Acute Radiation Syndrome: A Fact Sheet for Clinicians* defines 'acute radiation syndrome' as an acute 'illness' and states that this condition, which is also known as radiation toxicity and radiation sickness, occurs as the result of exposure to a high dose of penetrating radiation. The page cites the survivors of the Hiroshima and Nagasaki atomic bombs as people who would have suffered from this 'illness'; it is however, wholly inappropriate to describe the horrifying effects of ionising radiation from nuclear bombs as either an illness or a syndrome.

Unfortunately, the medical establishment operates from the basis of the idea that 'disease-causing entities' must be destroyed. Their arsenal of weapons to defeat these entities includes certain forms of ionising radiation that are used to treat certain diseases, especially cancers. Although the use of ionising radiation is believed to be 'beneficial', because it is said to destroy the cancer without killing the patient, the fact sheet nevertheless acknowledges that,

"Low doses of ionizing radiation can increase the risk of longer term effects such as cancer."

In other words, the treatment is recognised to cause the very 'disease' for which it is used as a remedy; however, no 'dose' of radiation has the ability to restore a person to health. The discussion in chapter six cites Dr Karl Z Morgan PhD, who stated in 1978 that,

"There is no safe level of exposure and there is no dose of radiation so low that the risk of a malignancy is zero."

Nevertheless, low doses or exposures do not inevitably lead to cancer. The likelihood that a person will develop cancer, or any other 'chronic disease', is not a matter of 'risk' or 'chance' or even 'genes'. It is entirely dependent on each individual's unique health status, which will be influenced by the degree to which they are affected by all of the 'four factors' discussed in this chapter.

In common with all other 'harmful substances and influences', electromagnetic radiation exerts its adverse effects through the mechanism of oxidative stress that induces free radical damage at the cellular level; EM radiation is, however, particularly detrimental to the organs and systems that operate electrically. One of the main organs that function electrically is the heart; it is therefore unsurprising that, as discussed in chapter seven, a relationship exists between exposures to EMFs, oxidative stress and cardiac problems. It is important to emphasise that the body's electrical system only requires very tiny amounts of electrical energy; as indicated by the previously cited statement by Dr Becker in *Cross Currents,*

"The body's internal energetic control systems are subtle, and they operate with minute amounts of electromagnetic energy."

The body's delicate electrical system can be, and invariably is, disrupted by unnatural electromagnetic fields.

The degree of harm that may result from exposures to low levels of non-ionising EM radiation will depend on each person's health status, which includes their unique body burden of toxins. Interestingly, there is evidence that a synergistic relationship exists between toxic chemicals and non-ionising EM radiation; as indicated by the EHT article entitled *Wireless Radiation/Electromagnetic Fields Increases Toxic Body Burden*, which refers to the known adverse health effects of toxic chemicals and states that,

"In addition, wireless and EMF radiation can synergistically increase the effect of these daily toxic exposures..."

The mechanism by which toxins and EM radiation interact synergistically is not known, but may relate to the fact that they both exert their effects through the generation of free radicals. Of particular concern, however, is that EM radiation has been shown to affect the blood-brain barrier, as the article also states,

"...replicated research shows that wireless radiation increases the permeability of the blood-brain barrier, allowing more movement of toxic chemicals into vulnerable organs."

The brain is extremely important; it is the other main organ that functions electrically. Many of the implications, and indeed some of the consequences, for the brain from the synergistic interactions between EM radiation and toxic chemicals were referred to in the discussion about autism. The most significant consequences will be for children, whose brains are particularly vulnerable as they are still undergoing development;

however, neurological problems are not exclusive to children; they can also affect adults.

It is important to emphasise that the body is not defenceless against 'harmful substances and influences'; it possesses many mechanisms that respond to their presence. One of these mechanisms, known as the 'cellular stress response', is discussed by Professor Martin Blank PhD, with particular reference to the cellular response to EM radiation, in his article entitled *The Cellular Stress Response: EMF-DNA Interaction* published in the BioInitiative Report 2012. In this article, which will be referred to as the *Stress Response* article, he states that,

> "The cellular stress response is a protective reaction of individual cells to potentially harmful stimuli in the environment. It is characterized by the synthesis of a class of proteins referred to as stress proteins."

The cellular stress response is not the same as the body's production of hormones in response to 'stress', which is discussed in the next section.

The first stimulus discovered to induce the cellular stress response is heating, which is the reason that these proteins were initially called heat shock proteins. These proteins are described in a 2004 article entitled *'The stress of dying': the role of heat shock proteins in the regulation of apoptosis*, which states that,

> "Heat shock proteins (Hsps) are a family of highly homologous chaperone proteins that are induced in response to environmental, physical and chemical stresses and that limit the consequences of damage and facilitate cellular recovery."

The acknowledgement that a variety of different 'stresses' induce the same cellular response further validates the 'new' explanation that asserts diseases are not separate 'entities', but merely different manifestations of cellular damage and the resulting bodily dysfunctions.

As the above article indicates, the cellular stress response can be induced by stimuli other than heating; however, non-thermal stimuli can induce this response at exposure levels that are orders of magnitude lower than those at which the tissues would be heated; as Professor Blank also states in his *Stress Response* article,

> "In fact, the cells were far more sensitive to EMF than to thermal stimuli, the threshold energy of the EMF stimulus being more than one billion times weaker than an effective thermal stimulus."

Despite this evidence, the WHO continues to assert that tissue heating is the main adverse health effect of non-ionising radiation; as indicated by the October 2014 fact sheet entitled *Electromagnetic fields and public health: mobile phones*, which, as previously cited, states that,

> "Tissue heating is the principal mechanism of interaction between radiofrequency energy and the human body."

The ICNIRP guidelines that claim to protect people from the effects of non-ionising radiation have set thresholds at levels that would prevent tissue heating on the basis that this is the only relevant adverse effect. The WHO web pages relating to the topic of *Electromagnetic fields* include an undated page entitled *Research*, which refers to research into the health effects of exposures to EM radiation and states that,

"All reviews conducted so far have indicated that exposures below the limits recommended in the ICNIRP (1998) guidelines, covering the full frequency range from 0-300 GHz, do not produce any known adverse health effects."

Although the page recognises the existence of some 'knowledge gaps' that need to be filled, the claim that there are no known adverse health effects is disingenuous. RF and ELF are both classified by the IARC as Group 2B carcinogens, which means they are both officially recognised as 'possible' human carcinogens. This classification challenges the claim that tissue heating is the only relevant adverse health effect.

The ICNIRP guidelines, now more than two decades old, are wholly inadequate to genuinely protect people, as they fail to reflect ongoing scientific research findings that continue to conclusively demonstrate the existence of serious non-thermal effects at exposure levels below those deemed to be safe by the governing bodies. Unfortunately, the WHO, ICNIRP and all other 'establishment' organisations that make pronouncements about the health effects of exposures to EM radiation, fail to acknowledge these non-thermal effects, mainly as the result of the influence of 'vested interests', especially those of the telecommunications and related industries.

A December 2018 article entitled *Planetary electromagnetic pollution: it is time to assess its impact* refers to the proliferation of artificial electromagnetic fields and states that,

"The most notable is the blanket of radiofrequency electromagnetic radiation, largely microwave radiation generated for wireless communication and surveillance technologies, as mounting scientific evidence suggests that prolonged exposure to radiofrequency electromagnetic radiation has serious biological and health effects."

The classification of RF and ELF as merely 'possible' carcinogens is no longer tenable; there is a large body of evidence, which demonstrates that a relationship exists between EM radiation and oxidative stress, cellular damage and cancer, and that this relationship is both direct and causal. A May 2018 article entitled *Radiofrequency radiation from nearby base stations gives high levels in an apartment in Stockholm, Sweden: A case report* states that,

"RF radiation leads to oxidative stress in biological systems, including the brain, due to an increase in free radicals and changes in antioxidant defence systems."

The article refers to studies that have shown radiofrequency radiation to increase the risk of cancer and have resulted in recommendations that RF radiation be upgraded from Group 2B to Group 1, the category for known human carcinogens.

The thresholds set by the ICNIRP guidelines are clearly in urgent need of revision, as Professor Blank emphasises in his *Stress Response* article,

"It should be obvious that EMF safety standards are based on false assumptions and must be revised to reflect the scientific evidence."

Unfortunately, the continually growing body of evidence that demonstrates exposures to non-ionising EM radiation to be associated with serious adverse health effects, is largely ignored by the telecommunications and related industries that are preparing for the imminent introduction of 5G, the fifth generation of wireless infrastructure, which is intended to facilitate the implementation of the Internet of Things (IoT). It must be emphasised that 5G will augment, not replace, existing 2G, 3G and 4G technologies.

There are many concerns about 5G and its related infrastructure and technologies, one of which is that it will raise the existing concentration of electromagnetic radiation in the environment to unacceptable levels. The frequencies to be used for 5G are at the high end of the radiofrequency section of the spectrum; these high frequency radio waves are also known as millimetre waves (MMW), due to their wavelength. But 5G will not be the first application of this range of frequencies, as MMWs are currently employed in airport body scanners used in a number of countries, most notably the US. These scanners are claimed to be 'safe' because they are low in energy; as indicated by the CDC web page entitled *Radiation from Airport Security Scanning*, which states that,

> "This form of technology uses low-energy non-ionizing radiation that releases thousands of times less energy than a cell phone."

This does not mean that they do not produce any adverse health effects. As discussed in chapter six, the military utilise MMWs in Active Denial Systems for applications such as crowd control, because they are known to produce extremely unpleasant sensations within the skin; sensations that are intended to discourage people from remaining within the vicinity of the source and to encourage them to disperse.

It is claimed that MMWs only heat the skin, but as has been repeatedly shown, adverse health effects from exposures to non-ionising radiation occur at levels orders of magnitude lower than those at which heating occurs. In his February 2019 article entitled *5G Wireless Technology: Millimeter Wave Health Effects*, Dr Joel Moskowitz PhD explains that MMWs are,

> "...mostly absorbed within 1-2 millimeters of human skin..."

This seemingly superficial level of absorption into the skin does not mean that the rest of the body will remain unaffected; as he further explains,

> "Since skin contains capillaries and nerve endings, MMW bio-effects may be transmitted through molecular mechanisms by the skin or through the nervous system."

The implementation of 5G, and its related infrastructure and technologies to facilitate the interconnection of all devices that utilise SMART (Self-Monitoring Analysis and Reporting Technologies) systems through the IoT, will clearly intensify the existing concentration of 'unnatural' EM radiation. In common with all previous generations of wireless technologies, however, 5G is to be implemented without a full investigation of the potential consequences for human health, as Dr Moskowitz states,

> "Unfortunately, few studies have examined prolonged exposure to low-intensity MMWs, and no research that I am aware of has focused on exposure to MMWs combined with other radiofrequency radiation."

Fortunately, 180 scientists concerned about the implementation of 5G in the absence of safety studies have signed a declaration addressed to the European Commission. The previously cited EHT web page entitled *Scientists And Doctors Demand Moratorium On 5G Warning of Health Effects* explains that this declaration requests the Commission to recommend a moratorium on the implementation of 5G,

"...until potential hazards for human health and the environment have been fully investigated by scientists independent from industry."

However, sufficient evidence has already accumulated to demonstrate that exposures to electromagnetic radiation in the radiofrequency range is extremely detrimental, not only to humans but to all living organisms, mainly as the result of oxidative stress, the underlying mechanism common to virtually all conditions of ill-health.

Although exposures to certain forms of EM radiation may be unavoidable, other sources of exposure can be avoided or minimised. According to the WHO, most exposures to ionising radiation are the result of medical examinations and diagnostic procedures; X-rays and CT scans for example; these exposures are avoidable. Other sources of exposure to ionising radiation, such as nuclear power plants and uranium mines for example, may not be so easy to avoid, particularly for people who work in these industries or live in their vicinity.

The phenomenal expansion in technologies that employ EM radiation in the radiofrequency range have profoundly changed the nature of the electromagnetic environment throughout the world. Although the wireless communications systems on which mobile phones and other devices depend are ubiquitous, they are higher within urban areas. Each person's exposure to non-ionising radiation will therefore depend, to a large extent, on where they live and work and on the nature of the devices, equipment and wireless systems they use, as well as those to which they are involuntarily exposed.

It is important to emphasise that the body's electrical system operates using currents that flow in only one direction, which is referred to as direct current (DC). Mains electricity, by contrast, operates with alternating current (AC) electricity, which means that electric current flows change direction. All electrical equipment and appliances produce electromagnetic fields in the ELF (extremely low frequency) range that interfere with the body's delicate electrical system and are associated with a number of adverse health effects, including leukaemia and brain tumours. As previously mentioned, the IARC has classified ELF EM radiation as a Group 2B 'possible' human carcinogen.

One particularly useful source of information about a wide variety of topics pertaining to EM radiation exposures is the Powerwatch website. In the section of the website labelled *Article library* are many different publications available for download. The *Child Cancer* section, for example, includes a publication entitled *Ionising radiation* that discusses diagnostic X-rays and CT scans and explains that CT scans give a higher dose of ionising radiation than X-rays.

In the section entitled *Powerfrequency EMFs and Health* is a publication entitled *Cellular changes and potential mechanisms* that refers to 'free radical effects' that can affect the 'brain oxidative balance' which could lead to the reduction of melatonin, a powerful antioxidant. The consequences of reduced melatonin levels are discussed by Dr Neil Cherry in his 2002 article entitled *EMF/EMR Reduces Melatonin in Animals and People*, which, although previously cited in chapter six, deserves repetition,

"...reduced melatonin output causes many serious biological effects in humans and other mammals, including sleep disturbance, chronic fatigue, DNA damage leading to cancer, cardiac, reproductive and neurological diseases and mortality."

The Powerwatch website also contains a number of other publications relating to exposures to EM radiation in the home from various appliances and equipment, as well as outside the home, from sources such as phone masts. In addition to information about the sources of exposure and the scientific studies that have investigated the effects, the website also offers advice about reducing exposures.

The most widely used device is the mobile phone, it is also the most widely studied; the adverse effects on the brain, especially tumours, are well documented. The EHT website is another source of useful information and downloadable documents, not only about the hazards but also advice about reducing exposures, such as the page entitled *10 Tips To Reduce Cell Phone Radiation*. The document entitled *What You Need To Know About 5G Wireless and 'Small Cells'* explains that safer alternatives exist and states that,

"Worldwide, many regions are investing in wired, fiberoptic connections which are safer, faster, more reliable, provide greater capacity and are more cyber-secure."

The body is an electrical system that needs to be maintained in the state of homeostasis, which can be assisted by making direct contact with the Earth; this is discussed in the *Earthing* book referred to at the beginning of this section. However, although the authors of *Earthing* do not claim that making direct contact with the Earth reduces the effects of EM radiation, they do claim that 'grounding' helps to restore electrical homeostasis and that,

"...Earthing naturally protects the body's delicate bioelectrical circuitry against static electrical charges and interference."

EM radiation mainly exerts its effects via oxidative stress that increases the generation of free radicals and reduces the effectiveness of the body's natural antioxidant system. These effects can, however, be mitigated by efforts to support the body, especially the regular consumption of antioxidant-rich foods. It is, of course, extremely important to pay attention not only to nutrition, but to all of the 'four factors' discussed in this book, including 'stress', the fourth factor and the topic of the next section.

Stress

The general understanding of stress is described by the Oxford Dictionary that refers to, "mental or emotional strain or tension."

In this context, stress is an effect. The establishment definition provided by the Oxford Concise Medical Dictionary, by contrast, describes stress as a cause; as indicated by the reference to stress as,

"any factor that threatens the health of the body or has an adverse effect on its functioning, such as injury, disease, or worry."

In addition to their descriptions of seemingly different phenomena, these definitions only refer to the 'negative' connotations of stress. But this is misleading; stress also has 'positive' connotations, as indicated by a 2005 article entitled *Stressed or stressed out: What is the difference?* which states that,

"For some, it means excitement and challenge ('good stress'); for many others, it reflects an undesirable state of chronic fatigue, worry, frustration and inability to cope ('bad stress')."

Dr Hans Selye MD, who is widely regarded as one of the key pioneers in this field of research, refers to stress as an effect; as indicated by his definition of the term in his book entitled *The Stress of Life* as,

"...the nonspecific response of the body to any demand, whether it is caused by, or results in, pleasant or unpleasant conditions."

In order to distinguish between causes and effects, Dr Selye created the term 'stressor' to refer to causal factors and retained the term 'stress' to refer to the effects, as indicated by his definition. In order to differentiate between its positive and negative connotations, he created the term 'eustress' to refer to 'good stress' and employed the term 'distress' to refer to 'bad stress'. These are the terms and the context in which they will be used in the ensuing discussion.

Distress is associated with emotions, such as fear, worry and the inability to cope, that arise as the result of tragic life events, such as the death of a loved one, or situations that pose a direct threat to life, such as a war, for example. Eustress is associated with emotions such as joy, excitement and exhilaration that can result from pleasantly challenging life events, such as a new career opportunity, although for some people events of this nature may generate 'distress'.

Dr Selye explains that any ordinary, everyday activity or emotion that places a demand on the body can be regarded as a stressor; the resulting 'stress' in this context, is therefore perfectly normal and unlikely to be detrimental to health. Eustress and distress are not the same as this normal stress; they represent a heightened level of stress caused by stressors that are not part of ordinary, everyday life. However, although eustress and distress represent increased demands on the body, they are not associated with the same effects; eustress is often regarded as beneficial, whereas distress is widely regarded as damaging to health, especially when prolonged.

The body's response to stressors is said to involve the 'fight or flight' response, also known as the 'acute stress response', which triggers the endocrine system to secrete high concentrations of certain hormones, especially cortisol and adrenaline (epinephrine), and the nervous system to release certain neurotransmitters, such as serotonin. Interestingly, adrenaline acts as a neurotransmitter and a hormone.

The purpose of these secretions is to provide a surge of energy to enable the body to react swiftly to a 'non-ordinary' stressor, especially a situation that induces emotions such as fear that can precipitate distress. When the stressor has been resolved or removed, the level of secretions gradually returns to normal and the body is restored to its normal state of homeostasis. If the stressor is not rapidly resolved or removed, the body will continue to release hormones and neurotransmitters, which, at certain elevated levels, are associated with adverse health effects, including neurological effects; an elevated cortisol level, for example, is associated with depression.

Neurological effects are not, however, solely the result of emotional stressors; they can also be caused by physical stressors, such as toxic chemicals and EM radiation, both of which are known to adversely affect the nervous system; as indicated by the 2014 Supplement to the BioInitiative Report entitled *Neurological Effects of Non-Ionizing Electromagnetic Fields*, which states that,

"Factors that act directly or indirectly on the nervous system causing morphological, chemical, or electrical changes in the nervous system can lead to neurological effects."

It is claimed that at certain low doses or exposures, toxic chemicals and EM radiation do not produce adverse effects, but this is misleading; claims of this nature completely ignore subtle effects at the cellular level; as Dr Blaylock MD explains in *Health and Nutrition Secrets*,

"...subtle toxicities can disrupt cellular function without producing obvious clinical toxicity – a condition known as subclinical toxicity."

Subclinical toxicity may also produce actual symptoms, but not of the type to be regarded as clinically significant. Symptoms of this nature are likely to be ignored on the grounds that they are not indicative of a 'disease' recognised by the medical establishment, whose attitude towards people with MCS and EHS was discussed in chapter seven. Dr Blaylock describes some of the symptoms that may be experienced,

"Rather than obvious signs such as nausea, vomiting and abdominal cramps, some people may experience no more than vague feelings of fatigue, cloudiness of thought, memory lapses, irritability, depression, or minor aches and pains..."

Sadly, few doctors are likely to recognise that obvious symptoms, such as nausea and vomiting, can result from the ingestion of toxins; most of them will ascribe such symptoms to a 'germ' of some description. Dr Blaylock also explains that doctors are largely unfamiliar with signs of 'subclinical toxicity'. This means that they are even less likely to associate subtle symptoms, such as 'cloudiness of thought' for example, with exposures to toxins or EM radiation; they are far more likely to associate these symptoms with a mental health problem.

The failure of physicians to recognise symptoms to be the result of exposures to 'harmful substances and influences' is due to their medical training, which only teaches them to recognise certain symptoms or symptom-complexes as indicative of the presence of a specific 'disease', the cause or causes of which may not even be known. Their training also extends to the recognition of certain symptoms and symptom-complexes as indicative of conditions referred to as 'mental illnesses', now known as 'mental disorders', the prevalence of which, according to the April 2018 WHO fact sheet entitled *Mental disorders*, is increasing,

"The burden of mental disorders continues to grow with significant impacts on health and major social, human rights and economic consequences in all countries around the world."

The fact sheet refers to some of the conditions included in this category and states that,

"Mental disorders include: depression, bipolar affective disorder, schizophrenia and other psychoses, dementia, intellectual disabilities and developmental disorders including autism."

The problems with the reference to depression as a 'mental disorder' were discussed in chapter one; the erroneous nature of the idea that autism is a 'mental disorder' was discussed in chapter seven. There are clearly similar problems with all of the other 'disorders' listed above; dementia is discussed later in this section.

The basic features of the conditions referred to as 'mental disorders' are described by the fact sheet that states,

"They are generally characterized by a combination of abnormal thoughts, perceptions, emotions, behaviour and relationships with others."

As discussed in chapter one, the reference to 'abnormal' presupposes the existence of a clearly defined description of 'normal'; but this is not the case. Although it may be appropriate to describe certain behaviours as unacceptable, it is inappropriate to attribute them to a mental illness. More importantly, it ought to be a matter of profound concern to everyone that any 'authority' possesses the right to determine the parameters of 'normal' in order to ascertain what can be described as 'abnormal'; especially with respect to people's thoughts, perceptions and emotions.

Interestingly, and as previously cited, the fact sheet claims that the factors that contribute to mental disorders also include stress and exposure to environmental hazards; the discussion in this section demonstrates these to be the major causal factors of neurological problems. The treatments recommended by the WHO for 'mental disorders' do not however, include measures to properly address these factors. Instead, treatments for many, but not all, of these conditions, include the use of psychoactive drugs to correct a 'chemical imbalance in the brain' that is claimed to be the main cause of these disorders; the erroneous nature of this claim was discussed in chapter one.

Psychoactive drugs are entirely inappropriate as treatments, not only because they are unable to correct a problem that has never been proven to exist, but also because they are known to cause severe harm to the brain. In his previously cited article entitled *Rational Principles of Psychopharmacology for Therapists, Healthcare Providers and Clients*, Dr Breggin refers to,

"...the brain-disabling principle, which states that all psychoactive substances work by causing dysfunctions of the brain and mind."

It can be seen that, yet again, medical 'treatments' have the ability to cause the very problems they are intended to remedy.

It is extremely important to reiterate that, as Dr Breggin states in his article,

"Withdrawing from psychiatric drugs can be emotionally and sometimes physically dangerous. It should be done carefully with experienced supervision."

Another reason that psychoactive drugs are an inappropriate remedy for 'mental disorders' is because they are utterly incapable of addressing any underlying emotional problems that may have precipitated the 'distress'. As previously stated, problems can only be resolved by addressing their cause or causes. Unfortunately, however, pharmaceuticals have become widely accepted as the panacea for many forms of 'distress'; as Dr Breggin explain in his article,

"A huge portion of the general population accepts that psychiatric drugs are the answer to everyday problems from fatigue and a broken heart to conflicts in the family between parents and their children."

Children who conflict with their parents, or other adults, may be diagnosed with a condition known as ODD (oppositional defiant disorder), which is generally described as a behavioural disorder, in which children display hostility, disobedience and defiance, often towards adult 'authority' figures. The medical establishment does not know what causes children to exhibit such behaviours, but a diagnosis of ODD requires the behaviours to have persisted for more than six months; temporary tantrums are therefore excluded.

Although children who exhibit these behaviours may have emotional problems that can be addressed through non-pharmaceutical-based therapies, they may also be affected by factors that are entirely unrelated to emotional problems. The most significant of these other factors are exposures to substances and influences that cause harm to the nervous system and produce neurological effects. The substances that can impair neurological functioning include various food additives, such as the chemicals used as food colourings and preservatives, as discussed in chapter six. Other sources of chemicals that impair neurological functioning, especially of children, include vaccines, many of which contain neurotoxic ingredients, as also previously discussed. The influences that can adversely affect the nervous system and cause neurological harm include RF-EMFs; children who use, or play with, mobile phones for example, will be exposed to the harmful radiofrequency EM radiation they emit.

Older people are another sector of the population claimed to be affected in large numbers by 'mental disorders'; the most common condition with which people over the age of 65 are diagnosed is dementia, which is described by the WHO May 2019 fact sheet entitled *Dementia* as,

"...a syndrome in which there is deterioration in memory, thinking, behaviour and the ability to perform everyday activities."

Although more common in older people, dementia is not solely a problem for people over the age of 65. More importantly, as the fact sheet acknowledges, dementia is not an inevitable consequence of ageing; many people older than 65 do not experience a deterioration in their mental faculties. The fact sheet does not identify the causes of dementia but instead, states that,

"Dementia results from a variety of diseases and injuries that primarily or secondarily affect the brain, such as Alzheimer's disease or stroke."

In addition to the statement that dementia can result from Alzheimer's disease, the fact sheet also states that Alzheimer's disease is the most common form of dementia. But this is highly anomalous because it suggests that one of the most common forms of dementia is a cause of dementia.

Interestingly, although unsurprisingly, the fact sheet attempts to associate cognitive impairments, including dementia, with the same 'risk factors' associated with 'physical' diseases, as indicated by the statement that,

"Studies show that people can reduce their risk of dementia by getting regular exercise, not smoking, avoiding harmful use of alcohol, controlling their weight, eating a healthy diet, and maintaining healthy blood pressure, cholesterol and blood sugar levels."

The problems with this statement have been discussed; however, the fact sheet claims that other 'risk factors' are also involved and states that,

"Additional risk factors include depression, low educational attainment, social isolation and cognitive inactivity."

In the same way that the medical establishment explanations about 'physical' diseases are flawed, those pertaining to 'cognitive impairments' are also flawed; they can however, be explained by reference to the 'new' explanation of disease. Cognitive impairments, including those referred to as 'mental disorders', are manifestations of dysfunctions, especially within the nervous system and the brain, resulting from exposures to 'harmful substances and influences'. In some instances, these exposures may have occurred prior to birth, as indicated by the discussions about the endocrine system and birth defects in chapter seven.

Significantly, the mechanism by which stressors exert their harmful effects is the same as all 'harmful substances and influences', namely, oxidative stress, which has been shown to be associated with a number of 'mental disorders', as discussed in a 2009 article entitled *Oxidative stress and anxiety* which states that,

"Oxidative damage in the brain causes nervous system impairment. Recently, oxidative stress has also been implicated in depression, anxiety disorder and high anxiety levels."

One of the most common symptoms caused by the tensions and anxieties associated with 'distress' is a headache. However, although headaches are recognised to be associated with the nervous system and neurological problems, they have been redefined as 'disorders'; as indicated by the April 2016 WHO fact sheet entitled *Headache disorders*, which states that,

"Headache disorders are among the most common disorders of the nervous system."

The fact sheet claims that there are four types of 'headache disorder': migraine; tension-type headache; cluster headache; and medication-overuse headache. Although persistent headaches are clearly debilitating, it is inappropriate to refer to them as 'disorders'. It is important to emphasise that headaches are one of the most common ailments for which people self-medicate; however, in common with all other 'medicines', over-the-counter pain-killers do not resolve or address the underlying problem. The category referred to as 'medication-overuse headache' is yet another demonstration that treatments are capable of causing the very problem they are intended to remedy.

An increasing number of studies have discovered that oxidative stress is a feature of the most common 'mental disorders'; as indicated by a 2014 article entitled *Oxidative Stress and Psychological Disorders*, which also states that,

"...the fact that oxidative stress is implicated in several mental disorders including depression, anxiety disorders, schizophrenia and bipolar disorder, is not surprising."

However, a 2013 article entitled *Good Stress, Bad Stress and Oxidative Stress: Insights from Anticipatory Cortisol Reactivity* makes the familiar statement that,

"...the mechanisms by which psychological stress promotes oxidative damage are poorly understood."

This statement is, however, rather surprising; Dr Russell Blaylock, a former neurosurgeon, explains in his 2006 book *Health and Nutrition Secrets* that stress increases the rate of metabolism and that increased metabolism increases the generation of free radicals. In the absence of adequate levels of antioxidants to counter them, free radicals will induce oxidative stress that can lead to free radical damage at the cellular level. Prolonged distress, therefore, will continue the process of free radical generation and cellular damage that will result in impaired functioning of tissues and organs, including those of the nervous system and brain.

This process is particularly significant with respect to the two most common neurodegenerative diseases; namely Alzheimer's disease (AD) and Parkinson's Disease (PD), both of which have been associated with high levels of oxidative stress; as reported in a 2017 article entitled *Oxidative Stress in Neurodegenerative Diseases: From Molecular Mechanisms to Clinical Applications*, which states that,

"The pathological mechanisms underlying the degeneration of dopaminergic neurons have been correlated to overaccumulation of ROS or other free radicals."

ROS are reactive oxygen species.

The WHO anticipates that dementia will continue to increase in incidence and prevalence into the foreseeable future; the fact sheet claims that there are approximately 50 million people around the world with dementia and that this number is predicted to reach 152 million by 2050. The reason that the incidence of dementia is anticipated to rise so dramatically in the next few decades is due to expectations that people will achieve ever-increasing lifespans, even though the WHO acknowledges that dementia is not an inevitable consequence of ageing. The credit for increased life expectancy is attributed to 'modern medicine', which is claimed to have reduced mortality, especially infant mortality, by successfully conquering deadly 'infectious diseases' through vaccination programmes; the erroneous nature of this claim has been discussed.

The real reasons that people, both young and old, experience cognitive impairments and neurological problems that may be diagnosed as 'mental disorders', are many and varied; but, like all other 'diseases', they are caused by exposures to various combinations of stressors, both physical and emotional.

It has been demonstrated in this discussion that stressors exert their harmful effects through the same mechanism as all other 'harmful substances and influences'; in other words, through the increased generation of free radicals that induce oxidative stress and lead to damage at the cellular level. It is clear therefore, that all stressors increase the utilisation of the body's supply of antioxidants. This inevitably places even greater emphasis on the importance of good nutrition and the regular intake of antioxidant-rich foods to 'scavenge' free radicals before they cause harm, and to provide support for the body's endogenous antioxidant production system. The nervous system, and especially the brain, can also be protected by avoiding or at least minimising exposures to substances and influences known to have harmful neurological effects.

Efforts to minimise exposures to stressors that can adversely impact the brain, and to increase the intake of protective antioxidants will not only help to slow down and prevent deterioration of cognitive functions, but they can also help to improve them. The reason for this is because another of the long-held beliefs of the medical establishment has been proven to be erroneous; this is the idea that new brain cells, also known as neurons, were not generated once they had been formed at the age of about 3 years old. In the 1970s, researchers discovered the presence of new neurons in certain parts of the adult brains of some animals. Continued research revealed that the generation of new neurons, also known as neurogenesis, occurs in many parts of the adult brain in many different animals, including humans. A 2008 article entitled *Estrogen and Adult Neurogenesis in the Amygdala and Hypothalamus* states that various factors may influence the rate at which new neurons may be generated. These factors include aspects of the external environment that can affect physiology and,

"...act on neurochemical and/or neurotransmitter systems to affect cellular proliferation and/or survival."

It should be clear from previous discussions that there are many 'environmental pollutants' that can act as physical stressors and contribute to neurological effects.

In the context of Dr Selye's definition, 'stress' is an inevitable aspect of life, but, as he explains,

"...we can learn a great deal about how to keep its damaging side-effects, 'distress', to a minimum."

Prolonged stress that has become 'distress' can clearly be debilitating and damaging to health. Although some stressors, such as the death of a loved one, may not be so easy to overcome, it is possible for people to take certain actions that will help to reduce their overall level of stress. The website of Dr Stephen Sinatra MD, for example, contains a page entitled *How to Handle Tension or Stress Headaches* that discusses strategies including diet, relaxation and sleep. On this page, Dr Sinatra, who is one of the co-authors of the previously cited *Earthing* book, refers to the practice of grounding that can 'de-stress' and help to re-balance the nervous system. He explains on the page entitled *What is Earthing or Grounding* that,

"Emerging science reveals that direct contact with the ground allows you to receive an energy infusion..."

He refers to this energy infusion as 'powerful stuff' that,

"...can restore and stabilize the bioelectrical circuitry that governs your physiology and organs, harmonize your basic biological rhythms, boost self-healing mechanisms..."

The human body clearly possesses mechanisms that are eminently capable of repairing damage to all areas of the body, including the brain, but this requires people to make every effort to avoid or minimise exposures to stressors that are harmful, as Dr Selye states,

"Only by intelligent adjustment of our conduct to the biologic rules is it possible to achieve full enjoyment of eustress without distress."

In Conclusion: How To Be Naturally Healthy

"Health is not something bestowed on you by beneficent nature at birth; it is achieved and maintained only by active participation in well-defined rules of healthful living..."

Henry Bieler

The health policy guidelines developed and issued by the WHO are recommended for implementation by all Member States; they therefore have the ability to affect the health of the entire world population. It may be assumed from the magnitude of this responsibility that the WHO possesses a thorough understanding of the problem it purports to be able to solve; it may also be assumed that the measures recommended for the treatment and prevention of illness are not only appropriate but are also safe and effective; these would however, be mistaken assumptions. As the discussions in this book have demonstrated, 'modern medicine' does not possess a thorough understanding of the nature of illness and has failed to correctly identify all of its causes. They have also demonstrated that the measures employed to treat and prevent disease, namely medicines and vaccines, are not only inappropriate, they are neither safe nor effective.

Although modern medicine is claimed to be founded on evidence-based science, it is abundantly obvious that it has failed to solve the problem of illness; this can be demonstrated by a substantial volume of evidence that shows ill-health to be a problem that continues to worsen rather than improve. It is clear that medicines and vaccines do not heal and prevent disease; but the problem with these measures is not merely their lack of efficacy. There is a large and growing body of evidence that shows pharmaceutical products to be toxic and therefore inimical to health, not supportive of it.

The main reason that 'modern medicine' has failed to solve the problem of illness is because it operates from the basis of fundamentally flawed theories; yet the medical establishment refuses to revise these theories, despite their obvious flaws.

In common with all other problems, that of 'illness' can only be solved by understanding its nature and correctly identifying its real causes. People can only be restored to good health when the causes of ill-health have been eliminated and therefore cease to exist; as indicated by Herbert Shelton who explains that,

736

"...full recovery cannot be expected so long as cause remains."

As stated in the Introduction to this book, health is the natural state of the human body, but achieving and retaining good health requires people to take certain actions. The main actions involve making conscious decisions, firstly, to avoid, or limit, exposures to the factors that adversely affect health and secondly, to increase exposures to the factors that improve health. In other words, it requires people to actively participate in 'healthful living', as explained by Dr Henry Bieler in the quote that opens this concluding section of the book.

Although most people trust the medical establishment as the 'authority' with respect to illness, especially in the treatment and prevention of disease, this is, unfortunately, a misplaced trust for reasons that have been discussed throughout this book. It must be emphasised that authority is not synonymous with 'truth'. Authority, when not based on truth, can impede progress and even prevent the discovery of truth; as indicated by a saying attributed to Albert Einstein,

"Unthinking respect for authority is the greatest enemy of truth."

It is likely that, at the beginning of this book, most readers would have considered the information in this book to have been controversial; it is however, appropriate at this juncture, to repeat the saying attributed to Arthur Schopenhauer,

"All truth passes through three stages. First, it is ridiculed. Second, it is violently opposed. Third, it is accepted as being self-evident."

It is sincerely hoped that, having reached the end of this book, you, the reader, will have attained the third stage and recognise the 'self-evident' nature of the information it contains. It is also hoped that, with your new understanding of what really makes you ill, you will feel you are now in possession of the information you require to make truly informed decisions about your healthcare.

References

The references and web pages listed below were correct at the time of preparing the book for publication; however, some web pages, especially WHO fact sheets, are dynamic and therefore subject to changes and updates.

All WHO fact sheets are available from this web page https://www.who.int/news-room/fact-sheets

Chapter One

WHO definition of health. www.who.int/about/mission/en

BMA founding principle. www.bma.org.uk

Bae YH, Park K. Targeted drug delivery to tumors: myths, reality and possibility. J Control Release. 2011 Aug 10;153(3):198-205. doi: 10.1016/j.jconrel.2011.06.001. Epub 2011 Jun 6. PMID: 21663778; PMCID: PMC3272876.

Where is the Wisdom...? The poverty of medical evidence www.bmj.com/content/bmj/303/6806/798.full.pdf

Pharmaceutical Waste Analysis www.blacksmithinstitute.org/files/FileUpload/files/Additional%20Reports/pwa1.pdf

Is US Health Really the Best in the World? www.jhsph.edu/research/centers-and-institutes/johns-hopkins-primary-care-policy-center/Publications_PDFs/A154.pdf

We're No. 26 US below average on most health measures www.nbcnews.com/health/were-number-20-us-below-average-most-health-measures-2d11635080

Gary Null et al – Death by Medicine www.webdc.com/pdfs/deathbymedicine.pdf

Rational Principles of Psychopharmacology for Therapists, Healthcare Providers and Clients www.breggin.com/wp-content/uploads/2008/06/Breggin2016_RationalPrinciples.pdf

SPRINT trial www.sprinttrial.org/public/dspHome.cfm

Landmark NIH study shows intensive blood pressure management may save lives. www.nhlbi.nih.gov/news/press-releases/2015/landmark-nih-study-shows-intensive-blood-pressure-management-may-save-lives

Chevalier G, Sinatra ST, Oschman JL, Delany RM. Earthing (grounding) the human body reduces blood viscosity-a major factor in cardiovascular disease. J Altern Complement Med. 2013 Feb;19(2):102-10. doi: 10.1089/acm.2011.0820. Epub 2012 Jul 3. PMID: 22757749; PMCID: PMC3576907.

High Blood Cholesterol: What You Need To Know. www.nhlbi.nih.gov/health/resources/heart/heart-cholesterol-hbc-what-html

Schreurs BG. The effects of cholesterol on learning and memory. Neurosci Biobehav Rev. 2010 Jul;34(8):1366-79. doi: 10.1016/j.neubiorev.2010.04.010. Epub 2010 May 12. PMID: 20470821; PMCID: PMC2900496.

Ramsden Christopher E, Zamora Daisy, Majchrzak-Hong Sharon, Faurot Keturah R, Broste Steven K, Frantz Robert P et al. Re-evaluation of the traditional diet-heart hypothesis: analysis of recovered data from Minnesota Coronary Experiment (1968-73) BMJ 2016;353:i1246

Statin Use and the Risk of Kidney Disease With Long-Term Follow-Up (8.4-Year Study) Acharya, Tushar et al. American Journal of Cardiology, Volume 117, Issue 4, 647 - 655

References

Cooper RJ. Over-the-counter medicine abuse - a review of the literature. J Subst Use. 2013 Apr;18(2):82-107. doi: 10.3109/14659891.2011.615002. Epub 2011 Oct 3. PMID: 23525509; PMCID: PMC3603170.

Drug Applications for Over-the-Counter (OTC) Drugs https://www.fda.gov/drugs/types-applications/drug-applications-over-counter-otc-drugs

Daily aspirin therapy: Understand the benefits and risks www.mayoclinic.org/diseases-conditions/heart-disease/in-depth/daily-aspirin-therapy/art-20046797

Chapter Two

Vaccines: A global health success story that keeps us on our toes www.who.int/mediacentre/commentaries/vaccines/en/

Global Vaccine Safety. Adverse Events Following Immunization (AEFI) www.who.int/vaccine_safety/initiative/detection/AEFI/en/

When vaccinations fail to cause response: Causes vary with vaccine and person https://medicalxpress.com/news/2013-08-vaccinations-response-vary-vaccine-person.html

Vaccines bring 7 diseases under control www.unicef.org/pon96/hevaccin.htm

Walter Hadwen 1896 address – The Case Against Vaccination www.bibliotecapleyades.net/salud/salud_vacunas24.htm#The_Case_Against_Vaccination

Vaccination greatly reduces disease, disability, death and inequity worldwide www.who.int/bulletin/volumes/86/2/07-040089/en/

WHO frequently asked questions and answers on smallpox www.who.int/csr/disease/smallpox/faq/en/

Dr Walter Hadwen's article in Truth magazine www.bibliotecapleyades.net/salud/salud_vacunas24.htm#THE_FRAUD_OF_VACCINATION

The Poison Cause of Poliomyelitis and Obstructions To Its Investigation www.whale.to/a/scobey2.html

Jim West's research on Polio http://harvoa.org/polio/overview.htm

Updates on CDC's Polio Eradication Efforts www.cdc.gov/polio/updates/

Polio free does not mean paralysis free www.thehindu.com/opinion/lead/polio-free-does-not-mean-paralysis-free/article4266043.ece

HPV Vaccine for Preteens and Teens www.cdc.gov/vaccines/parents/diseases/teen/hpv.html

Natural News interview with Dr Russell Blaylock about HPV vaccines www.naturalnews.com/036874_Dr_Russell_Blaylock_Gardasil_HPV_vaccines.html

Examining the FDA's HPV Vaccine Records www.judicialwatch.org/wp-content/uploads/2014/02/JW-Report-FDA-HPV-Vaccine-Records.pdf

JW Investigates HPV Compensation Program www.judicialwatch.org/press-room/press-releases/hpv-vaccine-injuries-and-deaths-is-the-government-compensating/

Emails from CDC and FDA on vaccines and mercury www.ageofautism.com/2007/12/emails-from-cdc.html

Bose-O'Reilly S, McCarty KM, Steckling N, Lettmeier B. Mercury exposure and children's health. Curr Probl Pediatr Adolesc Health Care. 2010 Sep;40(8):186-215. doi: 10.1016/j.cppeds.2010.07.002. PMID: 20816346; PMCID: PMC3096006.

Common Ingredients in U.S. Licensed Vaccines www.fda.gov/BiologicsBloodVaccines/SafetyAvailability/VaccineSafety/ucm187810.htm

Pontel LB, Rosado IV, Burgos-Barragan G, Garaycoechea JI, Yu R, Arends MJ, Chandrasekaran G, Broecker V, Wei W, Liu L, Swenberg JA, Crossan GP, Patel KJ. Endogenous Formaldehyde Is a Hematopoietic Stem Cell Genotoxin and Metabolic Carcinogen. Mol Cell. 2015 Oct 1;60(1):177-88. doi: 10.1016/j.molcel.2015.08.020. Epub 2015 Sep 24. PMID: 26412304; PMCID: PMC4595711.

Aluminium Adjuvants www.who.int/vaccine_safety/committee/topics/adjuvants/Jun_2012/en/

How Aluminium Affects Your Health www.thevaccinereaction.org/2016/06/how-aluminum-in-vaccines-affects-your-health/

Vaccine side effects www.nhs.uk/Conditions/vaccinations/Pages/reporting-side-effects.aspx

Multiple Vaccines and the Immune System www.cdc.gov/vaccinesafety/concerns/multiple-vaccines-immunity.html

No-fault compensation following adverse events attributed to vaccination: a review of international programmes www.who.int/bulletin/volumes/89/5/10-081901/en/

National Vaccine Injury Compensation Program www.hrsa.gov/vaccine-compensation/

Vaccine Injury Table https://www.hrsa.gov/sites/default/files/vaccinecompensation/vaccineinjurytable.pdf

Data and Statistics May 2019 https://www.hrsa.gov/sites/default/files/hrsa/vaccine-compensation/data/monthly-stats-may-2019.pdf

Transforming our world: the 2030 Agenda for Sustainable Development https://sustainabledevelopment.un.org/post2015/transformingourworld

Global Vaccine Action Plan 2011-2020 www.who.int/immunization/global_vaccine_action_plan/GVAP_doc_2011_2020/en/

PhRMA – Medicines in development Vaccines http://phrma-docs.phrma.org/sites/default/files/pdf/Vaccines_2013.pdf

Chapter Three

National Institutes of Health (US); Biological Sciences Curriculum Study. NIH Curriculum Supplement Series [Internet]. Bethesda (MD): National Institutes of Health (US); 2007. Understanding Emerging and Re-emerging Infectious Diseases. Available from: https://www.ncbi.nlm.nih.gov/books/NBK20370/

Dr ML Leverson MD May 1911 lecture http://www.whale.to/vaccine/shea1.html#Hume_

Disease is Remedial Action http://www.i-nhs.com/inhs/articles/classics1.html#0

Infectious Diseases https://www.mayoclinic.org/diseases-conditions/infectious-diseases/symptoms-causes/syc-20351173

WHO World Health Report 2007 – emerging diseases http://www.who.int/whr/2007/overview/en/index1.html

The Wisdom of Your Cells https://www.brucelipton.com/resource/article/the-wisdom-your-cells

Dr Harold Hillman's website is no longer active, some of his work is available on http://www.big-lies.org/harold-hillman-biology/

Are Viruses Alive? https://www.scientificamerican.com/article/are-viruses-alive-2004/

Introduction to Viruses http://www.ucmp.berkeley.edu/alllife/virus.html

Brandenburg B, Lee LY, Lakadamyali M, Rust MJ, Zhuang X, Hogle JM (2007) Imaging Poliovirus Entry in Live Cells. PLoS Biol 5(7): e183. https://doi.org/10.1371/journal.pbio.0050183

Ravindran MS, Bagchi P, Inoue T, Tsai B (2015) A Non-enveloped Virus Hijacks Host Disaggregation Machinery to Translocate across the Endoplasmic Reticulum Membrane. PLoS Pathog 11(8): e1005086. https://doi.org/10.1371/journal.ppat.1005086

Encyclopedia of Life – Viruses http://eol.org/info/458

Dr Stefan Lanka – Interview in Faktuell 2005 http://www.whale.to/b/lanka.html

Dr Stefan Lanka – Interview PRN http://prn.fm/infectious-myth-stefan-lanka-there-are-no-viruses-04-12-16/

Commensal-to-pathogen transition: One-single transposon insertion results in two pathoadaptive traits in Escherichia coli-macrophage interaction https://www.nature.com/articles/s41598-017-04081-1

References

McLaughlin RW, Vali H, Lau PC, Palfree RG, De Ciccio A, Sirois M, Ahmad D, Villemur R, Desrosiers M, Chan EC. Are there naturally occurring pleomorphic bacteria in the blood of healthy humans? J Clin Microbiol. 2002 Dec;40(12):4771-5. doi: 10.1128/jcm.40.12.4771-4775.2002. PMID: 12454193; PMCID: PMC154583.

Alberts B, Johnson A, Lewis J, et al. Molecular Biology of the Cell. 4th edition. New York: Garland Science; 2002. The Genetic Systems of Mitochondria and Plastids. Available from: https://www.ncbi.nlm.nih.gov/books/NBK26924/

Extreme Pleomorphism and the bacterial life cycle: a forgotten controversy http://www.whale.to/y/wainwright.html

Joshi HM, Toleti RS. Nutrition induced pleomorphism and budding mode of reproduction in Deinococcus radiodurans. BMC Res Notes. 2009 Jul 7;2:123. doi: 10.1186/1756-0500-2-123. PMID: 19583846; PMCID: PMC2714317.

Nilanjana Das and Preethy Chandran, "Microbial Degradation of Petroleum Hydrocarbon Contaminants: An Overview," Biotechnology Research International, vol. 2011, Article ID 941810, 13 pages, 2011. https://doi.org/10.4061/2011/941810.

S. S. BANG, M. PAZIRANDEH (1999) Physical properties and heavy metal uptake of encapsulated Escherichia coli expressing a metal binding gene (NCP), Journal of Microencapsulation, 16:4, 489-499, DOI: 10.1080/026520499288933

What are Escherichia coli? https://www.cdc.gov/ecoli/general/

Side effects of antibiotics https://www.nhs.uk/conditions/antibiotics/side-effects/

Antibiotic 'link to bowel cancer precursor' http://www.bbc.co.uk/news/health-39495192

Global antibiotics 'revolution' needed http://www.bbc.co.uk/news/health-36321394

Review on Antimicrobial Resistance https://amr-review.org/home.html

RHS – saprophytic fungi https://www.rhs.org.uk/advice/profile?pid=736

Kobayashi GS. Disease Mechanisms of Fungi. In: Baron S, editor. Medical Microbiology. 4th edition. Galveston (TX): University of Texas Medical Branch at Galveston; 1996. Chapter 74. Available from: https://www.ncbi.nlm.nih.gov/books/NBK8103/

Huffnagle GB, Noverr MC. The emerging world of the fungal microbiome. Trends Microbiol. 2013 Jul;21(7):334-41. doi: 10.1016/j.tim.2013.04.002. Epub 2013 May 17. PMID: 23685069; PMCID: PMC3708484.

Parfrey LW, Walters WA, Knight R. Microbial eukaryotes in the human microbiome: ecology, evolution, and future directions. Front Microbiol. 2011 Jul 11;2:153. doi: 10.3389/fmicb.2011.00153. PMID: 21808637; PMCID: PMC3135866.

WHO 2016 Malaria vaccine position paper http://www.who.int/wer/2016/wer9104.pdf?ua=1

NIH Medical Encyclopedia – antigen https://medlineplus.gov/ency/article/002224.htm

Breastfeeding provides passive and likely long-lasting active immunity https://www.ncbi.nlm.nih.gov/pubmed/9892025

The Bodyguard: Tapping the Immune System's Secrets http://sm.stanford.edu/archive/stanmed/2011summer/article7.html

Chapter Four

WHO Infectious diseases http://www.who.int/topics/infectious_diseases/en/

Morens DM, Fauci AS (2013) Emerging Infectious Diseases: Threats to Human Health and Global Stability. PLoS Pathog 9(7): e1003467. https://doi.org/10.1371/journal.ppat.1003467

Childhood Diseases – What Parents Need to Know https://medlineplus.gov/magazine/issues/spring08/articles/spring08pg5-6.html

Vaccinate Your Baby for Best Protection https://www.cdc.gov/features/infantimmunization/

Duthie MS, Gillis TP, Reed SG. Advances and hurdles on the way toward a leprosy vaccine. Hum Vaccin. 2011 Nov;7(11):1172-83. doi: 10.4161/hv.7.11.16848. Epub 2011 Nov 1. PMID: 22048122; PMCID: PMC3323495.

The Return of Syphilis https://www.theatlantic.com/health/archive/2015/12/the-return-of-syphilis/418170/

2015 STD Surveillance Report Press Release https://www.cdc.gov/nchhstp/newsroom/2016/std-surveillance-report-2015-press-release.html

The Influenza Pandemic of 1918 https://virus.stanford.edu/uda/

1918 Influenza: the Mother of All Pandemics https://wwwnc.cdc.gov/eid/article/12/1/05-0979_article

Byerly CR. The U.S. military and the influenza pandemic of 1918-1919. Public Health Rep. 2010 Apr;125 Suppl 3(Suppl 3):82-91. PMID: 20568570; PMCID: PMC2862337.

Death from 1918 pandemic influenza during the First World War http://onlinelibrary.wiley.com/doi/10.1111/irv.12267/abstract

Karen M. Starko, Salicylates and Pandemic Influenza Mortality, 1918–1919 Pharmacology, Pathology, and Historic Evidence, Clinical Infectious Diseases, Volume 49, Issue 9, 15 November 2009, Pages 1405–1410, https://doi.org/10.1086/606060

The fog of research: Influenza vaccine trials during the 1918-19 pandemic https://www.ncbi.nlm.nih.gov/pubmed/19525296

Eyler JM. The state of science, microbiology, and vaccines circa 1918. Public Health Rep. 2010 Apr;125 Suppl 3(Suppl 3):27-36. doi: 10.1177/00333549101250S306. PMID: 20568567; PMCID: PMC2862332.

Herbert Shelton – Contagion http://www.i-nhs.com/inhs/articles/classics4.html#18

Parallels between Neuroleptic Effects and Lethargic Encephalitis http://www.breggin.com/td-resources/Breggin-1993-antipsychotric-drugs-and-lethargic-encephalitis.pdf

Post-Vaccination Encephalitis http://annals.org/aim/article-abstract/669860/post-vaccination-encephalitis

Report about the University of Arizona study on the 1918 virus https://uanews.arizona.edu/story/mystery-of-1918-pandemic-flu-virus-solved-by-ua-researchers

The Plague http://www.livius.org/sources/content/thucydides/the-plague/

Justinian's Plague https://www.ancient.eu/article/782/justinians-plague-541-542-ce/

Can We Stop Blaming Rats for the Black Death? http://www.history.com/news/can-we-stop-blaming-rats-for-the-black-death

Herbert Shelton – Pestilence and Plagues http://www.i-nhs.com/inhs/articles/classics4.html#17

The Diary of Samuel Pepys – extract https://www.pepysdiary.com/diary/1664/12/24/

A Journal of the Plague Year – extract https://www.rc.umd.edu/editions/mws/lastman/defoe.htm

Pleomorphic appearance in Mycobacterium tuberculosis http://www.academicjournals.org/article/article1379341884_Malhotra%20et%20al.pdf

CDC questions about BCG vaccine https://www.cdc.gov/tb/publications/faqs/qa_latenttbinf.htm

Who should have the BCG (TB) vaccine? https://www.nhs.uk/conditions/vaccinations/when-is-bcg-tb-vaccine-needed/

AIDS and Poppers http://www.virusmyth.com/aids/hiv/tbpoppers.htm

The Drugs-AIDS Hypothesis http://www.virusmyth.com/aids/hiv/pddrdrugaids.htm

Kary Mullis interview http://www.virusmyth.com/aids/hiv/slquestions.htm

CDC Opportunistic infections https://www.cdc.gov/hiv/basics/livingwithhiv/opportunisticinfections.html

HIV Tests Are Not HIV Tests http://www.jpands.org/vol15no1/bauer.pdf

References

The Case Against HIV http://thecaseagainsthiv.net/

Management of Infants Born to Women with HIV Infection
https://aidsinfo.nih.gov/guidelines/html/3/perinatal/187/antiretroviral-management-of-newborns-with-perinatal-hiv-exposure-or-perinatal-hiv

The Yin & Yang of HIV http://www.whale.to/a/turner.html

Chapter Five

Managing public health risks at the human-Animal-environment interface
http://www.who.int/zoonoses/en/

FAO-OIE-WHO Collaboration document
http://www.who.int/foodsafety/zoonoses/final_concept_note_Hanoi.pdf?ua=1

Haydon DT, Cleaveland S, Taylor LH, Laurenson MK. Identifying reservoirs of infection: a conceptual and practical challenge. Emerg Infect Dis. 2002 Dec;8(12):1468-73. doi: 10.3201/eid0812.010317. PMID: 12498665; PMCID: PMC2738515.

Baum SG. Zoonoses-with friends like this, who needs enemies? Trans Am Clin Climatol Assoc. 2008;119:39-51; discussion 51-2. PMID: 18596867; PMCID: PMC2394705.

Emerging zoonotic viral diseases https://www.oie.int/doc/ged/D14089.PDF

Taylor LH, Latham SM, Woolhouse ME. Risk factors for human disease emergence. Philos Trans R Soc Lond B Biol Sci. 2001 Jul 29;356(1411):983-9. doi: 10.1098/rstb.2001.0888. PMID: 11516376; PMCID: PMC1088493.

The Wildlife Trusts – cattle vaccinations http://www.wildlifetrusts.org/badger-cull

Human Illness Associated with Use of Veterinary Vaccines
https://academic.oup.com/cid/article/37/3/407/437242

Jeong SH, Kang D, Lim MW, Kang CS, Sung HJ. Risk assessment of growth hormones and antimicrobial residues in meat. Toxicol Res. 2010 Dec;26(4):301-13. doi: 10.5487/TR.2010.26.4.301. PMID: 24278538; PMCID: PMC3834504.

Hormone Use in Food Animal Production: Assessing Potential Dietary Exposures and Breast Cancer Risk https://www.ncbi.nlm.nih.gov/pubmed/26231238

Landers TF, Cohen B, Wittum TE, Larson EL. A review of antibiotic use in food animals: perspective, policy, and potential. Public Health Rep. 2012 Jan-Feb;127(1):4-22. doi: 10.1177/003335491212700103. PMID: 22298919; PMCID: PMC3234384.

OIE – Animal Disease Information http://www.oie.int/for-the-media/animal-diseases/animal-disease-information-summaries/

Rabies Past Present in Scientific Review http://whale.to/vaccine/rabies.html

AVMA Vaccination FAQs https://www.avma.org/KB/Resources/FAQs/Pages/Vaccination-FAQs.aspx

Tuberculosis: a reemerging disease at the interface of domestic animals and wildlife
https://www.ncbi.nlm.nih.gov/pubmed/17848066

Badger cull kills more than 10,000 animals in three months
https://www.theguardian.com/environment/2016/dec/16/badger-cull-kills-more-than-10000-animals-three-months-bovine-tb

UK Government committed to badger culling
http://researchbriefings.parliament.uk/ResearchBriefing/Summary/SN06837

The Wildlife Trusts – Bovine Tuberculosis (bTB) http://www.wildlifetrusts.org/badger-cull

Tuberculin skin testing http://www.tbhub.co.uk/guidance/testing-and-compensation/tuberculin-skin-testing/

Studies in the Epidemiology of Infectious Myxomatosis – the series of seven papers
https://www.ncbi.nlm.nih.gov/pubmed/?term=Fenner%20F%5BAuthor%5D&cauthor=true&cauthor_uid=13439170

Rewilding Australia https://rewildingaustralia.org.au/

Use of OCPs in Australia http://www.environment.gov.au/protection/publications/ocp-trade-names

WHO Anthrax in humans and animals
http://www.who.int/csr/resources/publications/AnthraxGuidelines2008/en/

Anthrax Sterne strain (34F2) of Bacillus anthracis
https://www.cdc.gov/nczved/divisions/dfbmd/diseases/anthrax_sterne/

Guidance on anthrax: frequently asked questions
https://www.who.int/csr/disease/Anthrax/anthraxfaq/en/

Nass M. The Anthrax Vaccine Program: an analysis of the CDC's recommendations for vaccine use. Am J Public Health. 2002 May;92(5):715-21. doi: 10.2105/ajph.92.5.715. PMID: 11988433; PMCID: PMC1447151.

The history of woolsorters' disease: a Yorkshire beginning with an international future?
https://www.ncbi.nlm.nih.gov/pubmed/15486181

Arsenic and Old Wool http://allianceforcancerprevention.org.uk/wp-content/uploads/2012/01/ARSENICb-edited-and-tracked-changes-to-paper-30-June-20081.doc

Areas of Science that Use Animals https://www.navs.org/what-we-do/keep-you-informed/science-corner/areas-of-science-that-use-animals/#.WtIGrkxFzIU

Animals Used in Research https://www.navs.org/what-we-do/keep-you-informed/science-corner/areas-of-science-that-use-animals/animals-used-in-research/#.WtIHRUxFzIU

Chao Y, Zhang T. Optimization of fixation methods for observation of bacterial cell morphology and surface ultrastructures by atomic force microscopy. Appl Microbiol Biotechnol. 2011 Oct;92(2):381-92. doi: 10.1007/s00253-011-3551-5. Epub 2011 Sep 1. PMID: 21881891; PMCID: PMC3181414.

Vivisection Information Network
http://vivisectioninformation.com/index1945.html?p=1_14_Medical-quotes

Vivisection or Science: A Choice to Make
http://www.pnc.com.au/~cafmr/online/research/croce1.html

Chapter Six

WHO Preventing disease through healthy environments
http://www.who.int/quantifying_ehimpacts/publications/preventing-disease/en/

The Waning Days of Risk Assessment http://www.rachel.org/?q=en/node/4797

Environmental pollution and the global burden of disease
https://academic.oup.com/bmb/article/68/1/1/421204

Global rise in human infectious disease outbreaks
http://rsif.royalsocietypublishing.org/content/11/101/20140950

Carbon Dioxide in Greenhouses http://www.omafra.gov.on.ca/english/crops/facts/00-077.htm

Lead Poisoning http://rachel.org/files/document/Lead_Poisoning.pdf

How Far Is Too Far? http://naturalhygienesociety.org/articles/classics1.html#4

The Global Problem of Lead Arsenate Pesticides
http://www.lead.org.au/lanv10n3/lanv10n3-7.html

Health Effects of Uranium Mining http://www.ippnw.org/pdf/uranium-factsheet4.pdf

Nuclear Power's Other Tragedy
https://earthworks.org/publications/nuclear_powers_other_tragedy/

NIOSH Worker Health Study Uranium Miners (1)
https://www.cdc.gov/niosh/pgms/worknotify/uranium.html

Clean Up the Mines fact sheet http://www.cleanupthemines.org/facts/

How many chemicals are in use today? https://cen.acs.org/articles/95/i9/chemicals-use-today.html

TCSA Chemical Substance Inventory https://www.epa.gov/tsca-inventory

References

About the Office of Chemical Safety and Pollution Prevention (OCSPP) https://www.epa.gov/aboutepa/about-office-chemical-safety-and-pollution-prevention-ocspp

Where EPA Works Around the World https://www.epa.gov/international-cooperation/where-epa-works-around-world

Synergy: The Big Unknowns of Pesticide Exposure https://beyondpesticides.org/assets/media/documents/infoservices/pesticidesandyou/Winter%2003-04/Synergy.pdf

Methods for chemical assessment http://www.who.int/ipcs/methods/en/

Making Good Decisions https://www.ejnet.org/rachel/rehw470.htm

Colborn T. Neurodevelopment and endocrine disruption. Environ Health Perspect. 2004 Jun;112(9):944-9. doi: 10.1289/ehp.6601. PMID: 15198913; PMCID: PMC1247186.

Organic Chemistry https://www.acs.org/content/acs/en/careers/college-to-career/areas-of-chemistry/organic-chemistry.html

Chorine Chemistry: Providing Pharmaceuticals That Keep You and Your Family Healthy https://chlorine.americanchemistry.com/Chlorine/Pharmaceuticals/

Petrochemicals https://www.afpm.org/petrochemicals/

Organic Chemistry https://www.acs.org/content/acs/en/careers/college-to-career/areas-of-chemistry/organic-chemistry.html

What Are Rare Earths? http://www.rareearthchalliance.com/What-are-Rare-Earths

Effects of rare earth elements on the environment and human health: A literature review Rim, KT. Toxicol. Environ. Health Sci. (2016) 8: 189. https://doi.org/10.1007/s13530-016-0276-y

Rim KT, Koo KH, Park JS. Toxicological evaluations of rare earths and their health impacts to workers: a literature review. Saf Health Work. 2013 Mar;4(1):12-26. doi: 10.5491/SHAW.2013.4.1.12. Epub 2013 Mar 11. PMID: 23516020; PMCID: PMC3601293.

Radiation https://www.nirs.org/radiation/

No Such Thing as a Safe Dose of Radiation https://www.nirs.org/wp-content/uploads/factsheets/nosafedose.pdf

NIRS fact sheet Radiation Basics https://www.nirs.org/wp-content/uploads/radiation/radiationbasics.pdf

General Overview of the Effects of Nuclear Testing https://www.ctbto.org/nuclear-testing/the-effects-of-nuclear-testing/general-overview-of-theeffects-of-nuclear-testing/

Human Experimentation: An Overview of Cold War Programs https://www.gao.gov/products/T-NSIAD-94-266

Biological Effects of Ionizing Radiation http://webfiles.ehs.ufl.edu/rssc_stdy_chp_5.pdf

Dr John Gofman Synapse interview https://ratical.org/ratitorsCorner/09.23.15.html

Low Levels of Ionizing Radiation May Cause Harm http://www8.nationalacademies.org/onpinews/newsitem.aspx?RecordID=11340

Food Irradiation: What You Need to Know https://www.fda.gov/food/resourcesforyou/consumers/ucm261680.htm

About Food Irradiation https://www.centerforfoodsafety.org/issues/1039/food-irradiation/about-food-irradiation

Food Irradiation: A Gross Failure https://www.centerforfoodsafety.org/issues/1039/food-irradiation/reports/1398/food-irradiation-a-gross-failure

Objectives https://www.iaea.org/about/statute

Routine Radioactive Releases from US Nuclear Power Plants http://static1.1.sqspcdn.com/static/f/356082/21270648/1355504091613/Routine+Releases_Dec+2012.pdf?token=DiL5bs3e%2B9fw4Md9YdGV66gHHLg%3D

Report of the United Nations Scientific Committee on The Effects of Atomic Radiation to the General Assembly
http://www.unscear.org/docs/publications/2000/UNSCEAR_2000_Report_Vol.I.pdf

Treaty Adopted on 7th July https://www.un.org/disarmament/tpnw/

A Treaty Is Reached to Ban Nuclear Arms. Now Comes the Hard Part
https://www.nytimes.com/2017/07/07/world/americas/united-nations-nuclear-weapons-prohibition-destruction-global-treaty.html

Radiation non-ionizing http://www.who.int/topics/radiation_non_ionizing/en/

Safe Exposure Levels
http://www.weepinitiative.org/LINKEDDOCS/scientific/safe_exposure_levels_Dr._Cherry.pdf

The BioInitiative 2012 Report http://www.bioinitiative.org/table-of-contents/

Electromagnetic fields http://www.who.int/peh-emf/en/

The Biological Effects of Weak Electromagnetic Fields
https://ecfsapi.fcc.gov/file/7022311211.pdf

EMF/EMR Reduces Melatonin in Animals and People
http://www.neilcherry.nz/documents/90_b1_EMR_Reduces_Melatonin_in_Animals_and_People.pdf

Hyperthermia to Treat Cancer https://www.cancer.org/treatment/treatments-and-side-effects/treatment-types/hyperthermia.html

MRI scan https://www.nhs.uk/conditions/mri-scan/

How Does an MRI work?
https://www.hopkinsmedicine.org/healthlibrary/test_procedures/gynecology/breast_mri_92,P09110

Towards 5G communications systems: Are there health implications?
https://www.ncbi.nlm.nih.gov/pubmed/29402696

5G And The IOT: Scientific Overview of Human Health Risks https://ehtrust.org/key-issues/cell-phoneswireless/5g-networks-iot-scientific-overview-human-health-risks/

Theo Colborn, Carol Kwiatkowski, Kim Schultz & Mary Bachran (2011) Natural Gas Operations from a Public Health Perspective, Human and Ecological Risk Assessment: An International Journal, 17:5, 1039-1056, DOI: 10.1080/10807039.2011.605662

The Endocrine Disruption Exchange https://endocrinedisruption.org/

Fracking Linked to Cancer-Causing Chemicals, New YSPH Study Finds
https://publichealth.yale.edu/article.aspx?id=13714

Fracking: The New Global Water Crisis
https://www.foodandwaterwatch.org/insight/fracking-new-global-water-crisis

Hydraulic Fracturing for Oil and Gas: Impacts from the Hydraulic Fracturing Water Cycle on Drinking Water Resources in the United States
https://cfpub.epa.gov/ncea/hfstudy/recordisplay.cfm?deid=332990

Do fracking activities cause earthquakes? Seismologists and the state of Oklahoma say yes
https://www.cbc.ca/news/canada/edmonton/fracking-debate-earthquakes-oklahoma-1.3554275

Geoengineering the climate: Science, governance and uncertainty
https://royalsociety.org/topics-policy/publications/2009/geoengineering-climate/

CO2 is not a Greenhouse Gas that Raises Global Temperature. Period!
http://drtimball.com/2012/co2-is-not-a-greenhouse-gas-that-raises-global-temperature-period/

What in the World Are They Spraying? https://topdocumentaryfilms.com/what-in-the-world-are-they-spraying/

The Climate Engineers http://archive.wilsonquarterly.com/essays/climate-engineers

References

RAF rainmakers caused 1952 flood
https://www.theguardian.com/uk/2001/aug/30/sillyseason.physicalsciences

Impacts of Chemtrails in Human Health. Nanoaluminum: Neurodegenerative and Neurodevelopmental Effects https://www.globalresearch.ca/impacts-of-chemtrails-on-human-health-nanoaluminum-neurodegenerative-and-neurodevelopmental-effects/5342624

Elevated silver, barium and strontium in antlers, vegetation and soil sourced from CWD cluster areas: do Ag/Ba/Sr piezoelectric crystals represent the transmissible pathogenic agent in TSEs? https://www.ncbi.nlm.nih.gov/pubmed/15236778

Chemtrail Whistleblower Allan Buckmann: Some Thoughts on Weather Modification https://www.activistpost.com/2012/08/chemtrail-whistleblower-allan-buckmann.html

Ground Based 'Star Wars' https://earthpulse.com/haarp/

How To Wreck the Environment https://coto2.files.wordpress.com/2013/11/1968-macdonald-how-to-wreck-the-planet.pdf

Background on the HAARP Project
https://www.globalpolicy.org/component/content/article/212/45492.html

USAF Weather as a Force Multiplier
https://archive.org/details/WeatherAsAForceMultiplier/page/n0

Understanding Codex http://www.fao.org/3/a-i5667e.pdf

Chemicals in Foods https://www.efsa.europa.eu/en/topics/topic/chemicals-food

WHO International Food Standards (FAO/WHO Codex Alimentarius)
http://www.who.int/foodsafety/areas_work/en/

General Standard for Contaminants and Toxins in Food and Feed (Codex STAN 193-1995)
http://www.fao.org/fileadmin/user_upload/livestockgov/documents/1_CXS_193e.pdf

General Standard for the Labelling of Prepackaged Foods (Codex STAN 1-1985)
http://www.fao.org/docrep/005/Y2770E/y2770e02.htm

Guidelines on Nutrition labelling (CAC/GL 2-1985)
http://www.fao.org/docrep/005/y2770e/y2770e06.htm

Guidelines for Use of Nutrition Claims (CAC/GL 23-1997)
http://www.fao.org/docrep/005/Y2770E/y2770e07.htm

Food Additives https://www.efsa.europa.eu/en/topics/topic/food-additives

General Standard for Food Additives (Codex STAN 192-1995)
http://www.fao.org/gsfaonline/docs/CXS_192e.pdf

Crackdown on additives needed http://www.foodcomm.org.uk/press/additives_crackdown/

Chemical risks and JECFA http://www.fao.org/food/food-safety-quality/scientific-advice/jecfa/en/

JECFA Meeting re Aflatoxins http://www.fao.org/3/a-bq821e.pdf

Magnuson B, Munro I, Abbot P, Baldwin N, Lopez-Garcia R, Ly K, McGirr L, Roberts A, Socolovsky S. Review of the regulation and safety assessment of food substances in various countries and jurisdictions. Food Addit Contam Part A Chem Anal Control Expo Risk Assess. 2013;30(7):1147-220. doi: 10.1080/19440049.2013.795293. Epub 2013 Jun 20. PMID: 23781843; PMCID: PMC3725665.

Generally Recognized as Secret: Chemicals Added to Food in the United States
https://www.nrdc.org/resources/generally-recognized-secret-chemicals-added-food-united-states

Chemical risks http://www.who.int/foodsafety/areas_work/chemical-risks/en/

Additives https://www.firststepsnutrition.org/additives/

Food Dyes: A Rainbow of Risks https://cspinet.org/sites/default/files/attachment/food-dyes-rainbow-of-risks.pdf

Fact Sheet: The Science Linking Food Dyes with Impacts on Children's Behavior
https://cspinet.org/resource/science-linking-food-dyes-impacts-childrens-behavior

Major study indicates a link between hyperactivity in children and certain food additives
https://www.southampton.ac.uk/news/2007/09/hyperactivity-in-children-and-food-additives.page

CSPI Seeing Red: Time for Action on Food Dyes https://cspinet.org/resource/seeing-red-time-action-food-dyes

The cosmetic dye quinoline yellow causes DNA damage in vitro
https://www.ncbi.nlm.nih.gov/pubmed/25726175

Evaluation of certain food additives
http://apps.who.int/iris/bitstream/handle/10665/250277/9789241210003-eng.pdf;jsessionid=FCCB73E0FC8F0D265160DD3F790FE3DE?sequence=1

Food colours and hyperactivity https://www.nhs.uk/conditions/food-colours-and-hyperactivity/

A Question of Taste: A review of flavourings in food and drinks in the UK
https://static1.squarespace.com/static/59f75004f09ca48694070f3b/t/5a94002124a69489a7418287/1519648803309/questionoftaste.pdf

EFSA Flavourings https://www.efsa.europa.eu/en/topics/topic/flavourings

Guidelines for the Use of Flavourings (Codex CAC/GL 66-2008)
http://www.maff.go.jp/j/shokusan/seizo/pdf/66-2008.pdf

Extraction solvents
https://ec.europa.eu/food/safety/food_improvement_agents/extraction-solvents_en

Flavourings-related lung disease
https://www.cdc.gov/niosh/topics/flavorings/exposure.html

Questions and Answers on Monosodium glutamate (MSG)
https://www.fda.gov/food/ingredientspackaginglabeling/foodadditivesingredients/ucm328728.htm

On the Subject of Manufactured vs Natural Glutamic Acid
http://www.truthinlabeling.org/manufac.html

Effect of Storage on Nutritive Value of Food
https://onlinelibrary.wiley.com/doi/abs/10.1111/j.1745-4557.1977.tb00998.x

Nutritional aspects of food preservatives https://www.ncbi.nlm.nih.gov/pubmed/1298657

Preservatives to keep foods longer – and safer https://www.eufic.org/en/whats-in-food/article/preservatives-to-keep-foods-longer-and-safer

14th Report on Carcinogens https://ntp.niehs.nih.gov/pubhealth/roc/index-1.html

Institute of Medicine (US) Committee on Strategies to Reduce Sodium Intake; Henney JE, Taylor CL, Boon CS, editors. Strategies to Reduce Sodium Intake in the United States. Washington (DC): National Academies Press (US); 2010. Available from: https://www.ncbi.nlm.nih.gov/books/NBK50956/ doi: 10.17226/12818

WHO calls on countries to reduce sugars intake among
http://www.who.int/mediacentre/news/releases/2015/sugar-guideline/en/

141 Reasons Sugar Ruins Your Health https://nancyappleton.com/141-reasons-sugar-ruins-your-health/

Dooley KE, Chaisson RE. Tuberculosis and diabetes mellitus: convergence of two epidemics. Lancet Infect Dis. 2009 Dec;9(12):737-46. doi: 10.1016/S1473-3099(09)70282-8. PMID: 19926034; PMCID: PMC2945809.

Additional Information about High-Intensity Sweeteners Permitted for Use in Food in the United States
https://www.fda.gov/food/ingredientspackaginglabeling/foodadditivesingredients/ucm397725.htm#Saccharin

Aspartame https://www.efsa.europa.eu/en/topics/topic/aspartame

Genetically Engineered Crops: Experiences and Prospects
https://www.nap.edu/read/23395/chapter/3

References

GMO Myths and Truths: An evidence-based examination of the claims made for the safety and efficacy of genetically modified crops
https://earthopensource.org/wordpress/downloads/GMO-Myths-and-Truths-edition2.pdf

Failure to Yield: Evaluating the Performance of Genetically Engineered Crops
https://www.ucsusa.org/food_and_agriculture/our-failing-food-system/genetic-engineering/failure-to-yield.html#.W7DczvZFzIU

World Hunger Again On The Rise, Driven By Conflict And Climate Change, New UN Report Says https://www.wfp.org/news/news-release/world-hunger-again-rise-driven-conflict-and-climate-change-new-un-report-says

Patent 7851676 Stress tolerant plants and methods thereof
https://patents.google.com/patent/US7851676

The Case for a GM-Free Sustainable World http://www.i-sis.org.uk/TheCaseforAGM-FreeSustainableWorld.php

Debunking Popular Myths about GE Crops Portrayed in the Media
https://www.centerforfoodsafety.org/blog/3468/debunking-popular-myths-about-ge-crops-portrayed-in-the-media

Effects of diets containing genetically modified potatoes expressing Galanthus nivalis lectin on rat small intestine https://www.thelancet.com/journals/lancet/article/PIIS0140-6736(98)05860-7/fulltext

GMO Scandal: The Long Term Effects of Genetically Modified Food on Humans
https://www.globalresearch.ca/gmo-scandal-the-long-term-effects-of-genetically-modified-food-on-humans/14570

The GMO Emperor Has No Clothes
https://www.navdanyainternational.it/images/pubblicazioni/Full_Report_Rapporto_compl eto.pdf

Unraveling the DNA Myth: The spurious foundation of genetic engineering
https://pdfs.semanticscholar.org/3b1c/2f1dfoacf6a30beac244152fcof57f66523f.pdf

Study Shows Monsanto Roundup Herbicide Link to Birth Defects
https://www.globalresearch.ca/study-shows-monsanto-roundup-herbicide-link-to-birth-defects/21251

Glyphosate-based herbicides produce teratogenic effects on vertebrates by impairing retinoic acid signalling https://www.ncbi.nlm.nih.gov/pubmed/20695457

Largest international study into safety of GM food launched by Russian NGO
https://www.theguardian.com/environment/2014/nov/11/largest-international-study-into-safety-of-gm-food-launched-by-russian-ngo

How Much Water is There on Earth? https://water.usgs.gov/edu/earthhowmuch.html

WHO Guidelines for drinking-water quality, 4th edition, incorporating the 1st addendum
http://www.who.int/water_sanitation_health/publications/drinking-water-quality-guidelines-4-including-1st-addendum/en/

Water-related diseases https://www.who.int/water_sanitation_health/diseases-risks/diseases/diseasefact/en/

Water-related diseases Malnutrition
https://www.who.int/water_sanitation_health/diseases-risks/diseases/malnutrition/en/

National Primary Drinking Water Regulations https://www.epa.gov/ground-water-and-drinking-water/national-primary-drinking-water-regulations

Introduction To The Public Water System Supervision Program
https://cfpub.epa.gov/watertrain/pdf/modules/pwss.pdf

Water Fluoridation Data & Statistics https://www.cdc.gov/fluoridation/statistics/

Inadequate or excess fluoride
https://www.who.int/ipcs/assessment/public_health/fluoride/en/

The Phosphate Fertilizer Industry: An Environmental Overview
http://www.fluoridation.com/PhosphateFertilizer.htm

Fluoridation Chemicals https://fluoridealert.org/issues/water/fluoridation-chemicals/

Fluoride in Water https://www.ada.org/en/public-programs/advocating-for-the-public/fluoride-and-fluoridation

Sources of Fluoride https://fluoridealert.org/issues/sources/

Fluoride and Biochemistry https://fluoridealert.org/articles/fluoride-biochemistry/

Fluoride is not an Essential Element http://fluoridealert.org/studies/essential-nutrient/

Industrial Wastewater https://www.epa.gov/npdes/industrial-wastewater

Factory Farm Nation: 2015 Edition https://www.foodandwaterwatch.org/insight/factory-farm-nation-2015-edition

Persistent Organic Pollutants: A Global Issue, A Global Response https://www.epa.gov/international-cooperation/persistent-organic-pollutants-global-issue-global-response

Persistent organic pollutants (POPs) https://www.who.int/foodsafety/areas_work/chemical-risks/pops/en/

Just Say N2O: From manufactured fertiliser to biologically-fixed nitrogen https://www.soilassociation.org/media/4955/policy_2012_just_say_n2o.pdf

Dosed Without Prescription: Preventing Pharmaceutical Contamination of Our Nation's Drinking Water https://www.nrdc.org/resources/dosed-without-prescription-preventing-pharmaceutical-contamination-our-nations-drinking

Contaminants of Emerging Concern including Pharmaceuticals and Personal Care Products https://www.epa.gov/wqc/contaminants-emerging-concern-including-pharmaceuticals-and-personal-care-products

Only Half of Drugs Removed by Sewage Treatment https://www.scientificamerican.com/article/only-half-of-drugs-removed-by-sewage-treatment/

Unsafe levels of toxic chemicals found in drinking water for six million Americans https://www.hsph.harvard.edu/news/press-releases/toxic-chemicals-drinking-water/

Dermal Absorption http://www.inchem.org/documents/ehc/ehc/ehc235.pdf

Dermal Exposure http://www.who.int/ipcs/publications/ehc/ehc_242.pdf

Skin Exposures and Effects https://www.cdc.gov/niosh/topics/skin/default.html

Toxicity and Assessment of Chemical Mixtures http://ec.europa.eu/health/scientific_committees/environmental_risks/docs/scher_o_155.pdf

Household Hazardous Waste (HHW) https://www.epa.gov/hw/household-hazardous-waste-hhw

Phthalates https://www.fda.gov/cosmetics/productsingredients/ingredients/ucm128250.htm

Swan SH. Environmental phthalate exposure in relation to reproductive outcomes and other health endpoints in humans. Environ Res. 2008 Oct;108(2):177-84. doi: 10.1016/j.envres.2008.08.007. PMID: 18949837; PMCID: PMC2775531.

Pharmaceutical Excipients https://www.americanpharmaceuticalreview.com/25335-Pharmaceutical-Raw-Materials-and-APIs/25283-Pharmaceutical-Excipients/

PVC: The most widely used polymer in medical applications http://www.pvc.org/en/p/pvc---the-most-widely-used-polymer-in-medical-applications

EPA Phthalates Action Plan https://www.epa.gov/sites/production/files/2015-09/documents/phthalates_actionplan_revised_2012-03-14.pdf

Phthalates TEACH Chemical Summary https://archive.epa.gov/region5/teach/web/pdf/phthalates_summary.pdf

Bisphenol A (BPA): Use in Food Contact Application https://www.fda.gov/newsevents/publichealthfocus/ucm064437.htm

References

MSC unanimously agrees that Bisphenol A is an endocrine disruptor https://echa.europa.eu/-/msc-unanimously-agrees-that-bisphenol-a-is-an-endocrine-disruptor

Yang CZ, Yaniger SI, Jordan VC, Klein DJ, Bittner GD. Most plastic products release estrogenic chemicals: a potential health problem that can be solved. Environ Health Perspect. 2011 Jul;119(7):989-96. doi: 10.1289/ehp.1003220. Epub 2011 Mar 2. PMID: 21367689; PMCID: PMC3222987.

Fluorene-9-bisphenol is anti-oestrogenic and may cause adverse pregnancy outcomes in mice https://www.nature.com/articles/ncomms14585

How Toxic Are Your Household Cleaning Supplies? https://www.organicconsumers.org/news/how-toxic-are-your-household-cleaning-supplies

Severe Lung Injury after Exposure to Chloramine Gas from Household Cleaners https://www.nejm.org/doi/full/10.1056/NEJM199909093411115

Technical Fact Sheet – N-Nitroso-dimethylamine (NDMA) https://www.epa.gov/fedfac/technical-fact-sheet-n-nitroso-dimethylamine-ndma

Cleaning Supplies and Your Health https://www.ewg.org/guides/cleaners/content/cleaners_and_health#.W7Ifv_ZFzIU

Science & Safety Information https://cosmeticsinfo.org/science-of-safety

Parabens in Cosmetics https://www.fda.gov/cosmetics/productsingredients/ingredients/ucm128042.htm

Toxic effects of the easily avoidable phthalates and parabens https://www.ncbi.nlm.nih.gov/pubmed/21155623

Triclosan https://www.beyondpesticides.org/programs/antibacterials/triclosan

Number of cosmetic product recalls spikes 63% in 2016 https://www.cosmeticsbusiness.com/news/article_page/Number_of_cosmetic_product_recalls_spikes_63_in_2016/128534

Toxic Threads: The Big Fashion Stitch-Up https://www.greenpeace.org/international/publication/6889/toxic-threads-the-big-fashion-stitch-up/

The A-Z of Eco Fashion https://theecologist.org/2008/jan/10/z-eco-fashion

Polybrominated Diphenyl Ethers (PBDEs) https://www.epa.gov/assessing-and-managing-chemicals-under-tsca/polybrominated-diphenyl-ethers-pbdes

Mother's Milk: Health Risks of PBDEs https://www.ewg.org/research/mothers-milk/health-risks-pbdes#.W7IjnPZFzIU

PBDEs and their replacements: Does the benefit justify the harm? http://greensciencepolicy.org/wp-content/uploads/2013/12/22-PBDEs-and-replacements-benefits-v-harm.pdf

Toxic Threads: Putting Pollution on Parade https://www.greenpeace.org/international/publication/6925/toxic-threads-putting-pollution-on-parade/

Clement JL, Jarrett PS. Antibacterial silver. Met Based Drugs. 1994;1(5-6):467-82. doi: 10.1155/MBD.1994.467. PMID: 18476264; PMCID: PMC2364932.

What are potential harmful effects of nanoparticles? http://ec.europa.eu/health/scientific_committees/opinions_layman/en/nanotechnologies/l-2/6-health-effects-nanoparticles.htm

Permethrin https://www.beyondpesticides.org/assets/media/documents/pesticides/factsheets/permethrin.pdf

Mercury in Dental amalgam https://www.epa.gov/mercury/mercury-dental-amalgam

About Dental Amalgam Fillings https://www.fda.gov/medicaldevices/productsandmedicalprocedures/dentalproducts/dentalamalgam/ucm171094.htm#risks

WHO Mercury in Health Care
http://www.who.int/water_sanitation_health/medicalwaste/mercurypolpap230506.pdf

Fluoride https://www.nhs.uk/conditions/fluoride/

The Oceans Are Dying https://www.paulcraigroberts.org/2015/03/30/oceans-dying-paul-craig-roberts/

Chapter Seven

ICD Information Sheet https://www.who.int/classifications/icd/factsheet/en/

Global Action Plan for the Prevention and Control of Noncommunicable Diseases 2013-2020 http://apps.who.int/iris/bitstream/handle/10665/94384/9789241506236_eng.pdf;jsessionid=8BE1EDB6738CCF6B081E409801185203?sequence=1

Chen S, Kuhn M, Prettner K, Bloom DE (2018) The macroeconomic burden of noncommunicable diseases in the United States: Estimates and projections. PLoS ONE 13(11): e0206702. https://doi.org/10.1371/journal.pone.0206702

Sudden death warning over faulty heart gene https://www.bbc.co.uk/news/uk-politics-38809532

Nutrition, Methylation and Depression https://www.psychologytoday.com/gb/blog/health-matters/201011/nutrition-and-depression-nutrition-methylation-and-depression-part-2

Free Radicals and Reactive Oxygen http://www.vivo.colostate.edu/hbooks/pathphys/topics/radicals.html

Reactive oxygen species, vascular oxidative stress, and redox signalling in hypertension: what is the clinical significance? https://www.ncbi.nlm.nih.gov/pubmed/15262903

Pham-Huy LA, He H, Pham-Huy C. Free radicals, antioxidants in disease and health. Int J Biomed Sci. 2008 Jun;4(2):89-96. PMID: 23675073; PMCID: PMC3614697.

Damian G. Deavall, Elizabeth A. Martin, Judith M. Horner, and Ruth Roberts, "Drug-Induced Oxidative Stress and Toxicity," Journal of Toxicology, vol. 2012, Article ID 645460, 13 pages, 2012. https://doi.org/10.1155/2012/645460

Randomised controlled trial of Vitamin E in patients with coronary disease: Cambridge Heart Antioxidant Study (CHAOS) https://www.thelancet.com/journals/lancet/article/PIIS0140-6736(96)90866-1/abstract

Multiple Chemical Sensitivity https://www.multiplechemicalsensitivity.org/

Electromagnetic fields and public health http://www.who.int/peh-emf/publications/facts/fs296/en/

Chemical poisoning – general principles of diagnosis and treatment http://www.drmyhill.co.uk/wiki/Chemical_poisoning_-_general_principles_of_diagnosis_and_treatment

Gross L (2007) Diverse Toxic Chemicals Disrupt Cell Function through a Common Path. PLoS Biol 5(2): e41. https://doi.org/10.1371/journal.pbio.0050041

De Luca C, Raskovic D, Pacifico V, Thai JC, Korkina L. The search for reliable biomarkers of disease in multiple chemical sensitivity and other environmental intolerances. Int J Environ Res Public Health. 2011 Jul;8(7):2770-97. doi: 10.3390/ijerph8072770. Epub 2011 Jul 1. PMID: 21845158; PMCID: PMC3155329.

Electromagnetic Hypersensitivity report http://www.who.int/peh-emf/publications/reports/EHS_Proceedings_June2006.pdf?ua=1

Current science on Electromagnetic Sensitivity: an overview http://www.electrosensitivity.co/current-science-on-electromagnetic-sensitivity--overview.html

WHO Standards and Guidelines http://www.who.int/peh-emf/standards/en/

Evidence of Health Effects of Electromagnetic Radiation. To the Australian Senate Inquiry into electromagnetic Radiation http://www.neilcherry.nz/documents/90_m1_EMR_Australian_Senate_Evidence_8-9-2000.pdf

References

Everything You Need to Know About 5G
https://spectrum.ieee.org/video/telecom/wireless/everything-you-need-to-know-about-5g

Scientists and Doctors Demand Moratorium on 5G https://ehtrust.org/scientists-and-doctors-demand-moratorium-on-5g-warning-of-health-effects/

Reliable biomarkers characterizing and identifying electrohypersensitivity and multiple chemical sensitivity as two etiopathogenic aspects of a unique pathological disorder https://www.ncbi.nlm.nih.gov/pubmed/26613326

2015 Brussels International Scientific Declaration on EHS & MCS http://appel-de-paris.com/wp-content/uploads/2015/09/Press-Release-EN1.pdf

US Veterans Affairs Gulf War Veterans Medically Unexplained Illness https://www.publichealth.va.gov/exposures/gulfwar/medically-unexplained-illness.asp

Gulf War Exposures https://www.publichealth.va.gov/exposures/gulfwar/sources/index.asp

Vaccines Gulf-War Syndrome and Bio-defence http://www.i-sis.org.uk/VGWS.php

Health Effects of Serving in the Gulf War
https://www.federalregister.gov/documents/2011/04/14/2011-8937/determinations-concerning-illnesses-discussed-in-national-academy-of-sciences-reports-on-gulf-war

Gulf veterans' illnesses https://www.gov.uk/guidance/gulf-veterans-illnesses

Gulf War Illness and the Health of Gulf War Veterans https://www.va.gov/RAC-GWVI/docs/Committee_Documents/GWIandHealthofGWVeterans_RAC-GWVIReport_2008.pdf

NIAMS Autoimmune Diseases https://www.niams.nih.gov/health-topics/autoimmune-diseases#tab-causes

NIAID Autoimmune Diseases https://www.niaid.nih.gov/diseases-conditions/autoimmune-diseases

Pollard KM, Hultman P, Kono DH. Toxicology of autoimmune diseases. Chem Res Toxicol. 2010 Mar 15;23(3):455-66. doi: 10.1021/tx9003787. PMID: 20078109; PMCID: PMC3076021.

Environmental chemicals and autoimmune disease: cause and effect https://www.ncbi.nlm.nih.gov/pubmed/12505286

Understanding Autoinflammatory Diseases
https://www.niams.nih.gov/sites/default/files/catalog/files/understanding_inflammatory2.pdf

Are obesity-related insulin resistance and type 2 diabetes autoimmune diseases? http://diabetes.diabetesjournals.org/content/64/6/1886.long

Diabetes Education Online https://dtc.ucsf.edu/

Barry Eleanor, Roberts Samantha, Oke Jason, Vijayaraghavan Shanti, Normansell Rebecca, Greenhalgh Trisha et al. Efficacy and effectiveness of screen and treat policies in prevention of type 2 diabetes: systematic review and meta-analysis of screening tests and interventions BMJ 2017; 356 :i6538

A Comprehensive Review of Drug-Drug Interactions with Metformin https://www.ncbi.nlm.nih.gov/pubmed/25943187

Signs and symptoms https://www.mssociety.org.uk/about-ms/signs-and-symptoms

Multiple Sclerosis FAQs https://www.nationalmssociety.org/What-is-MS/MS-FAQ-s

Etemadifar M, Roomizadeh P, Abtahi SH, Sajjadi S, Abedini A, Golabbakhsh A, Fereidan-Esfahani M, Akbari M. Linkage of multiple sclerosis and guillain-barre syndrome: a population-based survey in isfahan, iran. Autoimmune Dis. 2012;2012:232139. doi: 10.1155/2012/232139. Epub 2012 Nov 4. PMID: 23198139; PMCID: PMC3501815.

Causes https://www.msif.org/about-ms/causes/

Mayo Clinic Multiple Sclerosis https://www.mayoclinic.org/diseases-conditions/multiple-sclerosis/symptoms-causes/syc-20350269

The Methylation Cycle https://www.dramyyasko.com/our-unique-approach/methylation-cycle/

O'Gorman C, Lucas R, Taylor B. Environmental risk factors for multiple sclerosis: a review with a focus on molecular mechanisms. Int J Mol Sci. 2012;13(9):11718-52. doi: 10.3390/ijms130911718. Epub 2012 Sep 18. PMID: 23109880; PMCID: PMC3472772.

The Connection Between MS and Aspartame https://rense.com/general53/ms.htm

Disproved Theories https://www.nationalmssociety.org/What-is-MS/What-Causes-MS/Disproved-theories

Methanol Institute https://www.methanol.org/about-methanol/

Teriflunomide https://www.mssociety.org.uk/about-ms/treatments-and-therapies/disease-modifying-therapies/teriflunomide

Effect of high-dose simvastatin on brain atrophy and disability in secondary progressive multiple sclerosis https://www.thelancet.com/journals/lancet/article/PIIS0140-6736(13)62242-4/fulltext

NINDS Guillain-Barré Syndrome Fact Sheet https://www.ninds.nih.gov/Disorders/Patient-Caregiver-Education/Fact-Sheets/Guillain-Barré-Syndrome-Fact-Sheet

Guillain-Barré syndrome and Flu Vaccine https://www.cdc.gov/flu/protect/vaccine/guillainbarre.htm

Vaccines and Guillain-Barré syndrome https://www.ncbi.nlm.nih.gov/pubmed/19388722

Guillain-Barré syndrome after Gardasil vaccination: data from Vaccine Adverse Event Reporting system 2006-2009 https://www.ncbi.nlm.nih.gov/pubmed/20869467

What causes allergies https://www.nhs.uk/conditions/allergies/

Allergic Reactions https://www.aaaai.org/conditions-and-treatments/library/allergy-library/allergic-reactions

Mechanisms of IgE-mediated allergy https://www.ncbi.nlm.nih.gov/pubmed/20211175

Galli SJ, Tsai M. IgE and mast cells in allergic disease. Nat Med. 2012 May 4;18(5):693-704. doi: 10.1038/nm.2755. PMID: 22561833; PMCID: PMC3597223.

Allergic rhinitis https://acaai.org/allergies/types/hay-fever-rhinitis

Food allergy https://aacijournal.biomedcentral.com/articles/10.1186/1710-1492-7-S1-S7

ACAAI Food allergy https://acaai.org/allergies/types/food-allergy

Food Allergy Research Funding https://www.foodallergy.org/education-awareness/advocacy-resources/food-allergy-research-funding

Peanut Allergy https://www.mayoclinic.org/diseases-conditions/peanut-allergy/symptoms-causes/syc-20376175

FARE Peanut Allergy https://www.foodallergy.org/common-allergens/peanut

NIH-sponsored expert panel issues clinical guidelines to prevent peanut allergy https://www.nih.gov/news-events/news-releases/nih-sponsored-expert-panel-issues-clinical-guidelines-prevent-peanut-allergy

LEAP study results http://www.leapstudy.com/leap-study-results#.W7SIjfZFzIU

Food Allergies: The Hidden Truth About Peanuts https://robynobrien.com/food-allergies-the-hidden-truth-about-peanuts/

FARE Symptoms of an allergic reaction to food https://www.foodallergy.org/life-with-food-allergies/food-allergy-101/symptoms-of-an-allergic-reaction-to-food

Skin Exposures and Effects https://www.cdc.gov/niosh/topics/skin/default.html

An Overview of the Different Types of Eczema https://nationaleczema.org/eczema/types-of-eczema/

Atopic Eczema https://www.nhs.uk/conditions/atopic-eczema/

NIOSH Allergic and Irritant Dermatitis https://www.cdc.gov/niosh/docs/96-115/diseas.html

Eczema Causes and Triggers https://nationaleczema.org/eczema/causes-and-triggers-of-eczema/

References

Atopic Dermatitis Found To Be an Immune-Driven Disease
https://www.mountsinai.org/about/newsroom/2014/atopic-dermatitis-found-to-be-an-immunedriven-disease

Demehri S, Morimoto M, Holtzman MJ, Kopan R (2009) Skin-Derived TSLP Triggers Progression from Epidermal-Barrier Defects to Asthma. PLoS Biol 7(5): e1000067. https://doi.org/10.1371/journal.pbio.1000067

Volatile Organic Compounds' Impact on Indoor Air Quality https://www.epa.gov/indoor-air-quality-iaq/volatile-organic-compounds-impact-indoor-air-quality

NHS drugs for asthma https://beta.nhs.uk/medicines/salbutamol-inhaler/

Chronic rheumatic conditions http://www.who.int/chp/topics/rheumatic/en/

Rheumatoid Arthritis (RA) https://www.cdc.gov/arthritis/basics/rheumatoid-arthritis.html

Arthritis Basics FAQs https://www.cdc.gov/arthritis/basics/faqs.htm#causes

Risk Factors https://www.cdc.gov/arthritis/basics/risk-factors.htm

Rheumatoid arthritis https://www.nhs.uk/conditions/rheumatoid-arthritis/causes/

Juvenile Arthritis https://www.arthritis.org/about-arthritis/types/juvenile-arthritis/

Drug Types https://www.arthritis.org/living-with-arthritis/treatments/medication/drug-types/

How to Prevent Arthritis https://www.arthritis.org/about-arthritis/understanding-arthritis/arthritis-prevention.php

Endocrine Disruption Overview https://endocrinedisruption.org/interactive-tools/endocrine-basics

NIDDK page Endocrine Diseases https://www.niddk.nih.gov/health-information/endocrine-diseases

Peace https://endocrinedisruption.org/assets/media/documents/peace.pdf

The endocrine system in diabetes mellitus https://www.ncbi.nlm.nih.gov/pubmed/12374457

Hormone replacement therapy (HRT) https://www.nhs.uk/conditions/hormone-replacement-therapy-hrt/side-effects/

Wingspread statement
https://endocrinedisruption.org/assets/media/documents/wingspread_consensus_statement.pdf

Vandenberg LN, Colborn T, Hayes TB, Heindel JJ, Jacobs DR Jr, Lee DH, Shioda T, Soto AM, vom Saal FS, Welshons WV, Zoeller RT, Myers JP. Hormones and endocrine-disrupting chemicals: low-dose effects and nonmonotonic dose responses. Endocr Rev. 2012 Jun;33(3):378-455. doi: 10.1210/er.2011-1050. Epub 2012 Mar 14. PMID: 22419778; PMCID: PMC3365860.

Endocrine Disrupting Chemicals: Science, Policy, and What You Can Do
https://endocrinedisruption.org/interactive-tools/endocrine-disruption-audio-and-video

TEDX List of Potential Endocrine Disruptors https://endocrinedisruption.org/interactive-tools/tedx-list-of-potential-endocrine-disruptors/search-the-tedx-list

About the TEDX List https://endocrinedisruption.org/interactive-tools/tedx-list-of-potential-endocrine-disruptors/about-the-tedx-list

CDC Facts about Birth Defects https://www.cdc.gov/ncbddd/birthdefects/facts.html

Marleen M.H.J. van Gelder, Iris A.L.M. van Rooij, Richard K. Miller, Gerhard A. Zielhuis, Lolkje T.W. de Jong-van den Berg, Nel Roeleveld, Teratogenic mechanisms of medical drugs, Human Reproduction Update, Volume 16, Issue 4, July-August 2010, Pages 378–394, https://doi.org/10.1093/humupd/dmp052

Winchester PD, Huskins J, Ying J. Agrichemicals in surface water and birth defects in the United States. Acta Paediatr. 2009 Apr;98(4):664-9. doi: 10.1111/j.1651-2227.2008.01207.x. Epub 2009 Jan 22. PMID: 19183116; PMCID: PMC2667895.

Study Shows Monsanto Roundup Herbicide Link to Birth Defects https://www.globalresearch.ca/study-shows-monsanto-roundup-herbicide-link-to-birth-defects/21251

Facts about Microcephaly https://www.cdc.gov/ncbddd/birthdefects/microcephaly.html

Planning for pregnancy https://www.cdc.gov/preconception/planning.html

Down Syndrome https://www.ndss.org/about-down-syndrome/down-syndrome/

The aneuploidy theory of cancer and the barriers to its acceptance http://www.davidrasnick.com/Cancer_files/Aneuploidy article.pdf

Facts about Down Syndrome https://www.cdc.gov/ncbddd/birthdefects/DownSyndrome.html

Spina Bifida Causes https://www.mayoclinic.org/diseases-conditions/spina-bifida/symptoms-causes/syc-20377860

Greene ND, Stanier P, Copp AJ. Genetics of human neural tube defects. Hum Mol Genet. 2009 Oct 15;18(R2):R113-29. doi: 10.1093/hmg/ddp347. PMID: 19808787; PMCID: PMC2758708.

Chromosomal abnormalities associated with neural tube defects (1): full aneuploidy https://www.ncbi.nlm.nih.gov/pubmed/18182338

Roy M Pitkin, Folate and neural tube defects, The American Journal of Clinical Nutrition, Volume 85, Issue 1, January 2007, Pages 285S–288S, https://doi.org/10.1093/ajcn/85.1.285S

Blom HJ, Shaw GM, den Heijer M, Finnell RH. Neural tube defects and folate: case far from closed. Nat Rev Neurosci. 2006 Sep;7(9):724-31. doi: 10.1038/nrn1986. PMID: 16924261; PMCID: PMC2970514.

Not all cases of neural tube defect can be prevented by increasing the intake of folic acid https://www.ncbi.nlm.nih.gov/pubmed/19079944

Why You Need Folate and Not Folic Acid https://www.drfuhrman.com/library/eat-to-live-blog/16/why-you-need-folate-and-not-folic-acid

How many people are affected by or at risk for spina bifida? https://www.nichd.nih.gov/health/topics/spinabifida/conditioninfo/affected-risk

Clinical care of pregnant women with epilepsy: neural tube defects and folic acid supplementation https://www.ncbi.nlm.nih.gov/pubmed/12790884

NHS epilepsy https://www.nhs.uk/conditions/epilepsy/

NHS Bipolar disorder https://www.nhs.uk/conditions/bipolar-disorder/causes/

Epstein RA, Moore KM, Bobo WV. Treatment of bipolar disorders during pregnancy: maternal and fetal safety and challenges. Drug Healthc Patient Saf. 2014 Dec 24;7:7-29. doi: 10.2147/DHPS.S50556. PMID: 25565896; PMCID: PMC4284049.

NHS Sudden infant death syndrome (SIDS) https://www.nhs.uk/conditions/sudden-infant-death-syndrome-sids/

CDC Sudden Infant Death Syndrome (SIDS) https://www.cdc.gov/vaccinesafety/concerns/sids.html

Six common misconceptions about immunization http://www.who.int/vaccine_safety/initiative/detection/immunization_misconceptions/en/index4.html

L. Matturri, G. Del Corno and A.M. Lavezzi, "Sudden Infant Death Following Hexavalent Vaccination: A Neuropathologic Study", Current Medicinal Chemistry (2014) 21: 941. https://doi.org/10.2174/09298673113206660289

Vaccinations for premature babies https://www.nhs.uk/conditions/vaccinations/when-to-get-your-child-vaccinated/

Vaccination and the Dynamics of Critical Days http://www.whale.to/v/scheibner.html

Cot Deaths Linked to Vaccinations http://www.whale.to/vaccines/cot_death.html

References

Duncan JR, Paterson DS, Hoffman JM, Mokler DJ, Borenstein NS, Belliveau RA, Krous HF, Haas EA, Stanley C, Nattie EE, Trachtenberg FL, Kinney HC. Brainstem serotonergic deficiency in sudden infant death syndrome. JAMA. 2010 Feb 3;303(5):430-7. doi: 10.1001/jama.2010.45. PMID: 20124538; PMCID: PMC3242415.

Adverse Effects on Infants of SSRI/SNRI Use During Pregnancy and Breastfeeding https://www.researchgate.net/publication/288761736_Adverse_Effects_on_Infants_of_SS RISNRI_Use_During_Pregnancy_and_Breastfeeding_A_report_on_the_evidence_linking _in-utero_exposure_to_antidepressants_and_sudden_infant_death_syndrome

The Pineal Gland and Melatonin http://www.vivo.colostate.edu/hbooks/pathphys/endocrine/otherendo/pineal.html

Melatonin concentrations in the sudden infant death syndrome https://www.ncbi.nlm.nih.gov/pubmed/2335331

What is Autism Spectrum Disorder? https://www.cdc.gov/ncbddd/autism/facts.html

Vaccines, neurodevelopment and Autism Spectrum Disorders https://vaccinechoicecanada.com/wp-content/uploads/blaylock-vaccines-neurodevelopment-autism-spectrum-disorders-2008.pdf

Data & Statistics on Autism Spectrum Disorder https://www.cdc.gov/ncbddd/autism/data.html

What Are Childhood Mental Disorders? https://www.cdc.gov/childrensmentalhealth/basics.html

Watchdog Says Report of 10,000 Toddlers on ADHD Drugs Tip of the Iceberg https://www.cchrint.org/2014/05/21/10000-toddlers-on-adhd-drugs-tip-of-the-iceberg/

$1.5 Million Award in Child Tardive Dyskinesia Malpractice https://breggin.com/peter-r-breggin-md-1-5-million-award-in-child-tardive-dyskinesia-malpractice/

Developmental Disabilities https://www.cdc.gov/ncbddd/developmentaldisabilities/index.html

Kern JK, Geier DA, Sykes LK, Geier MR. Evidence of neurodegeneration in autism spectrum disorder. Transl Neurodegener. 2013 Aug 8;2(1):17. doi: 10.1186/2047-9158-2-17. PMID: 23925007; PMCID: PMC3751488.

Al Backer NB. Developmental regression in autism spectrum disorder. Sudan J Paediatr. 2015;15(1):21-6. PMID: 27493417; PMCID: PMC4949854.

Miller NZ, Goldman GS. Infant mortality rates regressed against number of vaccine doses routinely given: is there a biochemical or synergistic toxicity? Hum Exp Toxicol. 2011 Sep;30(9):1420-8. doi: 10.1177/0960327111407644. Epub 2011 May 4. Erratum in: Hum Exp Toxicol. 2011 Sep;30(9):1429. PMID: 21543527; PMCID: PMC3170075.

İnci M, Zararsız İ, Davarcı M, Görür S. Toxic effects of formaldehyde on the urinary system. Turk J Urol. 2013 Mar;39(1):48-52. doi: 10.5152/tud.2013.010. PMID: 26328078; PMCID: PMC4548585.

Formaldehyde: A Poison and Carcinogen https://thevaccinereaction.org/2015/11/formaldehyde-a-poison-and-carcinogen/

Environmental neurotoxicants and developing brain https://www.ncbi.nlm.nih.gov/pubmed/21259263

Quaak I, Brouns MR, Van de Bor M. The dynamics of autism spectrum disorders: how neurotoxic compounds and neurotransmitters interact. Int J Environ Res Public Health. 2013 Aug 6;10(8):3384-408. doi: 10.3390/ijerph10083384. PMID: 23924882; PMCID: PMC3774444.

Pagan C, Delorme R, Callebert J, Goubran-Botros H, Amsellem F, Drouot X, Boudebesse C, Le Dudal K, Ngo-Nguyen N, Laouamri H, Gillberg C, Leboyer M, Bourgeron T, Launay JM. The serotonin-N-acetylserotonin-melatonin pathway as a biomarker for autism spectrum disorders. Transl Psychiatry. 2014 Nov 11;4(11):e479. doi: 10.1038/tp.2014.120. PMID: 25386956; PMCID: PMC4259991.

Veatch OJ, Goldman SE, Adkins KW, Malow BA. Melatonin in Children with Autism Spectrum Disorders: How Does the Evidence Fit Together? J Nat Sci. 2015;1(7):e125. PMID: 26120597; PMCID: PMC4478596.

ACOG Guidelines on Psychiatric Medication Use During Pregnancy and Lactation https://www.aafp.org/afp/2008/0915/p772.html

Pregnant mothers should not take antidepressants https://breggin.com/pregnant-mothers-should-not-take-ssri-antidepressants/

Autism, Antidepressants and Pregnancy: The Basics https://www.madinamerica.com/2014/08/autism-antidepressants-pregnancy-basics/

How Electromagnetically-Induced Cell Leakage May Cause Autism http://electromagnetichealth.org/wp-content/uploads/2011/05/Autism_2011_b.pdf

The Biological Effects of Weak Electromagnetic Fields http://stopsmartmeters.org.uk/dr-andrew-goldsworthy-the-biological-effects-of-weak-electromagnetic-fields/

Findings in Autism (ASD) Consistent with Electromagnetic Fields (EMF) and Radiofrequency Radiation (RFR) http://www.bioinitiative.org/report/wp-content/uploads/pdfs/sec20_2012_Findings_in_Autism_Consistent_with_EMF_and_RFR.pdf

Adolescents and Young Adults with Cancer https://www.cancer.gov/types/aya

The aneuploidy theory of cancer and the barriers to its acceptance http://www.davidrasnick.com/Cancer_files/Aneuploidy article.pdf

Infection and Cancer: Global Distribution and Burden of Disease https://www.ncbi.nlm.nih.gov/pubmed/25512154

Cancer and Environment https://www.jstor.org/stable/24945946?seq=1#page_scan_tab_contents

Do We Know What Causes Childhood Leukemia? https://www.cancer.org/cancer/leukemia-in-children/causes-risks-prevention/what-causes.html

Acute Lymphoblastic leukaemia https://www.thelancet.com/journals/lancet/article/PIIS0140-6736(12)62187-4/fulltext

Uncertain, unproven, or controversial risk factors https://www.cancer.org/cancer/leukemia-in-children/causes-risks-prevention/risk-factors.html

Electromagnetic fields, the modulation of brain tissue functions – A possible paradigm shift in biology http://www.emrpolicy.org/science/forum/adey_encneuro_emfs.pdf

Use of Wireless Phones and Evidence for Increased Risk of Brain Tumours http://www.bioinitiative.org/report/wp-content/uploads/2017/11/Hardell-2017-Sec11-Update-Use_of_Wireless_Phones.pdf

Acute Lymphoblastic Leukaemia https://www.childrenwithcancer.org.uk/childhood-cancer-info/cancer-types/acute-lymphoblastic-leukaemia/

The Chromosomal Imbalance Theory of Cancer http://www.davidrasnick.com/cancer/index.html

What is aneuploidy and why is it important http://www.ourstolenfuture.com/NewScience/oncompounds/bisphenola/2003/2003-0328aneuploidy.htm

Gene discovery could shed light on how cancer cells spread https://www.cancerresearchuk.org/about-us/cancer-news/news-report/2017-01-11-gene-discovery-could-shed-light-on-how-cancer-cells-spread?_ga=2.91830813.687432865.1538574081-447187103.1538574081

Cancer-fighting viruses win approval https://www.nature.com/news/cancer-fighting-viruses-win-approval-1.18651

Chapter Eight

UN What We Do https://www.un.org/en/sections/what-we-do/

About the UN – Overview http://www.un.org/en/sections/about-un/overview/index.html

References

UN Funds, Programmes, Specialized Agencies and Others
http://www.un.org/en/sections/about-un/funds-programmes-specialized-agencies-and-others/index.html

About UNCTAD https://unctad.org/en/Pages/aboutus.aspx

Club of Rome Limits to Growth https://www.clubofrome.org/report/the-limits-to-growth/

Agenda 21 https://sustainabledevelopment.un.org/outcomedocuments/agenda21

Millennium Development Goals http://www.un.org/millenniumgoals/

Millennium Development Goals 2015 Report
http://www.un.org/millenniumgoals/2015_MDG_Report/pdf/MDG%202015%20rev%20(J uly%201).pdf

Transforming Our World: the 2030 Agenda for Sustainable Development
https://sustainabledevelopment.un.org/post2015/transformingourworld

WHO Health and development http://www.who.int/hdp/en/

Aid for health https://www.who.int/hdp/aid/en/

The Epidemic of Sickness and Death from Prescription Drugs
http://www.asanet.org/sites/default/files/savvy/footnotes/nov14/prescription_1114.html

Downing NS, Shah ND, Aminawung JA, Pease AM, Zeitoun JD, Krumholz HM, Ross JS. Postmarket Safety Events Among Novel Therapeutics Approved by the US Food and Drug Administration Between 2001 and 2010. JAMA. 2017 May 9;317(18):1854-1863. doi: 10.1001/jama.2017.5150. PMID: 28492899; PMCID: PMC5815036.

FDA Safety Reviews on Drugs, Biologics and Vaccines: 2007-2013
http://pediatrics.aappublications.org/content/136/6/1125

Medicines in Development https://www.phrma.org/science/in-the-pipeline/medicines-in-development

Medicines in Development for Biologics 2013 Report
https://www.phrma.org/report/medicines-in-development-for-biologics-2013-report

Medicines in Development for Rare Diseases 2016 Report
https://www.phrma.org/report/medicines-in-development-for-rare-diseases-2016-report

Boosting drugs manufacture in developing countries will improve health outcome, UN investment forum told https://www.pharmaceutical-journal.com/news-and-analysis/boosting-drugs-manufacture-in-developing-countries-will-improve-health-outcomes-un-investment-forum-told/20066953.article?firstPass=false

WHO 10 Facts on Immunization
http://www.who.int/features/factfiles/immunization/facts/en/

2009 WHO Global Health Risks report
http://www.who.int/healthinfo/global_burden_disease/GlobalHealthRisks_report_full.pdf

UK Trends in Infectious Diseases
http://researchbriefings.files.parliament.uk/documents/POST-PN-0545/POST-PN-0545.pdf

About GAVI https://www.gavi.org/about/

WHO strives to provide universal access to immunization in the African Region by 2020
https://afro.who.int/news/who-strives-provide-universal-access-immunization-african-region-2020

Archie Kalokerinos interview 1995 https://www.vaccinationinformationnetwork.com/an-interview-with-dr-archie-kalokerinos-md/

Myths about children's vaccines https://www.nhs.uk/conditions/vaccinations/myths-truths-kids-vaccines/

Vaccines when your child is sick https://www.cdc.gov/vaccines/parents/visit/sick-child.html

Global Report for Research on Infectious Diseases of Poverty
http://www.who.int/tdr/capacity/global_report/en/

Children in Bangladesh to benefit from dual vaccine introduction
https://www.gavi.org/library/news/press-releases/2015/children-in-bangladesh-to-benefit-from-dual-vaccine-introduction/

Causes of childhood deaths in Bangladesh: an update
https://www.ncbi.nlm.nih.gov/pubmed/11440104

Polio in Pakistan http://www.endpolio.com.pk/polioin-pakistan

VASHISHT, Neetu ; PULIYE, Jacob Polio programme: let us declare victory and move on. Indian Journal of Medical Ethics, [S.l.], v. 9, n. 2, p. 114, nov. 2016. ISSN 0975-5691

Observed rate of Vaccine Reactions
https://www.who.int/vaccine_safety/initiative/tools/polio_vaccine_rates_information_she et.pdf

CDC Acute Flaccid Myelitis https://www.cdc.gov/acute-flaccid-myelitis/afm-surveillance.html

Paralytic poliomyelitis in a rural area of north India
http://archive.nmji.in/approval/archive/Volume-10/issue-1/original-articles-2.pdf

Lead poisoning affects 20% Kolkata kids
https://timesofindia.indiatimes.com/city/kolkata/Lead-poisoning-affects-20-Kolkata-kids/articleshow/21062303.cms

Vaccines for three deadly viruses fast-tracked https://www.bbc.co.uk/news/health-38669584

PhRMA Medicines in Development for Vaccines 2017 Update
https://www.phrma.org/report/medicines-in-development-vaccines-2017-update

WHO Risk factors http://www.who.int/topics/risk_factors/en/

Greenwood B. The contribution of vaccination to global health: past, present and future. Philos Trans R Soc Lond B Biol Sci. 2014 May 12;369(1645):20130433. doi: 10.1098/rstb.2013.0433. PMID: 24821919; PMCID: PMC4024226.

WHO World Health Statistics 2017
http://www.who.int/gho/publications/world_health_statistics/2017/en/

Hepatitis B Vaccine http://vk.ovg.ox.ac.uk/hepatitis-b-vaccine

AIDSinfo re Tenofovir https://aidsinfo.nih.gov/drugs/290/tenofovir-disoproxil-fumarate/0/patient

7 Million Deaths Averted through Hepatitis B Vaccination
http://www.wpro.who.int/mediacentre/releases/2016/20160621/en/

Delivering additional interventions to eliminate mother-to-child transmission of hepatitis B in the Western Pacific
http://www.wpro.who.int/hiv/media/features/addl_intervention_EMTCT_hepB_WPR/en/

Malaguarnera G, Cataudella E, Giordano M, Nunnari G, Chisari G, Malaguarnera M. Toxic hepatitis in occupational exposure to solvents. World J Gastroenterol. 2012 Jun 14;18(22):2756-66. doi: 10.3748/wjg.v18.i22.2756. PMID: 22719183; PMCID: PMC3374978.

McKenzie A. Anaesthetic and Other Treatments of Shell Shock: World War I and Beyond. Journal of the Royal Army Medical Corps 2012;158:29-33.

The evolution of pandemic influenza: evidence from India 1918-19
https://bmcinfectdis.biomedcentral.com/articles/10.1186/1471-2334-14-510

Lahariya C. A brief history of vaccines & vaccination in India. Indian J Med Res. 2014 Apr;139(4):491-511. PMID: 24927336; PMCID: PMC4078488.

Malaria's contribution to World war One – the unexpected adversary
https://malariajournal.biomedcentral.com/articles/10.1186/1475-2875-13-497

Chandra S. Mortality from the influenza pandemic of 1918-19 in Indonesia. Popul Stud (Camb). 2013 Jul;67(2):185-93. doi: 10.1080/00324728.2012.754486. Epub 2013 Jan 23. PMID: 23339482; PMCID: PMC3687026.

War Losses (Africa) https://encyclopedia.1914-1918-online.net/article/war_losses_africa

References

Reappraising AIDS in Africa http://www.virusmyth.com/aids/hiv/cgreappraising.htm

AIDS in Africa? http://www.virusmyth.com/aids/hiv/epvtafrica.htm

AIDS in Africa: distinguishing fact and fiction
http://www.virusmyth.com/aids/hiv/epafrica.htm

Demographic Patterns of HIV Testing Uptake in Sub-Saharan Africa
https://dhsprogram.com/pubs/pdf/CR30/CR30.pdf

Inungu J, Karl S. Understanding the scourge of HIV/AIDS in sub-Saharan Africa.
MedGenMed. 2006 Nov 9;8(4):30. PMID: 17415312; PMCID: PMC1868366.

Simplification of antiretroviral therapy: a necessary step in the public health response to
HIV/AIDS in resource-limited settings https://www.ncbi.nlm.nih.gov/pubmed/25310534

Kharsany AB, Karim QA. HIV Infection and AIDS in Sub-Saharan Africa: Current Status,
Challenges and Opportunities. Open AIDS J. 2016 Apr 8;10:34-48. doi:
10.2174/1874613601610010034. PMID: 27347270; PMCID: PMC4893541.

Accurate and Credible UNAIDS data on the HIV epidemic: the cornerstone of the AIDS
response
http://www.unaids.org/en/resources/presscentre/featurestories/2017/july/20170710_data

Bosamiya SS. The immune reconstitution inflammatory syndrome. Indian J Dermatol. 2011
Sep-Oct;56(5):476-9. doi: 10.4103/0019-5154.87114. PMID: 22121257; PMCID:
PMC3221202.

Lawn SD, Harries AD, Anglaret X, Myer L, Wood R. Early mortality among adults accessing
antiretroviral treatment programmes in sub-Saharan Africa. AIDS. 2008 Oct 1;22(15):1897-
908. doi: 10.1097/QAD.0b013e32830007cd. PMID: 18784453; PMCID: PMC3816249.

The ticking time bomb: toxic pesticide waste dumps
http://www.fao.org/News/2001/010502-e.htm

The world-wide increase in tuberculosis: how demographic changes, HIV infection and
increasing numbers in poverty are increasing tuberculosis
https://www.ncbi.nlm.nih.gov/pubmed/12846265

Sandhu GK. Tuberculosis: current situation, challenges and overview of its control programs
in India. J Glob Infect Dis. 2011 Apr;3(2):143-50. doi: 10.4103/0974-777X.81691. PMID:
21731301; PMCID: PMC3125027.

WHO Global Tuberculosis Report 2017 http://apps.who.int/medicinedocs/en/d/Js23360en/

Denholm JT, McBryde ES, Eisen DP, Penington JS, Chen C, Street AC. Adverse effects of
isoniazid preventative therapy for latent tuberculosis infection: a prospective cohort study.
Drug Healthc Patient Saf. 2014 Oct 20;6:145-9. doi: 10.2147/DHPS.S68837. PMID:
25364275; PMCID: PMC4211866.

Dooley KE, Chaisson RE. Tuberculosis and diabetes mellitus: convergence of two epidemics.
Lancet Infect Dis. 2009 Dec;9(12):737-46. doi: 10.1016/S1473-3099(09)70282-8. PMID:
19926034; PMCID: PMC2945809.

Balakrishnan S, Vijayan S, Nair S, Subramoniapillai J, Mrithyunjayan S, Wilson N, et al.
(2012) High Diabetes Prevalence among Tuberculosis Cases in Kerala, India. PLoS ONE
7(10): e46502. https://doi.org/10.1371/journal.pone.0046502

Gulati S, Misra A. Sugar intake, obesity, and diabetes in India. Nutrients. 2014 Dec
22;6(12):5955-74. doi: 10.3390/nu6125955. PMID: 25533007; PMCID: PMC4277009.

Highly evolvable malaria vectors: The genomes of 16 Anopheles mosquitoes
http://science.sciencemag.org/content/347/6217/1258522.full

Churcher TS, Sinden RE, Edwards NJ, Poulton ID, Rampling TW, Brock PM, et al. (2017)
Probability of Transmission of Malaria from Mosquito to Human Is Regulated by Mosquito
Parasite Density in Naïve and Vaccinated Hosts. PLoS Pathog 13(1): e1006108.
https://doi.org/10.1371/journal.ppat.1006108

Malaria in the UK https://blogs.lshtm.ac.uk/library/2014/04/25/malaria-in-the-uk/

From Shakespeare to Defoe: Malaria in England in the Little Ice Age
https://wwwnc.cdc.gov/eid/article/6/1/00-0101_article

Where Malaria Occurs https://www.cdc.gov/malaria/about/distribution.html

NHS Malaria https://www.nhs.uk/conditions/malaria/

Study: UK cities becoming mosquito-friendly habitats https://www.bbc.co.uk/news/science-environment-27491891

Elimination of Malaria in the United States (1947-1951) https://www.cdc.gov/malaria/about/history/elimination_us.html

Malaria in Europe: emerging threat or minor nuisance? https://www.sciencedirect.com/science/article/pii/S1198743X16301203

Life Cycle https://www.malariasite.com/life-cycle/

About Malaria – Biology https://www.cdc.gov/malaria/about/biology/index.html

How Mosquitoes Fight Malaria https://www.sciencemag.org/news/2010/09/how-mosquitoes-fight-malaria

Cox FE. History of the discovery of the malaria parasites and their vectors. Parasit Vectors. 2010 Feb 1;3(1):5. doi: 10.1186/1756-3305-3-5. PMID: 20205846; PMCID: PMC2825508.

Malaria Diagnosis (United States) https://www.cdc.gov/malaria/diagnosis_treatment/diagnosis.html

WHO World Malaria Report 2018 https://www.who.int/malaria/publications/world-malaria-report-2018/en/

Chai JY. Atlas of Human Malaria. Korean J Parasitol. 2008 Jun;46(2):113. doi: 10.3347/kjp.2008.46.2.113. Epub 2008 Jun 20. PMCID: PMC2532615.

Moody A. Rapid diagnostic tests for malaria parasites. Clin Microbiol Rev. 2002 Jan;15(1):66-78. doi: 10.1128/cmr.15.1.66-78.2002. PMID: 11781267; PMCID: PMC118060.

Malaria Diagnosis (United States) https://www.cdc.gov/malaria/diagnosis_treatment/diagnosis.html

Doolan DL, Dobaño C, Baird JK. Acquired immunity to malaria. Clin Microbiol Rev. 2009 Jan;22(1):13-36, Table of Contents. doi: 10.1128/CMR.00025-08. PMID: 19136431; PMCID: PMC2620631.

On Airs, Waters and Places http://classics.mit.edu/Hippocrates/airwatpl.mb.txt

What is David Livingstone's legacy, 200 years after his birth? https://www.newstatesman.com/sci-tech/sci-tech/2013/02/what-david-livingstones-legacy-200-years-after-his-birth

Bisoffi Z, Gobbi F, Buonfrate D, Van den Ende J. Diagnosis of Malaria Infection with or without Disease. Mediterr J Hematol Infect Dis. 2012;4(1):e2012036. doi: 10.4084/MJHID.2012.036. Epub 2012 May 9. PMID: 22708051; PMCID: PMC3375766.

Q&A on the malaria vaccine implementation programme (MVIP) http://www.who.int/malaria/media/malaria-vaccine-implementation-qa/en/

Beyond Pesticides fact sheet synthetic pyrethroids https://www.beyondpesticides.org/assets/media/documents/mosquito/documents/SyntheticPyrethroids.pdf

WHO Neglected tropical diseases (NTDs) http://www.who.int/neglected_diseases/diseases/en/

Alberts B, Johnson A, Lewis J, et al. Molecular Biology of the Cell. 4th edition. New York: Garland Science; 2002. Introduction to Pathogens. Available from: https://www.ncbi.nlm.nih.gov/books/NBK26917/

Global Leprosy Strategy 2016-2020 http://www.searo.who.int/entity/global_leprosy_programme/documents/global_leprosy_strategy_2020/en/

Leprosy Transmission https://www.cdc.gov/leprosy/transmission/index.html

Trivedi S, Pandit A, Ganguly G, Das SK. Epidemiology of Peripheral Neuropathy: An Indian Perspective. Ann Indian Acad Neurol. 2017 Jul-Sep;20(3):173-184. doi: 10.4103/aian.AIAN_470_16. PMID: 28904445; PMCID: PMC5586108.

References

High prevalence of vitiligo in lepromatous leprosy https://www.ncbi.nlm.nih.gov/pubmed/11123444

Bajaj AK, Saraswat A, Srivastav PK. Chemical leucoderma: Indian scenario, prognosis, and treatment. Indian J Dermatol. 2010 Jul-Sep;55(3):250-4. doi: 10.4103/0019-5154.70674. PMID: 21063517; PMCID: PMC2965911.

Promising New Leprosy Vaccine Moves into Human Trials https://www.idri.org/promising-new-leprosy-vaccine/

About Parasites https://www.cdc.gov/parasites/about.html

Intestinal Parasites http://naturalhygienesociety.org/articles/classics1.html#22

Arsenic - the 'Poison of kings' and the 'Saviour of Syphilis' https://jmvh.org/article/arsenic-the-poison-of-kings-and-the-saviour-of-syphilis/

The World's Worst Pollution Problems 2016 https://www.worstpolluted.org/

Global Burden of Disease of Mercury Used in Artisanal Small-Scale Gold Mining https://www.sciencedirect.com/science/article/pii/S2214999616308207?via%3Dihub

Leishmaniasis FAQs https://www.cdc.gov/parasites/leishmaniasis/gen_info/faqs.html

CDC Leishmaniasis Biology https://www.cdc.gov/parasites/leishmaniasis/biology.html

Aronson N, Herwaldt BL, Libman M, Pearson R, Lopez-Velez R, Weina P, Carvalho E, Ephros M, Jeronimo S, Magill A. Diagnosis and Treatment of Leishmaniasis: Clinical Practice Guidelines by the Infectious Diseases Society of America (IDSA) and the American Society of Tropical Medicine and Hygiene (ASTMH). Am J Trop Med Hyg. 2017 Jan 11;96(1):24-45. doi: 10.4269/ajtmh.16-84256. Epub 2016 Dec 7. PMID: 27927991; PMCID: PMC5239701.

CDC Schistosomiasis Biology https://www.cdc.gov/parasites/schistosomiasis/biology.html

Shen J, Lai DH, Wilson RA, Chen YF, Wang LF, Yu ZL, Li MY, He P, Hide G, Sun X, Yang TB, Wu ZD, Ayala FJ, Lun ZR. Nitric oxide blocks the development of the human parasite Schistosoma japonicum. Proc Natl Acad Sci U S A. 2017 Sep 19;114(38):10214-10219. doi: 10.1073/pnas.1708578114. Epub 2017 Sep 5. PMID: 28874579; PMCID: PMC5617295.

WHO Chronic respiratory diseases (CRDs) http://www.who.int/respiratory/en/

WHO Mental Health Action Plan 2013-2020 http://www.who.int/mental_health/publications/action_plan/en/

2017 World Population Data Sheet https://www.prb.org/2017-world-population-data-sheet/

Sexual and reproductive health https://www.unfpa.org/sexual-reproductive-health

International Programme on Chemical Safety http://www.who.int/ipcs/en/

Ten chemicals of major public health concern http://www.who.int/ipcs/assessment/public_health/chemicals_phc/en/

Guidelines for indoor air quality: selected pollutants http://www.euro.who.int/en/health-topics/environment-and-health/air-quality/publications/2010/who-guidelines-for-indoor-air-quality-selected-pollutants

Public health impact of chemicals: knowns and unknowns http://www.who.int/ipcs/publications/chemicals-public-health-impact/en/

UNEP About UN Environment https://www.unenvironment.org/about-un-environment

SAICM Overview http://www.saicm.org/About/SAICMOverview

Strategic Approach to International Chemicals Management: Good Chemistry, Together http://www.saicm.org/Portals/12/Documents/SAICM_Brochure-2015.pdf

WHO 10 facts on preventing disease through healthy environments http://www.who.int/features/factfiles/environmental-disease-burden/en/

Union Carbide's Disaster http://bhopal.org/what-happened/union-carbides-disaster/

FICCI http://ficci.in/sector.asp?sectorid=7

Indian Chemical Council – Responsible Care http://www.indianchemicalcouncil.com/responsible_care.htm

Chemicals and waste Management for Sustainable Development
http://www.undp.org/content/undp/en/home/librarypage/environment-
energy/chemicals_management/chemicals-and-waste-management-for-sustainable-
development.html
Introduction to UNIDO https://isid.unido.org/files/DG_Brochure_February_2015_Web.pdf
TATA group Business Profile https://www.tata.com/business/overview
Tuberculosis rates in England fall by third in six years https://www.bbc.co.uk/news/health-
43517246
Environmental Impacts of Mining and Smelting http://www.okinternational.org/mining
Effects of Quarry Activities on Some Selected Communities in the Lower Manya Krobo
District of the Eastern Region of Ghana
https://file.scirp.org/pdf/ACS20120300009_50914235.pdf
2016 World's Worst Pollution Problems: The Toxics Beneath Our Feet
https://www.worstpolluted.org/docs/WorldsWorst2016.pdf
Illegally Traded and Dumped E-Waste Worth up to $19 Billion Annually Poses Risks to
Health, Deprives Countries of Resources https://www.unenvironment.org/news-and-
stories/press-release/illegally-traded-and-dumped-e-waste-worth-19-billion-annually-poses
Daum K, Stoler J, Grant RJ. Toward a More Sustainable Trajectory for E-Waste Policy: A
Review of a Decade of E-Waste Research in Accra, Ghana. Int J Environ Res Public Health.
2017 Jan 29;14(2):135. doi: 10.3390/ijerph14020135. PMID: 28146075; PMCID:
PMC5334689.
World Bank Data Topics SDG 1 No poverty http://datatopics.worldbank.org/sdgatlas/SDG-
01-no-poverty.html
World Bank's New End-Poverty Tool: Surveys in Poorest Countries
http://www.worldbank.org/en/news/press-release/2015/10/15/world-bank-new-end-
poverty-tool-surveys-in-poorest-countries
61,000 Millionaires left India in the last 14 years
https://www.firstpost.com/business/61000-millionaires-left-india-in-the-last-14-years-why-
are-the-richie-rich-fleeing-the-country-2364766.html
The Egyptian Tinderbox: How Banks and Investors are Starving the Third World
http://www.webofdebt.com/articles/egyptian_tinderbox.php
The Global Crisis: Food, Water and Fuel. Three Fundamental Necessities of Life in Jeopardy
https://www.globalresearch.ca/the-global-crisis-food-water-and-fuel-three-fundamental-
necessities-of-life-in-jeopardy/9191
WHO Poverty and health http://www.who.int/hdp/poverty/en/
World Bank Poverty and health http://www.worldbank.org/en/topic/health/brief/poverty-
health
How the IMF Promotes Global Economic Stability
https://www.imf.org/en/About/Factsheets/Sheets/2016/07/27/15/22/How-the-IMF-
Promotes-Global-Economic-Stability
UN SDG 1 Progress of Goal 1 in 2017 https://sustainabledevelopment.un.org/sdg1
UN SDG 2 Progress of Goal 2 in 2017 https://sustainabledevelopment.un.org/sdg2
The state of food security and nutrition in the world 2017 http://www.fao.org/3/a-
I7695e.pdf
WHO page Micronutrients http://www.who.int/nutrition/topics/micronutrients/en/
WHO page 10 facts on nutrition http://www.who.int/features/factfiles/nutrition/en/
WFP Specialized nutritious foods https://www.wfp.org/nutrition/special-nutritional-
products
The Myth: Scarcity. The Reality: There IS Enough Food https://foodfirst.org/the-myth-
scarcity-the-reality-there-is-enough-food/

References

World Population projected to reach 9.8 billion in 2050, and 11.2 billion in 2100 https://www.un.org/development/desa/en/news/population/world-population-prospects-2017.html

WFP 11 Myths About Global Hunger https://www.wfp.org/stories/11-myths-about-global-hunger

Food First primer Green Revolution https://foodfirst.org/wp-content/uploads/2014/04/FoodFirst_primer_GreenRev_Final.pdf

The Farmers' Crisis https://navdanyainternational.org/the-farmers-crisis/

The Seeds of Suicide: How Monsanto Destroys Farming https://www.globalresearch.ca/the-seeds-of-suicide-how-monsanto-destroys-farming/5329947

World Hunger: Ten Myths https://foodfirst.org/publication/world-hunger-ten-myths/

Food First primer Land and Resources https://foodfirst.org/wp-content/uploads/2015/07/Land-and-Resources-FF-issue-primer1.pdf

Corporate Imperialism – The only reason for GMOs https://seedfreedom.info/corporate-imperialism-the-only-reason-for-gmos/

The new farm owners: Corporate investors lead the rush for control over overseas farmland https://www.grain.org/article/entries/4389-the-new-farm-owners-corporate-investors-lead-the-rush-for-control-over-overseas-farmland

Trends and impacts of foreign investment in developing country agriculture – Evidence from case studies http://www.fao.org/economic/est/publications/trends/en/

GMOs in Africa: Capturing frontier markets in the name of food security https://theafricacollective.com/2014/11/22/gmos-in-africa-capturing-frontier-markets-in-the-name-of-food-security/

AGRA Developing Africa's Seed Systems https://agra.org/program-development-and-innovation/developing-africas-seed-systems/

Food Wastage: key facts and figures http://www.fao.org/news/story/en/item/196402/icode/

Key facts on food loss and waste you should know! http://www.fao.org/save-food/resources/keyfindings/en/

The tremendous success of Agroecology in Africa https://theecologist.org/2015/nov/21/tremendous-success-agroecology-africa

Food First primer Agroecology https://foodfirst.org/wp-content/uploads/2014/04/FF_primer_Agroecology_Final.pdf

Organic Movement http://www.navdanya.org/organic-movement

Water Quality and Health Strategy 2013-2020 http://www.who.int/water_sanitation_health/publications/water_quality_strategy/en/

UN SDG 6 Progress of Goal 6 in 2016 https://sustainabledevelopment.un.org/sdg6

Global risk of pharmaceutical contamination from highly populated developing countries https://www.ncbi.nlm.nih.gov/pubmed/23535471

Effluent from drug manufacturers contain high levels of pharmaceuticals https://www.ncbi.nlm.nih.gov/pubmed/17706342

Chapter Nine

UN Charter http://www.un.org/en/charter-united-nations/

The American Century http://www.informationclearinghouse.info/article6139.htm

From Global Poverty to Exclusion and Despair: Reversing the Tide of War and Globalization https://www.globalresearch.ca/from-global-poverty-to-exclusion-and-despair-reversing-the-tide-of-war-and-globalization/5611619

UN Millennium Declaration http://www.un.org/millennium/declaration/ares552e.htm

Ruger JP, Yach D. The Global Role of the World Health Organization. Glob Health Gov. 2009 Apr 1;2(2):1-11. PMID: 24729827; PMCID: PMC3981564.

World Bank Development Report 1993: Investing in Health
https://openknowledge.worldbank.org/handle/10986/5976

Forbes Billionaires 2018: Meet The Richest People On The Planet
https://www.forbes.com/sites/luisakroll/2018/03/06/forbes-billionaires-2018-meet-the-richest-people-on-the-planet/

Eight people own same wealth as half the world https://www.oxfam.org.uk/media-centre/press-releases/2017/01/eight-people-own-same-wealth-as-half-the-world

An Economy for the 99% https://policy-practice.oxfam.org.uk/publications/an-economy-for-the-99-its-time-to-build-a-human-economy-that-benefits-everyone-620170

Reward Work, Not Wealth https://policy-practice.oxfam.org.uk/publications/reward-work-not-wealth-to-end-the-inequality-crisis-we-must-build-an-economy-fo-620396

Richest 1 percent bagged 82 percent of wealth created last year – poorest half of humanity got nothing https://www.oxfam.org/en/pressroom/pressreleases/2018-01-22/richest-1-percent-bagged-82-percent-wealth-created-last-year

Blood Money: These Companies and People Make Billions of Dollars from War
https://www.globalresearch.ca/blood-money-these-companies-and-people-make-billions-of-dollars-from-war/5438657

What Obama Told Us at West Point
https://www.foreignpolicyjournal.com/2014/06/03/what-obama-told-us-at-west-point/

Corporate Parasites and Economic Plunder: We Need a Genuine Green Revolution
http://rinf.com/alt-news/editorials/parasites-and-plunder-we-need-a-genuine-green-revolution/

Free Trade Agreements https://www.trade.gov/fta/

Global 500 http://fortune.com/global500/2016/

Confessions of an 'ex' Peak Oil Believer
http://www.engdahl.oilgeopolitics.net/Geopolitics___Eurasia/Peak_Oil___Russia/peak_oil___russia.html

An introduction to the modern petroleum science, and to the Russian-Ukrainian theory of deep, abiotic petroleum origins http://www.gasresources.net/introduction.htm

Russians and NASA Discredit 'Fossil Fuel' Theory https://principia-scientific.org/russians-nasa-discredit-fossil-fuel-theory-demise-of-junk-co2-science/

How Billionaires Become Billionaires https://www.globalresearch.ca/how-billionaires-become-billionaires/5612125

How Corporate Lobbyists Conquered American Democracy
https://www.theatlantic.com/business/archive/2015/04/how-corporate-lobbyists-conquered-american-democracy/390822/

USAID What We Do https://www.usaid.gov/what-we-do

NSSM 200 https://pdf.usaid.gov/pdf_docs/Pcaab500.pdf

Challenging Neoliberal Dogma: Pushing Indian Farmers into Bankruptcy Isn't 'Development'! https://www.globalresearch.ca/challenging-neoliberal-dogma-pushing-indian-farmers-into-bankruptcy-isnt-development/5594654

Neoliberalism and the Globalization of War: America's Hegemonic Project
https://www.globalresearch.ca/neoliberalism-and-the-globalization-of-war-americas-hegemonic-project/5531125

The WTO and the Sustainable Development Goals
https://www.wto.org/english/thewto_e/coher_e/sdgs_e/sdgs_e.htm

TTIP and CETA in detail https://stop-ttip.org/what-is-the-problem-ttip-ceta/faqs/

Austria's New Coalition Betrays on CETA Trade Agreement
https://www.globalresearch.ca/austrias-new-coalition-betrays-on-ceta-trade-agreement/5642134

Trade facilitation https://www.wto.org/english/tratop_e/tradfa_e/tradfa_e.htm

References

The Globalist Trade Agreement You Didn't Hear About
https://theinternationalforecaster.com/topic/international_forecaster_weekly/the_globalist
_trade_agreement_you_didnt_hear_about

Making Globalization Work for All
http://www.undp.org/content/dam/undp/library/corporate/UNDP-in-action/2007/UNDP-
in-action-2007-en-.pdf

WHO ICD-10 classification of diseases
http://apps.who.int/classifications/icd10/browse/2016/en

Development Approval Process (Drugs)
https://www.fda.gov/drugs/developmentapprovalprocess/default.htm

Light, D. W., Lexchin, J., & Darrow, J. J. (2013). Institutional Corruption of Pharmaceuticals
and the Myth of Safe and Effective Drugs. The Journal of Law, Medicine & Ethics, 41(3),
590–600. https://doi.org/10.1111/jlme.12068

Harmonisation for Better Health https://www.ich.org/about/mission.html

Brown TM, Cueto M, Fee E. The World Health Organization and the transition from
"international" to "global" public health. Am J Public Health. 2006 Jan;96(1):62-72. doi:
10.2105/AJPH.2004.050831. Epub 2005 Dec 1. PMID: 16322464; PMCID: PMC1470434.

WHO Model List of Essential Medicines http://www.who.int/selection_medicines/list/en/

WHO Collaborations and partnerships http://www.who.int/about/collaborations/en/

CDC Global Health Security Agenda https://www.cdc.gov/globalhealth/security/index.htm

Global Vaccine Action Plan 2011-2020
http://www.who.int/immunization/global_vaccine_action_plan/GVAP_doc_2011_2020/e
n/

Global Immunization Division
https://www.cdc.gov/globalhealth/resources/reports/annual/2017/global-immunization-
division-gid.html

USAID Promoting Global Health https://www.usaid.gov/promoting-global-health

WHO Health Security http://www.who.int/health-security/en/

WHO International Health Regulations (IHR)
http://www.who.int/topics/international_health_regulations/en/

Towards Access 2030
http://www.who.int/medicines/publications/towards_access2030/en/

UHC2030 Our mission https://www.uhc2030.org/our-mission/

WHO's engagement with non-State actors http://www.who.int/about/collaborations/non-
state-actors/en/

A Look Into the Petrochemical Industry https://www.americanlaboratory.com/914-
Application-Notes/37318-A-Look-Into-the-Petrochemicals-Industry/

Hess J, Bednarz D, Bae J, Pierce J. Petroleum and health care: evaluating and managing
health care's vulnerability to petroleum supply shifts. Am J Public Health. 2011
Sep;101(9):1568-79. doi: 10.2105/AJPH.2011.300233. Epub 2011 Jul 21. PMID: 21778473;
PMCID: PMC3154246.

Duffy TP. The Flexner Report--100 years later. Yale J Biol Med. 2011 Sep;84(3):269-76.
PMID: 21966046; PMCID: PMC3178858.

Funding for Medical Education: Maintaining a Healthy Separation from Industry
https://www.ahajournals.org/doi/full/10.1161/circulationaha.109.869636

UAEM Who We Are https://uaem.org/who-we-are/

Spithoff S. Industry involvement in continuing medical education: time to say no. Can Fam
Physician. 2014 Aug;60(8):694-6, 700-3. PMID: 25122806; PMCID: PMC4131951.

Epidemic Intelligence Service https://www.cdc.gov/eis/

Empathic Therapy: psychotherapy not psychoactive drugs https://breggin.com/empathic-
therapy/

Supporting the mental health of doctors and medical students
https://www.bma.org.uk/collective-voice/policy-and-research/education-training-and-workforce/supporting-the-mental-health-of-doctors-in-the-workforce

Medical schools should be prioritising nutrition and lifestyle education
https://blogs.bmj.com/bmj/2017/09/07/medical-schools-should-be-prioritising-nutrition-and-lifestyle-education/

What is the purpose of medical research?
https://www.thelancet.com/journals/lancet/article/PIIS0140-6736(13)60149-X/fulltext

Unethical Trials https://www.somo.nl/examples-of-unethical-trials/

What are medical journals for and how well do they fulfil those functions?
https://blogs.bmj.com/bmj/2016/04/19/richard-smith-what-are-medical-journals-for-and-how-well-do-they-fulfil-those-functions/

Ioannidis JPA (2005) Why Most Published Research Findings Are False. PLoS Med 2(8): e124. https://doi.org/10.1371/journal.pmed.0020124

Smith R (2005) Medical Journals Are an Extension of the Marketing Arm of Pharmaceutical Companies. PLoS Med 2(5): e138. https://doi.org/10.1371/journal.pmed.0020138

McHenry L. Of sophists and spin-doctors: industry-sponsored ghostwriting and the crisis of academic medicine. Mens Sana Monogr. 2010 Jan;8(1):129-45. doi: 10.4103/0973-1229.58824. PMID: 21327175; PMCID: PMC3031939.

Sismondo S (2007) Ghost Management: How Much of the Medical Literature Is Shaped Behind the Scenes by the Pharmaceutical Industry? PLoS Med 4(9): e286. https://doi.org/10.1371/journal.pmed.0040286

Rockefeller Foundation 1968 annual report https://www.rockefellerfoundation.org/about-us/governance-reports/annual-reports/

Functional and immunological relevance of the COOH-terminal extension of human chorionic gonadotropin beta: implications for the WHO birth control vaccine
https://www.fasebj.org/doi/abs/10.1096/fasebj.7.14.7693535

Talwar GP, Singh O, Pal R, Chatterjee N, Sahai P, Dhall K, Kaur J, Das SK, Suri S, Buckshee K. A vaccine that prevents pregnancy in women. Proc Natl Acad Sci U S A. 1994 Aug 30;91(18):8532-6. doi: 10.1073/pnas.91.18.8532. PMID: 8078917; PMCID: PMC44640.

What are genome editing and CRISPR-Cas9?
https://ghr.nlm.nih.gov/primer/genomicresearch/genomeediting

Genome editing and human reproduction: social and ethical issues
http://nuffieldbioethics.org/project/genome-editing-human-reproduction

Son of Frankenstein? UK Body Backs Human Embryo Gene Editing
http://www.williamengdahl.com/englishNEO23Jul2018.php

Global Goals https://www.globalgoals.org/

Project Everyone https://www.project-everyone.org/

New Thought Police Suppressing Dissent in Science http://www.i-sis.org.uk/isisnews/i-sisnews7-17.php

Healthy Not Hungry campaign http://www.project-everyone.org/case-studies/healthy-not-hungry/

IMPACT 2030 https://www.impact2030.com/

Sustainable Development Impact Summit 2018
https://www.weforum.org/events/sustainable-development-impact-summit/about

The Fourth Industrial Revolution: What it means, how to respond
https://www.weforum.org/agenda/2016/01/the-fourth-industrial-revolution-what-it-means-and-how-to-respond/

What is PR https://www.cipr.co.uk/content/policy/careers-advice/what-pr

New report shows that 400 million do not have access to essential health services
http://www.who.int/mediacentre/news/releases/2015/uhc-report/en/

References

UK doctors re-examine case for mandatory vaccination
https://www.bmj.com/content/358/bmj.j3414/rapid-responses

UK Vaccine Damage Payment https://www.gov.uk/vaccine-damage-payment

Wiedermann U, Garner-Spitzer E, Wagner A. Primary vaccine failure to routine vaccines: Why and what to do? Hum Vaccin Immunother. 2016;12(1):239-43. doi: 10.1080/21645515.2015.1093263. PMID: 26836329; PMCID: PMC4962729.

Recent charity register statistics: Charity Commission
https://www.gov.uk/government/publications/charity-register-statistics/recent-charity-register-statistics-charity-commission

Number of Charities and Foundations Passes 1.2 Million
https://www.philanthropy.com/article/Number-of-Charities-and/195165

Giving USA 2018: Americans Gave $410.02 Billion to Charity in 2017, Crossing the $400 Billion Mark for the First Time https://givingusa.org/giving-usa-2018-americans-gave-410-02-billion-to-charity-in-2017-crossing-the-400-billion-mark-for-the-first-time/

New global partnership to boost employee giving in the UK
https://www.charitiestrust.org.uk/news-blog/yourcause-partnership

Employees Teach the Global Goals https://www.impact2030.com/employeesforsdgs

The Global Goals Gateway https://solutions.yourcause.com/impact-2030/

SDG Watch Europe https://www.sdgwatcheurope.org/wp-content/uploads/2018/06/SDG-Watch-Europe-FINAL-16.05.18.pdf

Make Poverty History and G8 promises – was it worth it? https://www.oxfam.org.uk/media-centre/press-releases/2013/05/make-poverty-history-and-g8-promises-was-it-all-really-worth-it

War on Want: What We Do https://waronwant.org/what-we-do

Causes of cancer and reducing your risk https://www.cancerresearchuk.org/about-cancer/causes-of-cancer

Does This Cause Cancer? https://www.cancer.org/cancer/cancer-causes/general-info/does-this-cause-cancer.html

Bill Gates talks about 'vaccines to reduce population'
http://www.voltairenet.org/article164347.html

Working together for healthy vaccine markets
https://www.gavi.org/library/publications/gavi/market-shaping-brochure/

CGIAR Health https://www.cgiar.org/research/research-theme/health/

Syngenta Who We Are https://www.syngenta.com/who-we-are

'Fake news' inquiry launched https://www.parliament.uk/business/committees/committees-a-z/commons-select/culture-media-and-sport-committee/news-parliament-2015/fake-news-launch-16-17/

Access to medicines https://www.opensocietyfoundations.org/topics/access-medicines

Measles cases hit record high in Europe https://www.bbc.co.uk/news/health-45246049

Measles cases hit record high in the European Region http://www.euro.who.int/en/media-centre/sections/press-releases/2018/measles-cases-hit-record-high-in-the-european-region

Nkowane BM, Bart SW, Orenstein WA, Baltier M. Measles outbreak in a vaccinated school population: epidemiology, chains of transmission and the role of vaccine failures. Am J Public Health. 1987 Apr;77(4):434-8. doi: 10.2105/ajph.77.4.434. PMID: 3826461; PMCID: PMC1646939.

NHS Measles https://www.nhs.uk/conditions/measles/

Measles outbreak in Bristol prompts public health warning https://www.bbc.co.uk/news/uk-england-bristol-44669112

Ebola vaccine to help tackle DRC outbreak
https://www.gavi.org/library/news/statements/2018/ebola-vaccine-to-help-tackle-drc-outbreak/

Ebola vaccine praised as Congo outbreak declared over
https://www.gavi.org/library/news/statements/2018/ebola-vaccine-praised-as-congo-outbreak-declared-over/

Ebola situation reports: Democratic Republic of the Congo
http://www.who.int/ebola/situation-reports/drc-2018/en/

CDC Lyme disease https://www.cdc.gov/lyme/resources/brochure/lymediseasebrochure.pdf

CDC Study Finds Pesticide Ineffective at Stopping the Spread of Lyme Disease
https://beyondpesticides.org/dailynewsblog/2013/08/cdc-study-finds-pesticide-ineffective-at-stoping-the-spread-of-lyme-disease/

NPIC permethrin http://npic.orst.edu/ingred/permethrin.html

NPIC bifenthrin http://npic.orst.edu/ingred/bifenthrin.html

Chapter Ten

Navickas R, Petric VK, Feigl AB, Seychell M. Multimorbidity: What do we know? What should we do? J Comorb. 2016 Feb 17;6(1):4-11. doi: 10.15256/joc.2016.6.72. PMID: 29090166; PMCID: PMC5556462.

WHO 2016 Multimorbidity report https://apps.who.int/iris/handle/10665/252275

GBD 2017: a fragile world https://www.thelancet.com/journals/lancet/article/PIIS0140-6736(18)32858-7/fulltext

Multimorbidity: a priority for global health research https://acmedsci.ac.uk/policy/policy-projects/multimorbidity

Guidelines, polypharmacy and drug-drug interactions with multimorbidity
https://www.bmj.com/content/350/bmj.h1059

Artificial intelligence helps Stanford computer scientists predict the side effects of millions of drug combinations https://news.stanford.edu/press-releases/2018/07/10/ai-predicts-drug-pair-side-effects/

Systematic predictions of drug combinations based on clinical side-effects
https://www.nature.com/articles/srep07160

The evolution of free radicals and oxidative stress https://www.amjmed.com/article/S0002-9343(00)00412-5/fulltext

Introduction: oxidation and inflammation, a molecular link between non-communicable diseases https://www.ncbi.nlm.nih.gov/pubmed/25038988

The role of oxidative stress during inflammatory processes
https://www.ncbi.nlm.nih.gov/pubmed/24127541

Khanna RD, Karki K, Pande D, Negi R, Khanna RS (2014) Inflammation, Free Radical Damage, Oxidative Stress and Cancer. Microinflammation 1:109. doi: 10.4172/2381-8727.1000109

The role of oxidative stress in HIV disease https://www.ncbi.nlm.nih.gov/pubmed/7590404

Involvement of free radicals in parasitic infestations
https://www.tandfonline.com/doi/full/10.1080/09712119.2012.739093

Percário S, Moreira DR, Gomes BA, Ferreira ME, Gonçalves AC, Laurindo PS, Vilhena TC, Dolabela MF, Green MD. Oxidative stress in malaria. Int J Mol Sci. 2012 Dec 3;13(12):16346-72. doi: 10.3390/ijms131216346. PMID: 23208374; PMCID: PMC3546694.

Alexander V. Ivanov, Birke Bartosch, and Maria G. Isaguliants, "Oxidative Stress in Infection and Consequent Disease," Oxidative Medicine and Cellular Longevity, vol. 2017, Article ID 3496043, 3 pages, 2017. https://doi.org/10.1155/2017/3496043.

The role of free radicals in toxicity and disease
https://www.ncbi.nlm.nih.gov/pubmed/8852268

Pham-Huy LA, He H, Pham-Huy C. Free radicals, antioxidants in disease and health. Int J Biomed Sci. 2008 Jun;4(2):89-96. PMID: 23675073; PMCID: PMC3614697.

References

WHO Global action plan on physical activity 2018-2030: more active people for a healthier world https://www.who.int/ncds/prevention/physical-activity/global-action-plan-2018-2030/en/

Katritsis DG, Gersh BJ, Camm AJ. A Clinical Perspective on Sudden Cardiac Death. Arrhythm Electrophysiol Rev. 2016;5(3):177-182. doi: 10.15420/aer.2016:11:2. PMID: 28116082; PMCID: PMC5248660.

Sudden Cardiac Arrest https://www.nhlbi.nih.gov/health-topics/sudden-cardiac-arrest

Risk factors https://www.who.int/topics/risk_factors/en/

Epigenetics https://www.brucelipton.com/resource/article/epigenetics

WHO Nutrition https://www.who.int/topics/nutrition/en/

Campbell TC. Nutritional Renaissance and Public Health Policy. J Nutr Biol. 2017;3(1):124-138. doi: 10.18314/jnb.v3i1.145. Epub 2017 Aug 25. PMID: 29177204; PMCID: PMC5701757.

Tuso PJ, Ismail MH, Ha BP, Bartolotto C. Nutritional update for physicians: plant-based diets. Perm J. 2013 Spring;17(2):61-6. doi: 10.7812/TPP/12-085. PMID: 23704846; PMCID: PMC3662288.

WHO Micronutrients https://www.who.int/nutrition/topics/micronutrients/en/

WHO Micronutrient deficiencies https://www.who.int/nutrition/topics/vad/en/

The Truth About Vitamins in Supplements https://pdfs.semanticscholar.org/1ae0/608396d55120efcb6923c3d1dfa970f64bbb.pdf

NHS Food for strong bones https://www.nhs.uk/live-well/healthy-body/food-for-strong-bones/

Trace elements in human nutrition and health https://www.who.int/nutrition/publications/micronutrients/9241561734/en/

Global burden of protein-energy malnutrition in the year 2000 https://www.who.int/healthinfo/statistics/bod_malnutrition.pdf

Ready-to-use therapeutic food for children with severe acute malnutrition https://www.unicef.org/media/files/Position_Paper_Ready-to-use_therapeutic_food_for_children_with_severe_acute_malnutrition__June_2013.pdf

BNF Healthy hydration guide https://www.nutrition.org.uk/healthyliving/hydration/healthy-hydration-guide.html

Evolutionary Features in the Structure and Functions of Bacterial Toxins https://www.mdpi.com/2072-6651/11/1/15/htm

What is a Poison? https://soilandhealth.org/wp-content/uploads/02/0201hyglibcat/hygienic.review.articles.htm

Chapter 26 Anatomy and Physiology http://library.open.oregonstate.edu/aandp/chapter/26-0-introduction/

Free radicals and environmental toxins https://www.ncbi.nlm.nih.gov/pubmed/3526996

Free radicals in toxicology https://www.ncbi.nlm.nih.gov/pubmed/8511786

Michalopoulos GK. Liver regeneration. J Cell Physiol. 2007 Nov;213(2):286-300. doi: 10.1002/jcp.21172. PMID: 17559071; PMCID: PMC2701258.

The spectrum of hepatotoxicity due to drugs https://www.ncbi.nlm.nih.gov/pubmed/2874423

David S, Hamilton JP. Drug-induced Liver Injury. US Gastroenterol Hepatol Rev. 2010 Jan 1;6:73-80. PMID: 21874146; PMCID: PMC3160634.

Damian G. Deavall, Elizabeth A. Martin, Judith M. Horner, and Ruth Roberts, "Drug-Induced Oxidative Stress and Toxicity," Journal of Toxicology, vol. 2012, Article ID 645460, 13 pages, 2012. https://doi.org/10.1155/2012/645460.

Yew WW, Chang KC, Chan DP. Oxidative Stress and First-Line Antituberculosis Drug-Induced Hepatotoxicity. Antimicrob Agents Chemother. 2018 Jul 27;62(8):e02637-17. doi: 10.1128/AAC.02637-17. Erratum in: Antimicrob Agents Chemother. 2018 Sep 24;62(10):. PMID: 29784840; PMCID: PMC6105810.

Too Many Meds? America's Love Affair With Prescription Drugs
https://www.consumerreports.org/prescription-drugs/too-many-meds-americas-love-affair-with-prescription-medication/

Americans taking more prescription drugs than ever: a survey
https://www.webmd.com/drug-medication/news/20170803/americans-taking-more-prescription-drugs-than-ever-survey

Types of Pesticide Ingredients https://www.epa.gov/ingredients-used-pesticide-products/types-pesticide-ingredients

Basic Information about Pesticide Ingredients https://www.epa.gov/ingredients-used-pesticide-products/basic-information-about-pesticide-ingredients

Global Vector Control Response 2017-2030 https://www.who.int/vector-control/publications/global-control-response/en/

Aircraft Disinsection https://www.epa.gov/mosquitocontrol/aircraft-disinsection

Aircraft Disinsection Insecticides
https://www.who.int/ipcs/publications/ehc/ehc243.pdf?ua=1

WHO Aircraft disinsection
https://www.who.int/ith/mode_of_travel/aircraft_disinsection/en/

Methods and operating procedures for aircraft disinsection
https://www.who.int/whopes/resources/WHO-CDS-NTD-VEM-2018.07/en/

Permethrin-induced oxidative stress and toxicity and metabolism: A review
https://www.ncbi.nlm.nih.gov/pubmed/27183507

Hoffman JB, Petriello MC, Hennig B. Impact of nutrition on pollutant toxicity: an update with new insights into epigenetic regulation. Rev Environ Health. 2017 Mar 1;32(1-2):65-72. doi: 10.1515/reveh-2016-0041. PMID: 28076319; PMCID: PMC5489226.

10 Natural & Organic Makeup Brands Your Face Will Love You For
https://www.thegoodtrade.com/features/18-natural-organic-makeup-brands-your-face-will-love-you-for

Myths on cosmetics safety https://www.ewg.org/skindeep/myths-on-cosmetics-safety/

Volatile Organic Compounds' Impact on Indoor Air Quality https://www.epa.gov/indoor-air-quality-iaq/volatile-organic-compounds-impact-indoor-air-quality

Guide to Healthy Cleaning https://www.ewg.org/guides/cleaners

11 Natural & Eco-Friendly Cleaning Products For The Conscious Home
https://www.thegoodtrade.com/features/natural-eco-friendly-cleaning-products-for-the-conscious-home

How Toxic Are Your Household Cleaning Supplies?
https://www.organicconsumers.org/news/how-toxic-are-your-household-cleaning-supplies

35 Fair Trade & Ethical Clothing Brands Betting Against Fast Fashion
https://www.thegoodtrade.com/features/fair-trade-clothing

The Best Sustainable and Ethical European Fashion Brands https://ecocult.com/19-sustainable-european-fashion-brands-i-discovered-at-berlin-fashion-week/

10 Organic Sheets & Bedding Sources To Help You Sleep Sweetly
https://www.thegoodtrade.com/features/sleep-sweeter-with-these-natural-and-organic-bedding-brands

Kickstart your Zero Waste lifestyle https://www.recycling.com/zero-waste-store/

The Plastic Free Shop https://www.theplasticfreeshop.co.uk/

The Free-Radical fallacy about ionizing radiation
https://ratical.org/radiation/CNR/FreeRadFallacy.html

Acute Radiation Syndrome: A Fact Sheet for Clinicians
https://emergency.cdc.gov/radiation/arsphysicianfactsheet.asp

References

Wireless Radiation/Electromagnetic Fields Increases Toxic Body Burden https://ehtrust.org/key-issues/the-environment-and-health/wireless-radiationelectromagnetic-fields-increases-toxic-body-burden/

The Cellular Stress Response: EMF-DNA Interaction https://www.bioinitiative.org/wp-content/uploads/pdfs/sec07_2012_Evidence_for_Stress_Response_Cellular.pdf

`The stress of dying': the role of heat shock proteins in the regulation of apoptosis Helen M. Beere Journal of Cell Science 2004 117: 2641-2651; doi: 10.1242/jcs.01284

Electromagnetic fields – Research https://www.who.int/peh-emf/research/en/

Planetary electromagnetic pollution: it is time to assess its impact https://www.thelancet.com/journals/lanplh/article/PIIS2542-5196(18)30221-3/fulltext

Hardell L, Carlberg M, Hedendahl LK. Radiofrequency radiation from nearby base stations gives high levels in an apartment in Stockholm, Sweden: A case report. Oncol Lett. 2018 May;15(5):7871-7883. doi: 10.3892/ol.2018.8285. Epub 2018 Mar 16. PMID: 29725476; PMCID: PMC5920374.

Radiation from Airport Security Scanning https://www.cdc.gov/nceh/radiation/airport_scan.htm

5G Wireless Technology: Millimeter Wave Health Effects https://www.saferemr.com/2017/08/5g-wireless-technology-millimeter-wave.html

Powerwatch article library https://www.powerwatch.org.uk/library/index.asp

10 Tips To Reduce Cell Phone Radiation https://ehtrust.org/take-action/educate-yourself/10-things-you-can-do-to-reduce-the-cancer-risk-from-cell-phones/

What You Need To Know About 5G Wireless and "Small" Cells https://ehtrust.org/wp-content/uploads/5G_What-You-Need-to-Know.pdf

McEwen BS. Stressed or stressed out: what is the difference? J Psychiatry Neurosci. 2005 Sep;30(5):315-8. PMID: 16151535; PMCID: PMC1197275.

Neurological Effects of Non-Ionizing Electromagnetic Fields https://bioinitiative.org/wp-content/uploads/pdfs/sec09_2012_Evidence_Effects_Neurology_behavior.pdf

Bouayed J, Rammal H, Soulimani R. Oxidative stress and anxiety: relationship and cellular pathways. Oxid Med Cell Longev. 2009 Apr-Jun;2(2):63-7. PMID: 20357926; PMCID: PMC2763246.

Salim S. Oxidative stress and psychological disorders. Curr Neuropharmacol. 2014 Mar;12(2):140-7. doi: 10.2174/1570159X11666131120230309. PMID: 24669208; PMCID: PMC3964745.

Aschbacher K, O'Donovan A, Wolkowitz OM, Dhabhar FS, Su Y, Epel E. Good stress, bad stress and oxidative stress: insights from anticipatory cortisol reactivity. Psychoneuroendocrinology. 2013 Sep;38(9):1698-708. doi: 10.1016/j.psyneuen.2013.02.004. Epub 2013 Mar 13. PMID: 23490070; PMCID: PMC4028159.

Liu Z, Zhou T, Ziegler AC, Dimitrion P, Zuo L. Oxidative Stress in Neurodegenerative Diseases: From Molecular Mechanisms to Clinical Applications. Oxid Med Cell Longev. 2017;2017:2525967. doi: 10.1155/2017/2525967. Epub 2017 Jul 12. PMID: 28785371; PMCID: PMC5529664.

Fowler CD, Liu Y, Wang Z. Estrogen and adult neurogenesis in the amygdala and hypothalamus. Brain Res Rev. 2008 Mar;57(2):342-51. doi: 10.1016/j.brainresrev.2007.06.011. Epub 2007 Jul 27. PMID: 17764748; PMCID: PMC2373759.

How to Handle Tension, or Stress, Headaches https://heartmdinstitute.com/stress-relief/how-handle-tension-stress-headaches/

What is Earthing or Grounding? https://heartmdinstitute.com/alternative-medicine/what-is-earthing-or-grounding/

Bibliography

ANGELL, M. – *The Truth About the Drug Companies: How They Deceive Us and What To Do About It.* Random House Trade Paperback. 2005.

ASHFORD, N & Miller, C – *Chemical Exposures: Low Levels and High Stakes.* John Wiley & Sons, Inc. 1998.

BAILLIE, M. – *New Light on the Black Death: The Cosmic Connection.* Tempus Publishing. 2006.

BECKER, R. O. – *Cross Currents: The Perils of Electropollution, The Promise of Electromedicine.* Jeremy P. Tarcher/Penguin. 1990.

BECKER, R. O. & Selden, G. – *The Body Electric: Electromagnetism and the Foundation of Life.* Harper Collins 1985.

BEDDOW BAYLY, M – *The Case Against Vaccination.* 1936.

BEGICH, N & MANNING, J. – *Angels Don't Play This HAARP.* Earthpulse Press 2002.

BERTELL, R. – *No Immediate Danger: Prognosis for a Radioactive Earth.* The Women's Press. 1985.

BIELER, H. – *Food Is Your Best Medicine.* Ballantine Books. 1965.

BLAYLOCK, R. – *Health and Nutrition Secrets.* Health Press. 2006.

BLAYLOCK, R. – *Excitotoxins: The Taste That Kills.* Health Press. 1997.

BREGGIN, P. – *Toxic Psychiatry. Drugs and Electroconvulsive Therapy: The Truth and the Better Alternatives.* Harper Collins Publishers. 1993.

BREGGIN, P. & Cohen, D. – *Your Drug May Be Your Problem.* DaCapo Press. 1999.

BROWN, E. R. – *Rockefeller Medicine Men.* University of California Press. 1979.

BRYSON, C. – *The Fluoride Deception.* Seven Stories Press. 2004.

BUCHWALD, G. – *Vaccination: A Business Based in Fear.* Books on Demand GmbH. 1994.

CAMPBELL, T. C. & Campbell, T. M. – *The China Study: The Most Comprehensive Study of Nutrition Ever Conducted and the Startling Implications for Diet, Weight Loss and Long-Term Health.* BenBella Books. 2006.

CAMPBELL-MCBRIDE, N. – *Gut and Psychology Syndrome.* Medinform Publishing. 2010.

CARSON, R. – *Silent Spring.* Penguin Books. 1962.

CARTER, R. – *Climate: The Counter Consensus: A Palaeoclimatologist Speaks.* Stacey International. 2010.

CHOSSUDOVSKY, M. – *Globalization of Poverty and the New World Order.* Global Research. 2003.

CLEMENT, A. M. & Clement, B – *Killer Clothes: How Seemingly Innocent Clothing Choices Endanger Your Health…And How To Protect Yourself.* Hippocrates Publications. 2011.

COLBORN T., Dumanoski, D. & Meyers, J. P. – *Our Stolen Future: Are We Threatening Our Fertility, Intelligence, and Survival? – A Scientific Detective Story.* Little, Brown and Company. 1996.

COMMONER, B. – *Making Peace with the Planet.* The New Press. 1992.

DAVIES, N. – *Flat Earth News: An Award-winning Reporter Exposes Falsehood, Distortion and Propaganda in the Global Media.* Vintage Books. 2009.

DAVIS, D. – *The Secret History of the War on Cancer.* Perseus Books. 2007.

DEAN, C. – *Death by Modern Medicine.* Ebook www.drcarolyndean.com. 2012.

Bibliography

DEAN, C. – *The Magnesium Miracle*. Ballantine Books. 2007.

DOLE, L. – *The Blood Poisoners*. 1965.

DUESBERG, P. – *Inventing the AIDS Virus*. Regnery Publishing, Inc. 1996.

DUFTY, W. – *Sugar Blues*. Grand Central Life & Style. 1975.

ENGDAHL, F. W. – *Seeds of Destruction: The Hidden Agenda of Genetic Manipulation*. Global Research. 2007.

ENGDAHL, F. W. – *Gods of Money: Wall Street and the Death of the American Century*. Edition.engdahl. 2009.

ENGELBRECHT, T, & KOENLEIN, C. – *Virus Mania*. Trafford Publishing. 2007.

EPSTEIN, S. – *The Politics of Cancer Revisited*. East Ridge Press. 1998.

EPSTEIN, S. – *Toxic Beauty: How Cosmetics and Personal-Care Products Endanger Your Health...And What You Can Do About It*. BenBella Books. 2009

FREELAND, E. – *Chemtrails, HAARP and the Full Spectrum Dominance of Planet Earth*. Feral House. 2014.

GALEANO, E. – *Open Veins of Latin America: Five Centuries of the Pillage of a Continent*. Serpent's Tail. 2009.

HALE, A. R. – *The Medical Voodoo*. 1935.

HODGE, J. W. – *The Vaccination Superstition*. 1902.

HUGGINS, H. & Levy, T. – *Uninformed Consent: the hidden dangers in dental care*. Hampton Roads Publishing Company Inc. 1999.

KREMER, H. – *The Silent Revolution in Cancer and AIDS Medicine*. Xlibris. 2008.

KRIMSKY, S. – *Science in the Private Interest: Has the Lure of Profits Corrupted Biomedical Research?* Rowman & Littlefield Publishers, Inc. 2003.

LAPPE, F. & Collins, J. – *Food First: Beyond the Myth of Scarcity*. Ballantine Books. 1978.

LIPTON, B. – *The Biology of Belief*. Mountain of Love/Elite Books. 2005.

LOAT, L. – *The Truth About Vaccination and Immunization*. 1951.

MARGULIS, L. – *Symbiotic Planet: A New Look at Evolution*. Basic Book. 1998.

MCBEAN, E. – *The Poisoned Needle*. 1957.

MCBEAN, E. – *Swine Flu Exposé*. 1977.

MENDELSOHN, R. S. – *Confessions of a Medical Heretic*. McGraw-Hill. 1979.

MICHAELS, D. – *Doubt is Their Product: How Industry's Assault on Science Threatens Your Health*. Oxford University Press. 2008.

MONTE, W. – *While Science Sleeps: A sweetener kills*. Ebook. 2012.

MOORE, R. D – *The High Blood Pressure Solution: A Scientifically Proven Program for Preventing Strokes and Heart Disease*. Healing Arts Press. 2001.

NADER, R. – *In Pursuit of Justice*. Seven Stories Press. 2004.

NIGHTINGALE, F. – *Notes on Nursing: What it is, and what it is not*. Dover Publications. 1969.

OBER, C., Sinatra, S. & Zucker, M. – *Earthing: The Most Important Health Discovery Ever!* Basic Health Publications, Inc. 2014.

OVERELL, B. – *Animal Research Takes Lives*. 1993.

PAGE, T. – *Vivisection Unveiled: An Exposé of the Medical Futility of Animal Experimentation*. Jon Carpenter Publishing. 1997.

PEARSON, R B – *Pasteur: Plagiarist, Imposter: The Germ Theory Exploded*. 1942.

PHILIPS, A & Philips, J. – *The Powerwatch Handbook*. Piatkus Books. 2013.

PURDEY, M. – *Animal Pharm: One Man's Struggle to Discover the Truth About Mad Cow Disease and Variant CJD*. Clairview Books. 2007.

RAMPTON, S. & Stauber, J. – *Trust Us, We're Experts: How Industry Manipulates Science and Gambles with Your Future.* Jeremy P. Tarcher/Putnam. 2002.

ROWELL, A. – *Green Backlash: Global Subversion of the Environmental Movement.* Routledge. 1996.

RUESCH, H. – *1000 Doctors (and many more) Against Vivisection.* 1989.

SELYE, H. – *The Stress of Life.* McGraw-Hill. 1976.

SHELTON, H. – *Natural Hygiene: Man's Pristine Way of Life.* 1968.

SHELTON, H. – *The Hygienic System: Vol 1. The Science and Fine Art of Natural Hygiene.* 1953.

SHELTON, H. – *The Hygienic System: Vol II Orthotrophy.* 1975.

SHELTON, H. – *The Hygienic System: Vol VI Orthopathy.* 1939.

SHELTON, H. – *Syphilis: Is it a Mischievous Myth or a Malignant Monster.* 1962.

SMITH, J. M. – *Genetic Roulette: The Documented Health Risks of Genetically Engineered Foods.* Yes! Books. 2007.

SMITH, J. M. – *Seeds of Deception: Exposing Industry and Government Lies about the Safety of the Genetically Engineered Foods You're Eating.* Yes! Books. 2003.

STANNARD, D. – *American Holocaust: The Conquest of the New World.* Oxford University Press. 1992.

STERNGLASS, E. – *Secret Fallout.* McGraw-Hill Book Company. 1981.

STITT, P. – *Beating the Food Giants.* 1982.

TEBB, W. – *Leprosy and Vaccination.* 1893.

THORNTON, J. – *Pandora's Poison: Chlorine, Health, and a New Environmental Strategy.* MIT Press. 2000.

TILDEN, J. – *Toxemia Explained: The True Interpretation of the Cause of Disease.* 1926.

TILDEN, J. – *Impaired Health: Its Cause and Cure vol. 1.* 1921.

TILDEN, J. – *Impaired Health: Its Cause and Cure vol. 2.* 1921.

WAKEFIELD, A. – *Callous Disregard: Autism and Vaccines – The Truth Behind a Tragedy.* Skyhorse Publishing. 2010.

WALDBOTT, G. – *Fluoridation: The Great Dilemma.* Coronado Press. 1978.

WALLIN, I. – *Symbionticism and the origin of species.* The Williams & Wilkins Company. 1927.

WASSERMAN, H. & Solomon, N. – *Killing Our Own.* Dell Publishing Co, Inc. 1982.

WELSOME, E. – *The Plutonium Files.* Dell Publishing. 1999.

WHITE, W. – *The Story of a Great Delusion.* E, W, Allen. 1885.

WHORTON, J. – *The Arsenic Century: How Victorian Britain was Poisoned at Home, Work, & Play.* Oxford University Press. 2010.

About the Authors

Dawn Lester and David Parker have backgrounds in the fields of Accountancy and Electrical Engineering, respectively. These fields both require an aptitude for logic, which proved extremely useful for their investigation that has involved more than ten years continuous research to find answers to the question: what really makes people ill?

A popular saying, which is often attributed to Albert Einstein, claims that problems cannot be solved by using the same way of thinking that created them.

The concept underlying this saying can be extrapolated to indicate that a problem can often be better understood by people outside of the discipline in which it occurs because they are not bound by any dogma or biases inherent within that discipline.

The authors' investigation of why people become ill was conducted from a different perspective from that of the medical establishment; it was therefore free from the dogma and biases inherent within 'medical science'. This unbiased and logical approach enabled them to follow the evidence with open minds and led them to discover the flaws within the information about illness and disease that is promulgated by the medical establishment.

The results of their investigation are revealed within their book, *What Really Makes You Ill? Why Everything You Thought You Knew About Disease is Wrong.*